2008-2009

Clinical Guide to Pharmacotherapeutics for the Primary Care Provider

2008-2009
Clinical Guide to Pharmacotherapeutics for the Primary Care Provider

Mari J. Wirfs, MN, PhD, APRN, BC, FNP
Amelie Hollier, MSN, APRN, BC, FNP

Published by: Advanced Practice Education Associates, Inc.
103 Darwin Circle
Lafayette, Louisiana 70508 U.S.A.

Note: This book is a quick reference for health care providers practicing in primary care settings. The information has been extrapolated from a variety of sources and is presented in condensed and summary form. It is not intended to replace or substitute for complete and current manufacturer prescribing information, current research, or knowledge and experience of the user. For complete prescribing information, including toxicities, drug interactions, contraindications, and precautions, the reader is directed to the manufacturer's package insert and the published literature. The inclusion of a particular brand name neither implies nor suggests that the authors or publisher advise or recommend the use of that particular product or consider it superior to similar products available by other brand names. Neither the authors nor the publisher make any warranty, expressed or implied, with respect to the information, including any errors or omissions, herein.

ISBN 978-1-892418-14-2

All rights reserved. This book is protected by copyright. No part of this book may be reproduced or transmitted in any form or by any means including mechanical, electronic, photocopying, recording, or by information storage or retrieval systems without written permission.

Copyright © 2008 Advanced Practice Education Associates, Inc.
Printed in the United States of America.

2008-2009

Clinical Guide to Pharmacotherapeutics for the Primary Care Provider

Mari J. Wirfs, MN, PhD, APRN, BC, FNP

Amelie Hollier, MSN, APRN, BC, FNP

The Authors

Mari J. Wirfs, MN, PhD, APRN, BC, FNP is a nationally certified family nurse practitioner. She has over 30 years of experience in nursing education and practice and is Professor of Nursing at William Carey University in New Orleans, Louisiana. She is Clinical Director and sole primary care provider at Family Health Care serving the faculty, staff, students, and their families at William Carey University and the New Orleans Baptist Theological Seminary. She has co-authored six books for primary care providers and is a frequent guest lecturer on a variety of advanced practice topics to professional APRN groups.

Amelie Hollier, MSN, APRN, BC, FNP is a nationally certified family nurse practitioner. She is President and CEO of Advanced Practice Education Associates (APEA). She is a primary care provider serving the staff and their families at St. Clare's Employee Health Service at Our Lady of Lourdes Regional Medical Center in Lafayette, Louisiana. She has co-authored thirteen books for primary care providers. She travels extensively throughout the U.S. presenting on-site nurse practitioner certification exam review courses and lecturing on advanced pharmacology and other advanced practice topics to professional APRN groups.

Introduction

The *2008-2009 Clinical Guide to Pharmacotherapeutics for the Primary Care Provider* is a prescribing reference intended for use by health care providers in all clinical practice settings who are involved in the primary care management of patients with acute, episodic, and chronic health problems. It is presented in a concise and easy-to-read format. Comments are interspersed throughout, including such clinically useful information as laboratory values to be monitored, patient teaching points, and safety information.

The guide is divided into two sections. **Section I** presents pharmacotherapy regimens for over 300 clinical diagnoses. Each drug is listed alphabetically by generic name, followed by the FDA pregnancy category (in parentheses in bold font), adult dosing regimens, pediatric dosing regimens where applicable, brand names in bold font, and available dosage forms, identification of tablets and caplets that are scored (*), flavors of chewable and liquid forms, information regarding additives (e.g., dye-free, sugar-free, preservative-free or preservative type, alcohol-free or alcohol content), and generic availability.

Section II presents clinically useful information in convenient table format, including: the JNC-VII recommendations for hypertension management, descriptions of the U.S. schedule of controlled substances and FDA pregnancy categories, measurement conversions, childhood and adult immunization recommendations, brand-name drugs (with contents) for the management of common respiratory symptoms, anti-infectives by classification, pediatric dosing by weight for liquid forms, glucocorticosteroids by route of administration, contraceptives by route of administration and estrogen and/or progesterone content, and brand-name adult, pediatric, and prenatal vitamin and mineral supplements (with contents). An alphabetical cross reference index of drugs by generic and brand name, with FDA pregnancy category and controlled drug schedule, facilitates quick identification of drugs by alternate names and relative safety during pregnancy.

Selected diagnoses (e.g., angina, ADD/ADHD, growth failure, glaucoma, Parkinson's disease, HIV infection, CMV retinitis, multiple sclerosis, cystic fibrosis) and selected drugs (e.g., antineoplastics, antipsychotics, antiarrhythmics, anti-HIV drugs, and anticoagulants are included as often patients are referred to the primary care provider for follow up and/or maintenance therapies.

Safe and efficacious prescribing and monitoring of pharmacotherapy regimens requires adequate knowledge about a) the pharmacodynamics and pharmacokinetics of drugs and b) individual characteristics of the patient (e.g., current and past medical history, physical examination findings, hepatic and renal function, and comorbidities). Users of this guide are encouraged to utilize the manufacturer's package insert, recommendations and guidance of specialists, current research literature, and the referenced resources appended to this guide for more comprehensive information about specific drugs (e.g., special precautions, drug-drug and drug-food interactions, risks and benefits, age-related considerations, adverse reactions) and appropriate use with individual patients.

Note: This book is a quick reference for health care providers practicing in primary care settings. The information has been extrapolated from a variety of sources and is presented in condensed and summary form. It is not intended to replace or substitute for complete and current manufacturer prescribing information, current research, or knowledge and experience of the user. For complete prescribing information, including indications, toxicities, drug interactions, contraindications, and precautions, the reader is directed to the manufacturer's package insert and the published literature. The inclusion of a particular brand name neither implies nor suggests that the authors or publisher advise or recommend the use of that particular product or consider it superior to similar products available by other brand names. Neither the authors nor the publisher make any warranty, expressed or implied, with respect to the information, including any errors or omissions, herein.

Table of Contents

Section I: Pharmacotherapeutics by Clinical Diagnosis 27

Abscess (*see* Cellulitis) 98
Acetaminophen Overdose 29
Acne Rosacea 29
Acne Vulgaris 30
Acromegaly 35
Actinic Keratosis 35
Acute Exacerbation of Chronic Bronchitis (AECB)
    (*see* Bronchitis: Acute) 84
Alcohol Dependence 36
Allergic Reaction 37
Allergic Rhinitis (*see* Rhinitis: Allergic) 366
Allergic Sinusitis (*see* Rhinitis: Allergic) 366
Alzheimer's Disease 37
Amebic Dysentery (*see* Amebiasis) 38
Amebiasis 38
Amebic Liver Absess 39
Amenorrhea: Secondary 40
Anaphylaxis 41
Anemia of Chronic Renal Failure 41
Anemia: Folic Acid Deficiency 42
Anemia: Iron Deficiency 42
Anemia: Pernicious (Vitamin B-12 Deficiency) 45
Angina Pectoris: Stable 46
Ankylosing Spondylitis (*see* Osteoarthritis) 293
Anorexia/Cachexia 49
Anthrax 50
Anxiety Disorder: Generalized (GAD), Social (SAD) 51
Aphthous Stomatitis 55
Arterial Insufficiency (*see* Peripheral Vascular Disease) 327
Arthritis
    (*see* Osteoarthritis) 293
    (*see* Rheumatoid Arthritis) 363
Ascariasis (*see* Roundworm: Common, Intestinal 373
Aspergillosis (*Scedosporium apiospermum, Fusarium spp.*) 57

Asthma	57
Athlete's Foot (*see Tinea pedis*)	403
Atrophic Vaginitis	68
Attention Deficit Disorder (ADD)	68
Attention Deficit Hyperactivity Disorder (ADHD)	68
Bacterial Endocarditis: Prophylaxis	72
Bacterial Vaginosis (Gardnerella Vaginalis)	74
Baldness: Male Pattern	76
Bartonella Infection (*see* Cat Scratch Fever)	97
Basal Cell Carcinoma: Superficial (*see* Actinic Keratosis)	35
Bell's Palsy	76
Benign Essential Tremor	76
Benign Prostatic Hyperplasia (BPH)	76
Bile Acid Deficiency	77
Bipolar Disorder: Depression	77
Bipolar Disorder: Mania	78
Bite: Cat	78
Bite: Dog	79
Bite: Human	81
Blepharitis: Bacterial	82
Blepharoconjuctivitis (*see* Conjunctivitis/Blepharoconjunctivitis: Bacterial)	115
Bloating (*see Flatulence*)	173
Boil (*see* Skin Infection: Bacterial)	383
Bordetella pertussis (*see* Pertussis)	328
Breast Abscess (*see* Mastitis)	267
Breast Cancer Prophylaxis	83
Bronchiolitis	83
Bronchitis: Acute	84
Bronchitis: Chronic	89
Bulimia Nervosa	90
Burn: Minor	91
Bursitis	91
Cachexia (*see* Anorexia/Cachexia)	49
Calcium Deficiency (*see* Hypocalcemia)	232
Calloused Skin (*see* Skin: Calloused)	383
Candidiasis: Oral	92
Candidiasis: Skin	93
Candidiasis: Vulvovaginal (Moniliasis)	94
Canker Sore (*see* Aphthous Stomatitis)	55
Carbuncle (*see* Skin Infection: Bacterial)	383

Carpal Tunnel Syndrome (CTS) 96
Cat Scratch Fever (Bartonella Infection) 97
Cellulitis 98
Cerumen Impaction 100
Chalazion (*see* Stye) 391
Chancroid 101
Chest Wall Syndrome (*see* Costochondritis) 127
Chickenpox (*Varicella*) 101
Chlamydia (*Chlamydia Trachomatis*) 102
Cholelithiasis 104
Cholera 104
Chloasma (*see* Hyperpigmentation) 212
Chronic Obstructive Pulmonary Disease (COPD)
    (*see* Bronchitis: Chronic) 89
Cold Sore (*see* Herpes labialis) 206
Colic: Infantile 104
Colitis (*see* Ulcerative Colitis) 432
Colitis: Pseudomembranous (*see* Pseudomembranous Colitis) ..356
Common Cold (Upper Respiratory Infection) 105
Community Acquired Pneumonia (*see* Pneumonia:
    Community Acquired) 337
Condyloma Accuminata (*see* Wart: Venereal) 449
Congestive Heart Failure (CHF) 107
Conjunctivitis: Allergic 111
Conjunctivitis/Blepharoconjunctivitis: Bacterial 115
Conjunctivitis: Chlamydial 121
Conjunctivitis: Fungal 122
Conjunctivitis: Gonococcal 122
Conjunctivitis: Viral 123
Constipation 123
Contact Dermatitis (*see* Dermatitis: Allergic/Contact) 138
Corneal Edema 127
Corneal Ulceration 127
Costochondritis (Chest Wall Syndrome) 127
Crohn's Disease 127
Cradle Cap (*see* Dermatitis: Seborrheic) 139
Cryptosporidium parvum 129
Cystitis (*see* Urinary Tract Infection) 437
Cytomegalovirus Retinitis (*see* Retinitis: Cytomegalovirus) ...362
Dandruff (*see* Dermatitis: Seborrheic) 139
Decubitus Ulcer (*see* Ulcer: Pressure/Decubitus) 432

Deep Vein Thrombosis (DVT) 129
Dehydration 129
Dementia 130
Dental Abscess 130
Dental Procedure Prophylaxis (*see* **Bacterial Endocarditis: Prophylaxis**) 72
Denture Irritation 131
Depression 132
Dermatitis: Atopic 136
Dermatitis: Contact/Allergic 138
Dermatitis: Diaper (*see* **Diaper Rash**) 142
Dermatitis: Seborrheic 139
Diabetes Mellitus, Type 1 (*see* **Type 1 Diabetes Mellitus**) 419
Diabetes Mellitus, Type 2 (*see* **Type 2 Diabetes Mellitus**) 423
Diabetic Peripheral Neuropathy 141
Diaper Rash 142
Diarrhea: Acute 144
Diarrhea: Chronic 146
Diarrhea: Traveler's 148
Digitalis Toxicity 148
Diphtheria 149
Diverticulitis 149
Diverticulosis 150
Dry Eye Syndrome 150
Dry Mouth Syndrome (*see* **Sjogren's Syndrome**) 382
Dysentery (*see* **Amebiasis**) 38
Dyshidrosis 152
Dysfunctional Uterine Bleeding (DUB) 152
Dyslipidemia 152
Dyslipidemia, Mixed 152
Dysmenorrhea: Primary 157
Eczema (*see* **Dermatitis: Atopic**) 136
Edema 158
Emphysema 160
Encopresis 161
Endometriosis 162
Enterobiasis vermicularis (*see* **Pinworm**) 334
Enuresis: Primary, Nocturnal 163
Epicondylitis 163
Epididymitis 164
Erectile Dysfunction (Impotence) 165

Erysipelas 167
Erythema Infectiosum (*see* **Fifth Disease**) 173
Esophagitis 167
Exanthum Subitum (*see* **Roseola**) 372
Facial Hair: Excessive/Unwanted 168
Fecal Odor 168
Fever (Pyrexia) 168
Fever Blister (*see* *Herpes Labialis*) 206
Fibrocystic Breast Disease 172
Fibromyalgia 173
Fifth Disease (Erythema Infectiosum) 173
Flatulence 173
Flu (*see* **Influenza**) 245
Fluoridation, water (<0.6 ppm) 174
Folliculitis (*see* **Skin Infection: Bacterial**) 383
Folliculitis Barbae 176
Foreign Body: Esophagus 176
Foreign Body: Eye 176
Furuncle (*see* **Skin Infection: Bacterial**) 383
Fusarium spp. (*see* **Aspergillosis**) 57
Gardnerella Vaginalis (*see* **Bacterial Vaginosis**) 74
Gastritis 177
Gastroenteritis: Bacterial
    (*see* **Salmonellosis**) 375
    (*see* **Shigellosis**) 378
    (*see* **Nausea/Vomiting**) 282
    (*see* **Diarrhea: Acute**) 144
Gastroenteritis: Viral
    (*see* **Nausea/Vomiting**) 282
    (*see* **Diarrhea: Acute**) 144
    (*see* **Rotavirus Gastroenteritis**) 373
Gastroesophageal Reflux (GERD) 177
Generalized Anxiety Disorder (*see* **Anxiety**) 51
Genital Herpes: (*see* **Herpes Genitalis**) 205
Genital Warts (*see* **Wart: Venereal**) 449
German Measles (*see* **Rubella**) 374
Giardia lamblia (*see* **Giardiasis**) 182
Giardiasis (*see* *Giardia lamblia*) 182
Gingivitis/Periodontitis 183
Glaucoma: Open Angle 183
Golfer's Elbow (*see* **Epicondylitis**) 163

Gonorrhea	186
Gout	188
Gouty Arthritis (*see* Gout)	188
Growth Failure	188
Hair Loss (*see* Baldness: Male Pattern)	76
Hay Fever (*see* Sinusitis: Allergic)	366
Headache: Migraine	190
Headache: Tension	196
Heartburn (*see* GERD)	177
Helicobacter pylori infection	197
Hemorrhoids	199
Hepatitis A (HAV)	200
Hepatitis B (HBV)	200
Hepatitis C (HCV)	202
Herpangina	204
Herpes Genitalis	205
Herpes labialis (Cold Sore, Fever Blister)	206
Herpes Simplex Type I (*see* Herpes Labialis)	206
Herpes Simplex Type II (*see* Herpes Genitalis)	206
Herpes zoster (Shingles)	207
Hiccups: Intractable	208
Hidradenitis Suppurativa	208
HIV (*see* Human Immunodeficiency Virus)	210
Hives (*see* Urticaria)	446
Hookworm, Common American (Ucinariasis)	209
Hordeolum (*see* Stye)	391
H. pylori (*see* Helicobacter Pylori Infection)	197
Human Immunodeficiency Virus (HIV)	210
Human Papilloma Virus (*see* Wart: Venereal)	449
Hypercholesterolemia	152
Hyperhidrosis (Perspiration, Excesssive)	211
Hyperhomocysteinemia	211
Hyperlipidemia (*see* Dyslipidemia)	152
Hyperphosphatemia	211
Hyperpigmentation	212
Hypertension: Primary	213
Hyperthyroidism	229
Hypertriglyceridemia	230
Hypocalcemia	232
Hypokalemia	234
Hypomagnesemia	235

Hypoparathyrodism 235
Hypotension: Orthostatic 236
Hypothyroidism 236
Impetigo Contagiosa 238
Impotence (*see* **Erectile Dysfunction**) 165
Incontinence: Urinary 241
Indian Fire (*see* **Impetigo Contagiosa**) 238
Infectious Mononucleosis (*see* **Mononucleosis**) 275
Influenza (Flu) 245
Insect Bite/Sting 246
Insomnia 247
Intermittent Claudication (*see* **Peripheral Vascular Disease**) ...327
Interstitial Cystitis 249
Intertrigo 252
Iritis: Acute 252
Irritable Bowel Syndrome (IBS) 252
Iron Overload 252
Jock Itch (*see Tinea cruris*) 401
Juvenile Rheumatoid Arthritis (JRA)
    (*see* **Rheumatoid Arthritis**) 363
Keratitis/Keratoconjunctivitis: Herpes Simplex 256
Keratitis/Keratoconjunctivitis: Vernal 256
Labyrinthitis 257
Lactose Intolerance 257
Larva Migrans: Cutaneous or Visceral 257
Lead Encephalopathy (*see* **Lead Poisoning**) 258
Lead Poisoning 258
Lead Toxicity (*see* **Lead Poisoning**) 258
Leg Cramps: Nocturnal, Recumbency 259
Lentigines: Benign, Senile 259
Lice (*see* **Pediculosis**) 322
Lichen simplex chronicus (*see* **Dermatitis: Atopic**) 136
Listeriosis 259
Low Back Strain 260
Lyme Disease 260
Lymphadenitis 262
Lymphogranuloma Venereum 263
Magnesium Deficiency (*see* **Hypomagnesemia**) 235
Malaria (*P. falciparum, P. vivax malaria*) 264
Mask of Pregnancy (*see* **Hyperpigmentation**) 212
Mastitis (Breast Abscess) 267

Measles (*see* Rubeola) 375
Melanasia (*see* Hyperpigmentation) 212
Meniere's Disease 268
Meningitis 269
Menopause 270
Migraine Headache (*see* Headache: Migraine) 190
Mineral Deficiency (*see* Vitamin/Mineral Deficiency) 447
Mitral Valve Prolapse 274
Moniliasis (*see* Candidiasis: Vulvovaginal) 94
Mononucleosis 275
Motion Sickness 275
Mouth Ulcer (*see* Aphthous Stomatitis) 55
Multiple Sclerosis 276
Mumps (Infectious Parotitis) 276
Muscle Contraction Headache (*see* Headache: Tension) 196
Muscle Strain 277
Narcolepsy 279
Narcotic Dependence (*see* Opioid Dependence) 291
Nausea/Vomiting 282
Nerve Agent Poisoning 286
Nocturnal Enuresis (*see* Enuresis: Primary) 163
Obesity 286
Obsessive-Compulsive Disorder (OCD) 288
Odor: Fecal (*see* Fecal Odor) 168
Onychomycosis 289
Ophthalmia Neonatorum: Chlamydial 290
Ophthalmia Neonatorum: Gonococcal 291
Opioid Dependence 291
Opioid Overdose 292
Osgood-Schlatter Disease 292
Osteoarthritis (OA) 293
Osteoporosis 293
Osteoporosis Prophylaxis (*see* Osteoporosis) 293
Otitis Externa 296
Otitis Media: Acute 299
Otitis Media: Serous 304
Overdose: Opioid (*see* Opoid Overdose) 292
Paget's Disease: Bone 304
Pain 305
Pancreatic Enzyme Deficiency 316
Panic Disorder 317

Parkinson's Disease 320
Paronychia (Periungal Abscess) 322
Parotitis: Infectious (*see* Mumps) 276
Pediculosis Capitis (Head Lice), Phthirus (Pubic Lice),
    Corporis (Body Lice) 322
Pelvic Inflammatory Disease (PID) 323
Peptic Ulcer Disease (PUD) 325
Periodontitis (*see* Gingivitis/Periodontitis) 183
Peripheral Vascular Disease (PVD) 327
Periungal Abscess (*see* Paronychia) 322
Perspiration: Excesssive (*see* Hyperhidrosis) 211
Pertussis (Whooping Cough) 328
Pharyngitis: Gonococcal 329
Pharyngitis: Streptococcal 330
Pheochromocytoma 334
Pinworm Infection 334
Pityriasis Alba 335
Pityriasis Rosea 336
Plantar Wart (*see* Wart: Plantar) 448
Plague (*Yersinia pestis*) 336
Pneumococcal Pneumonia (*see* Pneumonia: Pneumococcal) ... 348
Pneumonia: Chlamydial 337
Pneumonia: Community Acquired (CAP) 337
Pneumonia: Legionella 346
Pneumonia: Mycoplasma 347
Pneumonia: Pneumococcal 348
Poliomyelitis 349
Polycystic Ovarian Syndrome (*see* Stein-Leventhal Disease) ... 349
Postherpetic Neuralgia 349
Posttraumatic Stress Disorder (PTSD) 350
Pregnancy 351
Premenstrual Dysphoric Disorder (PMDD)
    (Premenstrual Syndrome (PMS)) 351
Premenstrual Syndrome (PMS) (*see* Premenstrual
    Dysphoric Disorder (PMDD)) 351
Pressure Sore (*see* Ulcer: Pressure/Decubitus) 432
Prostatitis: Acute 353
Prostatitis: Chronic 353
Pruritus 354
Pruritus Ani (*see* Pruritis) 354
Pseudogout 356

Pseudomembranous Colitis	356
Psittacosis	357
Psoriasis	357
Psoriatic Arthritis	
(*see* **Osteoarthritis**)	293
(*see* **Rheumatoid Arthritis**)	363
Pyelonephritis: Acute	359
Pyrexia (*see* Fever)	168
Rabies	361
Respiratory Syncytial Virus (RSV)	361
Restless Leg Syndrome	362
Retinitis: Cytomegalovirus (CMV)	362
Rheumatoid Arthritis (RA)	363
Rhinitis: Allergic	366
Rhinitis Medicamentosa	370
Rhinitis: Vasomotor	372
Rhinosinusitis: Acute Bacterial (ABRS)	
(*see* **Sinusitis/Rhinosinusitis: Acute Bacterial**)	379
Rickettsia rickettseii (*see* **Rocky Mountain Spotted Fever**)	372
Rocky Mountain Spotted Fever (*Rickettsia rickettseii*)	372
Rosacea (*see* Acne Rosacea)	29
Roseola (Exanthum Subitum)	372
Rotavirus Gastroenteritis	373
Roundworm: Common, Intestinal (Ascariasis)	373
Rubella (German Measles)	374
Rubeola (Measles)	375
Salmonella typhi (*see* **Typhoid Fever**)	429
Salmonellosis	375
Sarcoptes scabei (Scabies)	376
Scabies (*see* *Sarcoptes scabei*)	376
Scarlatina (*see* Scarlet Fever)	376
Scarlet Fever (Scarlatina)	376
Sebaceous Cyst: Infected (*see* Skin Infection: Bacterial)	383
Seborrhea (*see* Dermatitis: Seborrheic)	139
Seizure Disorder	378
Shigellosis	378
Shingles (*see* *Herpes zoster*)	207
Sinusitis/Rhinosinusitis: Acute Bacterial	379
Sinusitis: Allergic (Hay Fever) (*see* Allergic Rhinitis)	366
Sjogren's Syndrome (Dry Mouth Syndrome)	382
Skin: Calloused	383

Skin Infection: Bacterial 383
Sleep Apnea 388
Sleepiness: Excessive 389
Smallpox 389
Solar Keratosis (*see* Actinic Keratosis) 35
Sprain 389
Status Asthmaticus 390
Status Epilepticus 390
Stein-Leventhal Disease (*see* Polycystic Ovarian Syndrome) 349
Stomatitis (*see* Aphthous Stomatitis) 55
Stress Incontinence (*see* Incontinence: Urinary) 241
Strongyloidiasis (*see* Threadworm) 397
Stye 391
Sunburn 392
Swimmer's Ear (*see* Otitis Externa) 296
Syphilis 392
Temporal Arteritis 395
Temporomandibular Joint Disorder (TMJ) 395
Tennis Elbow (*see* Epicondylitis) 163
Tension Headache (*see* Headache: Tension) 196
Testosterone Deficiency 395
Tetanus 397
Threadworm 397
Thrush (*see* Candidiasis: Oral) 92
Tic Douloureux (*see* Trigeminal Neuralgia) 415
Tinea Capitis 398
Tinea Corporis 399
Tinea Cruris (Jock Itch) 401
Tinea Pedis (Athlete's Foot) 403
Tinea Versicolor 406
Tobacco Dependence 408
Tonsillitis: Acute 410
Tremor: Benign Essential (*see* Benign Essential Tremor) 76
Trichinosis 413
Trichomoniasis (*Trichomonas vaginalis*) 414
Trichuriasis (*see* Whipworm) 449
Trigeminal Neuralgia (Tic Douloureux) 415
Tuberculosis (TB) 416
Type 1 Diabetes Mellitus 419
Type 2 Diabetes Mellitus 423
Typhoid Fever (*Salmonella typhi*) 429

Ucinariasis (*see* Hookworm: Common American) 209
Ulcer: Diabetic, Neuropathic (Lower Extremity) 432
Ulcer: Pressure/Decubitus 432
Ulcerative Colitis 432
Upper Respiratory Infection (*see* Common Cold) 105
Urethritis: Gonococcal 434
Urethritis: Nongonococcal 435
Urethritis: Recurrent/Persistent 436
Urinary Retention: Unobstructive 437
Urinary Tract Infection (UTI, Cystitis: Acute) 437
Urolithiasis 445
Urticaria: Chronic Idiopathic (CIU) 446
Urticaria: Acute (Hives) 446
Ucinariasis (Common American Hookworm) 209
Vaginal Irritation: External 447
Varicella (*see* Chickenpox) 101
Vascular Headache (*see* Headache: Migraine) 190
Vasomotor Rhinitis (*see* Rhinitis: Vasomotor) 372
Venereal Warts (*see* Wart: Venereal) 449
Verruca plantaris (*see* Wart: Plantar) 448
Verruca vulgaris (*see* Wart: Common) 448
Vertigo 447
Vitamin/Mineral Deficiency 447
Vitamin/Mineral Prophylaxis 447
Vitiligo 447
Vomiting (*see* Nausea/Vomiting) 282
Wart: Common (*Verruca vulgaris*) 448
Wart: Plantar (*Verruca plantaris*) 448
Wart: Venereal (Human Papilloma Virus (HPV),
    Condyloma Accuminata) 449
Whipworm (Trichuriasis) 449
Whooping Cough (*see* Pertussis) 328
Wound: Infected, Non-surgical, Minor 450
Wrinkles: Facial 453
Xerosis 454
Yersinia pestis (*see* Plague) 336
Zollinger-Ellison Syndrome 455

Section II: Appendixes 457

Appendix A: FDA Pregnancy Categories 459

Appendix B:	U.S. Schedule of Controlled Substances	460
Appendix C:	JNC-VII Hypertension Evaluation & Treatment Recommendations	462
Appendix C.1:	Blood Pressure Classification	462
Appendix C.2:	Identifiable Causes of Hypertension	462
Appendix C.3:	CVD Risk Factors	462
Appendix C.4:	Diagnostic Workup of Hypertension	462
Appendix C.5:	Compelling Indications for Individual Individual Drug Classes	463
Appendix C.6:	Initial Drug Choices Without Compelling Indications	463
Appendix D:	Target Lipid Recommendations	464
Appendix D.A:	Target TC, TG, HDL-C	464
Appendix D.B:	Target LDL-C	464
Appendix E:	Effects of Selected Drugs on Insulin Activity	465
Appendix F:	Glycosolated hemoglobin (HbA1C) & Average Blood Glucose Equivalents	465
Appendix G:	Childhood Immunizations	466
Appendix G.1:	Recommended Childhood Immunization Schedule	467
Appendix G.2:	Childhood Immunization Catch-up Schedule	467
Appendix G.3:	Contraindications to Vaccines	468
Appendix G.4:	Route of Administration & Dosage of Vaccines	469
Appendix G.5:	Adverse Reactions to Vaccines	469
Appendix H:	Contraceptives (Non-Barrier)	470
Appendix H.1:	Combined Oral Contraceptives	471
Appendix H.2:	Progesterone-only Contraceptives	475
Appendix H.3:	Injectable Contraceptives	476
Appendix H.4:	Transdermal Contraceptive	477
Appendix H.5:	Contraceptive Vaginal Ring	477
Appendix H.6:	Subdermal Contraceptive	478
Appendix H.7:	Emergency Contraception	478
Appendix I:	Anesthetic Agents for Local Infiltration & Dermal/Mucous Membrane Application	480
Appendix J:	Oral Non-Steroidal Antiinflammatory Drugs	481
Appendix K:	Topical Glucocorticosteroids	483
Appendix L:	Oral Glucocorticosteroids	487
Appendix M:	Parenteral Glucocorticosteroids	489
Appendix N:	Inhalational Glucocorticosteroids	491

Appendix O: Systemic Antiarrhythmic Drugs	494
Appendix P: Systemic Antineoplasia Drugs	497
Appendix Q: Antipsychosis Drugs	499
Appendix R: Anticonvulsant Drugs	501
Appendix S: Anti-HIV Drugs	503
Appendix T: Coumadin (Warfarin) Therapy	506
Appendix U: Low Molecular Weight Heparins	507
Appendix V: Vitamin & Mineral Supplements	508
Appendix V.1: Vitamin & Mineral Supplements for Adults	509
Appendix V.2: Vitamin & Mineral Supplements for Infants and Children	514
Appendix V.3: Prenatal Vitamin & Mineral Supplements	517
Appendix W: Oral Drugs for the Management of Common Respiratory Symptoms	523
Appendix X: Systemic Antiinfective Drugs	555
Appendix Y: Antiinfective Drug Dose by Weight for Liquid Forms	566
Appendix Z: Brand/Generic Drug Cross Reference	599

SECTION I

PHARMACOTHERAPEUTICS
by
CLINICAL DIAGNOSIS

Acetaminophen Overdose

Antidote/Chelating Agent
▶*acetylcysteine* **(B)**
>Loading Dose: 150 mg/kg administered over 15 minutes
>Maintenance: 50 mg/kg administered over 4 hours; then, 100 mg/kg administered over 16 hours
>*Pediatric:* same as adult
>**Acetadote®** *Soln for IV infusion after dilution:* 200 mg/ml (30 ml); dilute in D_5W; preservative-free)

Comment: Acetaminophen overdose is a medical emergency due to the risk of irreversible hepatic injury. An IV infusion of *acetylcysteine* should be started as soon as possible and within 24 hours if the exact time of ingestion is unknown. Use a serum *acetaminophen* nomogram to determine need for treatment. Extreme caution with concomitant hepatotoxic drugs.

Acne Rosacea

Comment: All products should be applied sparingly to clean, dry skin as directed. Avoid use of topical glucocorticosteroids.

Topical Antimicrobials
▶*azelaic acid* **(B)** apply bid in AM and PM
>**Azelex®** *Crm:* 20% (30, 50 g)
>**Finacea®** *Gel:* 15% (30 g)
>**Finevin®** *Crm:* 20% (30 g)

▶*metronidazole* **(B)**
>**MetroCream®** apply to affected area AM and PM
>*Emol crm:* 0.75% (45 g)
>**Metro-Gel®** apply to affected area q AM and PM
>*Gel:* 0.75, 10% (30, 45 g)
>**Metro-Lotion®** apply to affected area q AM and PM
>*Lotn:* 0.75% (2 oz)
>**Noritate®** apply to affected area daily
>*Emol crm:* 1% (30 g)

▶*sodium sulfacetamide* **(C)(G)** apply daily-tid
>**Klaron®** *Lotn:* 10% (2 oz)
>**Novacet®Lotion** *Lotn:* 10% (30, 60 g)

▶*sodium sulfacetamide/sulfur* **(C)**
>**Clenia®Emollient Cream** apply daily; max tid
>*Wash: sod sulfa* 10%/*sulfur* 5% (10 oz)

Acne Rosacea

    Clenia®Foaming Wash wash once or twice daily
        Wash: sod sulfa 10%/sulfur 5% (6, 12 oz)
    Rosula®Gel apply daily-tid
        Gel: sod sulfa 10%/sulfur 5% (45 ml)
    Rosula®Lotion apply daily-tid
        Lotn: sod sulfa 10%/sulfur 5% (45 ml; alcohol-free)
    Rosula®Wash wash 10-20 sec daily-bid
        Clnsr: sod sulfa 10%/sulfur 5% (335 ml)
    Sulfacet-R®Lotion apply daily-tid
        Lotn: sod sulfa 10%/sulfur 5% (25 g)
        Lotn (tint-free): sod sulfa 10%/sulfur 5% (25 g)

Oral Antimicrobials

▶*doxycycline* **(D)(G)** 40-100 mg daily-bid
        Pediatric: see page 587 for dose by weight
            <8 years: not recommended
            >8 years, <100 lb: 2 mg/lb on first day in 2 doses, followed by 1 mg/lb/day in 1-2 doses
            >8 years, >100 lb: same as adult
    Adoxa® *Tab:* 50, 100 mg ent-coat
    Doryx® *Cap:* 100 mg
    Monodox® *Cap:* 50, 100 mg
    Oracea® *Cap:* 40 mg
    Vibramycin® *Cap:* 50, 100 mg; *Syr:* 50 mg/5 ml (raspberry-apple, sulfites); *Oral susp:* 25 mg/5 ml (raspberry)
    Vibra-Tab® *Tab:* 100 mg film-coat

▶*minocycline* **(D)(G)** 200 mg on first day; then 100 mg q 12 hours x 9 more days
        Pediatric: <8 years: not recommended
            >8 years, <100 lb: 2 mg/lb on first day in 2 doses, followed by 1 mg/lb/ q 12 hours x 9 more days
            >8 years, >100 lb: same as adult
    Minocin® *Cap:* 100 mg ent-coat

Comment: Minocycline is contraindicated in pregnancy (discolors fetal tooth enamel).

Acne Vulgaris

Antibacterial Soaps
    Dial® (OTC) wash affected area bid
    Lever 2000®Antibacterial (OTC) wash affected area bid

Topical Antimicrobials

Acne Vulgaris

Comment: All products should be applied sparingly to clean, dry skin as directed.
▶*azelaic acid* **(B)** apply bid in AM and PM
  Azelex® *Crm:* 20% (30, 50 g)
  Finacea® *Gel:* 15% (30 g)
  Finevin® *Crm:* 20% (30 g)
▶*benzoyl peroxide* **(C)(G)**
Comment: May discolor clothing.
  Benzac® initially apply to affected area daily; increase to bid-tid as tolerated
    Gel: 2.5, 5, 10% (60 g; alcohol 12%); *Aqueous base gel:* 5, 10% (60, 90 g)
  Benzac®Wash wash affected area daily-bid; rinse and pat dry
    Wash: 5% (4, 8 oz); 10% (8 oz)
  Benzagel® apply to affected area one or more times/day
    Gel: 5, 10% (1.5, 3 oz; alcohol 14%)
  Benzagel®Wash wash affected area daily-bid; rinse and pat dry
    Gel: 10% (6 oz)
  Benziq®Gel wash affected area daily-bid; rinse and pat dry
    Gel: 5.2% (6 oz)
  Benziq®Gel wash affected area daily-bid; rinse and pat dry
    Gel: 5.2% (6 oz)
  Benziq®LS wash affected area daily-bid; rinse and pat dry
    Wash: 2.75% (6 oz)
  Brevoxyl® apply to affected area daily-bid
    Gel: 4, 8% (42.5, 90 g); *Cleansing lotn:* 4, 8% (10.5 oz)
  Desquam® apply to affected area daily-bid
    Gel: 2.5, 5, 10% (1.5, 3 oz); *Emol gel:* 2.5, 5, 10% (1.5, 3 oz); *Wash:* 5, 10% (5 oz); *Bar:* 10% (3.75 oz)
    Gel: 5, 10% (1 oz)
  Triaz®Gel apply daily-bid; cleanser: wash for 10-20 sec daily-bid
    Gel: 3, 6, 10% (42.5 oz); *Clnsr:* 3, 6% (3, 6 oz); 10% (3, 6, 12 oz)
  ZoDerm® apply daily-bid
    Gel: 4.5, 6.5, 8.5% (125 ml); *Crm:* 4.5, 6.5, 8.5% (125 ml); *Clnsr:* 4.5, 6.5, 8.5% (400 ml)
▶*benzoyl peroxide/hydrocortisone* **(C)** apply daily-tid
  Vanoxide®HC Lotion *Lotn:* benz 50 mg/*hydro* 5 mg (25 g)
▶*clindamycin topical* **(B)** apply bid
    Pediatric: not recommended
  Cleocin®T *Pad:* 1% (60/pck; alcohol 50%); *Lotn:* 1% (60 ml);

Acne Vulgaris

      Gel: 1% (30, 60 g); *Soln w. applicator:* 1% (30, 60 ml; alcohol 50%)
    Clindagel® *Gel:* 1% (42, 77 g)
    Clindets® *Pad:* 1% (60/pck)
▶ *clindamycin/benzoyl peroxide* topical **(C)**
    Pediatric: <12 years: not recommended
    BenzaClin®apply bid
        Gel: clin 1%/*benz* 5% (25, 50 g)
    Duac®apply daily in the evening
        Gel: clin 1%/*benz* 5% (45 g)
▶ *erythromycin* topical apply bid
    A/T/S® **(B)** *Soln:* 2% (60 ml); *Gel:* 2% (30 g)
    Emgel® **(B)** *Gel:* 2% (27, 50 g; alcohol 77%)
    Erycette® **(C)** *Swab:* 2% (60/pck; alcohol 66%)
    Eryderm® **(C)** *Soln:* 2% (60 ml w. applicator)
    Erygel® **(C)** *Gel:* 2% (30, 60 g)
    Erymax® **(C)** *Soln:* 2% (2, 4 oz w. applicator)
    Theramycin Z® **(C)** *Soln:* 2% (2 oz)
▶ *erythromycin/benzoyl peroxide* **(C)** initially apply daily; increase to bid as tolerated
    Benzamycin®Gel *Gel: eryth* 3%/*benz* 5% (23, 46 g)
    Benzamycin®Pak *Pak: eryth* 3%/*benz* 5% (60)
▶ *sodium sulfacetamide* **(C)(G)** apply daily-tid
    Klaron® *Lotn:* 10% (2 oz)
    Novacet®Lotion *Lotn:* 10% (30, 60 g)
▶ *sodium sulfacetamide/sulfur* **(C)**
    Clinia®Emollient Cream apply daily; max tid
        Wash: sod sulfa 10%/*sulfur* 5% (10 oz)
    Clinia®Foaming Wash wash once or twice daily
        Wash: sod sulfa 10%/*sulfur* 5% (6, 12 oz)
    Rosula®Gel apply daily-tid
        Gel: sod sulfa 10%/*sulfur* 5% (45 ml)
    Rosula®Lotion apply daily-tid
        Lotn: sod sulfa 10%/*sulfur* 5% (45 ml; alcohol-free)
    Rosula®Wash wash 10-20 sec daily-bid
        Clnsr: sod sulfa 10%/*sulfur* 5% (335 ml)
    Sulfacet-R®Lotion apply daily-tid
        Lotn: sod sulfa 10%/*sulfur* 5% (25 g); *Lotn (tint-free): sod sulfa* 10% /*sulfur* 5% (25 g)
▶ *tetracycline* **(D)** topical apply daily-bid
    Topicycline® *Soln:* 2.2% (70 ml)

Acne Vulgaris

Oral Antimicrobials

▶*doxycycline* **(D)(G)** 100 mg daily-bid
> *Pediatric: see page 587 for dose by weight*
>> <8 years: not recommended
>> >8 years, <100 lb: 2 mg/lb on first day in 2 doses, followed by 1 mg/lb/day in 1-2 doses
>> >8 years, >100 lb: same as adult

    Adoxa® *Tab:* 50, 100 mg ent-coat
    Doryx® *Cap:* 100 mg
    Monodox® *Cap:* 50, 100 mg
    Vibramycin® *Cap:* 50, 100 mg; *Syr:* 50 mg/5 ml (raspberry-apple, sulfites); *Oral susp:* 25 mg/5 ml (raspberry)
    Vibra-Tab® *Tab:* 100 mg film-coat

▶*erythromycin base* **(B)(G)** 250 mg qid, 333 mg tid, or 500 mg bid x 7-10 days; then taper to lowest effective dose
> *Pediatric: see page 588 for dose by weight*
>> <45 kg: 30-50 mg in 2-4 doses x 7-10 days
>> >45 kg: same as adult

    E-mycin® *Tab:* 250, 333 mg ent-coat
    Eryc® *Cap:* 250 mg ent-coat pellets
    Ery-Tab® *Tab:* 250, 333, 500 mg ent-coat
    PCE® *Tab:* 333, 500 mg

▶*minocycline* **(D)** initially 50-200 mg/day in 2 doses; reduce dose after improvement
> *Pediatric:* <8 years: not recommended
>> >8 years: same as adult

    Dynacin® *Cap:* 50, 100 mg
    Minocin® *Cap:* 50, 100 mg; *Oral susp:* 50 mg/5 ml (2 oz)

Comment: Minocycline is contraindicated in pregnancy (discolors fetal tooth enamel).

▶*tetracycline* **(D)(G)** initially 1 g/day in 2-4 doses; after improvement, 125-500 mg daily
> *Pediatric: see page 595 for dose by weight*
>> <8 years: not recommended
>> >8 years, <100 lb: 25-50 mg/kg/day in 2-4 doses
>> >8 years, >100 lb: same as adult

    Achromycin®V *Cap:* 250, 500 mg
    Sumycin® *Tab:* 250, 500 mg; *Cap:* 250, 500 mg; *Oral susp:* 125 mg/5 ml (100, 200 ml; fruit, sulfites)

Comment: Tetracycline is contraindicated in pregnancy (discolors fetal tooth enamel).

Acne Vulgaris

Topical Retinoids

Comment: Wash affected area with a soap-free cleanser; pat dry and wait 20 to 30 minutes; then apply sparingly to affected area; use only once daily in the evening. Avoid eyes, ears, nostrils, and mouth.

    Pediatric: <8 years: not recommended

▶*adapalene* **(C)** apply daily at HS

    Differin® *Crm:* 0.1% (15, 45 g); *Gel:* 0.1% (15, 45 g); *Pad:* 0.1% (30/pck; alcohol 30%)

    Differin®Solution *Soln:* 0.1% (30 ml; alcohol 30%)

▶*tazarotene* **(X)** apply daily at HS

    Pediatric: not recommended

    Avage®Cream *Crm:* 0.1% (30 g)

    Tazorac®Cream *Crm:* 0.05, 0.1% (15, 30, 60 g)

    Tazorac®Gel *Gel:* 0.05, 0.1% (30, 100 g)

▶*tretinoin* **(C)** apply daily at HS

    Pediatric: <12 years: not recommended

    Avita® *Crm:* 0.025% (20, 45 g); *Gel:* 0.025% (20, 45 g)

    Renova® *Crm:* 0.02% (40 g); 0.05% (40, 60 g)

    Retin-A®Cream *Crm:* 0.025, 0.05, 0.1% (20, 45 g)

    Retin-A®Gel *Gel:* 0.01, 0.025% (15, 45 g; alcohol 90%)

    Retin-A®Liquid *Soln:* 0.05% (alcohol 55%)

    Retin-A®Micro *Microspheres:* 0.04%, 0.1% (20, 45 g)

Oral Retinoid

Comment: Indicated only for severe recalcitrant nodular acne unresponsive to conventional therapy including systemic antibiotics.

▶*isotretinoin* **(X)** initially 0.5-1 mg/kg/day in 2 doses; maintenance 0.5-2 mg/kg/day in 2 doses x 4-5 months; repeat only if necessary 2 months following cessation of first treatment course

    Pediatric: not applicable

    Accutane® *Cap:* 10, 20, 40 mg (parabens)

Comment: Isotretinoin is highly teratogenic and, therefore, female patients should be counseled prior to initiation of treatment as follows:

    Two negative pregnancy tests are required prior to initiation of treatment and monthly thereafter. Not for use in females who are or who may become pregnant or who are breast feeding. Two effective methods of contraception should be used for 1 month prior to, during, and continuing for 1 month following completion of treatment. Low-dose *progestin*("mini-pill") may be an *inadequate* form of contraception. No refills; a new prescription is required every 30 days and prescriptions must be filled within 7 days. Serum lipids should be monitored until response is established (usually initially and again after 4 weeks). Bone growth, serum glucose, ESR, RBCs, WBCs, and liver enzymes should be monitored. Blood should not be donated during, or for 1 month after, completion of treatment. Avoid the sun and artificial UV

light.
Isotretinoin should be discontinued if any of the following occurs:
> visual disturbances, tinnitus, hearing impairment, rectal bleeding, pancreatitis, hepatitis, significant decrease in CBC, hyperlipidemia (particularly hypertriglyceridemia).

Oral Contraceptives
see **Combined Oral Contraceptives** *page 471*
see **Progesterone-only Contraceptives ("Mini-Pill")** *page 475*

Acromegaly

Growth Hormone Receptor Antagonist
▶*pegvisomant* **(B)**
> Loading dose: 40 mg SC
> Maintenance: 10 mg SC daily; titrate by 5 mg (increments or decrements, based on IGF-1 levels) every 4 to 6 weeks; max 30 mg/day
> *Pediatric:* not recommended
> **Somavert®** *Inj:* 10, 15, 20 mg

Actinic Keratosis

Comment: These treatments are also indicated for destroying superficial basal cell carcinoma (sBCC) lesions.

▶*diclofenac sodium* 3% **(B; not for use in 3rd)** apply to lesion(s) bid for 60-90 days
> *Pediatric:* not recommended
> **Solaraze®Gel** *Gel:* 3% (50 g)

Comment: Diclofenac sodium is contraindicated with *aspirin* allergy.

▶*fluorouracil* **(X)** apply to lesion(s) daily-bid until erosion occurs, usually 2-4 weeks
> *Pediatric:* not recommended
> **Carac®** *Crm:* 5% (30 g)
> **Efudex®** *Crm:* 5% (25 g); *Soln:* 2, 5% (10 ml w. dropper)
> **Fluoroplex®** *Crm:* 1% (30 g); *Soln:* 1% (30 ml w. dropper)

▶*imiquimod* **(B)** rub into lesion before bedtime and remove with soap and water 6-10 hours later; treat 3 times per week; max 16 weeks
> **Aldara®** *Crm:* 5% (250 mg single-use pkts; 12/box)

Alcohol Dependence
Alcohol Withdrawal Syndrome

Alcohol Withdrawal Syndrome
▶*clorazepate* **(D)(IV)(G)** in the following dosage schedule:
   Day 1: 30 mg initially, followed by 30-60 mg in divided doses
   Day 2: 45 to 90 mg in divided doses
   Day 3: 22.5 to 45 mg in divided doses
   Day 4: 15 to 30 mg in divided doses
   Thereafter, gradually reduce the daily dose to 7.5-15 mg then
   discontinue when patient's condition is stable; max dose 90 mg/day
   Tranxene® *Tab:* 3.75, 7.5, 15 mg
   Tranxene®SD *Tab:* 22.5 mg ext-rel
   Tranxene®SD Half Strength *Tab:* 11.25 mg ext-rel
   Tranxene®T-Tab *Tab:* 3.75*, 7.5*, 15*mg
▶*chlordiazepoxide* **(D)(IV)(G)**
   Librium® 50-100 mg q 6 hours x 24-72 hours; then q 8 hours
   x 24-72 hours; then q 12 hours x 24-72 hours; then daily x 24-72
   hours
      Cap: 5, 10, 25 mg
   Librium®Injectable 50-100 mg IM or IV, then 25-50 mg IM
   tid-qid prn; max 300 mg/day
      Inj: 100 mg
▶*diazepam* **(D)(IV)(G)** 2-10 mg q 6 hours x 24-72 hours; then q 8 hours
   x 24-72 hours; then q 12 hours x 24-72 hours; then daily x 24-72 hours
   Valium® *Tab:* 2*, 5*, 10*mg
▶*oxazepam* **(C)** 10-15 mg tid-qid x 24-72 hours; decrease dose and/or
   frequency every 24-72 hours; total length of therapy 5-14 days; max
   120 mg/day
   Serax® *Cap:* 10, 15, 30 mg

Abstinence Therapy
GABA Taurine Analogue
▶*acamprosate* **(C)** 666 mg tid; begin therapy during abstinence;
continue during relapse
   Campral® *Tab:* 333 mg ext-rel
Comment: Renal impairment, start ***Campral®*** at 333 mg tid.

Opioid Antagonist
▶*naltrexone* **(C)** 380 mg IM every 4 weeks; alternate buttocks
   Vivitrol® *Vial:* 380 mg (1 vial w. supplies)
Comment: Concomitant opoids, acute hepatitis, and liver failure are

contraindications for ***Vivitrol*®** therapy.

Aversion Therapy
▶*disulfiram* **(X)(G)**
> **Antabuse®** 500 mg daily x 1-2 weeks; then 250 mg daily
> *Tab:* 250, 500 mg

Comment: Requires informed consent. Contraindications: severe cardiac disease, psychosis, concomitant use of *isoniazid*, *phenytoin*, *paraldehyde*, and topical and systemic alcohol-containing products. Approximately 20% remains in the system for 1 week after discontinuation.

Nutritional Support
▶*thiamine* **(A)(G)** injectable 50-100 mg IM/IV daily (or tid if severely deficient)
> *Vial:* 100 mg/1 ml (1 ml)

Allergic Reaction

Parenteral Antihistamines
▶*diphenhydramine* **(C)(G)** 25-50 mg IM immediately; then q 6 hours
> *Pediatric:* 1.25 mg/kg up to 25 mg IM x 1 dose; then q 6 hours
>
> **Benadryl®Injectable** *Vial:* 50 mg/ml (1 ml single-use); 50 mg/ml (10 ml multidose); *Amp:* 10 mg/ml (1 ml); *Prefilled syringe:* 50 mg/ml (1 ml)

Oral Antihistamines
*see **1st Generation Antihistamines** page 525*
*see **2nd Generation Antihistamines** page 527*
Topical Glucocorticosteroids *see page 483*
Parenteral Glucocorticosteroids *see page 489*
Oral Glucocorticosteroids *see page 487*

Alzheimer's Disease

Reversible Anti-cholinesterase Inhibitors
Comment: These drugs do not halt disease progression. They are indicated for early stage disease; not effective for severe dementia. If treatment is stopped for more than several days, re-titrate from lowest dose. Side effects include nausea, anorexia, dyspepsia, diarrhea, headache, and dizziness. Side effects tend to resolve with continued treatment. Peak cognitive improvements are seen 12 weeks into therapy (increased spontaneity, reduced apathy, lessened confusion, and improved attention, conversational language, and performance of daily routines).
▶*donepezil* **(C)** initially 5 mg q HS, increase to 10 mg after 4-6 weeks

as needed; max 10 mg/day
> **Aricept®** *Tab:* 5, 10 mg
> **Aricept®ODT** *Tab:* 5, 10 mg orally disintegrating

▶*galantamine* **(B)** initially 4 mg bid x at least 4 weeks; usual maintenance 8 mg bid; max 16 mg bid
> **Razadyne®** *Tab:* 4, 8, 12 mg
> **Razadyne®ER** *Tab:* 8, 16, 24 mg ext-rel
> **Razadyne®Oral Solution** *Oral soln:* 4 mg/ml (100 ml w. cal pipette)

▶*rivastigmine* **(B)** initially 1.5 mg bid, increase every 2 weeks as needed; max 12 mg/day
> **Exelon®** *Cap:* 1.5, 3, 4.5, 6 mg
> **Exelon®Oral Solution** *Oral soln:* 2 mg/ml (120 ml w. dose syringe)

▶*tacrine* **(C)** initially 10 mg qid, increase 40 mg/day q 4 weeks as needed; max 160 mg/day
> **Cognex®** *Cap:* 10, 20, 30, 40 mg

Comment: Transaminase levels should be checked every 3 months.

N-Methyl-D-Aspartate (NMDA) Receptor Antagonist
▶*menantine* **(B)** initially 5 mg daily; may increase weekly by 5 mg increments given bid; maintenance 90 mg bid
> **Namenda®** *Tab:* 5, 10 mg
> **Namenda®Titration Pak** *Tab:* (28 x 5 mg + 21 x 10 mg)
> **Namenda®Oral Solution** *Oral soln:* 2 mg/ml (360 ml)(peppermint, sugar- and alcohol-free)

Comment: **Namenda®** does not halt disease progression. It is indicated for moderate to severe dementia.

Ergot alkaloid (Dopamine Agonist)
▶*ergoloid mesylate* **(C)** 1 mg tid
> **Hydergine®** *Tab:* 1 mg
> **Hydergine®LC** *Cap:* 1 mg
> **Hydergine®Liquid** *Liq:* 1 mg/ml (100 ml w. cal dropper; alcohol 28.5%)

Amebiasis

Amebiasis (Intestinal)
▶*diiodohydroxyquin (iodoquinol)* **(C)(G)** 650 mg tid pc x 20 days
> *Pediatric:* <6 years: 40 mg/kg/day in 3 doses pc x 20 days; max 1.95 g

6-12 years: 420 mg tid pc x 20 days
>	*Tab:* 210, 650 mg
▶ *furazolidone* **(C)** 100 mg qid; max 7 days
>	*Pediatric:* <1 month: not recommended
>	>1 month: 5 mg/kg/day in 4 doses; max 7 days
>	**Furoxone®** *Tab:* 100 mg; *Liq:* 50 mg/15 ml (60 ml; 8 oz)

▶ *metronidazole* **(not for use in 1st; B in 2nd, 3rd)(G)** 750 mg tid x 5-10 days
>	*Pediatric:* 35-50 mg/kg/day in 3 divided doses x 10 days
>	**Flagyl®375** *Cap:* 375 mg
>	**Flagyl®ER** *Tab:* 750 mg ext-rel
>	**Flagyl®, Protostat®** *Tab:* 250*, 500*mg

Comment: Alcohol is contraindicated during treatment with oral *metronidazole* and for 72 hours after therapy due to a possible *disulfiram*-like reaction (nausea, vomiting, flushing, headache).

▶ *tinidazole* **(not for use in 1st; B in 2nd, 3rd)** 2 g daily x 3 days; take with food
>	*Pediatric:* <3 years: not recommended
>	>3 years: 50 mg/kg daily x 3 days; take with food; max 2 g/day
>	**Tindamax®** *Tab:* 250*, 500*mg

▶ *paromomycin* 25-35 mg/kg/day in 3 divided doses x 5 to 10 days
>	*Pediatric:* same as adult
>	**Humatin®** *Cap:* 250 mg

Amebiasis (Extra-intestinal)
▶ *chloroquine phosphate* **(C)(G)** 1 g po daily x 2 days; then 500 mg daily x 2 to 3 weeks or 200-250 mg IM daily x 10 to 12 days (when oral therapy is impossible); use with intestinal amebicide
>	*Pediatric:* see mfr literature
>	**Aralen®** *Tab:* 500 mg; *Amp:* 50 mg/ml (5 ml)

Amebic Liver Abscess

Anti-infectives
▶ *metronidazole* **(not for use in 1st; B in 2nd, 3rd)(G)** 250 mg tid or 500 mg bid or 750 mg daily x 7 days
>	*Pediatric:* not recommended
>	**Flagyl®375** *Cap:* 375 mg
>	**Flagyl®ER** *Tab:* 750 mg ext-rel

Amebic Liver Abscess

Flagyl®, Protostat® *Tab:* 250*, 500*mg

Comment: Alcohol is contraindicated during treatment with oral *metronidazole* and for 72 hours after therapy due to a possible *disulfiram*-like reaction (nausea, vomiting, flushing, headache).

▶*tinidazole* **(not for use in 1st; B in 2nd, 3rd)** 2 g daily x 3-5 days; take with food

>   *Pediatric:* <3 years: not recommended
>   >3 years: 50 mg/kg daily x 3-5 days; take with food; max 2 g/day

Tindamax® *Tab:* 250*, 500*mg

Amenorrhea: Secondary

▶*estrogen/progesterone* **(X)**
>   **Premarin®** (*estrogen*) 0.625 mg daily x 25 days <u>with</u>
>   **Provera®** (*progesterone*) 5-10 mg last 10 days of cycle; repeat monthly

▶*estrogen replacement* **(X)**
see **Menopause** page 270

▶*human chorionic gonadotropin* 5,000-10,000 units IM x 1 dose following last dose of menotropins
>   **Pregnyl®** *Vial:* 10,000 units (10 ml) w. diluent (10 ml)

▶*medroxyprogesterone* **(X)**
>   Monthly: 5-10 mg last 5-10 days of cycle; begin on the 16th or 21st day of cycle; repeat monthly
>   One-time only: 10 mg daily x 10 days
>   **Amen®** *Tab:* 10 mg
>   **Cycrin®, Provera®** *Tab:* 2.5, 5, 10 mg

▶*norethindrone* **(X)**
>   **Aygestin®** 2.5-10 mg daily x 5-10 days
>   *Tab:* 5 mg

▶*progesterone, micronized* **(X)**
>   **Prometrium®** 400 mg q HS x 10 days
>   *Cap:* 100, 200 mg

Comment: Administration of *progesterone* induces optimum secretory transformation of the estrogen-primed endometrium. Administration of *progesterone* is contraindicated with breast cancer, undiagnosed vaginal bleeding, genital cancer, severe liver dysfunction or disease, missed abortion, thrombophlebitis, thromboembolic disorders, cerebral apoplexy, and as a diagnosis of pregnancy.

Anaphylaxis

▶*epinephrine* **(C)(G)** 0.3-0.5 mg (0.3-0.5 ml of a 1:1000 soln) SC q 20-30 minutes as needed up to 3 doses
    Pediatric: <2 years: 0.05-0.1 ml
              2-6 years: 0.1 ml
              6-12 years: 0.2 ml
              All: q 20-30 minutes as needed up to 3 doses
Parenteral Glucocorticosteroids *see page 489*
Oral Glucocorticosteroids *see page 487*
Anaphylaxis Emergency Treatment Kits
▶*epinephrine* **(C)** 0.3 ml IM in thigh; may repeat if needed
    Pediatric: 0.01 mg/kg IM in thigh; may repeat if needed
    EpiPen® *EpiPen 0.3 mg:* auto-injector with *epi* 1:1000, 0.3 ml (1, 2/box)
    EpiPen®Jr *EpiPen Jr 0.15 mg:* auto-injector with *epi* 1:2000, 0.3 ml (1, 2/box)
▶*epinephrine/chlorpheniramine* **(C)**
    Ana-Kit® 0.3 ml SC or IM <u>plus</u> 4 tabs *chlorpheniramine*
    Pediatric: infants-2 years: 0.05-0.1 ml SC or IM
                    2-6 years: 0.15 ml SC or IM <u>plus</u> 1 tab *chlor*
                    6-12 years: 0.2 ml SC or IM <u>plus</u> 2 tabs *chlor*
    Kit: two 0.3 ml syringes of *epi* 1:1000 for self-injection <u>plus</u> *chlor* 2 mg chewable tabs x 4

Anemia of Chronic Renal Failure

▶*darbepoetin alpha* (erythropoiesis stimulating protein) **(C)** administer IV or SC q 1-2 weeks; do not increase more frequently than once per month
    Not currently receiving epoetin alpha: initially 0.45 mcg/kg once weekly; adjust based on Hgb levels (target not to exceed 12 g/dL); reduce dose if Hgb increases more than 1 g/dL in any 2-week period; suspend therapy if polycythemia occurs
    Converting from epoetin alpha and for dose titration: see mfr literature
    Pediatric: not recommended
    Aranesp® *Vial:* 25, 40, 60, 100, 200, mcg/ml (single-dose) for IV

or SC administration (preservative-free, albumen [human] or polysorbate 80)

▶*epoetin alpha* (erythropoietin [human, recombinant]) **(C)** individualize; initially 50-100 units/kg 3 times/week IV (dialysis or non-dialysis) or SC (non-dialysis); usual max 200 units/kg 3 times/week (dialysis) or 150 units/kg 3 times/week (non-dialysis); target Hct 30-36%

>   *Pediatric:* <1 month: not recommended
>   >1 month: individualize; (dialysis) initially 50 units/kg 3 times/week IV or SC; target Hct 30-36%

Epogen® *Vial:* 2,000, 3,000, 4,000, 10,000, 40,000 units/ml (1 ml) single-use for IV or SC administration (albumin [human]; preservative-free)

Epogen®Multidose *Vial:* 10,000 units/ml (2 ml); 20,000 units/ml, (1 ml) for IV or SC administration (albumin [human]; benzoyl alcohol)

Procrit® *Vial:* 2,000, 3,000, 4,000, 10,000, 40,000 units/ml (1 ml) single-use for IV or SC administration (albumin [human]; preservative-free)

Procrit®Multidose *Vial:* 10,000 units/ml (2 ml); 20,000 units/ml, (1 ml) for IV or SC administration (albumin [human]; benzoyl alcohol)

Anemia: Folic Acid Deficiency

▶*folic acid* **(A)(OTC)** 0.4-1 mg daily
Comment: Folic acid (vitamin B-9) 1 mg daily is recommended during pregnancy to prevent neural tube defects.
see ***Vitamin & Mineral Supplements*** *page 508*

Anemia: Iron Deficiency

Comment: Iron supplements are best absorbed when taken between meals and with vitamin C rich foods. Excessive *iron* may be extremely hazardous to infants and young children. All vitamin and mineral supplements should be kept out of the reach of children.

Iron Preparations
▶*carbonyl iron* **(A)**
>   *Pediatric:* <12 years: 3-6 mg elemental iron/kg/day daily-tid;

Anemia: Iron Deficiency

max 15 mg/day
Icar®Pediatric Suspension *Oral susp:* 15 mg elemental iron per 1/4 tsp (15 ml); *Chew tab:* 15 mg elemental iron

▶*ferrous gluconate* **(A)(G)** 1 tab daily
   Fergon® (OTC)
     Pediatric: not recommended
     Tab: iron 27 mg (240 mg as gluconate)

▶*ferrous sulfate* **(A)(G)**
   Feosol®Tablets (OTC) 1 tab tid-qid pc and HS
     Pediatric: <6 years: use elixir
            6-12 years: 1 tab tid pc
     Tab: iron 65 mg (200 mg as sulfate)
   Feosol®Capsules (OTC) 1-2 caps daily
     Pediatric: not recommended
     Cap: iron 50 mg (169 mg as sulfate) sust-rel
   Feosol®Elixir (OTC) 5-10 ml tid
     Pediatric: >1 year: 2.5-5 ml tid between meals
     Elix: iron 44 mg (220 mg as sulfate) per 5 ml
   Fer-In-Sol® (OTC) 5 ml daily
     Pediatric: <4 years, use drops
            >4 years: 5 ml daily
     Syr: iron 18 mg (90 mg as sulfate) per 5 ml (480 ml)
   Fer-In-Sol®Drops (OTC)
     Pediatric: <4 years: 0.6 ml daily
            >4 years: use syrup
     Oral drops: iron 15 mg (75 mg as sulfate) per 5 ml (50 ml)
   Iberet®-500 Filmtab 1 tab daily
     Pediatric: not recommended
     Tab: iron 525 mg (as sulfate) cont-rel
   Slow Fe® (OTC) 1-2 tabs daily
     Pediatric: <6 years: not recommended
            6-12 years: 1 tab daily
     Tab: iron 50 mg, 160 mg (as sulfate) sust-rel

▶*polysaccharide iron complex* **(A)**
   Niferex® 1-2 tabs bid
     Pediatric: <6 years: not recommended
            6-12 years: 1-2 caps daily
     Tab: iron 50 mg (as cell-contracted akaganeite)
   Niferex®Elixir 5-10 ml daily
     Pediatric: 6-12 years: 5 ml daily
     Elix: iron 100 mg (as cell-contracted akaganeite) per 5 ml

Anemia: Iron Deficiency

(8 oz)

Niferex®-150 1-2 caps daily
- *Pediatric:* use elixir
- *Cap:* iron 150 mg (as cell-contracted akaganeite)

Iron and Vitamin/Mineral Preparations

Chromagen® (C) 1 cap daily
- *Pediatric:* not recommended
- *Cap:* iron 66 mg (200 mg as fumarate)/B-12, cyanocobalamin 10 mcg/C, ascorbic acid 250 mg/desiccated stomach substance 100 mg

Chromagen®FA (C) 1 cap daily
- *Pediatric:* not recommended
- *Cap:* iron 66 mg (200 mg as fumarate)/B-12, cyanocobalamin 10 mcg/C, ascorbic acid 250 mg/B-9, folic acid 1 mg

Chromagen®Forte (C) 1 cap daily
- *Pediatric:* not recommended
- *Cap:* iron 151 mg (460 mg as fumarate)/B-12, cyanocobalamin 10 mcg/C, ascorbic acid 60 mg/B-9, folic acid 1 mg

Fero-Folic-500® (C) 1 tab daily
- *Pediatric:* not recommended
- *Tab:* iron 105 mg (as sulfate)/C, ascorbic acid/B-9, folic acid 0.8 mg

Fero-Grad-500®Filmtab 1 tab daily
- *Pediatric:* not recommended
- *Tab:* iron 525 mg (as sulfate)/C, ascorbic acid 500 mg

Iberet®Liquid 2 tsp bid
- *Pediatric:* 1-3 years: 1 tsp bid
  >3 years: same as adult
- *Liq:* iron 26.25 mg (as sulfate)/B-1, thiamine 1.5 mg/B-2, riboflavin 1.5 mg/B-3, niacinamide 7.5 mg/B-6, pyridoxine 1.25 mg/B-12, cyanocobalamin 6.25 mg/C, ascorbic acid 37.5 mg/dexpantenol 2.5 mg per 5 ml (8 oz)

Iberet®-500 Liquid 2 tsp bid
- *Pediatric:* 1-3 years: 1 tsp bid
  >3 years: same as adult
- *Liq:* iron 26.25 mg (as sulfate)/B-1, thiamine 1.5 mg/B-2, riboflavin 1.5 mg/B-3, niacinamide 1.5 mg/B-6, pyridoxine 1.25 mg/B-12, cyanocobalamin 6.25 mg/C, ascorbic acid 125 mg per 5 ml (8 oz)

Iberet®-Folic-500 Filmtab (A) 1 tab daily
- *Pediatric:* not recommended

Tab: iron (525 mg as sulfate)/B-1, thiamine 6 mg/B-2, riboflavin 6 mg/B-3, niacinamide 30 mg/B-6, pyridoxine 5 mg/B-9, folic acid 800 mcg/B-12, cyanocobalamin 25 mcg/C, ascorbic acid 500 mg
Cont-rel tab: same as regular tab

Icar®-C Plus (A) 1 tab daily
Pediatric: <12 years: not recommended
Tab: iron 100 mg (as carbonyl)/B-9, folic acid 1 mg/B-12, cyanocobalamin 25 mcg/C, ascorbic acid 250 mg

Niferex®-150 Forte (A) 1 cap daily
Pediatric: not recommended
Cap: iron (as cell-contracted akaganeite) 150 mg/B-9, folic acid 1 mg/B-12, cyanocobalamin 25 mcg

Slow Fe®Plus Folic Acid (A)(OTC) 1 tab daily
Pediatric: not recommended
Tab: iron 50 mg (as sulfate) 160 mg/B-9, folic acid 400 mcg sust-rel

Trinsicon® (C) 1 cap bid
Pediatric: <10 years: not recommended
  >10 years: same as adult
Cap: iron (as fumarate) 110 mg/B-9, folic acid 0.5 mg/B-12, cyanocobalamin 15 mcg/C, ascorbic acid 75 mg/liver-stomach concentrate 240 mg

*For more oral iron-containing supplements, see **Vitamin & Mineral Supplements** page 508*

Anemia: Pernicious

Comment: Signs of vitamin B-12 deficiency include megaloblastic anemia, glossitis, paresthesias, ataxia, spastic motor weakness, and reduced mentation.
▶*vitamin B-12 (cyanocobalamin)* **(C)(G)**
  Injectable: 100 mcg SC daily x 1 week, then weekly x 1 month, then monthly for life

Nascobal®Gel 500 mcg intranasally once a week; may increase dose if serum B-12 levels decline; adjust dose in 500 mcg increments.

Intranasal gel: 500 mcg or 0.1 ml/actuation (2.3 ml)

Comment: For maintenance of hematologic remission following intramuscular B-12 therapy.
▶*vitamin complex with vitamin B-12 (cyanocobalamin)* **(C)(G)**

Anemia: Pernicious

Trinsicon® (C) 1 cap bid
> *Pediatric:* <10 years: not recommended
> >10 years: same as adult
> *Cap:* iron (as fumarate) 110 mg/B-9, folic acid 0.5 mg/B-12, cyanocobalamin 15 mcg/C, ascorbic acid 75 mg/liver-stomach concentrate 240 mg

*For more oral vitamin B-12-containing supplements, see **Vitamin & Mineral Supplements** page 508*

Angina Pectoris: Stable

▶*aspirin* **(D)** 325 mg daily

Calcium Antagonists
Comment: Calcium antagonists are contraindicated with history of ventricular arrhythmias, sick sinus syndrome, 2nd or 3rd degree heart block, cardiogenic shock, acute myocardial infarction, and pulmonary congestion.

▶*amlodipine* **(C)(G)** 5-10 mg daily
Norvasc® *Tab:* 2.5, 5, 10 mg

▶*bepridil* **(C)** initially 200 mg daily, titrate q 10 days; max 400 mg/day
Vascor® *Tab:* 200, 300, 400 mg

▶*diltiazem* **(C)(G)**
Cardizem® initially 30 mg qid; may increase gradually every 1 to 2 days; max 360 mg/day in divided doses
> *Pediatric:* not recommended
> *Tab:* 30, 60, 90, 120 mg

Cardizem®CD initially 120-180 mg daily; adjust at 1 to 2 week intervals; max 480 mg/day
> *Pediatric:* not recommended
> *Cap:* 120, 180, 240, 300, 360 mg ext-rel

Cardizem®LA initially 180-240 mg daily; titrate at 2 week intervals; max 540 mg/day
> *Pediatric:* not recommended
> *Tab:* 120, 180, 240, 300, 360, 420 mg ext-rel

Cardizem®SR initially 60-120 mg bid; adjust at 2 week intervals; max 360 mg/day
> *Pediatric:* not recommended
> *Cap:* 60, 90, 120 mg sust-rel

Dilacor®XR initially 120 mg q AM; may titrate over 7-14 days
> *Cap:* 120, 180, 240 mg ext-rel

Angina Pectoris: Stable

    Tiazac® initially 120-180 mg daily; max 540 mg/day
        Cap: 120, 180, 240, 300, 360, 420 mg ext-rel
▶*nicardipine* **(C)(G)** initially 20 mg tid; adjust q 3 days; max 120 mg/day
    Cardene® *Cap:* 20, 30 mg
▶*nifedipine* **(C)(G)**
    Adalat® initially 10 mg tid; usual range 10-20 mg tid; max 180 mg/day
        Cap: 10, 20 mg
    Procardia® initially 10 mg tid; titrate over 7-14 days: max 30 mg/dose and 180 mg/day in divided doses
        Cap: 10, 20 mg
    Procardia®XL initially 30-60 mg daily; titrate over 7-14 days; max dose 90 mg/day
        Tab: 30, 60, 90 mg ext-rel
▶*verapamil* **(C)(G)**
        Pediatric: not recommended
    Calan® 80-120 mg tid; increase daily or weekly if needed
        Tab: 40, 80*, 120*mg
    Covera®HS initially 180 mg q HS; titrate in steps to 240 mg; then to 360 mg; then to 480 mg if needed
        Tab: 180, 240 mg ext-rel
    Isoptin® initially 80-120 mg tid
        Tab: 40, 80, 120 mg
    Isoptin®SR initially 120-180 mg in the AM; may increase to 240 mg in the AM; then 180 mg q 12 hours or 240 mg in the AM and 120 mg in the PM, then 240 mg q 12 hours
        Tab: 120, 180*, 240*mg sust-rel

Beta-Blockers
Comment: Beta-blockers are contraindicated with history of ventricular arrhythmias, sick sinus syndrome, 2nd or 3rd degree heart block, cardiogenic shock, and pulmonary congestion.
▶*atenolol* **(D)(G)** initially 50 mg daily; increase weekly if needed; max 200 mg daily
    Tenormin® *Tab:* 25, 50, 100 mg
▶*metoprolol* **(C)(G)**
        Pediatric: not recommended
    Lopressor® initially 50 mg bid; increase weekly if needed;
        Tab: 50*, 100*mg
    Toprol®-XL initially 100 mg daily; increase weekly if needed; max 400 mg/day

Angina Pectoris: Stable

    Tab: 25*, 50*, 100*, 200*mg ext-rel
▶*nadolol* **(C)(G)** initially 40 mg daily; increase q 3-7 days; max 240 mg/day
    Corgard® *Tab:* 20*, 40*, 80*, 120*, 160*mg
▶*propranolol* **(C)(G)**
    Inderal® initially 80 mg in 2-4 doses; max 320 mg daily
        Tab: 10*, 20*, 40*, 60*, 80*mg
    Inderal®LA initially 80 mg daily in a single dose; increase q 3-7 days; usual range 120-160 mg/day; max 320 mg/day in a single dose
        Cap: 60, 80, 120, 160 mg sust-rel
    InnoPran®XL initially 80 mg q HS; max 120 mg/day
        Cap: 80, 120 mg ext-rel

Nitrates

Comment: Use a daily nitrate dose schedule that provides a dose-free period of 14 hours or more to prevent tolerance. *Aspirin* and *acetaminophen* may relieve nitrate-induced headache. *Isosorbide* is not recommended for use in MI and/or CHF. Nitrate use is a contraindication for using phosphodiesterase type 5 inhibitors: *sildenafil* (**Viagra®**), *tadalafil* (**Cialis®**), *vardinafil* (**Levitra®**).

▶*isosorbide dinitrate*
    Isordil®Sublingual 2.5-5 mg SL 15 minutes before activity
        SL tab: 2.5, 5, 10 mg
    Isordil®Tembids (B) initially 40 mg SL q 8-12 hours; maintenance 40-80 mg SL q 8-12 hours
        Cap: 40 mg sust-rel
    Isordil®Titradose (B) initially 5-20 mg q 6 hours; maintenance 10-40 mg q 6 hours
        Tab: 5, 10, 20, 30, 40 mg
    Sorbitrate® (C) 2.5-5 mg SL
        SL tab: 2.5, 5 mg
    Sorbitrate®Chewable (C) 5 mg 15 minutes before activity
        Chew tab: 5, 10 mg
    Sorbitrate®Oral Tab (B) initially 5-20 mg bid-tid; maintenance 10-4 mg bid-tid
        Tab: 5, 10, 20, 30, 40 mg
▶*isosorbide mononitrate*
    Dilatrate®-SR (C) *Cap:* 40 mg sust-rel
    Imdur® (C) initially 30-60 mg q AM; may increase to 120 mg daily; max 240 mg/day
        Tab: 30*, 60*, 120 mg ext-rel

Ismo® (C) 20 mg upon awakening; then 20 mg 7 hours later
  Tab: 20*mg
Monoket® (B) 20 mg upon awakening; then 20 mg 7 hours later
  Tab: 10*, 20*mg

▶*nitroglycerin* **(C)(G)**
  Deponit® initially 0.2 to 0.4 mg/hour patch on 12-14 hours and off 10-12 hours
    Transdermal patch: 0.2, 0.4 mg/hour
  Minitran®Transdermal initially 0.2 to 0.4 mg/hour patch with nitrate-free period of 10-12 hours/day
    Transdermal patch: 0.1, 0.2, 0.4, 0.6 mg/hour
  Nitro-Bid®Ointment initially 1/2 inch q 8 hours; titrate in 1/2 inch increments
    Oint: 2% (20, 60 g)
  Nitrodisc® initially one 0.2-0.4 mg/hour patch for 12-14 hours/day
    Transdermal disc: 0.2, 0.3, 0.4 mg/hour (30, 100/box)
  Nitro-Dur® initially 0.2-0.4 mg/hour patch for 12-14 hours/day
    Transdermal patch: 0.1, 0.2, 0.3, 0.4, 0.6, 0.8 mg/hour
  Nitrolingual® 1-2 sprays onto or under tongue; max 3 sprays/15 minutes
    Spray: 0.4 mg/dose (14.5 g, 200 doses)
  Nitrostat® 1 tab SL; may repeat q 5 minutes x 3
    SL tab: 0.3 ($^{1}/_{100}$ gr), 0.4 ($^{1}/_{150}$ gr), 0.6 ($^{1}/_{4}$ gr) mg
  Transderm-Nitro® initially one 0.2 mg/hour or 0.4 mg/hour patch for 12-14 hours/day
    Transdermal patch: 0.1, 0.2, 0.4, 0.6, 0.8 mg/hour

Non-nitrate Vasodilator
▶*hydralazine* **(C)(G)** initially 10 mg qid x 2-4 days, then increase to 25 mg qid for remainder of first week, then increase to 50 mg qid; max 300 mg/day
  Apresoline® *Tab:* 10, 25, 50, 100 mg

Non-nitrate Antianginal
▶*ranolazine* **(C)** initially 500 mg bid; may increase to max 1 g bid
  Ranexa® *Tab:* 500 mg ext-rel
Comment: **Ranexa®** is indicated for the treatment chronic angina that is inadequately controlled with other antianginals. Use with amlodipine, beta-blocker, or nitrate.

Anorexia/Cachexia

Appetite Stimulants

Anorexia/ Cachexia

▶*dronabinol* (cannabinoid) **(B)(III)** initially 2.5 mg bid before lunch and dinner; may reduce to 2.5 mg q HS or increase to 2.5 mg before lunch and 5 mg before dinner; max 20 mg/day in divided doses
    Pediatric: not recommended
  Marinol® *Cap:* 2.5, 5, 10 mg (sesame oil)

▶*megestrol* (progestin) **(X)** 40 mg qid
    Pediatric: not recommended
  Megace® *Tab:* 20*, 40*mg
  Megace®ES *Oral susp (concentrate):* 125 mg/ml; 625 mg/5 ml (5 oz; lemon-lime)
  Megace®Oral Suspension *Oral susp:* 40 mg/ml (8 oz); 820 mg/20 ml; lemon-lime)

Anthrax

Reference: MMWR, Vol. 50, No. 42 (Oct 26, 2001)
Post-exposure Prophylaxis of Inhalational Anthrax
and Treatment of Cutaneous Anthrax

▶*ciprofloxacin* **(C)(G)** 500 mg (or 10-15 mg/kg/day) po q 12 hours for 60 days (start as soon as possible after exposure)
    Pediatric: <18 years: usually not recommended
  Cipro® *Tab:* 100, 250, 500, 750 mg; *Oral susp:* 250 mg/5 ml (100 ml; strawberry)

▶*doxycycline* **(D)(G)** 100 mg daily-bid
    Pediatric: see page 587 for dose by weight
        <8 years: not recommended
        >8 years, <100 lb: 2 mg/lb on first day in 2 doses, followed by 1 mg/lb/day in 1-2 doses
        >8 years, >100 lb: same as adult
  Adoxa® *Tab:* 50, 100 mg ent-coat
  Doryx® *Cap:* 100 mg
  Monodox® *Cap:* 50, 100 mg
  Vibramycin® *Cap:* 50, 100 mg; *Syr:* 50 mg/5 ml (raspberry-apple, sulfites); *Oral susp:* 25 mg/5 ml (raspberry)
  Vibra-Tab® *Tab:* 100 mg film-coat

▶*minocycline* **(D)(G)** 100 mg q 12 hours
    Pediatric: <8 years: not recommended
        >8 years, <100 lb: 2 mg/lb on first day in 2 doses, followed by 1 mg/lb/ q 12 hours x 9 more days
        >8 years, >100 lb: same as adult

Minocin® *Cap:* 100 mg ent-coat
Comment: Minocycline is contraindicated in pregnancy (discolors fetal tooth enamel).

Treatment of Inhalational, GI, and Oropharyngeal Anthrax
▶ *ciprofloxacin* **(C)(G)** 400 mg IV q 12 hours (start as soon as possible); then switch to 500 mg po q 12 hours for total 60 days
> *Pediatric:* <18 years: usually not recommended
> 10-15 mg/kg IV q 12 hours (start as soon as possible); then switch to 10-15 mg/kg po q 12 hours for 60 days

Cipro® *Tab:* 100, 250, 500, 750 mg; *Oral susp:* 250 mg/5 ml (100 ml; srawberry); *IV conc:* 10 mg/ml after dilution (20, 40 ml); *IV premix:* 2 mg/ml (100, 200 ml)

Comment: Infuse IV *ciprofloxacin* over 60 minutes.

▶ *doxycycline* **(D)(G)** 100 mg daily-bid
> *Pediatric: see page 587 for dose by weight*
> <8 years: not recommended
> >8 years, <100 lb: 2 mg/lb on first day in 2 doses, followed by 1 mg/lb/day in 1-2 doses
> >8 years, >100 lb: same as adult

Adoxa® *Tab:* 50, 100 mg ent-coat
Doryx® *Cap:* 100 mg
Monodox® *Cap:* 50, 100 mg
Vibramycin® *Cap:* 50, 100 mg; *Syr:* 50 mg/5 ml (raspberry-apple, sulfites); *Oral susp:* 25 mg/5 ml (raspberry)
Vibra-Tab® *Tab:* 100 mg film-coat

▶ *minocycline* **(D)(G)** 100 mg q 12 hours
> *Pediatric:* <8 years: not recommended
> >8 years, <100 lb: 2 mg/lb on first day in 2 doses, followed by 1 mg/lb/ q 12 hours x 9 more days
> >8 years, >100 lb: same as adult

Minocin® *Cap:* 100 mg ent-coat

Comment: Minocycline is contraindicated in pregnancy (discolors fetal tooth enamel).

Anxiety Disorder: Generalized (GAD)
Anxiety Disorder: Social (SAD)

1st Generation Antihistamine
▶ *hydroxyzine* **(C)(G)** 50-100 mg qid; max 600 mg/day

Anxiety Disorder

        Pediatric: <6 years: 50 mg/day divided qid
                     >6 years: 50-100 mg/day divided qid
  Atarax® *Tab:* 10, 25, 50, 100 mg; *Syr:* 10 mg/5 ml (alcohol 0.5%)
  Vistaril® *Cap:* 25, 50, 100 mg; *Oral susp:* 25 mg/5 ml (4 oz; lemon)

Azapirones
▶*buspirone* **(B)** initially 7.5 mg bid; may increase by 5 mg/day q 2-3 days; max 60 mg/day
    Pediatric: <18 years: not recommended
  BuSpar® *Tab:* 5, 10, 15 mg

Benzodiazepines
Short-acting
▶*alprazolam* **(D)(IV)(G)**
    Pediatric: <18 years: not recommended
  Niravam®, Xanax® initially 0.25-0.5 mg tid; may titrate every 3-4 days; max 4 mg/day
    Tab: 0.25*, 0.5*, 1*, 2*mg
  Xanax®XR initially 0.5-1 mg once daily, preferably in the AM; increase at interals of at least 3-4 days by up to 1 mg/day. Taper no faster than 0.5 mg every 3 days; max 10 mg/day. When switching from immedate-release *alprazolam*, give total daily dose of immediate-release once daily.
    Tab: 0.5, 1, 2, 3 mg
▶*oxazepam* **(C)(IV)(G)** 10-15 mg tid-qid for moderate symptoms; 15-30 mg tid-qid for severe symptoms
    Pediatric: not recommended
  Serax® *Tab:* 15 mg; *Cap:* 10, 15, 30 mg

Intermediate-acting
▶*lorazepam* **(D)(IV)(G)** 1-10 mg/day in 2-3 divided doses
    Pediatric: not recommended
  Ativan® *Tab:* 0.5, 1*, 2*mg

Long-acting
▶*chlordiazepoxide* **(D)(IV)(G)**
    Pediatric: <6 years: not recommended
                    >6 years: 5 mg bid-qid; increase to 10 mg bid-tid
  Librium® 5-10 mg tid-qid for moderate symptoms; 20-25 mg tid-qid for severe symptoms
    Cap: 5, 10, 25 mg
  Librium®Injectable 50-100 mg IM or IV, then 25-50 mg IM tid-qid prn; max 300 mg/day
    Inj: 100 mg

Anxiety Disorder

▶*chlordiazepoxide/clidinium* **(D)(IV)** 1-2 caps tid-qid: max 8 caps/day
        Pediatric: not recommended
    Librax® *Cap:* chlor 5 mg/clid 2.5 mg
▶*clonazepam* **(D)(IV)(G)** initially 0.25 mg bid; increase to 1 mg/day after 3 days
        Pediatric: <18 years: not recommended
    Klonopin® *Tab:* 0.5*, 1, 2 mg
    Klonopin®Wafers dissolve in mouth with or without water
        Wafer: 0.125, 0.25, 0.5, 1, 2 mg orally-disintegrating
▶*clorazepate* **(D)(IV)(G)** 30 mg/day in divided doses; max 60 mg/day
        Pediatric: <9 years: not recommended
                 >9 years: same as adult
    Tranxene® *Tab:* 3.75, 7.5, 15 mg
    Tranxene®SD do not use for initial therapy
        Tab: 22.5 mg ext-rel
    Tranxene®SD Half Strength do not use for initial therapy
        Tab: 11.25 mg ext-rel
    Tranxene®T-Tab *Tab:* 3.75*, 7.5*, 15*mg
▶*diazepam* **(D)(IV)(G)** 2-10 mg bid-qid
        Pediatric: not recommended
    Valium® *Tab:* 2*, 5*, 10*mg
▶*prazepam* **(D)** 10 mg tid, 20-60 mg in divided doses or 20 mg q HS
        Pediatric: <18 years: not recommended
    Centrax® *Tab:* 10 mg; *Cap:* 5, 10, 20 mg

Mixed Neurotransmitter Reuptake Inhibitors
▶*venlafaxine* **(C)**
    Effexor® initially 75 mg/day in 2-3 doses; may increase at 4 day intervals in 75 mg increments to 150 mg/day; max 375 mg/day
        Pediatric: <18 years: not recommended
        Tab: 25, 37.5, 50, 75, 100 mg
    Effexor®XR initially 75 mg q AM; may start at 37.5 mg daily x 4-7 days, then increase by increments of up to 75 mg/day at intervals of at least 4 days; usual max 375 mg/day
        Pediatric: not recommended
        Cap: 37.5, 75, 150 mg ext-rel

Phenothiazines
▶*prochlorperazine* **(C)(G)**
    Compazine® 5 mg tid-qid
        Pediatric: not recommended
        Tab: 5 mg; *Syr:* 5 mg/5 ml (4 oz; fruit); *Rectal supp:*

2.5, 5, 25 mg

Compazine®Spansule 15 mg q AM or 10 mg q 12 hours
Pediatric: not recommended
Spansule: 10, 15 mg sust-rel

▶*trifluoperazine* **(C)(G)** 1-2 mg bid; max 6 mg/day; max 12 weeks
Pediatric: not recommended
Stelazine® *Tab:* 1, 2, 5, 10 mg

Selective Serotonin Reuptake Inhibitors (SSRIs)

▶*escitalopram* **(C)** initially 10 mg daily; may increase to 20 mg daily after 1 week
Pediatric: not recommended
Lexapro® *Tab:* 5, 10*, 20*mg
Lexapro®Oral Solution *Oral soln:* 1 mg/ml, 5 mg/tsp (240 ml; peppermint, parabens)

▶*fluoxetine* **(C)(G)**
Prozac® initially 20 mg daily; may increase after 1 week; doses >20 mg/day should be divided into AM and noon doses; max 80 mg/day
Pediatric: <8 years: not recommended
8-17 years: initially 10 or 20 mg/day; start lower weight children at 10 mg/day; if starting at 10 mg daily, may increase after 1 week to 20 mg daily
Tab: 10*mg; *Cap:* 10, 20, 40 mg; *Oral soln:* 20 mg/5 ml (4 oz; mint)

Prozac®Weekly following daily fluoxetine therapy at 20 mg/day for 13 weeks, may initiate **Prozac®Weekly** 7 days after the last 20 mg fluoxetine dose
Pediatric: not recommended
Cap: 90 mg ent-coat del-rel pellets

▶*paroxetine maleate* **(D)(G)**
Pediatric: not recommended
Paxil® initially 10-20 mg daily in AM; may increase by 10 mg/day at weekly intervals as needed; max 60 mg/day
Tab: 10*, 20*, 30, 40 mg
Paxil®CR initially 12.5-25 mg daily in AM; may increase by 12.5 mg at weekly intervals as needed; max 62.5 mg/day
Tab: 12.5, 25, 37.5 mg ent-coat cont-rel
Paxil®Suspension initially 10-20 mg daily in AM; may increase by 10 mg/day at weekly intervals as needed; max 60 mg/day
Oral susp: 10 mg/5 ml (250 ml; orange)

▶*sertraline* **(C)** initially 50 mg daily; increase at 1 week intervals if needed; max 200 mg daily
  Pediatric: <6 years: not recommended
  6-12 years: initially 25 mg daily; max 200 mg/day
  13-17 years: initially 50 mg daily; max 200 mg/day
  Zoloft® *Tab:* 15*, 50*, 100*mg; *Oral conc:* 20 mg per ml (60 ml, [dilute just before administering in 4 oz water, ginger ale, lemon-lime soda, lemonade, or orange juice]; alcohol 12%)

Combination Agents
▶*chlordiazepoxide/amitriptyline* **(D)(G)**
  Pediatric: not recommended
  Limbitrol® 3-4 tabs/day in divided doses
    Tab: chlor 5 mg/*amit* 12.5 mg
  Limbitrol®DS 3-4 tabs/day in divided doses; max 6 tabs/day
    Tab: chlor 10 mg/*amit* 25 mg
▶*perphenazine/amitriptyline* **(C)(G)**
  Pediatric: not recommended
  Etrafon® or **Triavil®2-10** initially 1 tab tid-qid; maintenance bid-qid
  Etrafon® or **Triavil®2-25** initially 1 tab tid-qid; maintenance bid-qid
  Triavil®4-10 initially 1 tab tid-qid; maintenance bid-qid
  Etrafon® or **Triavil®4-25** initially 1 tab tid-qid; maintenance bid-qid
  Triavil®4-50 initially 1 tab bid; maintenance bid
    Tab: **Etrafon®/Triavil®2-10**: *perph* 2 mg/*amit* 10 mg
    Etrafon®/Triavil®2-25: *perph* 2 mg/*amit* 25 mg
    Triavil®4-10: *perph* 4 mg/*amit* 10 mg
    Etrafon®/Triavil®4-25: *perph* 4 mg/*amit* 25 mg
    Triavil®4-50: *perph* 4 mg/*amit* 50 mg

Aphthous Stomatitis (Mouth Ulcer, Canker Sore)

Anti-inflammatory Agents
▶*amlexanox* **(B)** apply 1/4 inch to each ulcer qid until ulcer heals
  Pediatric: not recommended
  Aphthasol® *Adhesive oral paste:* 5% (5 g)
▶*dexamethasone* elixir **(B)** 5 ml swish and spit q 12 hours
  Pediatric: not recommended
  Elix: 0.5 mg/ml

Aphthous Stomatitis

▶*triamcinolone* 1% in **Orabase® (B)** apply 1/4 inch to each ulcer bid-qid
   until ulcer heals
   Pediatric: not recommended
   Kenalog® in Orabase *Crm:* 1% (15, 60, 80 g)

Topical Anesthetics
▶*benzocaine* **(C)(G)** topical gel apply tid-qid
▶**Chloraseptic®Spray**
▶*lidocaine* viscous soln **(B)(G)** 15 ml gargle or mouthwash; repeat after 3 hours; max 8 doses/day
   Pediatric: <3 years: 1.25 ml apply with cotton-tipped applicator; may repeat after 3 hours; max 8 doses/day
   Xylocaine®Viscous Solution *Viscous soln:* 2% (20, 100, 450 ml)
▶*triamcinolone* (**Kenalog®**) in **Orabase® (C)** apply with swab

Debriding Agent/Cleanser
▶*carbamide peroxide 10%* **(NR)(OTC)** apply 10 drops to affected area; swish x 2-3 minutes, then spit; do not rinse; repeat treatment qid
   Gly-Oxide® *Liq:* 10% (50, 60 ml squeeze bottle w. applicator)

Anti-infectives
▶*minocycline* **(D)** swish and spit 10 ml susp (50 mg/5 ml) or
   1-100 mg cap or 2-50 mg caps dissolved in 180 ml water, bid
   x 4-5 days
   Pediatric: <8 years: not recommended
      >8 years: same as adult
   Dynacin® *Cap:* 50, 100 mg
   Minocin® *Cap:* 50, 100 mg; *Oral susp:* 50 mg/5 ml (60 ml; custard, sulfites, alcohol 5%)
▶*tetracycline* **(D)** swish and spit 10 ml susp (125 mg/5 ml) or
   1-250 mg tab/cap dissolved in 180 ml water, qid x 4-5 days
   Pediatric: see page 595 for dose by weight
      <8 years: not recommended
      >8 years: same as adult
   Achromycin®V *Cap:* 250, 500 mg
   Sumycin® *Tab:* 250, 500 mg; *Cap:* 250, 500 mg; *Oral susp:* 125 mg/5 ml (100, 200 ml; fruit, sulfites)

Comment: Tetracycline is contraindicated in pregnancy (discolors fetal tooth enamel).

Aspergillosis (*Scedosporium, Apiospermum, Fusarium spp.*)

Invasive Infection
▶*posaconazole* **(D)** take with food
  Invasive fungal prophylaxis: 200 mg tid; refractory, 400 mg tids
    Pediatric: *<13 years:* not recommended
        ≥13 years: same as adult
   Noxafil® *Oral susp:* 40 mg/ml (cherry flavor)
▶*voriconazole* **(D)**
    Pediatric: not recommended
   IV: 6 mg/kg q 12 hours x 2 doses; then 4 mg/kg q 12 hour; max rate 3 mg/kg/hour over 1-2 hours
   PO: <40 kg: 100 mg q 12 hours; may increase to 150 mg q 12 hours if inadequate response
      >40 kg: 200 mg q 12 hours; may increase to 300 mg q 12 hours if inadequate response
   Vfend® *Tab:* 50, 200 mg
   Vfend®I.V. for Injection *Vial:* 200 mg pwdr for reconstitution (preservative-free)

Asthma

Leukotriene Receptor Antagonists
Comment: For prophylaxis and chronic treatment, only. Not for primary (rescue) treatment of acute asthma attack.
▶*montelukast* **(B)** 10 mg daily
    Pediatric: <2years: not recommended
        2-5 years: 1 chew tab or granule pkt daily
        6-14 years: 5 mg daily
        >14 years: same as adult
   Singulair® *Tab:* 10 mg
   Singulair®Chewable *Chew tab:* 4, 5 mg (cherry, phenylalanine)
   Singulair®Oral Granules take within 15 minutes of opening pkt; may mix with applesauce, carrots, rice, or ice cream
    Granules: 4 mg/pkt
▶*zafirlukast* **(B)** 20 mg bid, 1 hour ac or 2 hours pc
    Pediatric: <7 years: not recommended
        7-11 years: 10 mg bid 1 hour ac or 2 hours pc
   Accolate® *Tab:* 10, 20 mg
▶*zileuton* **(C)** 1 tab qid

Asthma

> *Pediatric:* <12 years: not recommended
>
> **Zyflo®** *Tab:* 600 mg

IgE Blocker (IgG1k Monoclonal Antibody)

▶*omalizumab* **(B)** 150-375 mg SC every 2-4 weeks based on body wt and pre-treatment serum total IgE level; max 150 mg/injection site

> *Pediatric:* <12 years: not recommended
>
> 30-90 kg + IgE >30-100 IU/ml 150 mg q 4 weeks
> 90-150 kg + IgE >30-100 IU/ml or
> 30-90 kg + IgE >100-200 IU/ml or
> 30-60 kg + IgE >200-300 IU/ml 300 mg q 4 hours
> >90-150 kg + IgE >100-200 IU/ml or
> >60-90 kg + IgE >200-300 IU/ml or
> 30-70 kg + IgE >300-400 IU/ml 225 mg q 2 weeks
> >90-150 kg + IgE >200-300 IU/ml or
> >70-90 kg + IgE >300-400 IU/ml or
> 30-70 kg + IgE >400-500 IU/ml or
> 30-60 kg + IgE >500-600 IU/ml or
> 30-60 kg + IgE >600-700 IU/ml 375 mg q 2 weeks
>
> **Xolair®** *Inj:* 150 mg (5 ml)

Inhaled Anticholinergics

▶*ipratropium bromide* **(C)(G)**

> **Atrovent®** 2 inhalations qid; additional inhalations as required; max 12 inhalations/day
>
> > *Pediatric:* not recommended
> >
> > *Inhaler:* 18 mcg/actuation (14 g, 200 inh)
>
> **Atrovent®Inhalation Solution** 500 mcg tid-qid prn by nebulizer
>
> > *Pediatric:* not recommended
> >
> > *Inhal soln:* 0.02% (500 mcg in 2.5 ml; 25/box)

Inhaled Anticholinergic/Beta₂-Agonist Combination

▶*ipratropium bromide/albuterol sulfate* **(C)** 2 inhalations qid

> **Combivent®** 2 inhalations qid; additional inhalations as required; max 12 inhalations/day
>
> > *Pediatric:* not recommended
> >
> > *Inhaler: ipra* 18 mcg/*albu* 90 mcg/actuation (14.7 g, 200 inh)

Inhaled Glucocorticosteroids

Comment: Instruct patient to rinse mouth after using an inhaled steroid to reduce risk of oral candidiasis. *Not* for primary (rescue) treatment of acute asthma attack.

▶*beclomethasone* **(C)(G)**

> **Beclovent®** 2 inhalations tid-qid or 4 inhalations bid; max 20 inhalations/day
>
> > *Pediatric:* <6 years: not recommended

Asthma

> 6-12 years: 1-2 inhalations tid-qid or 4 inhalations
> bid; max 10 inhalations/day
>
> *Inhaler:* 42 mcg/actuation (6.7 g, 80 inh); 16.8 g (200 inh)

Qvar®
> If previously using only bronchodilators, initiate 40-80 mcg bid; max 320 mcg bid
> If previously using inhaled corticosteroids, initiate 40-160 mcg bid; max 320 mcg/day
> If previously taking a systemic corticosteroid, attempt to wean off the systemic drug after approximately 1 week after initiating **Qvar®**
> *Pediatric:* not recommended
> *Inhaler:* 40, 80 mcg/actuation (7.3 g, 100 inh; 13.2 g, 200 inh) (chlorofluorocarbon [CFC]-free)

Vanceril® 2 inhalations tid-qid or 4 inhalations bid
> *Pediatric:* <6 years: not recommended
> 6-12 years: 1-2 inhalations tid-qid
> *Inhaler:* 42 mcg/actuation (16.8, 200 inh)

Vanceril®Double Strength 2 inhalations bid
> *Pediatric:* <6 years: not recommended
> 6-12 years: 1-2 inhalations bid
> *Inhaler:* 84 mcg/actuation (12.2 g, 120 inh)

▶*budesonide* **(B)**

Pulmicort®Respules adult use turbuhaler
> *Pediatric:* <6 months: not recommended
> 6 months-8 years:
> Previously using only bronchodilators: initiate 0.5 mg/day daily or in 2 divided doses; may start at 0.25 mg daily
> Previously using inhaled corticosteroids: initiate 0.5 mg/day daily or in 2 divided doses; max 1 mg/day
> Previously taking oral corticosteroids: initiate 1 mg/day daily or in 2 divided doses
> *Inhal susp:* 0.25 mg/2 ml (30/box)

Pulmicort®Turbuhaler 1-2 inhalations bid; if previously taking an oral corticosteroid, 2-4 inhalations bid
> *Pediatric:* <6 years: not recommended
> >6 years: 1-2 inhalations bid
> *Turbuhaler:* 200 mcg/actuation (200 inh)

▶*flunisolide* **(C)**

Asthma

AeroBid® and **AeroBid®-M** initially 2 inhalations bid; max 8 inhalations/day
> *Pediatric:* <6 years: not recommended
> 6-15 years: 2 inhalations bid
>
> *Inhaler:* 250 mcg/actuation (7 g, 100 inh)

▶*fluticasone* **(C)**

Flovent®HFA initially 88 mcg bid; if previously using an inhaled corticosteroid, initially 88-220 mcg bid; if previously taking an oral corticosteroid, 880 mcg bid
> *Pediatric:* use **Rotadisk®**: initially 2-50 mcg inh bid
> <4 years: not recommended
> 4-11 years: initially 50-88 mcg bid
> >11 years: initially 100 mcg bid; if previously using an inhaled glucocorticosteroid, initially 100-250 mcg bid; if previously taking an oral corticosteroid, 1000 mcg bid
>
> *Inhaler:* 44 mcg/actuation (7.9 g, 60 inh; 13 g, 120 inh); 110 mcg/actuation (13 g; 120 inh); 220 mcg/actuation (13 g; 120 inh)
>
> *Rotadisk:* 50 mcg/actuation (60 blisters/disk); 100 mcg/actuation (60 blisters/disk); 250 mcg/actuation (60 blisters/disk)

▶*triamcinolone* **(C)**

Azmacort® 2 inhalations tid-qid or 4 inhalations bid
> *Pediatric:* <6 years: not recommended
> 6-12 years: 1-2 inhalations tid or 2-4 inhalations bid
>
> *Inhaler:* 100 mcg/actuation (20 g, 240 inh)

Parenteral Glucocorticosteroids *see page 489*

Oral Glucocorticosteroids *see page 487*

Inhaled Mast Cell Stabilizers (Prophylaxis)

Comment: For prophylaxis and chronic treatment, only. Not for primary (rescue) treatment of acute asthma attack.

▶*cromolyn sodium* **(B)(G)**

Intal® 2 inhalations qid; 2 inhalations up to 10-60 minutes before precipitant as prophylaxis
> *Pediatric:* <2 years: not recommended
> 2-5 years: use inhal soln by nebulizer
> >5 years: 2 inhalations qid by inhaler
>
> *Inhaler:* 0.8 mg/actuation (8.1, 14.2 g; 112, 200 inh)

Intal®Inhalation Solution 20 mg by nebulizer qid; 20 mg up to 10-

Asthma

    60 minutes before precipitant as prophylaxis
        Pediatric: <2 years: not recommended
                >2 years: same as adult
        Inhal soln: 20 mg/2 ml (2 ml; 60, 120/box)

▶ *nedocromil sodium* **(B)**
    Tilade® 2 sprays qid
        Pediatric: <6 years: not recommended
                >6 years: 2 sprays qid
        Inhaler: 1.75 mg/spray (16.2 g; 104 sprays)
    Tilade®Nebulizer Solution 0.5% 1 amp qid by nebulizer
        Pediatric: <2 years: not recommended
                >2 years: initially 1 amp qid by nebulizer
                2-5 years: initially 1 amp tid by nebulizer
        Inhal soln: 11 mg/2.2 ml (2 ml; 60, 120/box)

Inhaled Beta$_2$-Agonists (Bronchodilators)

▶ *albuterol sulfate* **(C)(G)**
    AcuNeb®Inhalation Solution 1 unit-dose vial tid-qid prn by nebulizer; ages 2-12 years only; not for adult
        Pediatric: <2 years: not recommended
                2-12 years: initially 0.63 mg or 1.25 mg tid-qid
                6-12 years: with severe asthma, or >40 kg, or 11-12 years: initially 1.25 mg tid-qid
        Inhal soln: 0.63, 1.25 mg/3ml (3 ml, 25/box; preservative-free)
    Airet®Inhalation Solution 1 unit-dose vial tid-qid prn by nebulizer
        Pediatric: <12 years: not recommended
        Inhal soln: 0.083%/3ml (3 ml; 25/box)
    Proventil®HFA Inhaler 1-2 inhalations q 4-6 hours prn; 2 inhalations 15 minutes before exercise as prophylaxis for exercise-induced asthma
        Pediatric: <4 years: use syrup
                >4 years: same as adult
        Inhaler: 90 mcg/actuation (6.7 g, 200 inh)
    Proventil®Inhalation Solution 2.5 mg diluted to 3 ml with normal saline tid-qid prn by nebulizer
        Pediatric: use syrup
        Inhal soln: 0.5% (20 ml w. dropper); 0.083% (3 ml; 25/box)
    Ventolin®Inhaler 2 inhalations q 4-6 hours prn; 2 inhalations 15 minutes before exercise as prophylaxis for exercise-induced asthma

Asthma

    Pediatric: <2 years: not recommended
               2-4 years: use syrup
               >4 years: same as adult
    Inhaler: 90 mcg/actuation (17 g, 220 inh)

Ventolin®Rotacaps 1-2 cap inhalations q 4-6 hours prn; 2 inhalations 15 minutes before exercise as prophylaxis for exercise-induced asthma
    Pediatric: <4 years: not recommended
               >4 years 1-2 caps q 4-6 hours prn
    Rotacap: 200 mcg/rotacap (100 doses/Rotacap)

Ventolin®0.5% Inhalation Solution
    Pediatric: <2 years: not recommended
               >2 years: initially 0.1-0.15 mg/kg/dose tid-qid prn
               10-15 kg: 0.25 ml diluted to 3 ml with normal saline by nebulizer tid-qid prn
               >15 kg: 0.5 ml diluted to 3 ml with normal saline by nebulizer tid-qid prn
    Inhal soln: 20 ml w. dropper

Ventolin®Nebules
    Pediatric: <2 years: not recommended
               >2 years: initially 0.1-0.15 mg/kg/dose tid-qid prn
               10-15 kg: 1.25 mg or 1/2 nebule tid-qid prn
               >15 kg: 2.5 mg or 1 nebule tid-qid
    Inhal soln: 0.083% (3 ml; 25/box)

▶ *bitolterol mesylate* **(C)**
    Tornalate® 2 inhalations q 8 hours prn; max 2 inhalations q 4 hours prn or 3 inhalations q 6 hours prn
        Pediatric: not recommended
        Inhaler: 0.37 mg/actuation (16.4 g, 300 inh)
    Tornalate®Inhalation Solution 1 mg diluted to 2-4 ml by nebulizer bid-qid prn
        Pediatric: not recommended
        Inhal soln: 0.2% (10, 30, 60 ml w. dropper)

▶ *isoproterenol* **(B)**
   Rescue: 1 inhalation prn; repeat if no relief in 2-5 minutes
   Maintenance: 1-2 inhalations q 4-6 hours
        Pediatric: <12 years: not recommended
    Medihaler-1SO® *Inhaler:* 80 mcg/actuation (15 ml, 30 inh)

▶ *levalbuterol* **(C)** initially 0.63 mg tid q 6-8 hours prn by nebulizer; may increase to 1.25 mg tid at 6-8 hour intervals as needed
        Pediatric: not recommended

Xopenex® *Inhal soln:* 0.31, 0.63 mg/3 ml (3 ml; 24/box); 1.25 mg (3 ml; 96/box) (preservative-free)

▶ *metaproterenol* **(C)(G)**
Alupent® 2-3 inhalations tid-qid prn; max 12 inhalations/day
Pediatric: <6 years: use syrup
>6 years: by nebulizer 0.1-0.2 ml diluted with normal saline to 3 ml up to q 4 hours prn
Inhaler: 0.65 mg/actuation (14 g, 200 doses)
Alupent®Inhalation Solution 5-15 inhalations tid-qid prn; q 4 hours prn for acute attack
Pediatric: <6 years: use syrup
>6 years: by nebulizer 0.1-0.2 ml diluted with normal saline to 3 ml up to q 4 hours prn
Inhal soln: 5% (10, 30 ml w. dropper)

▶ *pirbuterol* **(C)** 1-2 inhalations q 4-6 hours prn; max 12 inhalations/day
Maxair®
Pediatric: <12 years: not recommended
Autohaler: 200 mcg/actuation (14 g, 400 inh); Inhaler: 200 mcg/actuation (25.6 g, 300 inh)

▶ *salmeterol* **(C)(G)** 2 inhalations q 12 hours prn; 2 inhalations at least 30-60 minutes before exercise as prophylaxis for exercise-induced asthma; do not use extra doses for exercise-induced bronchospasm if already using regular dose
Serevent®Diskus
Pediatric: <4 years: not recommended
>4 years: 1 inhalation q 12 hours prn;
1 inhalation at least 30-60 minutes before exercise as prophylaxis for exercise-induced asthma. Do not use extra doses for exercise-induced bronchospasm if already using regular dose
Diskus (pwdr): 50 mcg/actuation (60 doses/disk)

▶ *terbutaline* **(B)** 2 inhalations q 4-6 hours prn
Brethaire®
Pediatric: not recommended
Inhaler: 0.2 mg/actuation (10.5 g, 300 inh)

▶ *tiotropium* **(B)** 2 inhalations q 4-6 hours prn
Brethaire®
Pediatric: not recommended
Inhaler: 0.2 mg/actuation (10.5 g, 300 inh)

Inhaled Beta$_2$-Agonist (Long-Acting)/Corticosteroid Combinations
▶ *budesonide/formoterol* **(C)** 1 inhalation bid

Pediatric: <12 years: not recommended
Symbicort®80/4.5
> *Inhaler: bud* 160 mcg/*for* 4.5 mcg

Symbicort®160/4.5
> *Inhaler: bud* 80 mcg/*for* 4.5 mcg

▶*fluticasone propionate/salmeterol* **(C)** if insufficient response after 2 weeks, use next higher strength; max 1 inh 500/50 bid
Not previously using an inhaled steroid: start with 1 inh 100/50 bid
Already using an inhaled steroid: see mfr literature

Advair Diskus®100/50
> *Pediatric:* <4 years: not recommended
> 4-11 years: 1 inhalation bid
> >11 years: same as adult
>
> *Diskus: flu pro* 100 mcg/*sal* 50 mcg/actuation (60 blisters)

Advair Diskus®250/50
> *Pediatric:* 4-12 years: use 100/50 strength
>
> *Diskus: flu pro* 250 mcg/*sal* 50 mcg/actuation (60 blisters)

Advair Diskus®500/50
> *Pediatric:* 4-12 years: use 100/50 strength
>
> *Diskus:* fluticasone propionate 500 mcg/salmeterol 50 mcg/actuation (60 blisters)

Comment: **Advair Diskus®** is not a rescue inhaler.

Oral Beta$_2$-agonists (Bronchodilator)

▶*albuterol* **(C)(G)**

Proventil® 2-4 mg tid-qid prn
> *Pediatric:* <6 years: not recommended
> *Tab:* 2, 4 mg

Proventil®Repetabs 4-8 mg q 12 hours prn
> *Pediatric:* use syrup
> *Repetab:* 4 mg sust-rel

Proventil®Syrup 5-10 ml tid-qid prn; may increase gradually; max 20 ml qid prn
> *Pediatric:* <2 years: not recommended
> 2-6 years: 0.1 mg/kg tid prn; max initially 5 ml tid prn; may increase gradually to 0.2 mg/kg tid prn; max 10 ml tid
> 6-14 years: 5 ml tid-qid prn; may increase gradually; max 60 ml/day in divided doses
>
> *Syr:* 2 mg/5 ml

Ventolin® 2-4 mg tid-qid prn; may increase gradually; max 8 mg qid

Asthma

    Pediatric: <2 years: not recommended
                 2-6 years: 0.1 mg/kg tid prn; max initially 2 mg tid prn; may increase gradually to 0.2 mg /kg tid; max 4 mg tid
                   6-14 years: 2 mg tid-qid prn; may increase gradually; max 6 mg tid
    Tab: 2, 4 mg; *Syr:* 2 mg/5 ml (strawberry)

  Volmax® 4-8 mg q 12 hours prn; max 32 mg/day divided q 12 hours
    Pediatric: <6 years: not recommended
                 6-12 years: 4 mg q 12 hours; max 24 mg/day q 12 hours
    Tab: 4, 8 mg ext-rel

  VoSpire®ER 4-8 mg q 12 hours prn; max 32 mg/day divided q 12 hours
    Pediatric: <6 years: not recommended
                 6-12 years: 4 mg q 12 hours; max 24 mg/day q 12 hours
    Tab: 4, 8 mg ext-rel

▶ *metaproterenol* **(C)**
  Alupent® 20 mg tid-qid prn
    Pediatric: <6 years: not recommended (doses of 1.3-2.6 mg/kg/day have been used)
                 6-9 years (<60 lb): 10 mg tid-qid prn
                 9-12 years (>60 lb): 20 mg tid-qid prn
    Tab: 10, 20 mg; *Syr:* 10 mg/5 ml

▶ *oxtriphylline* **(C)**
  Choledyl® 200 mg qid prn
    Pediatric: 2-12 years: 4 mg/kg q 6 hours prn
    Tab: 100, 200, 400, 600 mg; *Elix:* 100 mg/5 ml
  Choledyl®SA 1 tab q 12 hours prn
    Pediatric: <12 years: not recommended
    Tab: 400, 600 mg ext-rel

▶ *terbutaline* **(B)(G)** 5 mg tid prn; may be initiated at 2.5 mg tid-qid prn; max 15 mg/day
    Pediatric: <12 years: not recommended
                 12-15 years: 2.5 mg tid prn at 6 hour intervals
                 >15 years: same as adult
  Brethine® *Tab:* 2.5*, 5*mg
  Bricanyl® *Tab:* 2.5, 5 mg

Asthma

Methylxanthines

Comment: Check serum theophylline level just before 5th dose is administered. Therapeutic theophylline level: 10-20 mcg/ml.

▶ *dyphylline* **(C)(G)** 200-800 mg q 6 hours; max 15 mg/kg q 6 hours
    Pediatric: <6 years: not recommended
               >6 years: 5 mg/kg/day in divided doses
  Dilor® *Tab:* 200, 400 mg; *Elix:* 100 mg/15 ml
  Lufyllin® *Tab:* 200, 400 mg; *Elix:* 100 mg/15 ml

▶ *theophylline* **(C)(G)**
    Pediatric: <6 years: not recommended
               >6 years: 5 mg/kg/day in divided doses
  Quibron® 1 tab bid
    Tab: 300 mg
  Quibron®**T/SR** 1 tab daily
    Tab: 300 mg sust-rel
  Respbid® initially 16 mg/kg/day or 400 mg daily (whichever is less) in 2-3 doses; max doses:
        6-9 years: 24 mg/kg/day
        9-12 years: 20 mg/kg/day
        12-16 years: 18 mg/kg/day
        >16 years: 13 mg/kg/day
    Tab: 50 mg
  Slo-Bid® 13 mg/kg/day in 2-3 doses
    Pediatric: <6 years (25 kg): not recommended
               6-9 years: 24 mg/kg/day in 2-3 doses
               9-12 years: 20 mg/kg/day in 2-3 doses
               12-16 years: 18 mg/kg/day in 2-3 doses
    Cap: 50, 75, 100, 125, 200, 300 mg ext-rel
  Slo-Phyllin® 13 mg/kg/day in 2-3 doses
    Pediatric: <6 years (25 kg): not recommended
               6-9 years: 24 mg/kg/day in 2-3 doses
               9-12 years: 20 mg/kg/day in 2-3 doses
               12-16 years: 18 mg/kg/day in 2-3 doses
    Tab: 100, 200, 300 mg ext-rel; *Syr:* 80 mg/15 ml
  Theo-24® initially 300-400 mg daily at HS; after 3 days increase to 400-600 mg daily at HS; max 600 mg/day
    Pediatric: <45 kg: initially 12-14 mg/kg/day; max 300 mg/day; increase after 3 days to 16 mg/kg/day to max 400 mg; after 3 more days increase to 30 mg/kg/day to max of 600 mg/day

Asthma

>45 kg: same as adult
Cap: 100, 200, 300, 400 mg ext-rel

Theo-Dur® initially 150 mg bid; increase to 200 mg bid after 3 days, then to 300 mg bid after 3 more days
Pediatric: <6 years: not recommended
6-15 years: initially 12-14 mg/kg/day in 2 doses; max 300 mg/day; then increase to 16 mg/kg in 2 doses; max of 400 mg/day; then to 20 mg/kg/day in 2 doses; max 600 mg/day
Tab: 100, 200, 300 mg ext-rel

Theolair®-SR *Tab:* 200, 250, 300, 500 mg sust-rel

Theo-X® 16 mg/kg/day or 400 mg/day (whichever is less) in 2 doses
Pediatric: <12 years: not recommended
Tab: 100, 200, 300 mg ext-rel

Uni-Dur® initially 300-400 mg daily; increase to 400-600 mg daily after 3 days
Pediatric: <12 years: not recommended
12-15 years: initially 12-14 mg/kg/day; (max 300 mg/day); increase to 16 mg/kg/day after 3 days (max 400 mg/day); then to 20 mg/kg/day (max 600 mg/day)
Tab: 400, 600 mg ext-rel

Uniphyl® 400-600 mg daily with meals
Pediatric: not recommended
Tab: 400*, 600*mg cont-rel

Methylxanthine/expectorant Combinations
▶*dyphylline/guaifenesin* **(C)** 1 tab or 30 ml qid
Pediatric: <6 years: not recommended
>6 years: ½-1 tab or 15-30 ml tid-qid

Dilor-G® *Tab: dyph* 200 mg/*guaif* 200 mg; *Liq: dyph* 100 mg/*guaif* 100 mg per 5 ml

Lufyllin®-GG *Tab: dyph* 200 mg/*guaif* 200 mg; *Elix: dyph* 100 mg/*guaif* 100 mg per 5 ml

▶*theophylline/guaifenesin* **(C)** 1 tab or 30 ml qid
Elixophyllin®-GG Liquid 30 ml qid
Elix: theo 100 mg/*guaif* 100 mg per 5 ml

Other Methylxanthine Combination
▶*theophylline/potassium iodide/ephedrine/phenobarbital* **(X)(IV)** 1 tab tid-qid prn; add an additional dose at HS as needed; dose may be increased to 1½ tab for severe attack

Asthma

> *Pediatric:* <6 years: not recommended
> 6-12 years: 1/2 tab tid

Quadrinal®
> *Tab:* theo 130 mg/*pot iod* 320 mg/*ephed* 24 mg/*pheno* 24 mg*

Atrophic Vaginitis

Vaginal Preparations
▶*estradiol* (X)
  Vagifem®Vaginal Tablet 1 tab intravaginally daily X 2 weeks, then 1 tab intravaginally twice weekly
  Vag tab: 25 mcg (15 tabs w. applicators)
▶*dienestrol* (X)
  Ortho-Dienestrol®Vaginal Cream 1-2 applicatorsful daily x 1-2 weeks, then reduce dose by half x 1-2 weeks; maintenance 1 applicatorful 1-3 times/week
  Vag crm: 0.01% (78 g w. cal applicator)
▶*estradiol* (X)
  Estrace®Vaginal Cream 2-4 g daily x 1-2 weeks, then gradually reduce to 1/2 initial dose x 1-2 weeks, then maintenance dose of 1 g 1-3 times/week
  Vag crm: 0.01% (1½ oz tube w. cal applicator)
▶*estrogens, conjugated* (X)
  Premarin®Cream ½-2 g/day intravaginally
  Vag crm: 1.5 oz w. applicator marked in 1/2 g increments to max 2 g
▶*estropriate* (X)
  Ogen®Cream 2-4 g intravaginally daily x 3 weeks; discontinue 4th week and continue in this cyclical pattern
  Vag crm: 1.5 mg/g (42.5 g w. cal applicator)

Oral Estrogens
see ***Menopause*** *page 270*

Attention Deficit Disorder (ADD)
Attention Deficit Hyperactivity Disorder (ADHD)

Selective Norepinephrine Reuptake Inhibitor (SNRI)
▶*atomoxetine* (C) take one dose daily in the morning or in two divided doses in the morning and late afternoon or early evening; initially 40

ADD & ADHD

mg/kg; increase after at least 3 days to 80 mg/kg; then after 2-4 weeks may increase to max 100 mg/day

> *Pediatric:* <6 years: not recommended
> >6 years, <70 kg: initially 0.5 mg/kg/day: increase after at least 3 days to 1.2 mg/kg/day; max 1.4 mg/kg/day or 100 mg/day (whichever is less)
> >6 years, >70 kg: same as adult

Strattera® *Cap:* 10, 18, 25, 40, 60, 80, 100 mg

Comment: Not associated with stimulant or euphoric effects. May discontinue without tapering.

Stimulants

▶*dextroamphetamine sulfate* **(C)(II)(G)** initially start with 10 mg daily; increase by 10 mg at weekly intervals if needed; may switch to daily dose with sust-rel spansules when titrated

> *Pediatric:* <3 years: not recommended
> 3-5 years: 2.5 mg daily; may increase by 2.5 mg daily at weekly intervals if needed
> 6-12 years: initially 5 mg daily-bid; may increase by 5 mg/day at weekly intervals; usual max 40 mg/day
> >12 years: initially 10 mg daily; may increase by 10 mg/day at weekly intervals; max 40 mg/day

Dexedrine® *Tab:* 5*mg (tartrazine)
Dexedrine®Spansule *Cap:* 5, 10, 15 mg sust-rel
Dextrostat® *Tab:* 5, 10 mg (tartrazine)

▶*dextroamphetamine saccharate/dextroamphetamine sulfate/ amphetamine aspartate/amphetamine sulfate* **(C)(II)**

Adderall® initially 10 mg daily; may increase weekly by 10 mg/day; usual max 60 mg/day in 2-3 divided doses; first dose on awakening and then q 4-6 hours prn

> *Pediatric:* <6 years: not indicated
> 6-12 years: initially 5 mg daily; may increase weekly by 5 mg/day

> *Tab:* 5**mg: 1.25 mg of each drug
> 7.5**mg: 1.875 mg of each drug
> 10**mg: 2.5 mg of each drug
> 12.5**mg: 3.125 mg of each drug
> 15**mg: 3.75 mg of each drug
> 20**mg: 5 mg of each drug
> 30**mg: 7.5 mg of each drug

Adderall®XR not recommended for adult

> *Pediatric:* <6 years: not recommended

ADD & ADHD

>6 years: initially 10 mg daily in the AM; may increase by 10 mg weekly; max 30 mg/day

Cap: 5 mg: 1.25 mg of each drug ext-rel
10 mg: 2.5 mg of each drug ext-rel
15 mg: 3.75 mg of each drug ext-rel
20 mg: 5 mg of each drug ext-rel
25 mg: 6.25 mg of each drug ext-rel
30 mg: 7.5 mg of each drug ext-rel
Do not chew; may sprinkle on apple sauce

▶ *dexmethylphenidate* **(C)(II)**

Pediatric: <6 years: not recommended
>6 years: initially 2.5 mg bid; allow at least 4 hours between doses; may increase at 1 week intervals; max 20 mg/day

Focalin® *Tab:* 2.5, 5, 10*mg (dye-free)
Focalin®XR *Cap:* 5, 10, 20 mg ext-rel

▶ *methamphetamine* **(C)(II)(G)**

Desoxyn®Granumets

Pediatric: <6 years: not recommended
>6 years: initially 5 mg daily-bid; may increase by 5 mg/day at weekly intervals; usual effective dose 20-25 mg/day

Tab: 5, 10, 15 mg sust-rel

▶ *methylphenidate* (regular-acting) **(C)(II)(G)**

Methylin®, Methylin®Chewable, Methylin®Oral Solution usual dose 20-30 mg/day in 2 or 3 divided doses 30-45 minutes before a meal; may increase to 60 mg/day

Pediatric: <6 years: not recommended
>6 years: initially 5 mg twice daily before breakfast and lunch; may increase 5-10 mg/week; max 60 mg/day

Tab: 5, 10*, 20*mg; *Chew tab:* 2.5, 5, 10 mg; (grape, phenylalanine); *Oral soln:* 5, 10 mg/5 ml (grape)

Ritalin® 10-60 mg/day in 2-3 divided doses 30-45 minutes ac; max 60 mg/day

Pediatric: <6 years: not recommended
>6 years: initially 5 mg bid ac (before breakfast and lunch); may gradually increase by 5-10 mg at weekly intervals as needed; max 60 mg/day

Tab: 5, 10*, 20*mg

▶ *methylphenidate* (long-acting) **(C)(II)**

ADD & ADHD

Concerta® initially 18 mg q AM; may increase in 18 mg increments as needed; max 54 mg/day
> *Tab:* 18, 27, 36, 54 mg sust-rel

Metadate®CD 1 cap daily in the AM
> *Pediatric:* <6 years: not recommended
> >6 years: initially 20 mg daily; may gradually increase by 20 mg/day at weekly intervals as needed; max 60 mg/day
>
> *Cap:* 10, 20, 30 mg immed- and ext-rel beads (dye-free)

Comment: May sprinkle on food, but do not crush or chew.

Metadate®ER 1 tab daily in the AM
> *Pediatric:* <6 years: not recommended
> >6 years: use in place of regular-acting *methylphenidate* when the 8-hour dose of Metadate®-ER corresponds to the titrated 8-hour dose of regular-acting *methylphenidate*
>
> *Tab:* 10, 20 mg ext-rel (dye-free)

Methylin®ER usual dose 20-30 mg/day in 2 or 3 divided doses 30-45 minutes before a meal; may increase to 60 mg/day
> *Pediatric:* <6 years: not recommended
> >6 years: initially 5 mg twice daily before breakfast and lunch; may increase by 5-10 mg/week; max 60 mg/day
>
> *Tab:* 10, 20 mg ext-rel

Ritalin®LA 1 cap daily in the AM
> *Pediatric:* <6 years: not recommended
> >6 years: use in place of regular-acting *methylphenidate* when the 8-hour dose of Ritalin®LA corresponds to the titrated 8-hour dose of regular-acting *meethylphenidate*; max 60 mg/day
>
> *Cap:* 10, 20, 30, 40 mg ext-rel (immed- and ext-rel beads)

Ritalin®SR 1 cap daily in the AM
> *Pediatric:* <6 years: not recommended
> >6 years: use in place of regular-acting *methylphenidate* when the 8-hour dose of Ritalin®SR corresponds to the titrated 8-hour dose of regular-acting *meethylphenidate*; max 60 mg/day
>
> *Tab:* 20 mg sust-rel (dye-free)

▶*methylphenidate* (transdermal patch) **(C)(II)(G)** 1 patch daily in the AM; apply to the hip up to 2 hours prior to desired effect; remove 9 hours after application

ADD & ADHD

>   *Pediatric:* <6 years: not recommended
>   >6 years: initially 10 mg patch daily in the AM; may
>   Increase by 5-10 mg/week; max 60 mg/day
>   **Daytrana®** *Transdermal patch:* 10, 15, 20, 30 mg

▶*pemoline* **(B)(IV)** 18.75-112.5 mg/day; usually start with 37.5 mg in AM; increase weekly by 18.75 mg/day if needed; max 112.5 g/day
>   **Cylert®**
>   *Pediatric:* <6 years: not recommended
>   >6 years: same as adult
>   *Tab:* 18.75*, 37.5*, 75*mg
>   **Cylert®Chewable** *Chew tab:* 37.5*mg

Comment: Monitor baseline serum ALT and repeat every 2 weeks thereafter.

Tricyclic Antidepressants
*see **Depression** page 132*

Other Agents
▶*clonidine* **(C)(G)** 4-5 mcg/kg/day
>   *Pediatric:* <12 years: not recommended
>   **Catapres®** *Tab:* 0.1*, 0.2*, 0.3*mg

Bacterial Endocarditis: Prophylaxis

Dental, Oral, Respiratory Track, or Esophageal Procedures
▶*amoxicillin* **(B)(G)** 3 g 1 hour before procedure and 1.5 g 6 hours later
>   *Pediatric: see page 569 for dose by weight*
>   <40 kg (88 lb): 50 mg/kg (max 3 g) 1 hour before
>   procedure and (max 1.5 g) 25 mg/kg 6 hours later
>   >40 kg: same as adult
>   **Amoxil®** *Cap:* 250, 500 mg; *Tab:* 875*mg; *Chew tab:* 125, 200, 250, 400 mg (cherry-banana-peppermint, phenylalanine); *Oral susp:* 125, 250 mg/5 ml (80, 100, 150 ml; strawberry); 200, 400 mg/5 ml (50, 75, 100 ml; bubble gum); *Oral drops:* 50 mg/ml (30 ml; bubble gum)
>   **Trimox®** *Cap:* 250, 500 mg; *Oral susp:* 125 mg/5 ml, 250 mg/5 ml (80, 100, 150 ml; raspberry-strawberry)

▶*ampicillin* **(B)(G)** 2 g IM 30 minutes before procedure
>   *Pediatric:* 50 mg/kg IM 30 minutes before procedure
>   **Omnipen®, Principen®** *Cap:* 250, 500 mg; *Oral susp:* 125, 250 mg/5 ml (100, 150, 200 ml; fruit)

Bacterial Endocarditis: Prophylaxis

▶*azithromycin* **(B)** 500 mg 1 hour before procedure
   Pediatric: see page 573 for dose by weight
      15 mg/kg 1 hour before procedure; max 500 mg
  Zithromax® *Tab:* 250, 500 mg; *Oral susp:* 100 mg/5 ml (15 ml); 200 mg/5 ml (15, 22.5, 30 ml) (cherry-vanilla-banana)

▶*cefadroxil* **(B)** 2 g 1 hour before procedure
   Pediatric: see page 576 for dose by weight
      50 mg/kg 1 hour before procedure
  Duricef® *Cap:* 500 mg; *Tab:* 1 g; *Oral susp:* 250 mg/5 ml (100 ml); 500 mg/5 ml (75, 100 ml) (orange-pineapple)

▶*cefazolin* **(B)** 1 g IM 30 minutes before procedure
   Pediatric: 25 mg/kg IM 30 minutes before procedure
  Ancef® *Vial:* 250, 500 mg; 1, 5 g
  Kefzol® *Vial:* 500 mg; 1 g

▶*cephalexin* **(B)(G)** 2 g 1 hour before procedure
   Pediatric: see page 582 for dose by weight
      50 mg/kg 1 hour before procedure
  Keflex® *Cap:* 250, 500, 750 mg; *Oral susp:* 125, 250 mg/5 ml (100, 200 ml)
  Keftab® *Tab:* 500 mg
  Keftab®K-pak *Tab:* 20-500 mg tabs/K-pak

▶*clarithromycin* **(C)** 500 mg or 500 mg ext-rel 1 hour before procedure
   Pediatric: see page 584 for dose by weight
      15 mg/kg 1 hour before procedure
  Biaxin® *Tab:* 250, 500 mg
  Biaxin®Oral Suspension *Oral susp:* 125, 250 mg/5 ml (50, 100 ml; fruit-punch)
  Biaxin®XL *Tab:* 500 mg ext-rel

▶*clindamycin* **(B)(G)** 300 mg 1 hour before procedure and 150 mg 6 hours later
   Pediatric: see page 585 for dose by weight
      20 mg/kg(max 300 mg) 1 hour before procedure and 10 mg/kg (max 150 mg) 6 hours later
  Cleocin® *Cap:* 75 (tartrazine), 150 (tartrazine), 300 mg
  Cleocin®Pediatric Granules
  Cleocin®T *Pad:* 1% (60/pck; alcohol 50%); *Lotn:* 1% (60 ml); *Gel:* 1% (30, 60 g); *Soln w. applicator:* 1% (30, 60 ml; alcohol 50%); 75 mg/5 ml (100 ml; cherry)

▶*erythromycin estolate* **(B)(G)** 1 g 1 hour before procedure and then 500 mg 6 hours later
   Pediatric: see page 589 for dose by weight

20 mg/kg 1 hour before procedure and then
10 mg/kg 6 hours later
  Ilosone® *Pulvule:* 250 mg; *Tab:* 500 mg; *Liq:* 125, 250 mg/5 ml (100 ml)
▶*penicillin v potassium* **(B)(G)** 2 g 1 hour before procedure and then 1 g 6 hours later or 2 g 1 hour before procedure and then 1 g q 6 hours X 8 doses
  Pediatric: see page 594 for dose by weight
    <60 lb: 1 g 1 hour before procedure and then 500 mg 6 hours later or 1 g 1 hour before procedure and then 500 mg q 6 hours x 8 doses
    >12 years: same as adult
  Pen-Vee®K *Tab:* 250, 500 mg; *Oral soln:* 125 mg/5 ml (100, 200 ml); 250 mg/5 ml (100, 150, 200 ml)
  Veetids® *Tab:* 250, 500 mg; *Oral soln:* 125, 250 mg/5 ml (100, 200 ml)

Bacterial Vaginosis (*Gardnerella vaginalis*)

Prophylaxis and Restoration of Vaginal Acidity
▶*acetic acid/oxyquinolone* **(C)** one full applicator intravaginally bid for up to 30 days
  Pediatric: not recommended
  Relagard® *Gel: acet acid* 0.9%/*oxyq* 0.025% (50 g tube w. applicator)
▶*glacial acetic acid/oxyquinolone/ricinoleic acid/glycerin* **(C)** one full applicator intravaginally bid
  Pediatric: not recommended
  Aci-Jel® *Gel: gla acet acid* 0.921%/*oxyquin* 0.025%/*ricin acid* 0.7%/*glycerin* 5% (85 g tube w. applicator)

Oral Anti-infectives
▶*metronidazole* (**not for use in 1st; B in 2nd, 3rd**) 250 mg tid or 500 mg bid or 750 mg daily x 7 days
  Pediatric: 35-50 mg/kg/day in 3 divided doses x 7 days
  Flagyl®375 *Cap:* 375 mg
  Flagyl®ER *Tab:* 750 mg ext-rel
  Flagyl®, Protostat® *Tab:* 250*, 500*mg
Comment: Alcohol is contraindicated during treatment with oral *metronidazole* and for 72 hours after therapy due to a possible *disulfiram*-like reaction (nausea,

vomiting, flushing, headache).
Vaginal Anti-infectives
▶*metronidazole* **(B)** one full applicator intravaginally q HS x 5 days
　　Pediatric: not recommended
　MetroGel ®-Vaginal, Vandazole *Vag gel:* 0.75% (70 g w. applicator; parabens)
▶*clindamycin* **(B)** 300 mg bid x 7 days
　　Pediatric: not recommended
　Cleocin® *Cap:* 75 (tartrazine), 150 (tartrazine), 300 mg
　Cleocin®Pediatric Granules *Oral susp:* 75 mg/5 ml (100 ml; cherry)
▶*clindamycin* **(B)** vaginal
　　Pediatric: premenarche: not recommended
　Cleocin®Vaginal Cream if non-pregnant, one full applicator intravaginally q HS x 3-7 days; during 2nd and 3rd trimester, 1 full applicator intravaginally q HS x 7 days
　　Vag crm: 2% (21, 40 g tubes w. applicator)
　Cleocin®Vaginal Ovules if non-pregnant, 1 suppository intravaginally q HS x 3 days
　　Vag supp: 100 mg
▶*sulfanilamide* **(C)(G)**
　AVC ® 1 applicatorful or one vaginal suppository q HS or bid for one complete menstrual cycle
　　Vag crm: 15% (70 g w. applicator); *Vag supp:* 1.05 g
▶*sulfathiazole/sulfacetamide/sulfabenzamide* **(C)(G)**
　　Vag crm: sulfathia 3.42%/*sulfaceta* 2.86%/*sulfabenza* 3.7% *urea* 0.64% (78 g) 1 applicatorful intravaginally bid x 4-6 days; repeat course if necessary reducing dosage by 1/2 to 1/4
　　Vag tab: sulfathia 172.5 mg/*sulfaceta* 143.75 mg/*sulfabenza* 184 mg 1 tab intravaginally bid x 10 days

Baldness: Male Pattern

▶*finasteride* **(X)** 1 mg daily
　Propecia® *Tab:* 1 mg
Comment: Pregnant persons should not touch broken **Propecia®** tabs.
▶*minoxidil* topical soln **(C)** 1 ml from dropper or 6 sprays bid
　　Pediatric: <18 years: not recommended
　Rogaine®for Men (OTC) *Regular soln:* 2% (60 ml w. applicator; alcohol 60%); *Extra strength soln:* 5% (60 ml w. applicator;

alcohol 30%)
Rogaine®for Women (OTC) Regular soln: 2% (60 ml w. applicator; alcohol 60%)

Comment: Do not use *minoxidil* on abraded or inflamed scalp.

Bell's Palsy

▶*prednisone* **(C)(G)** 80 mg daily x 3 days, then 60 mg daily x 3 days, then 40 mg daily x 3 days, then 20 mg daily, then discontinue

Benign Essential Tremor

▶*amantadine* **(C)(G)** 200 mg daily or 100 mg bid; 4 tsp of syrup daily or 2 tsp bid
    Symmetrel® *Tab:* 100 mg; *Syr:* 50 mg/5 ml (raspberry)
▶*propranolol* **(C)(G)**
    Inderal® initially 40 mg bid; usual range 160-240 mg/day
        Tab: 10*, 20*, 40*, 60*, 80*mg
    Inderal®LA initially 80 mg daily in a single dose; increase q 3-7 days; usual range 120-160 mg/day; max 320 mg/day in a single dose
        Cap: 60, 80, 120, 160 mg sust-rel
    InnoPran®XL initially 80 mg q HS; max 120 mg/day
        Cap: 80, 120 mg ext-rel

Benign Prostatic Hyperplasia (BPH)

Alpha-1 Blockers
Comment: Educate patient regarding potential side effect of hypotension especially with first dose. Start at lowest dose and titrate upward.
▶*terazosin* **(C)** initially 1 mg q HS; titrate up to 10 mg daily; max 20 mg/day
    Hytrin® *Cap:* 1, 2, 5, 10 mg
▶*doxazosin* **(C)** initially 1 mg daily; may double dose every 1-2 weeks; max 8 mg/day
    Cardura® *Tab:* 1*, 2*, 4*, 8*mg
    Cardura®XL *Tab:* 4, 8 mg
▶*tamsulosin* **(C)** initially 0.4 mg daily; may increase to 0.8 mg daily after 2-4 weeks if needed

Flomax® *Cap:* 0.4 mg
Type II 5 Alpha-Reductase Inhibitors
Comment: Pregnant women and women of child-bearing age should not handle *alfuzosin* or *finasteride*. Monitor for potential side effects of decreased libido and/or impotence.
▶ *alfuzosin* **(X)** 10 mg daily taken immediately after the same meal each day
    UroXatral® *Tab:* 10 mg ext-rel
▶ *finasteride* **(X)** 5 mg daily
    Proscar® *Tab:* 5 mg
Type I & II 5 Alpha-Reductase Inhibitor
Comment: Pregnant women and women of child-bearing age should not handle *dutasteride*. Monitor for potential side effects of decreased libido and/or impotence.
▶ *dutasteride* **(X)** 0.5 mg daily
    Avodart® *Cap:* 0.5 mg

Bile Acid Deficiency

▶ *ursodiol* **(B)**
    Dissolution of radiolucent non-calcified gallstones <20 mm diameter: 8-10 mg/kg/day in 2-3 divide doses
    Prevention: 13-15 mg/kg/day in 4 divided doses
        Pediatric: not recommended
    Actigall® *Cap:* 300 mg

Bipolar Disorder: Depression

▶ *olanzapine/fluoxetine* **(C)** initially one 6/25 cap q PM; titrate; max 18mg/75 mg/day
        Pediatric: <18 years: not recommended
    Symbyax®
        Cap: **Symbyax®6/25**: *olan* 6 mg/*fluo* 25 mg
            Symbyax®6/50: *olan* 6 mg/*fluo* 50 mg
            Symbyax®12/25: *olan* 12 mg/*fluo* 25 mg
            Symbyax®12/50: *olan* 12 mg/*fluo* 50 mg
Comment: **Symbyax®** is a *thienobenzodiazepine*-selective serotonin reuptake inhibitor indicated for the treatment of depressive episodes associated with bipolar disorder.

Bipolar Disorder: Mania

▶*aripiprazole* **(C)** 15 mg daily; usual maintenance 15 mg/day; may increase at 2 week intervals; max 30 mg/day
    Abilify® *Tab:* 2, 5, 10, 15, 20, 30 mg
▶*clanzapine* **(C)** initially 2.5-10 mg daily; increasing to 10 mg/day within a few days; then by 5 mg/day at weekly intervals; max 20 mg/day
    Zyprexa® *Tab:* 2.5, 5, 7.5, 10 mg; *Vial:* 10 mg/ml (1 ml)
▶*quetiapine fumarate* **(C)** initially 25 mg bid, titrate q 2nd or 3rd day in increments of 25-50 mg bid-tid; max range 100-800 mg/day in 2-3 doses
    SeroQUEL® *Tab:* 25, 100, 200, 300 mg
▶*risperidone* **(C)** 0.5 mg bid x 1 day; adjust in increments of 0.5 mg bid to usual range of 0.5-5 mg/day
    Risperdal® *Tab:* 1, 2, 3, 4 mg; *Oral soln:* 1 mg/ml (100 ml)
    Risperdal®M-Tab *Tab:* 0.5, 1, 2 mg
▶*thioridazine* **(C)** 10-25 mg bid

Bite: Cat

Tetanus Prophylaxis
▶*tetanus toxoid* vaccine **(C)** 0.5 cc IM x 1 dose if previously immunized
    Vial: 5 Lf units/0.5 ml (0.5, 5 ml); *Prefilled syringe:* 5 Lf units/0.5 ml (0.5 ml)
see **Tetanus** page 397 for patients not previously immunized
Anti-infectives
▶*amoxicillin/clavulanate* **(B)(G)** 500 mg tid or 875 mg bid x 10 days
    Pediatric: see pages 571-572 for dose by weight
        40-45 mg/kg/day divided tid x 10 days or
        90 mg/kg/day divided bid x 10 days
    Augmentin® *Tab:* 250, 500, 875 mg; *Chew tab:* 125, 250 mg (lemon-lime); 200, 400 mg (cherry-banana, phenylalanine) *Oral susp:* 125 mg/5 ml (banana), 250 mg/5 ml (orange) (75, 100, 150 ml); 200, 400 mg/5 ml (50, 75, 100 ml; orange-raspberry, phenylalanine)
    Augmentin®ES-600 *Oral susp:* 600 mg/5 ml (50, 75, 100, 150 ml; orange-raspberry, phenylalanine)
    Augmentin®XR 2 tabs q 12 hours x 10 days
        Pediatric: <16 years: use other forms

Tab: 1000 mg ext-rel
▶*cefuroxime axetil* **(B)(G)** 500 mg bid x 10 days
> *Pediatric: see page 581 for dose by weight*
> 15 mg/kg bid x 10 days

Ceftin® *Tab:* 125, 250, 500 mg; *Oral susp:* 125, 250 mg/5 ml (50, 100 ml; tutti-frutti)

▶*doxycycline* **(D)(G)** 100 mg daily-bid
> *Pediatric: see page 587 for dose by weight*
> <8 years: not recommended
> >8 years, <100 lb: 2 mg/lb on first day in 2 doses, followed by 1 mg/lb/day in 1-2 doses
> >8 years, >100 lb: same as adult

Adoxa® *Tab:* 50, 100 mg ent-coat
Doryx® *Cap:* 100 mg
Monodox® *Cap:* 50, 100 mg
Vibramycin® *Cap:* 50, 100 mg; *Syr:* 50 mg/5 ml (raspberry-apple, sulfites); *Oral susp:* 25 mg/5 ml (raspberry)
Vibra-Tab® *Tab:* 100 mg film-coat

▶*penicillin v* **(B)(G)** 500 mg po qid x 3 days
> *Pediatric: see page 594 for dose by weight*
> 50 mg/kg/day in 4 doses x 3 days
> >12 years: same as adult

Pen-Vee®K *Tab:* 250, 500 mg; *Oral soln:* 125 mg/5 ml (100, 200 ml); 250 mg/5 ml (100, 150, 200 ml)
Veetids® *Tab:* 250, 500 mg; *Oral soln:* 125, 250 mg/5 ml (100, 200 ml)

Bite: Dog

Tetanus prophylaxis
▶*tetanus toxoid* vaccine **(C)** 0.5 cc IM x 1 dose if previously immunized
> *Vial:* 5 Lf units/0.5 ml *(0.5, 5 ml)*
> *Prefilled* syringe: 5 Lf units/0.5 ml (0.5 ml)

see **Tetanus** page 397 for patients not previously immunized

Anti-infectives
▶*amoxicillin/clavulanate* **(B)(G)** 500 mg tid or 875 mg bid x 10 days
> *Pediatric: see pages 571-572 for dose by weight*
> 40-45 mg/kg/day divided tid x 10 days or
> 90 mg/kg/day divided bid x 10 days

Augmentin® *Tab:* 250, 500, 875 mg; *Chew tab:* 125, 250 mg

Bite: Dog

>　　　(lemon-lime), 200, 400 mg (cherry-banana, phenylalanine); *Oral susp:* 125 mg/5 ml (banana), 250 mg/5 ml (orange) (75, 100, 150 ml); 200, 400 mg/5 ml (50, 75, 100 ml; orange-raspberry, phenylalanine)
>　　　**Augmentin®ES-600** *Oral susp:* 600 mg/5 ml (50, 75, 100, 150 ml; orange-raspberry, phenylalanine)
>　　　**Augmentin®XR** 2 tabs q 12 hours x 10 days
>　　　　　*Pediatric:* <16 years: use other forms
>　　　　　*Tab:* 1000 mg ext-rel
>▶*clindamycin* **(B)** (administer with fluoroquinolone in adult and TMP-SMX in children) 300 mg qid x 10 days
>　　　　　*Pediatric: see page 585 for dose by weight*
>　　　　　　　　8-16 mg/kg/day in 3-4 doses x 10 days
>　　　**Cleocin®** *Cap:* 75 (tartrazine), 150 (tartrazine), 300 mg
>　　　**Cleocin®Pediatric Granules** *Oral susp:* 75 mg/5 ml (100 ml; cherry)
>▶*doxycycline* **(D)(G)** 100 mg daily-bid
>　　　　　*Pediatric: see page 587 for dose by weight*
>　　　　　　　　<8 years: not recommended
>　　　　　　　　>8 years, <100 lb: 2 mg/lb on first day in 2 doses, followed by 1 mg/lb/day in 1-2 doses
>　　　　　　　　>8 years, >100 lb: same as adult
>　　　**Adoxa®** *Tab:* 50, 100 mg ent-coat
>　　　**Doryx®** *Cap:* 100 mg
>　　　**Monodox®** *Cap:* 50, 100 mg
>　　　**Vibramycin®** *Cap:* 50, 100 mg; *Syr:* 50 mg/5 ml (raspberry-apple, sulfites); *Oral susp:* 25 mg/5 ml (raspberry)
>　　　**Vibra-Tab®** *Tab:* 100 mg film-coat
>▶*penicillin v* **(B)(G)** 500 mg po qid x 3 days
>　　　　　*Pediatric: see page 594 for dose by weight*
>　　　　　　　　50 mg/kg/day in 4 doses x 3 days
>　　　　　　　　>12 years: same as adult
>　　　**Pen-Vee®K** *Tab:* 250, 500 mg; *Oral soln:* 125 mg/5 ml (100, 200 ml); 250 mg/5 ml (100, 150, 200 ml)
>　　　**Veetids®** *Tab:* 250, 500 mg; *Oral soln:* 125 mg/5 ml, 250 mg/5 ml (100, 200 ml)

Bite: Human

Tetanus prophylaxis
▶ *tetanus toxoid* vaccine **(C)** 0.5 cc IM x 1 dose if previously immunized
> *Vial:* 5 Lf units/0.5 ml (0.5, 5 ml)
> *Prefilled syringe:* 5 Lf units/0.5 ml (0.5 ml)

see **Tetanus** *page 397* for patients not previously immunized

Anti-infectives
▶ *amoxicillin/clavulanate* **(B)(G)** 500 mg tid or 875 mg bid x 10 days
> *Pediatric: see pages 571-572 for dose by weight*
> 40-45 mg/kg/day divided tid x 10 days or
> 90 mg/kg/day divided bid x 10 days

Augmentin® *Tab:* 250, 500, 875 mg; *Chew tab:* 125, 250 mg (lemon-lime), 200, 400 mg (cherry-banana, phenylalanine); *Oral susp:* 125 mg/5 ml (banana), 250 mg/5 ml (orange) (75, 100, 150 ml); 200, 400 mg/5 ml (50, 75, 100 ml; orange-raspberry, phenylalanine)

Augmentin®ES-600 *Oral susp:* 600 mg/5 ml (50, 75, 100, 150 ml; orange-raspberry, phenylalanine)

Augmentin®XR 2 tabs q 12 hours x 10 days
> *Pediatric:* <16 years: use other forms
> *Tab:* 1000 mg ext-rel

▶ *cefoxitin* **(B)** 80-160 mg/kg/day IM in 3-4 doses x 10 days; max 12 g/day
> *Pediatric:* <3 months: not recommended

Mefoxin®Injectable *Vial:* 1, 2 g

▶ *ciprofloxacin* **(C)** 500 mg bid x 10 days
> *Pediatric:* <18 years: not recommended

Cipro® *Tab:* 100, 250, 500, 750 mg; *Oral susp:* 250 mg/5 ml (100 ml; strawberry)

▶ *erythromycin base* **(B)(G)** 250 mg qid x 10 days
> *Pediatric: see page 588 for dose by weight*
> <45 kg: 30-40 mg/kg/day in 4 doses x 10 days
> >45 kg: same as adult

E-mycin® *Tab:* 250, 333 mg ent-coat
Eryc® *Cap:* 250 mg ent-coat
Ery-Tab® *Tab:* 250, 333, 500 mg ent-coat
PCE® *Tab:* 333, 500 mg

▶ *trimethoprim/sulfamethoxazole* **(C)(G)** bid x 10 days

Bite: Human

>
> *Pediatric: see page 596 for dose by weight*
> >   <2 months: not recommended
> >   >2 months: 40 mg/kg/day of *sulfamethoxazole*
> >   in 2 doses bid x 10 days
>
> **Bactrim®, Septra®** 2 tabs bid x 10 days
> >   *Tab: trim* 80 mg/*sulfa* 400 mg*
>
> **Bactrim®DS, Septra®DS** 1 tab bid x 10 days
> >   *Tab: trim* 160 mg/*sulfa* 800 mg*
>
> **Bactrim®Pediatric Suspension, Septra®Pediatric Suspension** 20 ml bid x 10 days
> >   *Oral susp: trim* 40 mg/*sulfa* 200 mg per 5 ml (100 ml; cherry, alcohol 0.3%)

Comment: Trimethoprim/sulfamethoxazole is not recommended in pregnancy or lactation.

Blepharitis

Ophthalmic Agents

▶*erythromycin* ophthalmic ointment **(B)** apply 1/2 inch bid-qid x 14 days, then q HS
>   *Pediatric:* same as adult
>
>   **Ilotycin®** *Oint:* 5 mg/g (1/2 oz)

▶*polymyxin/bacitracin* ophthalmic ointment **(C)** apply 1/2 inch bid-qid x 14 days, then q HS
>   *Pediatric:* same as adult
>
>   **Polysporin®** *Oint: poly B* 10,000 U/*baci* 500 U (3.75 g)

▶*polymyxin B/bacitracin/neomycin* ophthalmic ointment **(C)** apply 1/2 inch bid-qid x 14 days, then q HS
>   *Pediatric:* same as adult
>
>   **Neosporin®** *Oint: poly B* 10,000 U/*baci* 400 U/*neo* 3.5 mg/g 3.75 g)

▶*sodium sulfacetamide* **(C)**
>   **Bleph-10®Ophthalmic Solution** 2 drops q 4 hours x 7-14 days
> >   *Pediatric:* <2 years: not recommended
> >   >2 years: 1-2 drops q 2-3 hours during the day
> >   x 7-14 days
>
>   *Ophth soln:* 10% (2.5, 5, 15 ml; benzalkonium chloride)
>
>   **Bleph-10®Ophthalmic Ointment** apply 1/2 inch qid and HS x 7-14 days
> >   *Pediatric:* <2 years: not recommended

>2 years: same as adult
Ophth oint: 10% (3.5 g; phenylmercuric acetate)

Sulamyd®Ophthalmic Solution 1 drop of 30% soln or 1-2 drops of 10% soln q 2 hours while awake
Pediatric: same as adult
Ophth oint: 10% (5, 15 ml); 30% (15 ml) (parabens)

Sulamyd®Ophthalmic Ointment apply 1/2 inch qid and HS x 7-14 days
Pediatric: same as adult
Ophth oint: 10% (3.5 g; parabens)

Systemic Agents

▶*tetracycline* **(D)(G)** 250 mg qid x 7 days
Pediatric: see page 595 for dose by weight
<8 years: not recommended
>8 years, <100 lb: 25-50 mg/kg/day in 2-4 doses x 7-10 days

Achromycin®V *Cap:* 250, 500 mg

Sumycin® *Tab:* 250, 500 mg; *Cap:* 250, 500 mg; *Oral susp:* 125 mg/5 ml (100, 200 ml; fruit, sulfites)

Comment: Tetracycline is contraindicated in pregnancy (discolors fetal tooth enamel).

Breast Cancer: Prophylaxis

▶*fulvestrant* **(D)** 250 mg IM once monthly; administer 2.5 ml IM in each buttock concurrently
Faslodex® *Prefilled syringe:* 50 mg/ml (2 x 2.5 ml, 1 x 5 ml)

▶*tamoxifen* **(D)** 20 mg daily x 5 years
Nolvadex® *Tab:* 10, 20 mg

Comment: Cautious use with concomitant coumarin-type anticoagulation therapy, history of DVT, or history of pulmonary embolus.

Bronchiolitis

Inhaled Bronchodilators *see Asthma page 61*
Oral Beta$_2$-Agonists *see Asthma page 64*
Inhaled Anti-cholinergic/Beta$_2$-Agonist Combinations *see Asthma page 61*
Inhaled Glucocorticosteroids *see Asthma page 58*
Parenteral Glucocorticosteroids *see page 389*

Bronchiolitis

Oral Glucocorticosteroids *see page 387*

Bronchitis: Acute

Inhaled Bronchodilators *see Asthma page 61*
Systemic Bronchodilators *see Asthma page 64*
Decongestants *see page 528*
Expectorants *see page 529*
Antitussives *see page 530*
Combination Oral Agents
*see **Oral Drugs for Management of Common Respiratory Symptoms** page 523*
Anti-infectives for Secondary Bacterial Infection
▶*amoxicillin* **(B)(G)** 500-875 mg bid or 250-500 mg tid x 10 days
    Pediatric: see page 569 for dose by weight
        <40 kg (88 lb): 20-40 mg/kg/day in 3 doses x 10
        days or 25-45 mg/kg/day in 2 doses x 10 days
        >40 kg: same as adult
  Amoxil® *Cap:* 250, 500 mg; *Tab:* 875*mg; *Chew tab:* 125, 200, 250, 400 mg (cherry-banana-peppermint, phenylalanine); *Oral susp:* 125, 250 mg/5 ml (80, 100, 150 ml; strawberry); 200, 400 mg/5 ml (50, 75, 100 ml; bubble gum); *Oral drops:* 50 mg/ml (30 ml; bubble gum)
  Trimox® *Cap:* 250, 500 mg; *Oral susp:* 125 mg/5 ml, 250 mg/5 ml (80, 100, 150 ml; raspberry-strawberry)
▶*amoxicillin/clavulanate* **(B)(G)** 500 mg tid or 875 mg bid x 10 days
    Pediatric: see pages 571-572 for dose by weight
        40-45 mg/kg/day divided tid x 10 days or
        90 mg/kg/day divided bid x 10 days
  Augmentin® *Tab:* 250, 500, 875 mg; *Chew tab:* 125, 250 mg (lemon-lime), 200, 400 mg (cherry-banana, phenylalanine); *Oral susp:* 125 mg/5 ml (banana), 250 mg/5 ml (orange) (75, 100, 150 ml); 200, 400 mg/5 ml (50, 75, 100 ml; orange-raspberry, phenylalanine)
  Augmentin®ES-600 *Oral susp:* 600 mg/5 ml (50, 75, 100, 150 ml; orange-raspberry, phenylalanine)
  Augmentin®XR 2 tabs q 12 hours x 10 days
    Pediatric: <16 years: use other forms
    Tab: 1000 mg ext-rel

Bronchitis: Acute

▶*ampicillin* **(B)** 250-500 mg qid x 10 days
    Pediatric: not recommended for bronchitis in children
    Omnipen®, Principen® *Cap:* 250, 500 mg; *Oral susp:* 125, 250 mg/5 ml (100, 150, 200 ml; fruit)

▶*azithromycin* **(B)** 500 mg x 1 dose on day 1, then 250 mg daily on days 2-5 or 500 mg daily x 3 days or 2 g in a single dose
    Pediatric: not recommended for bronchitis in children
    Zithromax® *Tab:* 250, 500 mg; *Oral susp:* 100 mg/5 ml (15 ml); 200 mg/5 ml (15, 22.5, 30 ml) (cherry-vanilla-banana); *Pkt:* 1 g for reconstitution (cherry-banana)
    Zithromax®Tri-pak *Tab:* 3-500 mg tabs/pck
    Zithromax®Z-pak *Tab:* 6-250 mg tabs/pck
    Zmax® *Oral susp:* 2 g ext rel (cherry-banana)

▶*cefaclor* **(B)(G)**
    Ceclor® 250 mg tid x 7 days
        Pediatric: see page 575 for dose by weight
            20-40 mg/kg/day in 3 doses x 10 days
        Pulvule: 250, 500 mg; *Oral susp:* 125, 250 mg/5 ml (75, 150 ml); 187, 375 mg/5 ml (50, 100 ml) (strawberry)
    Ceclor®CD 500 mg q 12 hours x 7 days
        Pediatric: <16 years: not recommended
        Tab: 375, 500 mg ext-rel
    Ceclor®CDpak 500 mg q 12 hours x 7 days
        Pediatric: <16 years: not recommended
        Tab: 500 mg (14 tabs/CDpak)
    Raniclor® 500 mg q 12 hours x 7 days
        Pediatric: 20-40 mg/kg/day in 3 doses x 10 days
        Chew tab: 125, 187, 250, 375 mg

▶*cefadroxil* **(B)** 1-2 g in 1-2 doses x 10 days
    Pediatric: see page 576 for dose by weight
        30 mg/kg/day in 2 doses x 10 days
    Duricef® *Tab:* 1 g; *Cap:* 500 mg; *Oral susp:* 250 mg/5 ml (100 ml); 500 mg/5 ml (75, 100 ml) (orange-pineapple)

▶*cefdinir* **(B)** 300 mg bid x 5-10 days or 600 mg daily x 10 days
    Pediatric: see page 574 for dose by weight
        <6 months: not recommended
        6 months-12 years: 14 mg/kg/day in 1-2 doses x 10 days
    Omnicef® *Cap:* 300 mg; *Oral susp:* 125 mg/5 ml (60, 100 ml; strawberry)

Bronchitis: Acute

▶ *cefditoren pivoxil* **(B)** 400 mg bid x 10 days
  Pediatric: not recommended
 Spectracef® *Tab:* 200 mg
Comment: Contraindicated with milk protein allergy or carnitine deficiency.
▶ *cefixime* **(B)(G)**
  Pediatric: see page 577 for dose by weight
    <6 months: not recommended
    6 months-12 years, <50 kg: 8 mg/kg/day in 1-2
    doses x 10 days
    >12 years, >50 kg: same as adult
 Suprax®Oral Suspension *Oral susp:* 100 mg/5 ml (50, 75, 100 ml; strawberry)
▶ *cefpodoxime proxetil* **(B)** 200 mg bid x 10 days
  Pediatric: see page 578 for dose by weight
    <2 months: not recommended
    2 months-12 years: 10 mg/kg/day (max 400 mg/
    dose) or 5 mg/kg/day bid (max 200 mg/dose)
    x 10 days
 Vantin® *Tab:* 100, 200 mg; *Oral susp:* 50, 100 mg/5 ml (50, 75, 100 mg; lemon-creme)
▶ *cefprozil* **(B)** 500 mg bid x 10 days
  Pediatric: see page 579 for dose by weight
    2-12 years: 7.5 mg/kg bid x 10 days
 Cefzil® *Tab:* 250, 500 mg; *Oral susp:* 125, 250 mg/5 ml (50, 75, 100 ml; bubble gum, phenylalanine)
▶ *ceftibuten* **(B)** 400 mg daily x 10 days
  Pediatric: see page 580 for dose by weight
   9 mg/kg daily x 10 days; max 400 mg/day
 Cedax® *Cap:* 400 mg; *Oral susp:* 90 mg/5 ml (30, 60, 90, 120 ml); 180 mg/5 ml (30, 60, 120 ml; cherry)
▶ *ceftriaxone* **(B)** 1-2 gm IM daily continued 2 days after signs of infection have disappeared; max 4 g/day
  Pediatric: 50 mg/kg IM daily continued 2 days after signs of
    infection have disappeared
 Rocephin® *Vial:* 250, 500 mg; 1, 2 g

Bronchitis: Acute

▶*cefuroxime axetil* **(B)(G)** 250-500 mg bid x 10 days
    Pediatric: see page 581 for dose by weight
        15 mg/kg bid x 10 days
  Ceftin® *Tab:* 125, 250, 500 mg; *Oral susp:* 125, 250 mg/5 ml (50, 100 ml; tutti-frutti)

▶*cephalexin* **(B)(G)** 250-500 mg qid or 500 mg bid x 10 days
    Pediatric: see page 581 for dose by weight
        25-50 mg/kg/day in 4 doses x 10 days
  Keflex® *Cap:* 250, 500, 750 mg; *Oral susp:* 125, 250 mg/5 ml (100, 200 ml)
  Keftab® *Tab:* 500 mg
  Keftab®K-pak *Tab:* 20-500 mg tabs/K-pak

▶*cephradine* **(B)** 250 mg q 6 hours or 500 mg q 12 hours; max 4 g/day
    Pediatric: see page 583 for dose by weight
        <9 months: not recommended
        >9 months: 25-50 mg/kg/day divided q 6-12 hours; max 4 g/day
  Velosef® *Cap:* 250, 500 mg; *Oral susp:* 125, 250 mg/5 ml (100, 200 ml)

▶*clarithromycin* **(C)(G)** 500 mg or 500 mg ext-rel daily x 7 days
    Pediatric: see page 584 for dose by weight
        <6 months: not recommended
        >6 months: 7.5 mg/kg bid x 7 days
  Biaxin® *Tab:* 250, 500 mg
  Biaxin®Oral Suspension *Oral susp:* 125, 250 mg/5 ml (50, 100 ml; fruit-punch)
  Biaxin®XL *Tab:* 500 mg ext-rel

▶*dirithromycin* **(C)** 500 mg daily x 7 days
    Pediatric: <12 years: not recommended
  Dynabac® *Tab:* 250 mg

▶*doxycycline* **(D)(G)** 100 mg daily-bid x 10 days
    Pediatric: see page 587 for dose by weight
        <8 years: not recommended
        >8 years, <100 lb: 2 mg/lb on first day in 2 doses, followed by 1 mg/lb/day in 1-2 doses
        >8 years, >100 lb: same as adult
  Adoxa® *Tab:* 50, 100 mg ent-coat
  Doryx® *Cap:* 100 mg

Bronchitis: Acute

Monodox® *Cap:* 50, 100 mg
Vibramycin® *Cap:* 50, 100 mg; *Syr:* 50 mg/5 ml (raspberry-apple, sulfites); *Oral susp:* 25 mg/5 ml (raspberry)
Vibra-Tab® *Tab:* 100 mg film-coat

▶*erythromycin ethylsuccinate* **(B)(G)** 400 mg po qid x 7 days
    Pediatric: see page 589 for dose by weight
        30-50 mg/kg/day in 4 divided doses x 7 days; may double dose with severe infection; max 100 mg/kg/day

Ery-Ped® *Oral susp:* 200 mg/5 ml (100, 200 ml; fruit); 400 mg/5 ml (60, 100, 200 ml; banana); *Oral drops:* 200, 400 mg/5 ml (50 ml; fruit); *Chew tab:* 200 mg wafer (fruit)
E.E.S.® *Oral susp:* 200, 400 mg/5 ml (100 ml; fruit)
E.E.S.®Granules *Oral susp:* 200 mg/5 ml (100, 200 ml; cherry)
E.E.S.®400 Tablets *Tab:* 400 mg

▶*levofloxacin* **(C)**
    Uncomplicated: 500 mg daily x 7 days
    Complicated: 750 mg daily x 7 days
    Pediatric: <18 years: not recommended

Levaquin® *Tab:* 250, 500, 750 mg

▶*loracarbef* **(B)** 200-400 mg bid x 7 days
    Pediatric: see page 593 for dose by weight
        30 mg/kg/day in 2 doses x 7 days

Lorabid® *Pulvule:* 200, 400 mg; *Oral susp:* 100 mg/5 ml (50, 100 ml); 200 mg/5 ml (50, 75, 100 ml) (strawberry bubble gum)

▶*moxifloxacin* **(C)** 400 mg daily x 5 days
    Pediatric: <18 years: not recommended

Avelox® *Tab:* 400 mg

▶*ofloxacin* **(C)(G)** 400 mg bid x 10 days
    Pediatric: <18 years: not recommended

Floxin® *Tab:* 200, 300, 400 mg

▶*sparfloxacin* **(C)** 400 mg daily in a single dose on day 1, then 200 mg in a single dose on days 2-10
    Pediatric: <18 years: not recommended

Zagam® *Tab:* 200 mg

▶*telithromycin* **(C)** 2-400 mg tabs in a singe dose daily x 5 days
    Pediatric: <18 years not recommended

▶*tetracycline* **(D)(G)** 250-500 mg qid x 7 days

Pediatric: see page 595 for dose by weight
>   <8 years: not recommended
>   >8 years, <100 lb: 25-50 mg/kg/day in 2-4 doses x 7 days
>   >8 years, >100 lb: same as adult

Achromycin®V *Cap:* 250, 500 mg

Sumycin® *Tab:* 250, 500 mg; *Cap:* 250, 500 mg; *Oral susp:* 125 mg/5 ml (100, 200 ml; fruit, sulfites)

Comment: Tetracycline is contraindicated in pregnancy (discolors fetal tooth enamel).

▶*trimethoprim/sulfamethoxazole* **(C)(G)** bid x 10 days
>   *Pediatric: see page 596 for dose by weight*
>   <2 months: not recommended
>   >2 months: 40 mg/kg/day of *sulfamethoxazole* in 2 doses bid x 10 days

Bactrim®, Septra® 2 tabs bid x 10 days
   Tab: trim 80 mg/*sulfa* 400 mg*

Bactrim®DS, Septra®DS 1 tab bid x 10 days
   Tab: trim 160 mg/*sulfa* 800 mg*

Bactrim®Pediatric Suspension, Septra®Pediatric Suspension 20 ml bid x 10 days
   Oral susp: trim 40 mg/*sulfa* 200 mg per 5 ml (100 ml; cherry, alcohol 0.3%)

Comment: Trimethoprim/sulfamethoxazole is not recommended in pregnancy or lactation.

▶*trovafloxacin* **(C)** 100 mg daily x 7-10 days
>   *Pediatric:* <18 years: not recommended

Trovan® *Tab:* 100, 200 mg

Comment: Trovafloxacin is indicated only for life- or limb-threatening infection.

Bronchitis: Chronic

Inhaled Bronchodilators *see Asthma page 61*
Systemic Bronchodilators *see Asthma page 64*
Inhaled Glucocorticosteroids *see Asthma page 58*
Parenteral Glucocorticosteroids *see page 489*
Oral Glucocorticosteroids *see page 487*
Inhaled Anticholinergics

Bronchitis: Chronic

▶ *ipratropium* **(B)(G)**
    Atrovent® 2 inhalations qid; max 12 inhalations/day
        Inhaler: 14 g (200 inh)
    Atrovent®Inhaled Solution 500 mcg by nebulizer tid-qid
        Inhal soln: 0.02% (2.5 ml)
Comment: Contraindicated with allergy to atropine or its derivatives.

Inhaled Long-Acting Anti-cholinergic
▶ *tiotropium (as bromide monohydrate)* **(C)** 1 inhalation daily using inhaler; do not swallow caps
    Pediatric: not recommended
    Spiriva®HandiHaler *Inhaler:* 18 mcg/cap (6, 30 caps w device)
Comment: For prophylaxis and chronic treatment, only. Not for primary (rescue) treatment of acute attack. Avoid getting powder in eyes. Precaution with narrow-angle glaucoma, BPH, bladder neck obstruction, and pregnancy. Contraindicated with allergy to atropine or its derivatives (e.g., ipratropium)

Beta$_2$-Agonist/Anti-cholinergic Combination
▶ *ipratropium/albuterol* **(C)** 2 inhalations qid; max 12 inhalations/day
    Combivent® *Inhaler:* 14.7 g (200 inh)

Methylxanthines
see Asthma page 66

Methylxanthine/Expectorant Combinations
▶ *dyphylline/guaifenesin* **(C)**
    Lufyllin®GG 1 tab qid
        Tab: dyphy 200 mg/*guaif* 200 mg
    Lufyllin®GG Elixir 30 ml qid
        Elix: dyphy 100 mg/*guaif* 100 mg per 15 ml

Other Methylxanthine Combination
▶ *theophylline/potassium iodide/ephedrine/phenobarbital* **(X)(IV)** 1 tab tid-qid prn; add an additional dose at HS as needed; dose may be increased to 1½ tab for severe attack
    Pediatric: <6 years: not recommended
                  6-12 years: 1/2 tab tid
    Quadrinal® *Tab: theo* 130 mg/*pot iod* 320 mg/*ephed* 24 mg/*phenol* 24 mg

Expectorants *see page 529*

Anti-infectives for Acute Exacerbations
see Bronchitis: Acute page 84

Bulimia Nervosa

▶ *fluoxetine* **(C)(G)**

Prozac® initially 20 mg daily; may increase after 1 week; doses >20 mg/day should be divided into AM and noon doses; max 80 mg/day
> *Pediatric:* <8 years: not recommended
> 8-17 years: initially 10 or 20 mg/day; start lower weight children at 10 mg/day; if starting at 10 mg daily, may increase after 1 week to 20 mg daily
>
> *Tab:* 10*mg; *Cap:* 10, 20, 40 mg; *Oral soln:* 20 mg/5 ml (4 oz; mint)

Prozac®Weekly following daily *fluoxetine* therapy at 20 mg/day for 13 weeks, may initiate **Prozac®Weekly** 7 days after the last 20 mg *fluoxetine* dose
> *Pediatric:* not recommended
> *Cap:* 90 mg ent-coat del-rel pellets

Burn: Minor

▶*silver sulfadiazine* **(C)(G)** apply topically to burn daily-bid
> *Pediatric:* not recommended
>
> **Silvadene®** *Crm:* 1% (20, 50, 85, 400, 1000 g jar; 20 g tube)

Topical anesthetics
▶*lidocaine* 3% cream **(B)** apply bid-tid prn
> *Pediatric:* reduce dosage commensurate with age, body weight, and physical condition
>
> **LidaMantle®** *Crm:* 3% (1 oz)

Bursitis

NSAIDs *see **Pain** page 305*
Oral Non-narcotic Analgesics *see **Pain** page 308*
Oral Narcotic Analgesics *see **Pain** page 308*
Topical Analgesics *see **Pain** page 308*
Parenteral Glucocorticosteroids *see page 389*
Oral Glucocorticosteroids *see page 387*
Topical Anesthetics *see page 383*
Topical Anesthetics/Steroid Combinations *see page 480*

Candidiasis: Oral (Thrush)

▶*amphotericin B* **(C)** 1 ml swish and swallow qid
    Pediatric: same as adult
  Fungizone® *Oral susp:* 100 mg/ml (24 ml w. dropper)

▶*clotrimazole* **(C)**
    Prophylaxis: 1 troche dissolved in mouth tid
    Treatment: 1 troche dissolved in mouth 5 times/day x 10-14 days
    Pediatric: <3 years: not recommended
              >3 years: same as adult
  Mycelex®Troches Troches: 10 mg

▶*fluconazole* **(C)** 200 mg x 1 dose first day, then 100 mg daily x 13 days
    Pediatric: see page 591 for dose by weight
           >2 weeks: 6 mg/kg x 1 day; then 3 mg/kg/day for at least 3 weeks
  Diflucan® *Tab:* 50, 100, 150, 200 mg; *Oral susp:* 10, 40 mg/ml (35 ml; orange)

▶*gentian violet* **(NR)(G)** apply to oral mucosa with a cotton swab tid x 3 days

▶*itraconazole* **(C)** 200 mg daily x 7-14 days
    Pediatric: see page 592 for dose by weight
    5 mg/kg daily x 7-14 days; max 200 mg/day
  Sporanox® *Oral soln:* 10 mg/ml (150 ml) (cherry-caramel)

▶*nystatin* **(C)(G)**
  Mycostatin® 1-2 pastilles dissolved slowly in mouth 4-5 times/day x 10-14 days; max 14 days
    Pediatric: same as adult
    Pastille: 200,000 units/pastille (30 pastilles/pck)
  Mycostatin®Suspension 4-6 ml qid swish and swallow
    Pediatric: infants: 1 ml in each cheek qid after feedings
              older children: same as adult
    Oral susp: 100,000 units/ml (60 ml w. dropper)

Invasive Infection

▶*posaconazole* **(D)** take with food; 100 mg bid on day one; then, 100 mg once daily x 13 days; refractory, 400 mg bid
    Pediatric: <13 years: not recommended
            ≥*13 years:* same as adult
  Noxafil® *Oral susp:* 40 mg/ml (cherry flavor)

Candidiasis: Skin

Topical Anti-fungals

▶*amphotericin B* **(B)** apply tid-qid x 7-14 days
    Fungizone® *Oral susp:* 100 mg/ml (24 ml w. dropper)

▶*butenafine* **(B)** apply bid x 1 week or daily x 4 weeks
    Pediatric: <12 years: not recommended
    Lotrimin®Ultra (C)(OTC) *Crm:* 1% (12, 24 g)
    Mentax® *Crm:* 1% (15, 30 g)

Comment: Butenafine is a benzylamine, not an "azole." Fungicidal activity continues for at least 5 weeks after the last application.

▶*ciclopirox* **(B)**
    Loprox®Cream apply bid; max 4 weeks
        Pediatric: <10 years: not recommended
                >10 years: same as adult
    Crm: 0.77% (15, 30, 90 g)
    Loprox®Lotion apply bid; max 4 weeks
        Pediatric: <10 years: not recommended
                >10 years: same as adult
    Lotn: 0.77% (30, 60 ml)
    Loprox®Gel apply bid; max 4 weeks
        Pediatric: <16 years: not recommended
                >16 years: same as adult
    Gel: 0.77% (30, 45 g)

▶*clotrimazole* **(B)** apply to affected area bid x 7 days
    Pediatric: same as adult
    Fungoid® *Crm:* 1% (45 g); *Soln:* 1% (1 oz w. dropper)
    Lotrimin® *Crm::* 1% (15, 30, 45 g)
    Lotrimin®AF (OTC) *Crm:* 1% (12 g); *Lotn:* 1% (10 ml); *Soln:* 1% (10 ml)

▶*econazole* **(C)** apply bid x 14 days
    Spectazole® *Crm:* 1% (15, 30, 85 g)

▶*ketoconazole* **(C)** apply daily x 14 days
    Nizoral®Cream *Crm:* 2% (15, 30, 60 g)

▶*miconazole 2%* **(C)** apply daily x 2 weeks
    Pediatric: same as adult
    Lotrimin®AF Spray Liquid (OTC) *Spray liq:* 2% (113 g; alcohol 17%)
    Lotrimin®AF Spray Powder (OTC) *Spray pwdr:* 2% (90 g; alcohol 10%)

Candidiasis: Skin

>   **Monistat-Derm®** *Crm:* 2% (1, 3 oz); *Spray liq:* 2% (3.5 oz); *Spray pwdr:* 2% (3 oz)

▶*nystatin* **(C)**
>   **Nystop®Powder** dust freely bid-tid to affected skin
>   *Pwdr: nystatin* 100,000 U/g (15 g)

Oral Anti-fungals
▶*ketoconazole* **(C)** 400 mg daily x 1-2 weeks
>   *Pediatric:* <2 years: not recommended
>   >2 years: 3.3-6.6 mg/kg daily
>   **Nizoral®** *Tab:* 200 mg

Candidiasis: Vulvovaginal (Moniliasis)

Prophylaxis
▶*acetic acid/oxyquinolone* **(C)** one full applicator intravaginally bid for up to 30 days
>   *Pediatric:* not recommended
>   **Relagard®** *Gel: acetic acid* 0.9%/*oxyquin* 0.025% (50 g tube w. applicator)

Vaginal Anti-fungals
▶*butoconazole* **(C)**
>   *Pediatric:* not recommended
>   **Gynazole-1 2% Vaginal Cream** 1 applicatorful x 1 dose
>   *Prefilled vag applicator:* 5 g
>   **Femstat®3 Vaginal Cream (OTC)** 1 applicatorful q HS x 3 days
>   *Vag crm:* 2% (20 g w. 3 applicators)
>   *Prefilled vag applicator:* 5 g (3/pck)

▶*clotrimazole* **(B)**
>   *Pediatric:* not recommended
>   **Gyne-Lotrimin®Vaginal Cream (OTC)** 1 applicatorful q HS x 7-14 days
>   *Vag crm:* 1% (45 g w. applicator)
>   **Gyne-Lotrimin® Vaginal Suppository (OTC)** 1 supp q HS x 7 days
>   *Vag supp:* 100 mg (7/pck)
>   **Gyne-Lotrimin®3 Vaginal Suppository (OTC)** 1 supp q HS x 3 days
>   *Vag supp:* 200 mg (3/pck)
>   **Gyne-Lotrimin®Combination Pack (OTC)** 1 vaginal supp q HS x 7 days; apply cream prn to vulval area

Candidiasis: Vulvovaginal

Combination pck: 7-100 mg supp <u>with</u> 7 g 1% cream
Gyne-Lotrimin®3 Combination Pack (OTC) 1 vaginal supp q HS x 3 days; apply cream to vulval area prn
Combination pck: 200 mg supp (7/pck) <u>plus</u> 1% cream (7 g)
Mycelex®-G Vaginal Cream 1 applicatorful q HS x 7-14 days
Vag crm: 1% (45, 90 g w. applicator)
Mycelex®-G Vaginal Tab 1 at HS x 1 dose
Tab: 500 mg (1/pck)
Mycelex®Twin Pack 1 vaginal tablet at HS x 1 dose; apply cream to vulval area bid x 7 days
Twin pck: 500 mg tab (7/pck) <u>with</u> 1% crm (7 g)
Mycelex®-7 Vaginal Cream (OTC) 1 applicatorful q HS x 7 days
Vag crm: 1% (45 g w. applicator)
Mycelex®-7 Vaginal Inserts (OTC) 1 insert q HS x 7 days
Vag insert: 100 mg insert (7/pck)
Mycelex®-7 Combination Pack (OTC) 1 vaginal insert q HS x 7 days; apply cream to vulval area daily-bid as needed for up to 7 days
Combination pck: 100 mg inserts (7/pck) <u>plus</u> 1% crm (7 g)

▶*miconazole* **(B)**
Pediatric: not recommended
Monistat® -3 Combination Pack (OTC) 1 vaginal supp q HS x 3 days; cream apply bid prn for up to 7 days
Combination pck: 200 mg supp (3/pck) <u>plus</u> 2% crm (9 g)
Monistat®-7 Combination Pack (OTC) 1 vaginal supp q HS x 7 days; apply cream bid prn for up to 7 days
Combination pck: 100 mg supp (7/pck) <u>plus</u> 2% crm (9 g)
Monistat®-7 Vaginal Cream (OTC) 1 applicatorful q HS x 7 days
Vag crm: 2% (45 g w. applicator)
Monistat®-7 Vaginal Suppositories (OTC) 1 supp q HS x 7 days
Vag supp: 100 mg supp (7/pck)
Monistat®-3 Vaginal Suppositories (OTC) 1 supp q HS x 3 days
Vag supp: 200 mg supp (3/pck)

▶*nystatin* **(C)**
Mycostatin® 1 vaginal tablet daily x 14 days
Vag tab: 100,000 U (1/pck)

▶*terconazole* **(C)**
Pediatric: not recommended
Terazol®-3 Vaginal Cream 1 applicatorful q HS x 3 days
Vag crm: 0.8% (20 g w. applicator)
Terazol®-3 Vaginal Suppositories 1 supp q HS x 3 days

Candidiasis: Vulvovaginal

>   *Vag supp:* 80 mg supp (3/pck)
>   **Terazol®-7 Vaginal Cream** 1 applicatorful q HS x 7 days
>   *Vag crm:* 0.4% (45 g w. applicator)

▶ *tioconazole*
>   *Pediatric:* not recommended
>   **1-Day® (OTC)** 1 applicatorful at HS x 1 dose
>   *Vag oint:* 6.5% (prefilled applicator x 1)
>   **Monistat®1 Vaginal Ointment (OTC)** 1 applicatorful at HS x 1 dose
>   *Vag oint:* 6.5% (Prefilled applicator x 1)
>   **Vagistat®-1 Vaginal Ointment (OTC)** 1 applicatorful q HS x 1 dose
>   *Vag oint:* 6.5% (prefilled applicator x 1)

Vaginal Sulfonamide

▶ *sulfanilamide* **(C)(G)** one full applicator or 1 suppository intravaginally daily-bid for up to 30 days
>   *Pediatric:* not recommended
>   **AVC®** *Vag crm:* 15% (4 oz tube w. applicator); *Vag supp:* 1.05 g

Oral Anti-fungal

▶ *fluconazole* **(C)** 150 mg x 1 dose
>   *Pediatric:* not recommended
>   **Diflucan®** *Tab:* 50, 100, 150, 200 mg; *Oral susp:* 10, 40 mg/ml (35 ml; orange)

Comment: For recurrent episodes (4 or more per year), initiate an intensive regimen with vaginal anti-fungal preparation q HS x 10-14 days, then follow with a maintenance regimen for 6 months. Resistant cases may require sexual partner treatment.

Carpal Tunnel Syndrome (CTS)

NSAIDs *see **Pain** page 305*
Oral Non-narcotic Analgesics *see **Pain** page 308*
Oral Narcotic Analgesics *see **Pain** page 308*
Topical Analgesics *see **Pain** page 308*
Parenteral Glucocorticosteroids *see page 389*
Oral Glucocorticosteroids *see page 387*
Topical Anesthetics *see page 383*
Topical Anesthetics/Steroid Combination *see page 480*

Cat Scratch Fever (*Bartonella* Infection)

▶*erythromycin base* **(B)(G)** 500-1000 mg qid x 4 weeks
    Pediatric: see page 588 for dose by weight
        <45 kg: 30-50 mg in 2-4 doses x 4 weeks
        >45 kg: same as adult
  E-mycin® *Tab:* 250, 333 mg ent-coat
  Eryc® *Cap:* 250 mg ent-coat pellets
  Ery-Tab® *Tab:* 250, 333, 500 mg ent-coat
  PCE® *Tab:* 333, 500 mg

▶*doxycycline* **(D)(G)** 100 mg daily-bid
    Pediatric: see page 587 for dose by weight
        <8 years: not recommended
        >8 years, <100 lb: 2 mg/lb on first day in 2 doses,
        followed by 1 mg/lb/day in 1-2 doses
        >8 years, >100 lb: same as adult
  Adoxa® *Tab:* 50, 100 mg ent-coat
  Doryx® *Cap:* 100 mg
  Monodox® *Cap:* 50, 100 mg
  Vibramycin® *Cap:* 50, 100 mg; *Syr:* 50 mg/5 ml (raspberry-apple, sulfites); *Oral susp:* 25 mg/5 ml (raspberry)
  Vibra-Tab® *Tab:* 100 mg film-coat

▶*trimethoprim/sulfamethoxazole* **(C)(G)** bid x 10 days
    Pediatric: see page 597 for dose by weight
        <2 months: not recommended
        >2 months: 40 mg/kg/day of *sulfamethoxazole*
        in 2 doses bid x 10 days
  Bactrim®, Septra® 2 tabs bid x 10 days
    Tab: trim 80 mg/*sulfa* 400 mg*
  Bactrim®DS, Septra®DS 1 tab bid x 10 days
    Tab: trim 160 mg/*sulfa* 800 mg*
  Bactrim®Pediatric Suspension, Septra®Pediatric Suspension 20 ml bid x 10 days
    Oral susp: trim 40 mg/*sulfa* 200 mg per 5 ml (100 ml; cherry, alcohol 0.3%)

Comment: Trimethoprim/sulfamethoxazole is not recommended in pregnancy or lactation.

Cellulitis

Comment: Duration of treatment should be 10-30 days. Obtain culture from site. Consider blood cultures.

▶ *amoxicillin* **(B)(G)** 500-875 mg bid or 250-500 mg tid x 10 days
> *Pediatric: see page 569 for dose by weight*
>> <40 kg (88 lb): 20-40 mg/kg/day in 3 doses x 10 days or 25-45 mg/kg/day in 2 doses x 10 days
>> >40 kg: same as adult

> **Amoxil®** *Cap:* 250, 500 mg; *Tab:* 875*mg; *Chew tab:* 125, 200, 250, 400 mg (cherry-banana-peppermint, phenylalanine); *Oral susp:* 125, 250 mg/5 ml (80, 100, 150 ml; strawberry); 200, 400 mg/5 ml (50, 75, 100 ml; bubble gum); *Oral drops:* 50 mg/ml (30 ml; bubble gum)

> **Trimox®** *Cap:* 250, 500 mg; *Oral susp:* 125 mg/5 ml, 250 mg/5 ml (80, 100, 150 ml; raspberry-strawberry)

▶ *amoxicillin/clavulanate* **(B)(G)** 500 mg tid or 875 mg bid x 10 days
> *Pediatric: see pages 571-572 for dose by weight*
>> 40-45 mg/kg/day divided tid x 10 days or
>> 90 mg/kg/day divided bid x 10 days

> **Augmentin®** *Tab:* 250, 500, 875 mg; *Chew tab:* 125, 250 mg (lemon-lime), 200, 400 mg (cherry-banana, phenylalanine); *Oral susp:* 125 mg/5 ml (banana), 250 mg/5 ml (orange) (75, 100, 150 ml); 200, 400 mg/5 ml (50, 75, 100 ml; orange-raspberry, phenylalanine)

> **Augmentin®ES-600** *Oral susp:* 600 mg/5 ml (50, 75, 100, 150 ml; orange-raspberry, phenylalanine)

> **Augmentin®XR** 2 tabs q 12 hours x 10 days
>> *Pediatric:* <16 years: use other forms
>> *Tab:* 1000 mg ext-rel

▶ *azithromycin* **(B)** 500 mg x 1 dose on day 1, then 250 mg daily on days 2-5 or 500 mg daily x 3 days or 2 g in a single dose
> *Pediatric: see page 573 for dose by weight*
>> 12 mg/kg/day x 5 days; max 500 mg/day

> **Zithromax®** *Tab:* 250, 500 mg; *Oral susp:* 100 mg/5 ml (15 ml); 200 mg/5 ml (15, 22.5, 30 ml) (cherry-vanilla-banana); *Pkt:* 1 g for reconstitution (cherry-banana)

> **Zithromax®Tri-pak** *Tab:* 3-500 mg tabs/pck

> **Zithromax®Z-pak** *Tab:* 6-250 mg tabs/pck

> **Zmax®** *Oral susp:* 2 g ext rel (cherry-banana)

Cellulitis

▶*cefaclor* **(B)(G)**
    Ceclor® 250 mg tid x 7 days
        Pediatric: see page 575 for dose by weight
            20-40 mg/kg/day in 3 doses x 10 days
        Pulvule: 250, 500 mg; *Oral susp:* 125, 250 mg/5 ml (75, 150 ml); 187, 375 mg/5 ml (50, 100 ml) (strawberry)
    Ceclor®**CD** 500 mg q 12 hours x 7 days
        Pediatric: <16 years: not recommended
        Tab: 375, 500 mg ext-rel
    Ceclor®**CDpak** 500 mg q 12 hours x 7 days
        Pediatric: <16 years: not recommended
        Tab: 500 mg (14 tabs/CDpak)
    Raniclor® 500 mg q 12 hours x 7 days
        Pediatric: 20-40 mg/kg/day in 3 doses x 10 days
        Chew tab: 125, 187, 250, 375 mg
▶*cefpodoxime proxetil* **(B)** 400 mg bid x 7-14 days
        Pediatric: see page 578 for dose by weight
            <2 months: not recommended
            2 months-12 years: 10 mg/kg/day (max 400 mg/dose) or 5 mg/kg/day bid (max 200 mg/dose) x 7-14 days
    Vantin® *Tab:* 100, 200 mg; *Oral susp:* 50, 100 mg/5 ml (50, 75, 100 mg; lemon-creme)
▶*ceftriaxone* **(B)** 1-2 g daily IM; max 4 g
        Pediatric: 50-75 mg/kg IM in 1-2 doses; max 2 g/day
    Rocephin® *Vial:* 250, 500 mg; 1, 2 g
▶*cefuroxime axetil* **(B)(G)** 250-500 mg bid x 10 days
        Pediatric: Pediatric: see page 581 for dose by weight
            <3 months: not recommended
            >3 months: 30 mg/kg/day in 2 doses x 10 days
    Ceftin® *Tab:* 125, 250, 500 mg; *Oral susp:* 125, 250 mg/5 ml (50, 100 ml; tutti-frutti)
▶*cephalexin* **(B)(G)** 500 mg bid x 10 days
        Pediatric: see page 582 for dose by weight
            25-50 mg/kg/day in 4 doses x 10 days
    Keflex® *Cap:* 250, 500, 750 mg; *Oral susp:* 125, 250 mg/5 ml (100, 200 ml)
    Keftab® *Tab:* 500 mg
    Keftab®**K-pak** *Tab:* 20-500 mg tabs/K-pak
▶*clarithromycin* **(C)** 500 mg q 12 hours or 500 mg ext-rel daily x 10 days

Cellulitis

> *Pediatric: see page 584 for dose by weight*
> > <6 months: not recommended
> > >6 months: 7.5 mg/kg bid x 10 days

Biaxin® *Tab:* 250, 500 mg

Biaxin®**Oral Suspension** *Oral susp:* 125, 250 mg/5 ml (50, 100 ml; fruit-punch)

Biaxin®**XL** *Tab:* 500 mg ext-rel

▶ *dicloxacillin* **(B)(G)** 500 mg q 6 hours x 10 days
> *Pediatric: see page 586 for dose by weight*
> > 12.5-25 mg/kg/day in 4 doses x 10 days

Dynapen® *Cap:* 125, 250, 500 mg; *Oral susp:* 62.5 mg/5 ml (80, 100, 200 ml)

▶ *dirithromycin* **(C)** 500 mg daily x 5-7 days
> *Pediatric:* <12 years: not recommended

Dynabac® *Tab:* 250 mg

▶ *erythromycin base* **(B)(G)** 250 mg qid, or 333 mg tid, or 500 mg bid x 7-10 days, then taper to lowest effective dose
> *Pediatric: see page 588 for dose by weight*
> > <45 kg: 30-50 mg in 2-4 doses x 7-10 days
> > >45 kg: same as adult

E-mycin® *Tab:* 250, 333 mg ent-coat
Eryc® *Cap:* 250 mg ent-coat pellets
Ery-Tab® *Tab:* 250, 333, 500 mg ent-coat
PCE® *Tab:* 333, 500 mg

▶ *loracarbef* **(B)** 200 mg bid x 10 days
> *Pediatric: see page 593 for dose by weight*
> > 15 mg/kg/day in 2 doses x 10 days

Lorabid® *Pulvule:* 200, 400 mg; *Oral susp:* 100 mg/5 ml (50, 100 ml); 200 mg/5 ml (50, 75, 100 ml) (strawberry bubble gum)

▶ *trovafloxacin* **(C)** 100 mg x 7-10 days
> *Pediatric:* <18 years: not recommended

Trovan® *Tab:* 100, 200 mg

Comment: Trovafloxacin is indicated only for life- or limb-threatening infection.

Cerumen Impaction

Ceruminolytics

▶ *triethanolamine* **(NR)(G)**

Cerumenex® fill ear canal and insert cotton plug for 15-30 minutes before irrigating with warm water

Soln: 10% (6, 12 ml)
▶ *carbamide peroxide*
Debrox® (OTC) instill 5-10 drops in ear canal; keep drops in ear several minutes; then irrigate with warm water; repeat bid for up to 4 days
Soln: 15, 30 ml squeeze bottles w. applicator

Chancroid

▶ *azithromycin* **(B)** 1 g x 1 dose
Pediatric: see page 573 for dose by weight
>45 kg: 1 g x 1 dose
Zithromax® *Tab:* 250, 500 mg; *Oral susp:* 100 mg/5 ml (15 ml); 200 mg/5 ml (15, 22.5, 30 ml) (cherry-vanilla-banana); *Pkt:* 1 g for reconstitution (cherry-banana)
▶ *ceftriaxone* **(B)** 250 mg IM x 1 dose
Pediatric: <45 kg: 125 mg IM x 1 dose
>45 kg: same as adult
Rocephin® *Vial:* 250, 500 mg; 1, 2 g
▶ *ciprofloxacin* **(C)** 500 mg bid x 3 days
Pediatric: <18 years: not recommended
Cipro® *Tab:* 100, 250, 500, 750 mg; *Oral susp:* 250 mg/5 ml (100 ml; strawberry)
▶ *erythromycin base* **(B)(G)** 500 mg qid x 7 days
E-mycin® *Tab:* 250, 333 mg ent-coat
Eryc® *Cap:* 250 mg ent-coat pellets
Ery-Tab® *Tab:* 250, 333, 500 mg ent-coat
PCE® *Tab:* 333, 500 mg

Chickenpox (*Varicella*)

Prophylaxis
▶ *Varicella virus* vaccine, live, attenuated **(C)**
Varivax® 0.5 ml SC; repeat 4-8 weeks later
Pediatric: <12 months: not recommended
12 months-12 years: 1 dose of 0.5 ml SC
Vial: 1350 PFU/0.5 ml single-dose w. diluent (preservative-free)
Comment: Administer SC in the deltoid for adult and children.

Chickenpox

Treatment
Antipyretics
see Fever page 168
Antivirals
▶*acyclovir* **(B)(G)** 800 mg qid x 5 days
    Pediatric: see page 568 for dose by weight
        <2 years: not recommended
        >2 years, <40 kg: 20 mg/kg qid x 5 days
        >2 years, >40 kg: 800 mg qid x 5 days
  Zovirax® *Cap:* 200 mg; *Tab:* 400, 800 mg
  Zovirax®Oral Suspension *Oral susp:* 200 mg/5 ml (banana)

Chlamydia Trachomatis

Comment: Empiric treatment requires concomitant treatment of gonorrhea. Treat all sexual contacts

Primary Therapy
▶*amoxicillin* **(B)(G)** 500-875 mg bid or 250-500 mg tid x 7 days
    Pediatric: see page 569 for dose by weight
        <40 kg (88 lb): 20-40 mg/kg/day in 3 doses x 7 days
        or 25-45 mg/kg/day in 2 doses x 7 days
        >40 kg: same as adult
  Amoxil® *Cap:* 250, 500 mg; *Tab:* 875*mg; *Chew tab:* 125, 200, 250, 400 mg (cherry-banana-peppermint, phenylalanine); *Oral susp:* 125, 250 mg/5 ml (80, 100, 150 ml; strawberry); 200, 400 mg/5 ml (50, 75, 100 ml; bubble gum); *Oral drops:* 50 mg/ml (30 ml; bubble gum)
  Trimox® *Cap:* 250, 500 mg; *Oral susp:* 125, 250 mg/5 ml (80, 100, 150 ml; raspberry-strawberry)
▶*azithromycin* **(B)** 1 g x 1 dose
    Pediatric: see page 573 for dose by weight
        <45 kg: not recommended
        >45 kg: 1 g x 1 dose
  Zithromax® *Tab:* 250, 500 mg; *Oral susp:* 100 mg/5 ml (15 ml); 200 mg/5 ml (15, 22.5, 30 ml) (cherry-vanilla-banana); *Pkt:* 1 g for reconstitution (cherry-banana)
▶*doxycycline* **(D)(G)** 100 mg daily-bid
    Pediatric: <8 years: not recommended
        >8 years, <100 lb: 2 mg/lb on first day in 2 doses, followed by 1 mg/lb/day in 1-2 doses

Chlamydia Trachomatis

>8 years, >100 lb: same as adult

Adoxa® *Tab:* 50, 100 mg ent-coat
Doryx® *Cap:* 100 mg
Monodox® *Cap:* 50, 100 mg
Vibramycin® *Cap:* 50, 100 mg; *Syr:* 50 mg/5 ml (raspberry-apple, sulfites); *Oral susp:* 25 mg/5 ml (raspberry)
Vibra-Tab® *Tab:* 100 mg film-coat

Alternative Therapy

▶*erythromycin base* **(B)(G)** 500 mg qid x 14 days
        Pediatric: see page 588 for dose by weight
            <45 kg: 50 mg/kg/day in 4 doses x 14 days
            >45 kg: same as adult

E-mycin® *Tab:* 250, 333 mg ent-coat
Eryc® *Cap:* 250 mg ent-coat pellets
Ery-Tab® *Tab:* 250, 333, 500 mg ent-coat
PCE® *Tab:* 333, 500 mg

▶*erythromycin ethylsuccinate* **(B)(G)** 800 mg po qid x 7 days
        Pediatric: see page 589 for dose by weight
            30-50 mg/kg/day in 4 divided doses x 7 days; may double dose with severe infection; max 100 mg/kg/day

Ery-Ped® *Oral susp:* 200 mg/5 ml (100, 200 ml; fruit); 400 mg/5 ml (60, 100, 200 ml; banana); *Oral drops:* 200, 400 mg/5 ml (50 ml; fruit); *Chew tab:* 200 mg wafer (fruit)
E.E.S.® *Oral susp:* 200, 400 mg/5 ml (100 ml; fruit)
E.E.S.®Granules *Oral susp:* 200 mg/5 ml (100, 200 ml; cherry,
E.E.S.®400 Tablets *Tab:* 400 mg

▶*erythromycin* estolate **(B)(G)** 500 mg qid x 7 days or 250 mg qid x 14 days
        Pediatric: see page 588 for dose by weight
            20 mg/kg q 6 hours x 14 days

Ilosone® *Pulvule:* 250 mg; *Tab:* 500 mg; *Liq:* 125, 250 mg/5 ml; 100 ml)

▶*ofloxacin* **(C)** 300 mg bid x 7 days
        Pediatric: <18 years: not recommended
Floxin® *Tab:* 200, 300, 400 mg

▶*tetracycline* **(D)(G)** 500 mg qid x 7 days
        Pediatric: Pediatric: see page 595 for dose by weight
            <8 years: not recommended
            >8 years, <100 lb: 25-50 mg/kg/day in 2-4 doses

Chlamydia Trachomatis

        x 7 days
        >8 years, >100 lb: same as adult
Achromycin®V *Cap:* 250, 500 mg
Sumycin® *Tab:* 250, 500 mg; *Cap:* 250, 500 mg; *Oral susp:* 125 mg/5 ml (100, 200 ml; fruit, sulfites)

Comment: Tetracycline is contraindicated in pregnancy (discolors fetal tooth enamel).

Cholelithiasis

▶*ursodiol* **(B)** 8-10 mg/kg/day in 2 or 3 divided doses
    Pediatric: not recommended
Actigall® *Cap:* 300 mg

Comment: **Actigall®** is indicated for the dissolution of radiolucent, non-calciferous, gallstones <20 mm in diameter and for prevention of gall stones during rapid weight loss.

Cholera

▶*tetracycline* **(D)(G)** 250-500 mg qid x 7 days
    Pediatric: see page 595 for dose by weight
        <8 years: not recommended
        >8 years, <100 lb: 25-50 mg/kg/day in 2-4 doses x 7 days
        >8 years, >100 lb: same as adult
Achromycin®V *Cap:* 250, 500 mg
Sumycin® *Tab:* 250, 500 mg; *Cap:* 250, 500 mg; *Oral susp:* 125 mg/5 ml (100, 200 ml; fruit, sulfites)

Comment: Tetracycline is contraindicated in pregnancy (discolors fetal tooth enamel).

Colic: Infantile

▶*dicyclomine* **(B)**
    Pediatric: <6 months: not recommended
        6 months-2 years: 5-10 mg tid-qid
Antispas® *Liq:* 10 mg/5 ml (118, 473, 946 ml)
▶*hyoscyamine* **(C)(G)**
Levsin®Drops

Pediatric: 3.4 kg: 4 drops q 4 hours prn; max 24 drops/day
5 kg: 5 drops q 4 hours prn; max 30 drops/day
7 kg: 6 drops q 4 hours prn; max 36 drops/day
10 kg: 8 drops q 4 hours prn; max 40 drops/day
Oral drops: 0.125 mg/ml (15 ml; orange, alcohol 5%)

Levsin®Elixir
Pediatric: <10 kg: use drops
10-19 kg: 1.25 ml q 4 hours prn
20-39 kg: 2.5 ml q 4 hours prn
40-49 kg: 3.75 ml q 4 hours prn
>50 kg: 5 ml q 4 hours prn
Elix: 0.125 mg/5 ml (orange, alcohol 20%)

▶*simethicone* **(C)** 0.3 ml qid pc and HS
Mylicon®Drops (OTC)
Oral drops: 40 mg/0.6 ml (30 ml)

Common Cold

Oral Drugs for the Treatment of Common Respiratory Symptoms
see page 523

Nasal Saline Drops/Sprays
Comment: Homemade saline nose drops: 1/4 tsp salt added to 8 oz boiled water, then cool water.

▶*saline* nasal spray **(G)**
Afrin®Saline Mist w/Eucalyptol and Menthol (OTC) 2-6 sprays in each nostril prn
Pediatric: 1 month-2 years: 1-2 sprays in each nostril prn
2-12 years: 1-4 sprays in each nostril prn
Squeeze bottle: 45 ml

Afrin® Moisturizing Saline Mist (OTC) 2-6 sprays in each nostril prn
Pediatric: 1 month-2 years: 1-2 sprays in each nostril prn
2-12 years: 1-4 sprays in each nostril prn
Squeeze bottle: 45 ml

Ocean Mist® (OTC) 2-6 sprays in each nostril prn
Pediatric: same as adult
Squeeze bottle: saline 0.65% (45 ml; alcohol-free)

Pediamist® (OTC) 2-6 sprays in each nostril prn
Pediatric: 1 month-2 years: 1-2 sprays in each nostril prn
2-12 years: 1-4 sprays in each nostril prn

Squeeze bottle: saline 0.5% (15 ml; alcohol-free)

Nasal Sympathomimetics

▶*oxymetazoline* **(C) (OTC)**

12-hour formulation: 2-3 drops or sprays in each nostril q 10-12 hours prn; max 2 doses/day
> *Pediatric:* <6 years: not recommended
> >6 years: same as adult

4-hour formulation: 2-3 drops or sprays q 4 hours prn
> *Pediatric:* not recommended

Afrin®12-Hour Extra Moisturizing Nasal Spray
Afrin®12-Hour Nasal spray Pump Mist
Afrin®12-Hour Original Nasal spray
Afrin®12-Hour Original Nose Drops
Afrin®12-Hour Severe Congestion Nasal Spray
Afrin®12-Hour Sinus Nasal Spray
Nasal spray: 0.05% (45 ml); *Nasal drops:* 0.05% (45 ml)

Afrin®4-Hour Nasal Spray
Neo-Synephrine®12 Hour Nasal Spray
Neo-Synephrine®12 Hour Extra Moisturizing Nasal Spray
Nasal spray: 0.05% (15 ml)

▶*phenylephrine* **(C)**

Afrin®Allergy Nasal Spray (OTC) 2-3 sprays in each nostril q 4 hours prn
> *Pediatric:* <12 years: not recommended
> *Nasal spray:* 0.5% (15 ml)

Afrin®Nasal Decongestant Children's Pump Mist (OTC)
> *Pediatric:* <6 years: not recommended
> >6 years: 2-3 sprays in each nostril q 4 hours prn
> *Nasal spray:* 0.25% (15 ml)

Neo-Synephrine®Extra Strength (OTC) 2-3 sprays or drops in each nostril q 4 hours prn
> *Pediatric:* <12 years: not recommended
> *Nasal spray:* 0.1% (15 ml); *Nasal drops:* 0.1% (15 ml)

Neo-Synephrine®Mild Formula (OTC) 2-3 sprays or drops in each nostril q 4 hours prn
> *Pediatric:* <6 years: not recommended
> >6 years: same as adult
> *Nasal spray:* 0.25% (15 ml)

Neo-Synephrine®Regular Strength (OTC) 2-3 sprays or drops in each nostril q 4 hours prn
> *Pediatric:* <12 years: not recommended

Nasal spray: 0.5% (15 ml); *Nasal drops:* 0.5% (15 ml)
- ▶*tetrahydrozoline* **(C)**
  Tyzine® 2-4 drops or 3-4 sprays in each nostril q 3-8 hours prn
  Pediatric: <6 years: not recommended
  >6 years: same as adult
  Nasal spray: 0.1% (15 ml); *Nasal drops:* 0.1% (30 ml)
  Tyzine®Pediatric Nasal Drops 2-3 sprays or drops in each nostril q 3-6 hours prn
  Nasal drops: 0.05% (15 ml)

Congestive Heart Failure (CHF)

ACE Inhibitors
- ▶*captopril* **(C; D in 2nd, 3rd)(G)** initially 25 mg tid; after 1-2 weeks may increase to 50 mg tid; max 450 mg/day
  Pediatric: not recommended
  Capoten® *Tab:* 12.5*, 25*, 50*, 100*mg
- ▶*enalapril* **(C; D in 2nd, 3rd)** initially 5 mg daily; usual dosage range 10-40 mg/day; max 40 mg/day
  Pediatric: not recommended
  Vasotec® *Tab:* 2.5*, 5*, 10, 20 mg
- ▶*fosinopril* **(C; D in 2nd, 3rd)** initially 10 mg daily, usual maintenance 20-40 mg/day in 1 or more doses
  Pediatric: <6 years, <50 kg: not recommended
  6-12 years, >50 kg: 5-10 mg daily
  Monopril® *Tab:* 10*, 20, 40 mg
- ▶*lisinopril* **(C; D in 2nd, 3rd)** initially 5 mg daily
  Pediatric: not recommended
  Prinivil® *Tab:* 2.5, 5*, 10, 20, 40 mg
  Zestril® *Tab:* 2.5, 5, 10, 20, 40 mg
- ▶*quinapril* **(C; D in 2nd, 3rd)** initially 5 mg bid; increase weekly to 10-20 mg bid
  Pediatric: not recommended
  Accupril® *Tab:* 5*, 10, 20, 40 mg
- ▶*ramipril* **(C; D in 2nd, 3rd)** initially 2.5 mg bid; usual maintenance 5 mg bid
  Pediatric: not recommended
  Altace® *Cap:* 1.25, 2.5, 5, 10 mg
- ▶*trandolapril* **(C; D in 2nd, 3rd)** initially 1 mg daily; titrate to dose of 4 mg daily as tolerated

Congestive Heart Failure

    Pediatric: not recommended
  Mavik® *Tab:* 1*, 2, 4 mg
Beta-Blocker, Cardioselective
▶*metoprolol* (C) initially 20-200 mg daily
    Pediatric: not recommended
  Toprol®-XL *Tab:* 25*, 50*, 100*, 200*mg ext-rel

Comment: **Toprol®-XL** is indicated for the treatment of stable, symptomatic, heart failure in patients already taking an ACE inhibitor, diuretic, and usually digitalis.

Diuretics
Thiazide Diuretics
▶*chlorthalidone* **(B)(G)** 12.5-200 mg daily
  Hygroton®, Hylidon®, Novothalidone® *Tab:* 12.5, 25 mg
  Thalitone® *Tab:* 15 mg
▶*chlorothiazide* **(C)(G)** 0.5-1 g/day in single or divided doses; max 2 g/day
    Pediatric: <6 months: up to 15 mg/lb/day in 2 doses
              >6 months: 10 mg/lb/day in 2 doses
  Diuril® *Tab:* 250*, 500*mg; *Oral susp:* 250 mg/5 ml (237 ml)
▶*hydrochlorothiazide* **(B)(G)**
    Pediatric: not recommended
  Esidrix® 25-100 mg daily
    Tab: 25, 50, 100 mg
  Hydrodiuril® initially 50-100 mg/day in single or divided doses; max 200 mg/day
    Tab: 25*, 50*mg
  Microzide® 12.5 mg daily; usual max 50 mg/day
    Cap: 12.5 mg
  Oretic® 25-50 mg bid; max 100 mg bid
    Tab: 25, 50 mg
▶*hydroflumethiazide* **(B)** 50-100 mg/day
    Pediatric: not recommended
  Diucardin® *Tab:* 50 mg
▶*methyclothiazide* **(B)** initially 2.5 mg daily; max 5 mg daily
    Pediatric: not recommended
  Enduron® *Tab:* 2.5, 5 mg
▶*polythiazide* **(C)** 2-4 mg daily
    Pediatric: not recommended
  Renese® *Tab:* 1, 2, 4 mg
Potassium-Sparing Diuretics
▶*amiloride* **(B)** initially 5 mg; may increase to 10 mg; max 20 mg

Congestive Heart Failure

    Pediatric: not recommended

  Midamor® *Tab:* 5 mg

▶ *spironolactone* **(D)(G)** initially 50-100 mg in 1 or more doses; titrate at 2 week intervals

    Pediatric: not recommended

  Aldactone® *Tab:* 25, 50*, 100*mg

▶ *triamterene* **(B)** 100 mg bid; max 300 mg

  Dyrenium®

    Pediatric: not recommended

    Cap: 50, 100 mg

Loop Diuretics

▶ *bumetanide* **(C)(G)** 0.5-2 mg daily; may repeat at 4-5 hour intervals; max 10 mg/day

    Pediatric: <18 years: not recommended

  Bumex® *Tab:* 0.5*, 1*, 2*mg

▶ *ethacrynic acid* **(B)** initially 50-200 mg/day

    Pediatric: infants: not recommended

              >1 month: initially 25 mg/day; then adjust dose in 25 mg increments

  Edecrin® *Tab:* 25, 50 mg

▶ *furosemide* **(C)(G)** initially 40 mg bid

    Pediatric: not recommended

  Lasix® *Tab:* 20, 40*, 80 mg; *Oral soln:* 10 mg/ml (2, 4 oz w. dropper)

Comment: Furosemide is contraindicated with sulfa drug allergy.

▶ *torsemide* **(B)** 5 mg daily; may increase to 10 mg daily

    Pediatric: not recommended

  Demadex® *Tab:* 5*, 10*, 20*, 100*mg

Other Diuretics

▶ *indapamide* **(B)** initially 1.25 mg daily; may titrate dosage upward q 4 weeks if needed; max 5 mg/day

  Lozol® *Tab:* 1.25, 2.5 mg

Comment: Indapamide is contraindicated with sulfa drug allergy.

▶ *metolazone* **(B)**

    Pediatric: not recommended

  Mykrox® initially 0.5 mg q AM; max 1 mg/day

    Tab: 0.5 mg

  Zaroxolyn® 2.5-5 mg daily

    Tab: 2.5, 5, 10 mg

Comment: Metolazone is contraindicated with sulfa drug allergy.

Diuretic Combinations

Congestive Heart Failure

▶ *amiloride/hydrochlorothiazide* **(B)(G)** initially 1 tab daily; may increase to 2 tabs/day in single or divided doses
> *Pediatric:* not recommended

Moduretic® *Tab: amil* 5 mg/*hydro* 50 mg*

▶ *spironolactone/hydrochlorothiazide* **(D)(G)**
> *Pediatric:* not recommended

Aldactazide®**25** usual maintenance 50-100 mg in 1 or more doses
Tab: spiro 25 mg/*hydro* 25 mg

Aldactazide®**50** usual maintenance 50-100 mg each in 1 or more doses
Tab: spiro 50 mg/*hydro* 50 mg

▶ *triamterene/hydrochlorothiazide* **(C)(G)**
> *Pediatric:* not recommended

Dyazide® 1-2 caps daily
Cap: triam 37.5 mg/*hydro* 25 mg

Maxzide® 1 tab daily
Tab: triam 75 mg/*hydro* 50 mg*

Maxzide®**-25** 1-2 daily
Tab: triam 37.5 mg/*hydro* 25 mg*

Nitrate/Direct Vasodilator Combination

▶ *isosorbide dinitrate/hydralazine* **(C)** initially 1 tab tid; may reduce to 1/2 tab tid if not tolerated; titrate as tolerated after 3-5 days; max 2 tabs tid
> *Pediatric:* not recommended

BiDil® *Tab: isosor* 20 mg/*hydral* 37.5 mg

Comment: **BiDil**® is an adjunct to standard therapy in self-identified black persons to improve survival, to prolong time to hospitalization for heat failure, and to improve patient-reported functional status.

Cardiac Glycosides

Comment: Therapeutic serum level of *digoxin* is 0.8-2 mcg/ml.

▶ *digoxin* **(C)(G)** 1-1.5 mg IM, IV, or po in divided doses over 1-3 days as a loading dose; then 0.125-0.5 mg/day is usual maintenance
> *Pediatric:* <1 month: initially 25-35 mcg/kg/day, then 20-30% of digitalizing dose
> 1-24 months: initially 35-60 mcg/kg/day, then 20-30% of digitalizing dose
> 2-5 years: initially 30-40 mcg/kg/day, then 25-35% of digitalizing dose
> 5-10 years: initially 20-35 mcg/kg/day, then 25-35% of digitalizing dose
> >10 years: initially 10-15 mcg/kg/day, then 25-35%

of digitalizing dose

Lanoxicaps®
> *Pediatric:* <10 years: use elixir or parenteral form
> *Cap:* 0.05, 0.1, 0.2 mg soln-filled (alcohol)

Lanoxin®
> *Pediatric:* <10 years: use elixir or parenteral form
> *Tab:* 0.125*, 0.25*mg; *Elix:* 0.05 mg/ml (2 oz w. dropper; lime, alcohol 10%)

Lanoxin®Injection *Amp:* 0.25 mg/ml (2 ml)
Lanoxin®Injection Pediatric *Amp:* 0.1 mg/ml (1 ml)

Conjunctivitis: Allergic

Oral 1st Generation Antihistamines *see page 525*
Oral 2nd Generation Antihistamines *see page 527*
Ophthalmic Glucocorticosteroids
Comment: Concomitant contact lens wear is contraindicated during therapy. Ophthalmic steroids are contraindicated with ocular, fungal, mycobacterial, viral (except herpes zoster), and untreated bacterial infection. Ophthalmic steroids may mask or exacerbate infection, and may increase intraocular pressure, optic nerve damage, cataract formation, or corneal perforation.

▶*dexamethasone* **(C)** initially 1-2 drops hourly during the day and q 2 hours at night; then prolong dose interval to 4-6 hours as condition improves
> *Pediatric:* not recommended

Maxidex® *Ophth susp:* 0.1% (5, 15 ml; benzalkonium chloride)

▶*dexamethasone phosphate* **(C)** initially 1-2 drops hourly during the day and q 2 hours at night; then 1 drop q 4-8 hours or more as condition improves
> *Pediatric:* not recommended

Decadron® *Ophth soln:* 0.1% (5 ml; sulfites)

▶*fluorometholone* **(C)** 1 drop bid-qid or 1/2 inch of ointment daily-tid; may increase dose frequency during initial 24-48 hours
> *Pediatric:* <2 years: not recommended
> >2 years: same as adult

FML® *Ophth susp:* 0.1% (5, 10, 15 ml; benzalkonium chloride)
FML®Forte *Ophth susp:* 0.25% (5, 10, 15 ml; benzalkonium chloride)
FML®S.O.P. Ointment *Ophth oint:* 0.1% (3.5 g)

▶*fluorometholone acetate* **(C)** initially 2 drops q 2 hours during the first 24-48 hours; then 1-2 drops qid as condition improves

Conjunctivitis: Allergic

>*Pediatric:* not recommended

Flarex® *Ophth susp:* 0.1% (2.5, 5 10 ml; benzalkonium chloride)

▶ *loteprednol etabonate* **(C)**
>*Pediatric:* not recommended

Alrex® 1 drop qid
>*Ophth susp:* 0.2% (5, 10 ml; benzalkonium chloride)

Lotemax® 1-2 drops qid
>*Ophth susp:* 0.5% (5, 10, 15 ml; benzalkonium chloride)

▶ *medrysone* **(C)** 1 drop up to q 4 hours
>*Pediatric:* not recommended

HMS® *Ophth susp:* 1% (5, 10 ml; benzalkonium chloride)

▶ *rimexolone* **(C)** initially 1-2 drops hourly while awake x 1 week; then 1 drop q 2 hours while awake x 1 week; then taper as condition improves
>*Pediatric:* not recommended

Vexol® *Ophth susp:* 0.1% (5, 10 ml; benzalkonium chloride)

▶ *prednisolone acetate* **(C)**
>*Pediatric:* not recommended

Econopred® 2 drops qid
>*Ophth susp:* 0.125% (5, 10 ml)

Pred®Forte initially 2 drops hourly x 24-48 hours; then 1-2 drops bid-qid
>*Ophth susp:* 1% (1, 5, 10, 15 ml; benzalkonium chloride, sulfites)

Pred®Mild® initially 2 drops hourly x 24-48 hours; then 1-2 drops bid-qid
>*Ophth susp:* 0.12% (5, 10 ml; benzalkonium chloride)

▶ *prednisolone sodium phosphate* **(C)** initially 1-2 drops hourly during the day and q 2 hours at night; then 1 drop q 4 hours; then 1 drop tid-qid as condition improves
>*Pediatric:* not recommended

Inflamase®Forte *Ophth soln:* 1% (5, 10, 15 ml; benzalkonium chloride)

Inflamase®Mild® *Ophth soln:* 1/8% (5, 10 ml; benzalkonium chloride)

Ophthalmic H₁ Antagonists (Antihistamines)

Comment: May insert contact lens 10 minutes after administration.

▶ *emedastine* **(C)** 1 drop qid
>*Pediatric:* <3 years: not recommended
>>3 years: same as adult

Emadine® *Ophth soln:* 0.05% (5 ml; benzalkonium chloride)

Conjunctivitis: Allergic

▶ *epinastine* **(C)** 1 drop bid
    Pediatric: <3 years: not recommended
              >3 years: same as adult
  Elestat® *Ophth soln:* 0.05% (5 ml; benzalkonium chloride)

▶ *levocabastine* **(C)** 1 drop qid
    Pediatric: not recommended
  Livostin® *Ophth susp:* 0.05% (2.5, 5, 10 ml; benzalkonium chloride)

Ophthalmic Mast Cell Stabilizers
Comment: Concomitant contact lens wear is contraindicated during therapy.

▶ *cromolyn sodium* **(B)** 1-2 drops 4-6 times/day at regular intervals
    Pediatric: <4 years: not recommended
              >4 years: same as adult
  Crolom®, Opticrom® *Ophth soln:* 4% (10 ml; benzalkonium chloride)

▶ *lodoxamide tromethamine* **(B)** 1-2 drops qid up to 3 months
    Pediatric: <2 years: not recommended
              >2 years: same as adult
  Alomide® *Ophth soln:* 1% (10 ml)

▶ *nedocromil* **(B)** 1-2 drops bid
    Pediatric: <3 years: not recommended
              >3 years: same as adult
  Alocril® *Ophth soln:* 2% (5 ml; benzalkonium chloride)

▶ *pemirolast potassium* **(C)** 1-2 drops qid
    Pediatric: <3 years: not recommended
              >3 years: same as adult
  Alamast® *Ophth soln:* 0.1% (10 ml; lauralkonium chloride)

Ophthalmic Anti-histamine/Mast Cell Stabilizer Combinations

▶ *azelastine* **(C)** 1 drop bid
    Pediatric: <3 years: not recommended
              >3 years: same as adult
  Optivar® *Ophth soln:* 0.05% (6 ml; benzalkonium chloride)
Comment: May insert contact lens 10 minutes after administration.

▶ *ketotifen fumarate* **(C)** 1 drop q 8-12 hours
    Pediatric: <3 years: not recommended
              >3 years: 1 drop qid
  Zaditor® *Ophth soln:* 0.025% (5 ml; benzalkonium chloride)

▶ *olopatadine* **(C)** 1 drop bid
    Pediatric: <3 years: not recommended
              >3 years: same as adult
  Patanol® *Ophth soln:* 0.1% (5 ml; benzalkonium chloride)

Conjunctivitis: Allergic

Comment: May insert contact lens 10 minutes after administration.
Ophthalmic Vasoconstrictors
Comment: Concomitant contact lens wear is contraindicated during therapy.
▶*naphazoline* **(C)** 1-2 drops qid prn
    Pediatric: not recommended
  Vasocon-A® *Ophth soln:* 0.1% (15 ml; benzalkonium chloride)
▶*oxymetazoline* **(NR)(OTC)** 1-2 drops qid prn
    Pediatric: <6 years: not recommended
        >6 years: same as adult
  Visine®**L-R** *Ophth soln:* 0.025% (15, 30 ml)
▶*tetrahydrozoline* **(NR)(OTC)(G)** 1-2 drops qid prn
    Pediatric: <6 years: not recommended
        >6 years: same as adult
  Visine® *Ophth soln:* 0.05% (15, 22.5, 30 ml)

Ophthalmic Vasoconstrictor/Moisturizer Combination
Comment: Concomitant contact lens wear is contraindicated during therapy.
▶*tetrahydrozoline/polyethylene glycol 400/povidone/dextran 70* **(NR)(OTC)** 1-2 drops qid prn
    Pediatric: <6 years: not recommended
        >6 years: same as adult
  Advanced Relief Visine® *Ophth soln:* tetra 0.025%/poly 1%/pov 1%/dex 0.1% (15, 30 ml)

Ophthalmic Vasoconstrictor/Astringent Combination
Comment: Concomitant contact lens wear is contraindicated during therapy.
▶*tetrahydrozoline/zinc sulfate* **(NR)(OTC)** 1-2 drops qid prn
    Pediatric: <6 years: not recommended
        >6 years: same as adult
  Visine®**AC** *Ophth soln:* tetra 0.025%/zinc 0.05% (15, 30 ml)

Ophthalmic Vasoconstrictor/Anti-histamine Combinations
Comment: Concomitant contact lens wear is contraindicated during therapy.
▶*naphazoline/pheniramine* **(C)** 1-2 drops qid
    Pediatric: <6 years: not recommended
        >6 years: 1-2 drops qid
  Naphcon A® **(OTC)** *Ophth soln:* naph 0.025%/phen 0.3% (15 ml; benzalkonium chloride)
  Ocuhist® **(OTC)** *Ophth soln:* naph 0.025%/phen 0.3% (15 ml)

Ophthalmic NSAIDs
Comment: Concomitant contact lens wear is contraindicated during therapy.
▶*diclofenac* **(B)** 1 drop qid
    Pediatric: not recommended
  Voltaren®**Ophthalmic Solution** *Ophth soln:* 0.1% (2.5, 5 ml)

▶*ketorolac tromethamine* **(C)** 1 drop qid for up to 4 days
>   *Pediatric:* <3 years: not recommended
>   >3 years: same as adult

Acular® *Ophth soln:* 0.5% (3, 5, 10 ml; benzalkonium chloride)
Acular®LS *Ophth soln:* 0.4% (5 ml; benzalkonium chloride)
Acular®PF *Ophth soln:* 0.5% (0.4 ml; 12 single-use vials/box) (preservative-free)

Conjunctivitis/Blepharoconjunctivitis: Bacterial

Ophthalmic Anti-infectives

▶*chloramphenicol* ophthalmic ointment and drops **(C)** apply 1/2 inch to the lower conjunctival sac q 3 hours x 48 hours or 1-2 drops 4-6 times daily for the first 72 hours, then prolong the dose interval and continue for 48 hours after the eye appears normal

Chloroptic®Ophthalmic Ointment *Ophth oint:* 0.1% (3.5 g)
Chloroptic®Ophthalmic Drops *Ophth drops:* 0.5% (2.5, 7.5 ml)

Comment: Avoid prolonged continuous or intermittent use with *chloramphenicol*. The ophthalmic ointment may retard corneal healing. Should only be used if safer agents are unavailable or the infective organism is resistant. Associated with hematologic toxicity including bone marrow depression and aplastic anemia.

▶*ciprofloxacin* ophthalmic ointment **(C)** apply 1/2 inch to the lower conjunctival sac tid x 2 days, then bid x 5 days
>   *Pediatric:* <2 years: not recommended
>   >2 years: same as adult

Ciloxan®Ophthalmic Ointment *Ophth oint:* 0.3% (3.5 g)

▶*ciprofloxacin* ophthalmic solution **(C)** 1-2 drops q 2 hours while awake x 2 days, then q 4 hours while awake x 5 days
>   *Pediatric:* <1 year: not recommended
>   >1 year: same as adult

Ciloxan®Ophthalmic Solution *Ophth soln:* 0.3% (2.5, 5, 10 ml; benzalkonium chloride)

▶*erythromycin* ophthalmic ointment **(B)** apply 1/2 inch to the lower conjunctival sac up to 6 times/day
>   *Pediatric:* same as adult

E-mycin®Ophthalmic Ointment *Ophth oint:* 0.5%/g (3.5 g)
Ilotycin®Ophthalmic Ointment *Ophth oint:* 5 mg/g (1/8 oz)

▶*erythromycin* ophthalmic solution **(B)** initially 1-2 drops q 1-2 hours; then increase dose interval as condition improves
>   *Pediatric:* same as adult

Isopto Cetamide®Ophthalmic Solution *Ophth soln:* 15% (15 ml)

Conjunctivitis/Blepharoconjunctivitis

▶ *gatifloxacin* ophthalmic solution **(C)** initially 1 drop q 2 hours while awake; then up to 8 times/day for 2 days; then 1 drop up to qid while awake x 5 days
> *Pediatric:* <1 year: not recommended
> >1 year: same as adult

    Zymar®Ophthalmic Solution *Ophth soln:* 0.03% (2.5, 5 ml)

▶ *gentamicin sulfate* ophthalmic ointment **(C)** apply 1/2 inch to the lower conjunctival sac bid-tid
> *Pediatric:* same as adult

    Garamycin®Ophthalmic Ointment *Ophth oint:* 3 mg/g (3.5 g)
    Genoptic®Ophthalmic Ointment *Ophth oint:* 3 mg/g (3.5 g)
    Gentacidin®Ophthalmic Ointment *Ophth oint:* 3 mg/g (3.5 g)

▶ *gentamicin sulfate* ophthalmic solution **(C)** 2 drops q 4 hours x 7-14 days; max 2 drops q 1 h
> *Pediatric:* same as adult

    Garamycin®Ophthalmic Solution *Ophth soln:* 0.3% (5 ml; benzalkonium chloride)
    Genoptic®Ophthalmic Solution *Ophth soln:* 0.3% (3, 5 ml)
    Gentacidin®Ophthalmic Solution *Ophth soln:* 0.3% (3, 5 ml)

▶ *levofloxacin* ophthalmic solution **(C)** 1-2 drops q 2 hours while awake on days 1 and 2 (max 8 times/day); then 1-2 drops q 4 hours while awake on days 3 to 7; max 4 times/day
> *Pediatric:* <1 year: not recommended
> >1 year: same as adult

    Quixin®Ophthalmic Solution *Ophth soln:* 0.5% (2.5, 5 ml; benzalkonium chloride)

▶ *moxifloxacin* ophthalmic solution **(C)** 1 drop tid x 7 days
> *Pediatric:* <1 year: not recommended
> >1 year: same as adult

    Vigamox®Ophthalmic Solution *Ophth soln:* 0.5% (3 ml)

▶ *norfloxacin* ophthalmic drops **(C)** 1-2 drops qid x 7 days
> *Pediatric:* <1 year: not recommended
> >1 year: same as adult

    Chibroxin®Ophthalmic Drops *Ophth drops:* 0.3% (5 ml)

▶ *ofloxacin* ophthalmic solution **(C)** 1-2 drops q 2-4 hours x 2 days, then qid x 5 days
> *Pediatric:* <1 year: not recommended
> >1 year: same as adult

    Ocuflox®Ophthalmic Solution *Ophth soln:* 0.3% (5, 10 ml; benzalkonium chloride)

▶ *sulfacetamide* ophthalmic solution and ointment **(C)**

Bleph-10®Ophthalmic Solution 1-2 drops q 2-3 hours x 7-10 days
Pediatric: <2 months: not recommended
>2 months: 1-2 drops q 2-3 hours during the day x 7-10 days
Ophth soln: 10% (2.5, 5, 15 ml; benzalkonium chloride)

Bleph-10®Ophthalmic Ointment apply 1/2 inch to the lower conjunctival sac q 3-4 hours and HS x 7-10 days
Pediatric: <2 years: not recommended
>2 years: same as adult
Ophth oint: 10% (3.5 g; phenylmercuric acetate)

Cetapred®Ophthalmic Ointment apply 1/2 inch to the lower conjunctival sac qid and HS
Pediatric: <6 years: not recommended
>6 years: same as adult
Ophth oint: 10% (3.5 g)

Sulamyd®Ophthalmic Solution 1 drop of 30% soln or 1-2 drops of 10% soln q 2 hours
Pediatric: same as adult
Ophth soln: 10% (5, 15 ml); 30% (15 ml; parabens)

Sulamyd®Ophthalmic Ointment apply 1/2 inch to the lower conjunctival sac qid and HS
Pediatric: same as adult
Ophth oint: 10% (3.5 g; parabens)

▶ *tobramycin* **(B)**
Tobrex®Ophthalmic Solution 1-2 drops q 4 hours
Pediatric: same as adult
Ophth soln: 0.3% (5 ml; benzalkonium chloride)

Tobrex®Ophthalmic Ointment apply 1/2 inch to the lower conjunctival sac bid-tid
Pediatric: same as adult
Ophth oint: 0.3% (3.5 g; chlorobutanol)

Ophthalmic Anti-infective Combinations

▶ *polymixin B sulfate/bacitracin* ophthalmic ointment **(C)** apply 1/2 inch to the lower conjunctival sac q 3-4 hours x 7-10 days
Pediatric: same as adult
Polysporin®Ophthalmic Ointment *Ophth oint: poly B* 10,000 U/*bac* 500 U (3.75 g)

▶ *polymyxin B sulfate/bacitracin zinc/neomycin sulfate* ophthalmic ointment **(C)** apply 1/2 inch to the lower conjunctival sac q 3-4 hours x 7-10 days
Pediatric: same as adult

Conjunctivitis/Blepharoconjunctivitis

    Neosporin®Ophthalmic Ointment *Ophth oint: poly B* 10,000 U/*bac* 400 U/*neo* 3.5 mg/g (3.75 g)

▶*polymyxin B sulfate/gramicidin/neomycin* ophthalmic solution **(C)** 1-2 drops q 1 hour 2-3 times, then 1-2 drops bid-qid x 7-10 days
       Pediatric: not recommended
    Neosporin®Ophthalmic Solution *Ophth soln: poly B* 10,000 U/*gram* 0.025 mg/*neo* 1.7 mg/g (10 ml)

▶*trimethoprim*/polymyxin B sulfate ophthalmic solution **(C)** 1 drop q 3 hours x 7-10 days; max 6 doses/day
       Pediatric: <2 months: not recommended
                 >2 months: same as adult
    Polytrim® *Ophth soln: trim* 1 mg/*poly B* 10,000 U/ml (10 ml; benzalkonium chloride)

Ophthalmic Anti-infective/Steroid Combinations

Comment: Ophthalmic glucocorticosteroids are contraindicated after removal of a corneal foreign body, epithelial herpes simplex keratitis, *varicella*, other viral infections of the cornea or conjunctiva, fungal ocular infections, and mycobacterial ocular infections.

▶*gentamicin sulfate/prednisolone acetate* ophthalmic suspension **(C)**
       Pediatric: not recommended
    Pred-G®Ophthalmic Suspension 1 drop bid-qid; max 20 ml/therapeutic course
       Ophth susp: gent 3%/*pred* 1%/ml (2, 5, 10 ml; benzalkonium chloride)
    Pred-G®Ophthalmic Ointment apply 1/2 inch to the lower conjunctival sac daily-tid; max 8 g/therapeutic course
       Ophth oint: gent 0.3%/*pred* 0.6%/g (3.5 g)

▶*neomycin base/dexamethasone* ophthalmic solution and ointment **(C)**
       Pediatric: not recommended
    NeoDecadron®Ophthalmic Solution 1-2 drops hourly during the day and q 2 hours during the night; then 1 drop q 4 hours; then 1 drop tid-qid as condition improves; max 20 ml/therapeutic course
       Ophth soln: neo 0.35%/*dexa* 1 mg/ml (5 ml)
    NeoDecadron®Ophthalmic Ointment 1-2 drops hourly during the day and q 2 hours during the night; then 1 drop q 4 hours; then 1 drop tid-qid as condition improves; max 8 g/therapeutic course
       Ophth oint: neo base 0.35%/*dexa* 0.5 mg/g (3.5 g)

▶*neomycin sulfate/polymixin B sulfate/dexamethasone* ophthalmic suspension **(C)**

Conjunctivitis/Blepharoconjunctivitis

  Pediatric: not recommended
 Maxitrol®Ophthalmic Suspension 1-2 drops q 1 hour (severe infection) or 4-6 times/day (mild-moderate infection)
  Ophth susp: neo 0.35%/poly B 10,000 U/dexa 1%/ml (5 ml; benzalkonium chloride)
 Maxitrol®Ophthalmic Ointment apply 1/2 inch to the lower conjunctival sac q 1 hour (severe infection) or 4-6 times/day (mild-moderate infection)
  Ophth oint: neo 0.35%/poly B 10,000 U/dexa 1%/g (3.5 g)

▶*neomycin sulfate/polymixin B sulfate/prednisolone acetate* ophthalmic suspension **(NR)**
  Pediatric: same as adult
 Poly-Pred®Ophthalmic Suspension 1-2 drops q 3-4 hours or more often as necessary; max 20 ml/therapeutic course.
  Ophth susp: neo 0.35%/poly B 10,000 U/pred 0.5%/ml (5, 10 ml)

▶*polymixin B sulfate/neomycin sulfate/hydrocortisone* ophthalmic suspension **(C)**
  Pediatric: same as adult
 Cortisporin®Ophthalmic Suspension 1-2 drops tid-qid; more often if necessary; max 20 ml/therapeutic course
  Ophth susp: poly B 10,000 U/neo 0.35%/hydro 1%/ml (7.5 ml; thimerosal)

▶*polymixin B sulfate/neomycin sulfate/bacitracin zinc/ hydrocortisone* ophthalmic ointment **(C)**
  Pediatric: same as adult
 Cortisporin®Ophthalmic Ointment apply 1/2 inch to the lower conjunctival sac tid-qid; more often if necessary; max 8 g/ therapeutic course
  Ophth oint: poly B 10,000 U/neo 0.35%/bac 400 U/hydro 1%/ g (3.5 g)

▶*sulfacetamide sodium/fluorometalone* suspension **(C)** 1 drop qid; max 20 ml/therapeutic course
  Pediatric: not recommended
 FML-S® *Ophth susp: sulfa 10%/flouro 0.1%/ml (5, 10, 15 ml; benzalkonium chloride)*

▶*sulfacetamide sodium/prednisolone acetate* ophthalmic suspension and ointment **(C)**
  Pediatric: <6 years: not recommended
     >6 years: same as adult
 Blephamide®Liquifilm 2 drops qid and HS and 1-2 times during

Conjunctivitis/Blepharoconjunctivitis

the night
> *Ophth susp: sulfa* 10%/*pred* 0.2%/ml (2.5, 5, 10 ml; benzalkonium chloride)

Blephamide®S.O.P. Ophthalmic Ointment apply 1/2 inch to the lower conjunctival sac tid-qid and 1-2 times during the night
> *Ophth oint: sulfa* 10%/*pred* 0.2%/g (3.5 g; benzalkonium chloride)

Isopto-Cetapred® 2-3 drops q 1-2 hours during the day and at HS; may prolong dose interval as condition improves; max 20 ml/therapeutic course
> *Ophth susp: sulfa* 10%/*pred* 0.25%/ml (2.5, 5, 10 ml; benzalkonium chloride)

Metimyd®Ophthalmic Suspension 2-3 drops q 1-2 hours during the day and at HS; may prolong dose interval as condition improves; max 8 g/therapeutic course
> *Ophth susp: sulfa* 10%/*pred* 0.5% (5 ml)

Metimyd®Ophthalmic Ointment apply 1/2 inch to the lower conjunctival sac tid-qid and once at HS; max 8 g/therapeutic course
> *Ophth oint: sulfa* 10%/*pred* 0.5%/g (3.5 g)

▶ *sulfacetamide sodium/prednisolone acetate* ophthalmic ointment **(C)** apply 1/2 inch to the lower conjunctival sac tid-qid
> *Pediatric:* <6 years: not recommended
> >6 years: same as adult

Vasocidin®Ophthalmic Ointment *Ophth oint: sulfa* 10%/*pred* 0.5%/g (3.5 g)

▶ *sulfacetamide sodium/prednisolone sodium phosphate* ophthalmic solution **(C)** 2 drops q 4 hours
> *Pediatric:* <6 years: not recommended
> >6 years: same as adult

Vasocidin®Ophthalmic Solution *Ophth soln: sulfa* 10%/*pred* 0.25%/ml (5, 10 ml)

▶ *tobramycin/dexamethasone* ophthalmic solution and ointment **(C)**
> *Pediatric:* not recommended

TobraDex®Ophthalmic Solution 1-2 drops q 2-6 hours x 24-48 hours; then 4-6 hours; reduce frequency of dose as condition improves; max 20 ml per therapeutic course
> *Ophth susp: tobra* 0.3%/*dexa* 0.1%/ml (2.5, 5, 10 ml; benzalkonium chloride)

TobraDex®Ophthalmic Ointment apply 1/2 inch to the lower conjunctival sac up to tid-qid; may use at bedtime in conjunction

with daytime drops; max 8 g/therapeutic course
> *Ophth oint:* tobra 0.3%/dexa 0.1%/g (3.5 g; chlorobutanol chloride)

Ophthalmic Anti-infective/Vasoconstrictor Combination
▶*sulfacetamide sodium/phenylephrine* ophthalmic solution **(C)**
1-2 drops q 2-3 hours during the day and less often at night; prolong dose intervals as condition improves
> *Pediatric:* not recommended
> **Vasosulf®** *Ophth soln:* sulfa15%/phenyle 0.125%/ml (5, 15 ml)

Conjunctivitis: Chlamydial

▶*azithromycin* **(B)** 500 mg x 1 dose on day 1, then 250 mg daily on days 2-5 or 500 mg daily x 3 days or 2 g in a single dose
> *Pediatric:* not recommended for bronchitis in children
> **Zithromax®** *Tab:* 250, 500 mg; *Oral susp:* 100 mg/5 ml (15 ml); 200 mg/5 ml (15, 22.5, 30 ml); (cherry-vanilla-banana); *Pkt:* 1 g for reconstitution (cherry-banana)
> **Zithromax®Tri-pak** *Tab:* 3-500 mg tabs/pck
> **Zithromax®Z-pak** *Tab:* 6-250 mg tabs/pck
> days 2-5 or 500 mg daily x 3 days
> **Zmax®** *Oral susp:* 2 g ext rel (cherry-banana)

▶*doxycycline* **(D)(G)** 100 mg bid x 2-3 weeks
> *Pediatric:* see page 587 for dose by weight
>> <8 years: not recommended
>> >8 years, <100 lb: 2 mg/lb on first day in 2 doses, followed by 1 mg/lb/day in 1-2 doses
>> >8 years, >100 lb: same as adult

> **Adoxa®** *Tab:* 50, 100 mg ent-coat
> **Doryx®** *Cap:* 100 mg
> **Monodox®** *Cap:* 50, 100 mg
> **Vibramycin®** *Cap:* 50, 100 mg; *Syr:* 50 mg/5 ml (raspberry-apple, sulfites); *Oral susp:* 25 mg/5 ml (raspberry)
> **Vibra-Tab®** *Tab:* 100 mg film-coat

Comment: Doxycycline is contraindicated in pregnancy (discolors fetal tooth enamel).

▶*erythromycin base* **(B)(G)** 250 mg qid x 10-14 days
> *Pediatric:* see page 588 for dose by weight
>> <45 kg: 50 mg/kg/day in 4 doses x 10-14 days
>> >45 kg: same as adult

Conjunctivitis: Chlamydial

    E-Mycin® *Tab:* 250 mg ent-coat
    Eryc® *Cap:* 250 mg ent-coat
    Ery-Tab®*Tab:* 250, 333, 500 mg ent-coat
    PCE® *Tab:* 333, 500 mg
▶*minocycline* **(D)(G)** 100 mg q 12 hours x 10 days
    Pediatric: <8 years: not recommended
               >8 years, <100 lb: 2 mg/lb on first day in 2 doses, followed by 1 mg/lb/ q 12 hours x 9 more days
               >8 years, >100 lb: same as adult
    Minocin® *Cap:* 100 mg ent-coat
Comment: Minocycline is contraindicated in pregnancy (discolors fetal tooth enamel).
▶*tetracycline* **(D)(G)** 250 mg qid x 2-3 weeks
    Pediatric: Pediatric: see page 595 for dose by weight
            <8 years: not recommended
            >8 years, <100 lb: 25-50 mg/kg/day in 2-4 doses x 2-3 weeks
    Achromycin®V *Cap:* 250, 500 mg
    Sumycin® *Tab:* 250, 500 mg; *Cap:* 250, 500 mg; *Oral susp:* 125 mg/5 ml (100, 200 ml; fruit, sulfites)
Comment: Tetracycline is contraindicated in pregnancy (discolors fetal tooth enamel).

Conjunctivitis: Fungal

▶*natamycin* ophthalmic suspension **(C)** 1 drop q 1-2 hours x 3-4 days; then 1 drop every 6 hours; treat for 14-21 days; withdraw dose gradually at 4-7 day intervals
    Pediatric: <1 year: not recommended
            >1 year: same as adult
    Natacyn®Ophthalmic Suspension *Ophth susp:* 0.5% (15 ml; benzalkonium chloride)

Conjunctivitis: Gonococcal

▶*ceftriaxone* **(B)** 250 mg IM x 1 dose
    Pediatric: <45 kg: 125 mg or 50 mg/kg IM x 1 dose
            >45 kg: same as adult
    Rocephin® *Vial:* 250, 500 mg; 1, 2 g

Conjunctivitis: Viral

Comment: For prevention of secondary bacterial infection, see agents listed under bacterial conjunctivitis. Ophthalmic corticosteroids are contraindicated with herpes simplex, keratitis, *Varicella*, and other viral infections of the cornea.
▶*trifluridine* ophthalmic suspension **(C)** 1 drop q 2 hours while awake; max 9 drops/day; after re-epithelialization, 1 drop q 4 h x 7 days (at least 5 drops/day); max 21 days of therapy
    Pediatric: <6 years: not recommended
              >6 years: same as adult
  Viroptic® Ophthalmic Solution *Ophth soln:* 1% (7.5 ml; thimerosal)

Constipation

Chronic Idiopathic Constipation
▶*lubiprostone* **(C)** (Chloride Chanel Activator [GI Motility Enhancer]) 1 cap bid with food
    Pediatric: not recommended
  Amitiza® *Cap:* 24 mcg

Bulk-Forming Agents
▶*calcium polycarbophil* **(C)**
  FiberCon® (OTC) 2 tabs daily-qid
    Pediatric: <6 years: not recommended
              6-12 years: 1 tab daily-qid
  Cplt: 625 mg
  Konsyl®Fiber Tablets (OTC) *Tab:* 625 mg
▶*methylcellulose*
  Citrucel® 1 heaping tblsp in 8 oz cold water daily-tid
    Pediatric: <6 years: not recommended
              6-12 years: 1/2 adult dose
  Oral pwdr: 16, 24, 30 oz and single-dose pkts (orange)
  Citrucel®Sugar-Free 1 heaping tblsp in 8 oz cold water daily-tid
    Pediatric: <6 years: not recommended
              6-12 years: 1/2 adult dose
  Oral pwdr: 16, 24, 30 oz and single-dose pkts (orange, sugar-free, phenylalanine)
▶*psyllium husk* **(B)**
    Pediatric: <6 years: not recommended

6-12 years: 1/2 adult dose in 8 oz liquid daily-tid
Metamucil® (OTC) wafer or cap or 1 pkt or 1 rounded tsp (1 rounded tblsp for sugar-containing form) in 8 oz liquid daily-tid
Cap: psyllium husk 5.2 g (100, 150/box); *Wafer: psyllium husk* 3.4 g/rounded tsp (24/box) (apple crisp or cinnamon spice; *Plain and flavored pwdr:* 3.4 g/rounded tsp (15, 20, 24, 29, 30, 36, 44, 48 oz); *Efferv sugar-free flav pkts:* 3.4 g/pkt (30/pkt; phenylalanine)

▶*psyllium* hydrophilic mucilloid **(B)** 2 rounded tsp in 8 oz water daily-qid

Pediatric: <6 years: not recommended
6-12 years: 1 rounded tsp in 8 oz liquid daily-tid

Konsyl® (OTC) *Pwdr:* 6 g/rounded tsp (10.6, 15.9 oz); *Pwdr pkt:* 6 g/rounded tsp (30/box)

Konsyl®-D (OTC) *Pwdr:* 3.4 g/rounded tsp (11.5, 17.59 oz); *Pwdr pkt:* 3.4 g/rounded tsp (30/box)

Konsyl®Easy Mix Formula (OTC) *Pwdr:* 3.4 g/rounded tsp (8 oz; sugar-free, low sodium)

Konsyl®Orange (OTC) *Pwdr:* 3.4 g/rounded tsp (19 oz); *Pwdr pkt:* 3.4 g/rounded tsp (30/box)

Konsyl®Orange SF (OTC) *Pwdr:* 3.5 g/rounded tsp (15 oz; (phenylalanine); *Pwdr pkt:* 3.5 g/rounded tsp (30/box; phenylalanine)

Stool Softeners

▶*docusate sodium* **(OTC)** 50-200 mg/day

Pediatric: <3 years: 10-40 mg/day
3-6 years: 20-60 mg/day
>6 years: 40-120 mg/day

Cap: 50, 100 mg; *Liq:* 10 mg/ml (30 ml w. dropper); *Syr:* 20 mg/5 ml (8 oz; alcohol $\leq$1%)

Dialose® 1 tab q HS

Pediatric: <6 years: not recommended
>6 years: same as adult

Tab: 100 mg

Surfak® (OTC) 240 mg/day

Pediatric: not recommended
Cap: 240 mg

Osmotic Laxatives

▶*lactulose* **(B)(G)**

Pediatric: not recommended

Duphalac® 15-30 ml/day; max 60 ml/day

Constipation

    Syr: 10 g/15 ml (8, 16, 32 oz)
  Kristalose® 10-20 g/day; max 40 g/day
    Crystals for oral soln: 10, 20 g
▶ *magnesium citrate* **(B)(G)** ½-1 full bottle (120-300 ml)
    Pediatric: 2-6 years: 4-12 ml
              6-12 years: 50-100 ml
  Citrate of Magnesia® **(OTC)** *Oral soln:* 300 ml
▶ *magnesium hydroxide* **(B)** 30-60 ml/day in 1 or more divided doses
    Pediatric: 2-5 years: 5-15 ml/day in 1 or more divided doses
              6-11 years: 15-30 ml/day in 1 or more divided doses
  Milk of Magnesia® *Liq:* 390 mg/5 ml (10, 15, 20, 30, 100, 120, 180, 360, 720 ml)
▶ *polyethylene glycol* **(C)** 1 tblsp (17 g) dissolved in 8 oz water per day x 1-4 days; max 2 weeks
    Pediatric: not recommended
  MiraLax® *Oral pwdr:* 255, 527 g/bottle

Stimulants
▶ *bisacodyl* **(B)** 2-3 tabs or 1 suppository bid
    Pediatric: <12 years: 1/2 suppository daily
              6-12 years: 1 tablet or 1/2 suppository daily
  Dulcolax®, Gentlax® *Tab:* 5 mg; *Rectal supp:* 10 mg
Tab: 5 mg; *Rectal supp:* 10 mg
  Senokot® (OTC) initially 2-4 tabs or 1 level tsp at HS; max 4 tabs or 2 tsp bid
    Pediatric: <2 years: not recommended
             2-6 years: 1/4 tab or 1/2 tsp daily; max 1 tab or 1/2 tsp bid
            6-12 years: 1 tab or 1/2 tsp daily; max 2 tabs or 1 tsp daily
    Tab: 8.6*mg; *Granules:* 15 mg/tsp (2, 6, 12 oz; cocoa)
  Senokot®Syrup (OTC) initially 10-15 ml at HS; max 15 ml bid
    Pediatric: use Children's Syrup
    Syr: 8.8 mg/5 ml (2, 8 oz; chocolate, alcohol-free)
  Senokot®Children's Syrup (OTC)
    Pediatric: <2 years: not recommended
             2-6 years: 2.5-3.75 ml daily; max 3.75 ml bid
            6-12 years: 5-7.5 ml daily; max 7.5 ml bid
    Syr: 8.8 mg/5 ml (2.5 oz; chocolate, alcohol-free)
  Senokot®Xtra (OTC) 1 tab at HS; max 2 tabs bid
    Pediatric: <2 years: not recommended
             2-6 years: use Children's Syrup

Constipation

                6-12 years: 1/2 tab daily; max 1 tab bid
    Tab: 17*mg

Bulk Forming Agent/Stimulant Combinations

▶*psyllium/senna* **(B)**

    Perdiem® (OTC) 1-2 rounded tsp swallowed with 8 oz cool liquid daily-bid
        Pediatric: <7 years: not recommended
                7-11 years: 1 rounded tsp swallowed with 8 oz cool liquid daily-bid
    Canister: 8.8, 14 oz; *Individual pkt:* 6 g (6/pck)

    SennaPrompt® (OTC) initially 2-5 caps daily-bid;
        Pediatric: not recommended
    Cap: psyl 500 mg/*senna* 9 mg

Stool Softener/Stimulant Combinations

▶*docusate/casanthranol* **(C)**

    Doxidan® (OTC) 1-3 caps/day; max 1 week
        Pediatric: <2 years: not recommended
                >2 years: 1 cap/day
    Cap: doc 60 mg/*cas* 30 mg

    Peri-Colace® (OTC) 1-2 caps or 15-30 ml q HS; max 2 caps or 30 ml bid or 3 caps q HS
        Pediatric: 5-15 ml q HS
    Cap: doc 100 mg/*cas* 30 mg; *Syr: doc* 60 mg/*cas* 30 mg per 15 ml (8, 16 oz)

▶*docusate/senna* concentrate **(C)**

    Senokot®S (OTC) 2 tabs q HS; max 4 tabs bid
        Pediatric: <2 years: not recommended
                2-6 years: 1/2 tab daily; max 1 tab bid
                6-12 years: 1 tab daily; max 2 tabs bid
    Tab: doc 50 mg/*senna* 8.6 mg

Enemas and Other Agents

▶*sodium biphosphate/sodium phosphate* enema **(C)(OTC)**

    Fleets®Adult 59-118 ml rectally
        Pediatric: <2 years: not recommended
                2-12 years: 59 ml rectally
    Enema: Na biphos 19 g/ *Na phos* 7 g (59, 118 ml w. applicator)

    Fleets®Pediatric
        Pediatric: rectally
    Enema: Na biphos 19 g/ *Na phos* 7 g (59 ml w. applicator)

▶*glycerin* suppositories **(C)(OTC)**

Pediatric: <6 years: 1 pediatric suppository
>6 years: 1 adult suppository

Corneal Edema

▶*sodium chloride* **(NR)(G)**
  Pediatric: same as adult
  Muro®128 Ophthalmic Solution (OTC) 1-2 drops q 3-4 hours prn; reduce frequency as edema subsides
   Ophth soln: 2, 5% (15, 30 ml)
  Muro®128 Ophthalmic Ointment (OTC) small amount 1 or more times daily; reduce frequency as edema subsides
   Ophth oint: 5% (3.5 g)

Corneal Ulceration

Anti-bacterial Ophthalmic Solution/Ointment
see ***Conjunctivitis/Blepharoconjunctivitis: Bacterial** page 115*

Costochondritis (Chest Wall Syndrome)

NSAIDs see ***Pain** page 305*
Oral Non-narcotic Analgesics see ***Pain** page 308*
Oral Narcotic Analgesics see ***Pain** page 308*
Topical Analgesics see ***Pain** page 308*
Parenteral Glucocorticosteroids *see page 389*
Oral Glucocorticosteroids *see page 387*
Topical Anesthetics *see page 383*
Topical Anesthetics/Steroid Combinations *see page 480*

Crohn's Disease

Comment: Standard treatment regimen is antibiotic, anti-spasmodic, and bowel rest; progress to clear liquids; then progress to high fiber diet.
▶*azathioprine* **(D)(G)**
  Imuran® *Tab:* 50*mg; *Injectable:* 100 mg
▶*infliximab* **(B)** (tumor necrosis factor-alpha blocker)
  Administer 5 mg/kg/dose by IV infusion over at least 2 hours

Crohn's Disease

Fistulizing disease: initial dose; repeat dose at 2 weeks and 6 weeks (total 3 doses); then repeat dose every 8 weeks
Maintenance: usually 5 mg/kg/dose every 8 weeks; may increase to 10 mg/kg/dose
> *Pediatric:* not recommended

Remicade® *Vial:* 100 mg pwdr for IV infusion single-use (preservative-free)

▶ *mesalamine* **(B)**

Asacol® 800 mg tid x 6 weeks; maintenance 1.6 g/day in divided doses
> *Pediatric:* not recommended
>
> *Tab:* 400 mg del-rel

Pentasa® 1 g qid for up to 8 weeks
> *Pediatric:* not recommended
>
> *Cap:* 250 mg cont-rel

Rowasa®Enema 4 g rectally by enema q HS; retain for 8 hours x 3-6 weeks
> *Enema:* 4 g/60 ml (7/pck; sulfites)

Rowasa®Suppository 1 suppository rectally bid x 3-6 weeks; retain for 1-3 hours or longer
> *Rectal supp:* 500 mg

▶ *olsalazine* **(C)**

Dipentum® 1 g/day in 2 doses; max 2 g/day
> *Cap:* 250 mg

Comment: Indicated in persons who cannot tolerate *sulfasalazine*.

▶ *sulfasalazine* **(B; D if near term)(G)** initially 0.5 g bid; gradually increase q 4 days up to 1 g qid; max 4 g/day
> *Pediatric:* <2 years: not recommended
> >2 years: initially 40-60 mg/kg/day in 3-6 doses; maintenance 30 mg/kg/day in 4 doses

Azulfidine® *Tab:* 500 mg
Azulfidine®EN *Tab:* 500 mg ent-coat

Parenteral Glucocorticosteroids *see page 489*
Oral Glucocorticosteroids *see also page 487*

▶ *budesonide* **(C)** 9 mg daily in the AM up to 8 weeks; may taper to 6 mg/day for last 2 weeks; may repeat an 8-week course

Entocort® EC *Cap:* 3*mg ent-coat granules in caps

Comment: Taper other systemic steroids when transferring to **Entocort®EC**.

Oral Antibiotics

▶ *metronidazole* **(not for use in 1st; B in 2nd, 3rd)(G)** 500 mg tid or 750 mg bid; max 8 weeks

Pediatric: 35-50 mg/kg/day in 3 divided doses x 10 days
Flagyl®375 *Cap:* 375 mg
Flagyl®ER *Tab:* 750 mg ext-rel
Flagyl®, Protostat® *Tab:* 250*, 500*mg
Comment: Alcohol is contraindicated during treatment with oral *metronidazole* and for 72 hours after therapy due to a possible *disulfiram*-like reaction (nausea, vomiting, flushing, headache).

Cryptosporidium parvum

▶*nitazoxanide* **(B)** dose by age q 12 hours x 3 days
    Pediatric: 12 -47 months: 5 ml q 12 hours x 3 days
              4-11 years: 10 ml q 12 hours x 3 days
Alinia® *Oral susp:* 100 mg/5 ml (60 ml)
Comment: **Alinia®** is intended for pediatric use only.

Deep Vein Thrombosis (DVT)

Anti-coagulation Therapy *see pages 506-507*

Dehydration

Oral Rehydration and Electrolyte Replacement Therapy
▶*oral electrolyte replacement* **(NR)(OTC)(G)**
    KaoLectrolyte® 1 pkt dissolved in 8 oz water q 3-4 hours
        Pediatric: not indicated <2 years
        Pkt: sod 12 mEq/*pot* 5 mEq/*chlor* 10 mEq/*citrate* 7 mEq/
        dextrose 5 g/*calories* 22 per 6.2 g
    Pedialyte®
        Pediatric: <2 years: as desired and as tolerated
                    >2 years: 1-2 L/day
        Oral soln: dextrose 20 g/*fructose* 5 g/*sodium* 25 mEq/
        potassium 20 mEq/*chloride* 35 mEq/*citrate* 30 mEq/*calories*
        100 per liter (8 oz, 1 L)
    Pedialyte®Freezer Pops
        Pediatric: as desired and as tolerated
        Pops: dextrose 1.6 g/*sodium* 2.8 mEq/*potassium* 1.25 mEq/

chloride 2.2 mEq/*citrate* 1.88 mEq/*calories* 6.25 per 6.25 ml pop (8 oz, 1 L)

Dementia

Comment: Underlying cause should be explored and addressed.
Antidepressants see ***Depression*** *page 132*
Hypnotics/Sedatives see ***Insomnia*** *page 247*
Antipsychotics
▶*haloperidol* **(C)(G)** 0.5-1 mg q HS
  Haldol® *Tab:* 0.5, 1, 2, 5, 10, 20 mg
▶*mesoridazine* **(C)** initially 25 mg tid; max 300 mg/day
  Serentil® *Tab:* 10, 25, 50, 100 mg; *Conc:* 25 mg/ml (118 ml)
▶*clanzapine* **(C)** initially 2.5-10 mg daily; increasing to 10 mg/day within a few days; then by 5 mg/day at weekly intervals; max 20 mg/day
  Zyprexa® *Tab:* 2.5, 5, 7.5, 10 mg; *Vial:* 10 mg/ml (1 ml)
▶*quetiapinefumarate* **(C)** initially 25 mg bid, titrate q 2nd or 3rd day in increments of 25-50 mg bid-tid; max range 100-800 mg/day in 2-3 doses
  SeroQUEL® *Tab:* 25, 100, 200, 300 mg
▶*risperidone* **(C)** 0.5 mg bid x 1 day; adjust in increments of 0.5 mg bid to usual range of 0.5-5 mg/day
  Risperdal® *Tab:* 1, 2, 3, 4 mg; *Oral soln:* 1 mg/ml (100 ml)
  Risperdal®**M-Tab** *Tab:* 0.5, 1, 2 mg
▶*thioridazine* **(C)(G)** 10-25 mg bid
  Mellaril® *Tab:* 10, 15, 25, 50, 100, 150, 200 mg; *Oral susp:* 25 mg/5 ml, 100 mg/5 ml; *Oral conc:* 30 mg/ml, 100 mg/ml (4 oz)

Dental Abscess

▶*amoxicillin/clavulanate* **(B)(G)** 500 mg tid or 875 mg bid x 10 days
  Pediatric: see pages 571-572 for dose by weight
    40-45 mg/kg/day divided tid x 10 days or
    90 mg/kg/day divided bid x 10 days
  Augmentin® *Tab:* 250, 500, 875 mg; *Chew tab:* 125, 250 mg (lemon-lime), 200, 400 mg (cherry-banana, phenylalanine); *Oral susp:* 125 mg/5 ml (banana), 250 mg/5 ml (orange) (75, 100, 150 ml); 200, 400 mg/5 ml (50, 75, 100 ml; orange-raspberry, phenylalanine)

Augmentin®ES-600 *Oral susp:* 600 mg/5 ml (50, 75, 100, 150 ml; orange-raspberry, phenylalanine)

Augmentin®XR 2 tabs q 12 hours x 10 days
  Pediatric: <16 years: use other forms
  Tab: 1000 mg ext-rel; *Oral susp:* 600 mg/5 ml (50, 75, 100, 150 ml; orange-raspberry, phenylalanine)

▶*clindamycin* **(B)** (administer with fluoroquinolone in adult and TMP-SMX in children) 300 mg qid x 10 days
  Pediatric: see page 585 for dose by weight
      8-16 mg/kg/day in 3-4 doses x 10 days
  Cleocin® *Cap:* 75 (tartrazine), 150 (tartrazine), 300 mg
  Cleocin®Pediatric Granules *Oral susp:* 75 mg/5 ml (100 ml; cherry)

▶*erythromycin base* **(B)(G)** 500 mg q 6 hours x 10 days
  Pediatric: see page 588 for dose by weight
      30-40 mg/kg/day in 4 doses x 10 days
  E-mycin® *Tab:* 250, 333 mg ent-coat
  Eryc® *Cap:* 250 mg ent-coat
  Ery-Tab® *Tab:* 250, 333, 500 mg ent-coat
  PCE® *Tab:* 333, 500 mg

▶*penicillin v* **(B)** 250-500 mg q 6 hours x 5-7 days
  Pediatric: see page 594 for dose by weight
      <60 lb: 1 g 1 hour before procedure and then
      500 mg 6 hours later or 1 g 1 hour before procedure
      and then 500 mg q 6 hours x 8 doses
      >12 years: same as adult
  Pen-Vee®K *Tab:* 250, 500 mg; *Oral soln:* 125 mg/5 ml (100, 200 ml); 250 mg/5 ml (100, 150, 200 ml)
  Veetids® *Tab:* 250, 500 mg; *Oral soln:* 125, 250 mg/5 ml (100, 200 ml)

Denture Irritation

Debriding Agent/Cleanser
▶*carbamide peroxide 10%* **(NR)(OTC)** apply 10 drops to affected area; swish x 2-3 minutes, then spit; do not rinse; repeat treatment qid
  Pediatric: with adult supervision only
  Gly-Oxide® *Liq:* 10% (15, 60 ml, squeeze bottle w. applicator)

Depression

Selective Serotonin Reuptake Inhibitors (SSRIs)
Comment: Co-administration of SSRIs and TCAs should be done cautiously. Concomitant use of MAOIs and SSRIs is contraindicated.

▶ *citalopram* **(C)(G)** initially 20 mg daily; increase after one week to 40 mg

    Pediatric: not recommended

  Celexa® *Tab:* 20, 40mg; *Oral soln:* 10 mg/5 ml (120 ml)

▶ *escitalopram* **(C)** initially 10 mg daily; may increase to 20 mg daily after 1 week

    Pediatric: not recommended

  Lexapro® *Tab:* 5, 10*, 20*mg

  Lexapro®Oral Solution *Oral soln:* 1 mg/ml, 5 mg/tsp (240 ml) (peppermint, parabens)

▶ *fluoxetine* **(C)(G)**

  Prozac® initially 20 mg daily; may increase after 1 week; doses >20 mg/day should be divided into AM and noon doses; max 80 mg/day

    Pediatric: <8 years: not recommended
               8-17 years: initially 10 or 20 mg/day; start lower weight children at 10 mg/day; if starting at 10 mg daily, may increase after 1 week to 20 mg daily

  Tab: 10*mg; *Cap:* 10, 20, 40 mg; *Oral soln:* 20 mg/5 ml (4 oz; mint)

  Prozac®Weekly following daily fluoxetine therapy at 20 mg/day for 13 weeks, may initiate **Prozac®Weekly** 7 days after the last 20 mg fluoxetine dose

    Pediatric: not recommended

  Cap: 90 mg ent-coat del-rel pellets

▶ *paroxetine maleate* **(D)(G)**

    Pediatric: not recommended

  Paxil® initially 20 mg daily in AM; may increase by 10 mg/day at weekly intervals as needed; max 60 mg/day

    Tab: 10*, 20*, 30, 40 mg

  Paxil®CR initially 25 mg daily in AM; may increase by 12.5 mg at weekly intervals as needed; max 62.5 mg/day

    Tab: 12.5, 25, 37.5 mg cont-rel ent-coat

  Paxil®Suspension initially 20 mg daily in AM; may increase by 10 mg/day at weekly intervals as needed; max 60 mg/day

Oral susp: 10 mg/5 ml (250 ml; orange)
▶*sertraline* **(C)(G)** initially 50 mg daily; increase at 1 week intervals if needed; max 200 mg daily; dilute oral concentrate immediately prior to administration in 4 oz water, ginger ale, lemon/lime soda, lemonade, or orange juice
> *Pediatric:* <6 years: not recommended
> 6-12 years: initially 25 mg daily; max 200 mg/day
> 13-17 years: initially 50 mg daily; max 200 mg/day

Zoloft® *Tab:* 15*, 50*, 100*mg; *Oral conc:* 20 mg per ml (60 ml, [dilute just before administering in 4 oz water, ginger ale, lemon-lime soda, lemonade, or orange juice]; alcohol 12%)

Serotonin-Norepinephrine Reuptake Inhibitor (Mixed Neurotransmitter Reuptake Inhibitor)
▶*venlafaxine* **(C)**
Effexor® initially 75 mg/day in 2-3 doses; may increase at 4 day intervals in 75 mg increments to 150 mg/day; max 375 mg/day
> *Pediatric:* <18 years: not recommended
> *Tab:* 25, 37.5, 50, 75, 100 mg

Effexor®**XR** initially 75 mg q AM; may start at 37.5 mg daily x 4-7 days, then increase by increments of up to 75 mg/day at intervals of at least 4 days; usual max 375 mg/day
> *Pediatric:* not recommended
> *Cap:* 37.5, 75, 150 mg ext-rel

Tricyclic Antidepressants
Comment: Coadministration of SSRIs and TCAs requires extreme caution.
▶*amitriptyline* **(C)(G)** initially 75 mg/day in divided doses of 50-100 mg/day q HS; max 300 mg/day
> *Pediatric:* not recommended

Amitryl®, **Endep**® *Tab:* 10, 25, 50, 75, 100, 150 mg
▶*amoxapine* **(C)** initially 50 mg bid-tid; after 1 week may increase to 100 mg bid-tid; usual effective dose 200-300 mg/day; if total dose exceeds 300 mg/day, give in divided doses (max 400 mg/day); may give as a single bedtime dose (max 300 mg q HS)
> *Pediatric:* not recommended

Ascendin® *Tab:* 25, 50, 100, 150 mg
▶*clomipramine* **(C)** initially 25 mg q HS with food; max 250 mg/day
> *Pediatric:* <10 years: not recommended
> >10 years: initially 25 mg q HS with food; increase gradually over first 2 weeks to 3 mg/kg/day or 200 mg/day in divided doses or q HS

Anafranil® *Tab:* 25, 50, 75 mg

Depression

▶ *desipramine* **(C)(G)** 100-200 mg/day in single or divided doses; max 300 mg/day
    Pediatric: not recommended
  Norpramin®, **Pertofrane**® *Tab:* 10, 25, 50, 75, 100, 150 mg
▶ *doxepin* **(C)(G)** 75 mg/day; max 150 mg/day
    Pediatric: not recommended
  Adapin®, **Sinequan**® *Cap:* 10, 25, 50, 75, 100, 150 mg; *Oral conc:* 10 mg/ml (4 oz w. dropper)
▶ *imipramine* **(C)(G)**
    Pediatric: not recommended
  Tofranil® initially 75 mg daily (max 200 mg); adolescents initially 30-40 mg daily (max 100 mg/day); if maintenance dose exceeds 75 mg daily, may switch to **Tofranil**®**PM** for divided or bedtime dose
    Tab: 10, 25, 50 mg
  Tofranil®**PM** initially 75 mg daily 1 hour before HS; max 200 mg
    Cap: 75, 100, 125, 150
  Tofranil®**Injection** 50 mg IM; lower dose for adolescents; switch to oral form as soon as possible
    Amp: 25 mg/2 ml (2 ml)
▶ *nortriptyline* **(D)(G)** initially 25 mg tid-qid; max 150 mg/day
    Pediatric: not recommended
  Aventyl®, **Pamelor**® *Cap:* 10, 25, 50, 75 mg; *Oral soln:* 10 mg/5 ml (16 oz)
▶ *protriptyline* **(C)** initially 5 mg tid; usual dose 15-40 mg/day in 3-4 doses; max 60 mg/day
    Pediatric: <12 years: not recommended
  Vivactyl® *Tab:* 5, 10 mg
▶ *trimipramine* **(C)** initially 75 mg/day in divided doses; max 200 mg/day
    Pediatric: not recommended
  Surmontil® *Cap:* 25, 50, 100 mg

Aminoketones
▶ *bupropion* **(B)(G)**
    Pediatric: <18 years: not recommended
  Wellbutrin® initially 100 mg bid for at least 3 days; may Increase to 375 or 400 mg/day after several weeks; then after at least 3 more days, 450 mg in 4 doses; max 450 mg/day, 150 mg/single-dose
    Tab: 75, 100 mg
  Wellbutrin®**SR** initially 150 mg in AM for at least 3 days;

Depression

increase to 150 mg bid if well tolerated; usual dose 300 mg/day; max 400 mg/day
   Tab: 100, 150 mg sust-rel
Wellbutrin®XL initially 150 mg in AM for at least 3 days; increase to 150 mg bid if well tolerated; usual dose 300 mg/day; max 450 mg/day
   Tab: 150, 300 mg sust-rel

Monoamine Oxidase Inhibitors (MAOI)
Comment: Many drug and food interactions with this class of drugs, use cautiously. Should be reserved for refractory depression that has not responded to other classes of antidepressants. Concomitant use of MAOIs and SSRIs is contraindicated.

▶*phenelzine* **(C)** initially 15 mg tid; max 90 mg/day
   Nardil®
      Pediatric: <16 years: not recommended
      Tab: 15 mg
▶*selegeline* **(C)** initially 10 mg tid; max 60 mg/day
   Emsam® *Transdermal patch:* 6 mg/24 hrs, 9 mg/24 hrs, 12 mg/24 hrs
Comment: At the **Emsam®** transdermal patch 6 mg/24 hrs dose, the dietary restrictions commonly required when using nonselective MAOIs are not necessary.
▶*tranylcypromine* **(C)** initially 10 mg tid; max 60 mg/day
   Parnate® *Tab:* 10 mg

Tetracyclics
▶*maprotiline* **(B)(G)** initially 75 mg/day for 2 weeks then change Gradually as needed in 25 mg increments; max 225 mg/day
      Pediatric: <18 years: not recommended
   Ludiomil® *Tab:* 25, 50, 75 mg
▶*mirtazepine* **(C)** initially 15 mg q HS; increase at intervals of 1-2 weeks; usual range 15-45 mg/day; max 45 mg/day
      Pediatric: not recommended
   Remeron® *Tab:* 15, 30, 45 mg
   Remeron®SolTab *Tab:* 15, 30, 45 mg orally-disintegrating

Other Agents
▶*amoxapine* **(C)(G)** initially 50 mg bid-tid or as a single dose q HS; may increase weekly as needed; usual range 200-300 mg q HS; max 300 mg/single-dose
      Pediatric: not recommended
   Asendin® *Tab:* 25, 50, 100, 150 mg
▶*chlordiazepoxide/amitriptyline* **(C)(IV)**

Depression

    Pediatric: not recommended
Limbitrol® 3-4 tabs in divided doses
    Tab: chlor 5 mg/*amit* 12.5 mg
Limbitrol®DS 3-4 tabs in divided doses; max 6 tabs/day
    Tab: chlor 10 mg/*amit* 25 mg
▶*trazodone* **(C)** initially 150 mg/day in divided doses with food; increase by 50 mg/day q 3-4 days; max 400 mg/day in divided doses
    Pediatric: <18 years: not recommended
Desyrel® *Tab:* 50, 100, 150, 300 mg

Bipolar Disorder: Depression
▶*olanzapine/fluoxetine* **(C)** initially one 6/25 cap q PM; titrate; max 18mg/75 mg/day
    Pediatric: <18 years: not recommended
Symbyax®
    Cap: **Symbyax®6/25**: *olan* 6 mg/*fluo* 25 mg
          Symbyax®6/50: *olan* 6 mg/*fluo* 50 mg
          Symbyax®12/25: *olan* 12 mg/*fluo* 25 mg
          Symbyax®12/50: *olan* 12 mg/*fluo* 50 mg

Comment: **Symbyax®** is a thienobenzodiazepine/selective serotonin reuptake inhibitor indicated for the treatment of depressive episodes associated with bipolar disorder.

Dermatitis: Atopic (Eczema)

Moisturizing Agents
    Aquaphor®Healing Ointment (OTC) *Oint:* 1.75, 3.5, 14 oz (alcohol)
    Eucerin®Daily Sun Defense (OTC) *Lotn:* 6 oz (fragrance-free)
Comment: **Eucerin®Daily Sun Defense** is a moisturizer with SPF 15 sunscreen.
    Eucerin®Facial Lotion (OTC) *Lotn:* 4 oz
    Eucerin®Light Lotion (OTC) *Lotn:* 8 oz
    Eucerin®Lotion (OTC) *Lotn:* 8, 16 oz
    Eucerin®Original Creme (OTC) *Crm:* 2, 4, 16 oz (alcohol)
    Eucerin®Plus Creme (OTC) *Crm:* 4 oz
    Eucerin®Plus Lotion (OTC) *Lotn:* 6, 12 oz
    Eucerin®Protective Lotion (OTC) *Lotn:* 4 oz (alcohol)
Comment: **Eucerin®Protective Lotion** is a moisturizer with SPF 25 sunscreen.
    Lac-Hydrin®Cream (OTC) *Crm:* 280, 385 g
    Lac-Hydrin®Lotion (OTC) *Lotn:* (25, 400 g
    Lubriderm®Dry Skin Scented (OTC) *Lotn:* 6, 10, 16, 32 oz

Dermatitis: Atopic

Lubriderm®Dry Skin Unscented (OTC) *Lotn:* 3.3, 6, 10, 16 oz (fragrance-free)
Lubriderm®Sensitive Skin Lotion (OTC) *Lotn:* 3.3, 6, 10, 16 oz (lanolin-free)
Lubriderm®Dry Skin (OTC) *Lotn (scented):* 2.5, 6, 10, 16 oz; *Lotn (fragrance-free):* 1, 2.5, 6, 10, 16 oz
Lubriderm®Bath & Shower Oil (OTC) 1-2 capsful in bath or rub onto wet skin as needed, then rinse
  Oil: 8 oz
Moisturel® apply as needed
  Crm: 4, 16 oz; *Lotn:* 8, 12 oz; *Clnsr:* 8.75 oz

Oatmeal Colloids
  Aveeno® (OTC) add to bath as needed
    Regular: 1.5 oz (8/pck); *Moisturizing:* 0.75 oz (8/pck)
  Aveeno® Oil (OTC) add to bath as needed
    Oil: 8 oz
  Aveeno®Moisturizing (OTC) apply as needed
    Lotn: 2.5, 8, 12 oz; *Crm:* 4 oz
  Aveeno®Cleansing Bar (OTC) *Bar:* 3 oz
  Aveeno®Gentle Skin Cleanser (OTC) *Liq clnsr:* 6 oz

Topical Oil
▶*fluocinolone acetomide* 0.01% topical oil **(C)**
  Pediatric: <6 years: not recommended
  >6 years: apply sparingly bid for up to 4 weeks
  Derma-Smoothe®/FS Topical Oil apply sparingly tid
    Topical oil: 0.01% (4 oz; peanut oil)

Topical Analgesics
▶*capsaicin* cream **(NR)(G)** apply tid-qid prn
  Pediatric: <2 years: not recommended
  >2 years: apply sparingly tid-qid prn
  Axsain® *Crm:* 0.075% (1, 2 oz)
  Capin® *Lotn:* 0.025, 0.075% (59 ml)
  Capzasin®-P (OTC) *Crm:* 0.025% (1.5 oz); *Lotn:* 0.025% (2 oz)
  Capzasin®-HP (OTC) *Crm:* 0.075% (1.5 oz); *Lotn:* 0.075% (2 oz)
  Dolorac® *Crm:* 0.025% (28 g)
  DoubleCap® (OTC) *Crm:* 0.05% (2 oz)
  R-Gel® *Gel:* 0.025% (15, 30 g)
  Zostrix® (OTC) *Crm:* 0.025% (0.7, 1.5, 3 oz)
  Zostrix®HP (OTC) *Emol crm:* 0.075% (1, 2 oz)
Comment: Provides some relief by 1-2 weeks; optimal benefit may take 4-6 weeks.

Dermatitis: Atopic

▶*doxepin* **(B)** cream apply to affected area qid at intervals of at least 3-4 hours; max 8 days
        Pediatric: not recommended
  Prudoxin® *Crm:* 5% (45 g)
  Zonalon® *Crm:* 5% (30, 45 g)

▶*tacrolimus* **(C)** apply to affected area bid; continue for 1 week after clearing
        Pediatric: <2 years: not recommended
                2-15 years: use 0.03% strength; apply to affected area bid; continue for 1 week after clearing
  Protopic® *Oint:* 0.03, 0.1% (30, 60 g)

Topical Anesthetic
▶*lidocaine* 3% cream **(B)** apply to affected area bid-tid prn
        Pediatric: reduce dosage commensurate with age, body weight, and physical condition
  LidaMantle® *Crm:* 3% (1 oz)

Miscellaneous Topical Agent
▶*pimecrolimus* 1% cream **(C)** apply to affected area bid
        Pediatric: <2 years: not recommended
                >2 years: same as adult
  Elidel® *Crm:* 1% (30, 60, 100 g)

Comment: Pimecrolimus is indicated for short-term and intermittent long-term use. Discontinue use when resolution occurs. Contraindicated if the patient is immunosuppressed or if secondary bacterial infection is present.

Oral 1st Generation Antihistamines *see page 525*
Oral 2nd Generation Antihistamines *see page 527*
Topical Glucocorticosteroids *see page 483*
Parenteral Glucocorticosteroids *see page 389*
Oral Glucocorticosteroids *see page 387*

Dermatitis: Contact

Prophylaxis
▶*bentoquatam* **(NR)** apply as a wet film to exposed skin at least 15 minutes prior to possible contact; reapply at least q 4 hours; remove with soap and water
        Pediatric: <6 years: not recommended
                >6 years: same as adult
  IvyBlock® **(OTC)** *Soln:* 120 ml

Comment: Provides protection against genus rhus (poison ivy, oak, and sumac).

Treatment

Oatmeal Colloids
- **Aveeno® (OTC)** add to bath as needed
  - *Regular:* 1.5 oz (8/pck); *Moisturizing:* 0.75 oz (8/pck)
- **Aveeno®Oil (OTC)** add to bath as needed
  - *Oil:* 8 oz
- **Aveeno®Moisturizing (OTC)** apply as needed
  - *Lotn:* 2.5, 8, 12 oz; *Crm:* 4 oz
- **Aveeno®Cleansing Bar (OTC)** *Bar:* 3 oz
- **Aveeno®Gentle Skin Cleanser (OTC)** *Liq clnsr:* 6 oz

Oral 1st Generation Antihistamines *see page 525*
Oral 2nd Generation Antihistamines *see page 527*
Topical Glucocorticosteroids *see page 483*
Parenteral Glucocorticosteroids *see page 389*
Oral Glucocorticosteroids *see page 387*

Dermatitis: Seborrheic

Shampoos

▶*chloroxine* shampoo **(C)** massage onto wet scalp; wait 3 minutes, rinse, repeat, and rinse thoroughly; use twice weekly
  Pediatric: not recommended
  Capitrol®Shampoo *Shampoo:* 2% (4 oz)

▶*ciclopirox* shampoo **(B)** massage onto wet scalp; wait 3 minutes, rinse, repeat, and rinse thoroughly; use twice weekly
  Pediatric: <16 years: recommended
  Loprox®Shampoo *Shampoo:* 1% (120 ml)

▶*coal tar* shampoo **(C)** use at least twice weekly x 2 weeks, then regularly thereafter
  DHS®Zinc Shampoo (OTC) *Shampoo:* 2% (8, 12 oz)

▶*fluocinolone acetomide* shampoo **(C)**
  Pediatric: not recommended
  Derma-Smoothe®/FS Shampoo apply up to 1 oz to scalp daily, lather, and leave on x 5 minutes, then rinse twice
  Shampoo: 0.01% (4 oz)

▶*ketoconazole* shampoo **(C)** daily x 4 weeks
  Pediatric: not recommended
  Nizoral®Shampoo *Shampoo:* 2% (4 oz)

Dermatitis: Seborrheic

▶*selenium sulfide* shampoo **(C)** massage into wet scalp; wait 2-3 minutes, rinse, repeat; use twice weekly x 2 weeks, then as needed
    Pediatric: not recommended
   Exsel®Shampoo *Shampoo:* 2.5% (4 oz)
   Selsun®Shampoo *Shampoo:* 1% (120, 210, 240, 330 ml); 2.5% (120 ml)

Topical Anti-fungal Preparation
▶*ciclopirox* **(B)**
   Loprox®Cream apply bid; max 4 weeks
    Pediatric: <10 years: not recommended
             >10 years: same as adult
    Crm: 0.77% (15, 30, 90 g)
   Loprox®Lotion apply bid; max 4 weeks
    Pediatric: <10 years: not recommended
             >10 years: same as adult
    Lotn: 0.77% (30, 60 ml)
   Loprox®Gel apply bid; max 4 weeks
    Pediatric: <16 years: not recommended
    Gel: 0.77% (30, 45 g)

Topical Steroid Preparation
▶*betamethasone valerate* 0.12% foam **(C)** apply twice daily in the AM and PM; invert can and dispense a small amount of foam onto a clean saucer or other cool surface (do not apply directly to hand) and massage a small amount into affected area until foam disappears
    Pediatric: not recommended
   Luxiq® *Foam:* 100 g

Other Topical Agents
▶*ketoconazole* **(C)(G)** apply bid x 4 weeks
    Pediatric: not recommended
   Nizoral®Cream *Crm:* 2% (15, 30, 60 g)
▶*fluocinolone acetomide* 0.01% topical oil **(C)** apply sparingly tid; for scalp psoriasis wet or dampen hair or scalp, then apply a thin film, massage well, cover with a shower cap and leave on for at least 4 hours or overnight, then wash hair with regular shampoo and rinse
    Pediatric: <6 years: not recommended
            >6 years: apply sparingly bid for up to 4 weeks
   Derma-Smoothe®/FS Topical Oil
    Topical oil: 0.01% (4 oz; peanut oil)
▶*selenium sulfide* lotion **(C)** massage into wet scalp, wait 2-3 minutes, rinse; repeat; use twice weekly for 2 weeks; then as needed

Selsun®Rx *Lotn:* 2.5% (4 oz)
▶ *sodium sulfacetamide/sulfur* **(C)**
    Clinia®Emollient Cream apply daily-tid
        Wash: sod sulfa 10%/*sulfur* 5% (10 oz)
    Clinia®Foaming Wash wash once or twice daily
        Wash: sod sulfa 10%/*sulfur* 5% (6, 12 oz)
    Rosula®Gel apply daily-tid
        Gel: sod sulfa 10%/*sulfur* 5% (45 ml)
    Rosula®Lotion apply daily-tid
        Lotn: sod sulfa 10%/*sulfur* 5% (45 ml; alcohol-free)
    Rosula®Wash wash 10-20 sec daily-bid
        Clnsr: sod sulfa 10%/*sulfur* 5% (335 ml)
    Sulfacet-R®Lotion apply daily-tid
        Lotn: sod sulfa 10%/*sulfur* 5% (25 g); *Lotn (tint-free): sod sulfa* 10%/*sulfur* 5% (25 g)
Topical Glucocorticosteroids *see page 483*

Diabetic Peripheral Neuropathy

▶ *gabapentin* **(C)(G)** 100 mg daily x 1 day, then 100 mg bid x 1 day, then 100 mg tid continuously; max 900 mg tid
    Pediatric: <3 years: not recommended
        3-12 years: initially 10-15 mg/kg/day in 3 divided doses; max 12 hours between doses; titrate over 3 days
        3-4 years: titrate to 40 mg/kg/day
        5-12 years: titrate to 25-35 mg/kg/day; max 50 mg/kg/day
    Neurontin® *Cap:* 100, 300, 400 mg; *Tab:* 600*, 800* mg; *Oral soln:* 250 mg/5 ml (480 ml; strawberry-anise)
Comment: Avoid abrupt cessation of *gabapentin*.
▶ *pregabalin* **(C)(V)(GABA analog)** initially 50 mg tid; may titrate to 100 mg tid within one week; max 600 mg divided tid; discontinue over one week
    Pediatric: <18 years: not recommended
    Lyrica® *Cap:* 25, 50, 75, 100, 150, 200, 225, 300 mg
Topical Analgesics
▶ *capsaicin* cream **(NR)** apply tid-qid after lesions have healed
    Pediatric: <2 years: not recommended
        >2 years: same as adult

Diabetic Peripheral Neuropathy

    Axsain® *Crm:* 0.075% (1, 2 oz)
    Capin® *Lotn:* 0.025, 0.075% (59 ml)
    Capasicin®**-P (OTC)** *Crm:* 0.025% (1.5 oz); *Lotn:* 0.025% (2 oz)
    Capasicin®**-HP (OTC)** *Crm:* 0.075% (1.5 oz); *Lotn:* 0.075% (2 oz); *Crm:* 0.025% (45, 90 g)
    Dolorac® *Crm:* 0.025% (28 g)
    DoubleCap® **(OTC)** *Crm:* 0.05% (2 oz)
    R-Gel® *Gel:* 0.025% (15, 30 g)
    Zostrix® **(OTC)** *Crm:* 0.025% (0.7, 1.5, 3 oz)
    Zostrix®**HP** *Emol crm:* 0.075% (1, 2 oz)

▶ *lidocaine* 5% patch **(B)** apply up to 3 patches at one time for up to 12 hours/24 hour period (12 hours on/12 hours off); patches may be cut into smaller sizes before removal of the release liner; do not reuse
    Pediatric: not recommended
    Lidoderm® *Patch:* 5% 10x14 cm (5 patches/pck)

Oral Analgesics

▶ *acetaminophen* **(B)(G)** see **Fever** page 168

▶ *aspirin* **(D)(G)** see **Fever** page 169

Comment: Aspirin-containing medications are contraindicated with history of allergic-type reaction to *aspirin*, children and adolescents with *Varicella* or other viral illness, and 3rd trimester pregnancy.

▶ *tramadol* **(C)(G)** 50-100 mg q 4-6 hours prn
    Pediatric: <16 years: not recommended
    Ultram® *Tab:* 50*mg

▶ *tramadol/acetaminophen* **(C)(G)** 2 tabs q 4-6 hours; max 8 tabs/day; max 5 days
    CrCl <30 ml/min: max 2 tabs q 12 hours; max 5 days
    Pediatric: not recommended
    Ultracet® *Tab: tram* 37.5/*acet* 325 mg

Oral Narcotic Analgesics see **Pain** page 308

Diaper Rash

Protective Barriers

▶ *aloe/vitamin E/zinc oxide* **(NR)** ointment apply at each diaper change after thoroughly cleansing skin
    Balmex® *Oint:* 2, 4 oz tube; 16 oz jar

▶ *vitamin A&D* **(NR)(G)** ointment apply at each diaper change after thoroughly cleansing skin
    A&D®**Ointment** *Oint:* 1.5, 4 oz

Diaper Rash

▶ *zinc oxide* **(NR)(G)** cream and ointment apply at each diaper change after thoroughly cleansing the skin
    A&D®Ointment with Zinc Oxide *Oint:* 10% (1.5, 4 oz)
    Desitin® *Oint:* 40% (1, 2, 4, 9 oz)
    Desitin®Creamy *Crm:* 10% (2, 4 oz)

Topical Glucocorticosteroids *see page 483*
Comment: Low to intermediate potency topical glucocorticosteroids are indicated if inflammation is present.

Topical Anti-fungals
Comment: Use if caused by *Candida albicans*.

▶ *butenafine* **(B)(G)** apply bid x 1 week or daily x 4 weeks
       Pediatric: <12 years: not recommended
    Lotrimin®Ultra (C)(OTC) *Crm:* 1% (12, 24 g)
    Mentax® *Crm:* 1% (15, 30 g)
Comment: Butenafine is a benzylamine, not an "azole." Fungicidal activity continues for at least 5 weeks after last application.

▶ Clotrimazole **(B)** apply to affected area bid x 7 days
       Pediatric: same as adult
    Fungoid® *Crm:* 1% (45 g); *Soln:* 1% (1 oz w. dropper)
    Lotrimin® **(OTC)** *Crm:* 1% (15, 30, 45 g)
    Lotrimin®AF (OTC) *Crm:* 1% (12 g); *Lotn:* 1% (10 ml); *Soln:* 1% (10 ml)

▶ *econazole* **(C)** apply bid x 7 days
    Spectazole® *Crm:* 1% (15, 30, 85 g)

▶ *ketoconazole* **(C)(G)**
    Nizoral®Cream *Crm:* 2% (15, 30, 60 g)

▶ *miconazole* 2% **(C)(G)** apply bid x 7 days
       Pediatric: same as adult
    Lotrimin®AF Spray Liquid (OTC) *Spray liq:* 2% (113 g;alcohol 17%)
    Lotrimin®AF Spray Powder (OTC) *Spray pwdr:* 2% (90 g; alcohol 10%)
    Monistat-Derm® *Crm:* 2% (1, 3 oz); *Spray liq:* 2% (3.5 oz); *Spray pwdr:* 2% (3 oz)

▶ *nystatin* **(C)(G)** apply bid x 7 days
    Mycostatin® *Crm:* 100,000 U/g (15, 30 g)

Combination Agent
▶ *clotrimazole/betamethasone* **(C)** cream apply bid x 7 days
    Lotrisone® *Crm:* 15, 45 g

Diarrhea: Acute

▶ *attapulgite* **(C)**
Donnagel® (OTC) 30 ml after each loose stool; max 7 doses/day x 2 days
> *Pediatric:* <3 years: not recommended
> 3-6 years: 7.5 ml
> 6-12 years: 15 ml
> *Liq:* 600 mg/15 ml (120, 240 ml)

Donnagel®Chewable Tab (OTC) 2 tabs after each loose stool; max 14 tabs/day
> *Pediatric:* <3 years: not recommended
> 3-6 years: 1/2 tab after each loose stool; max 7 doses/day
> 6-12 years: 1 tab after each loose stool; max 7 tabs/day
> *Chew tab:* 600 mg

Kaopectate® (OTC) 30 ml after each loose stool; max 7 doses/day x 2 days
> *Pediatric:* <3 years: not recommended
> 3-6 years: 7.5 ml after each loose stool
> 6-12 years: 15 ml after each loose stool
> *Liq:* 600 mg/15 ml (120, 240 ml)

▶ *bismuth subsalicylate* **(C; D in 3rd)(G)**
Pepto-Bismol® (OTC) 2 tabs or 30 ml q 30-60 minutes as needed; max 8 doses/day
> *Pediatric:* <3 years (14-18 lb): 2.5 ml q 4 hours; max 6 doses/day
> <3 years (18-28 lb): 5 ml q 4 hours; max 6 doses/day
> 3-6 years: 1/3 tab or 5 ml q 30-60 minutes; max 8 doses/day
> 6-9 years: 2/3 tab or 10 ml q 30-60 minutes; max 8 doses/day
> 9-12 year: 1 tab or 15 ml q 30-60 minutes; max 8 doses/day
> *Chew tab:* 262 mg; *Liq:* 262 mg/15 ml (4, 8, 12, 16 oz)

Pepto-Bismol®Maximum Strength (OTC) 30 ml q 60 minutes; max 4 doses/day
> *Pediatric:* <3 years: not recommended
> 3-6 years: 5 ml q 60 minutes; max 4 doses/day

Diarrhea: Acute

> 6-9 years: 10 ml q 60 minutes; max 4 doses/day
> 9-12 years: 15 ml q 60 minutes; max 4 doses/day

Liq: 525 mg/15 ml (4, 8, 12, 16 oz)

Comment: Aspirin-containing medications are contraindicated with history of allergic-type reaction to aspirin, children and adolescents with *Varicella* or other viral illness, and 3rd trimester pregnancy.

▶*calcium polycarbophil* **(C)**
    Fibercon® **(OTC)** 2 tabs daily-qid
        Pediatric: <6 years: not recommended
            6-12 years: 1 tab daily-qid
    Cplt: 625 mg

▶*difenoxin/atropine* **(C)**
    Motofen® 2 tabs, then 1 tab after each loose stool or 1 tab q 3-4 hours as needed; max 8 tab/day x 2 days
        Pediatric: <2 years: not recommended
    Tab: dif 1 mg/*atro* 0.025 mg

▶*diphenoxylate/atropine* **(C)(V)(G)**
    Lomotil® 2 tabs or 10 ml qid until diarrhea is controlled
        Pediatric: <2 years: not recommended
            2-12 years: initially 0.3-0.4 mg/kg/day in 4 doses
    Tab: diphen 2.5 mg/*atrop* 0.025 mg; *Liq: diphen* 2.5 mg/*atrop* 0.025 mg per 5 ml (2 oz)

▶*loperamide* **(B)(OTC)(G)**
    Imodium® 4 mg initially, then 2 mg after each loose stool; max 16 mg/day
        Pediatric: <5 years: not recommended
    Cap: 2 mg
    Imodium®A-D 4 mg initially, then 2 mg after each loose stool; usual max 8 mg/day x 2 days
        Pediatric: <2 years: not recommended
            2-5 years (24-47 lb): 1 mg up to tid x 2 days
            6-8 years (48-59 lb): 2 mg initially, then 1 mg after after each loose stool; max 4 mg/day x 2 days
            9-11 years (60-95 lb): 2 mg initially, then 1 mg after after each loose stool; max 6 mg/day x 2 days
    Cplt: 2 mg; *Liq:* 1 mg/5 ml (2, 4 oz; cherry-mint, alcohol 0.5%)

▶*loperamide/simethicone* **(B)(OTC)(G)**
    Imodium®Advanced 2 tabs chewed after loose stool, then 1 after the next loose stool; max 4 tabs/day
        Pediatric: 9-11 years: 1 tab chewed after loose stool, then 1/2 after next loose stool; max 3 tabs/day

Diarrhea: Acute

>6-8 years: 1 tab chewed after loose stool, then 1/2 after next loose stool
>
>*Chew tab: loper* 2 mg/*simeth* 125 mg (vanilla-mint)

Oral Rehydration and Electrolyte Replacement Therapy

▶*oral electrolyte replacement* **(NR)(OTC)**

>**CeraLyte®50** dissolve in 8 oz water
>>*Pediatric:* not indicated <4 years
>>>*Pkt: sod* 50 mEq/*pot* 20 mEq/*chlor* 40 mEq/*citrate* 30 mEq/*rice syrup solids* 40 g/*calories* 190 per liter (mixed berry, gluten-free)
>
>**CeraLyte®70** dissolved in 8 oz water
>>*Pediatric:* not indicated <4 years
>>>*Pkt: sod* 70 mEq/*pot* 20 mEq/*chlor* 60 mEq/*citrate* 30 mEq/*rice syrup solids* 40 g/*calories* 165 per liter (natural or lemon, gluten-free)
>
>**KaoLectrolyte®** 1 pkt dissolved in 8 oz water q 3-4 hours
>>*Pediatric:* not indicated <2 years
>>>*Pkt: sod* 12 mEq/*pot* 5 mEq/*chlor* 10 mEq/*citrate* 7 mEq/*dextrose* 5 g/calories 22 per 6.2 g
>
>**Pedialyte®**
>>*Pediatric:* <2 years: as desired and as tolerated
>>>\>2 years: 1-2 L/day
>>
>>*Oral soln: dextrose* 20 g/*fructose* 5 g/*sodium* 25 mEq/ *Potassium* 20 mEq/*chloride* 35 mEq/*citrate* 30 mEq/*calories* 100 per liter (8 oz, 1 L)
>
>**Pedialyte®Freezer Pops**
>>*Pediatric:* as desired and as tolerated
>>
>>*Pops: dextrose* 1.6 g/*sodium* 2.8 mEq/*potassium* 1.25 mEq/ *chloride* 2.2 mEq/*citrate* 1.88 mEq/*calories* 6.25 per 6.25 ml pop (8 oz, 1 L)

Diarrhea: Chronic

▶*cholestyramine* **(C)**

>**Questran®Powder for Oral Suspension** initially 1 pkt or scoop daily; usual maintenance 2-4 pkts or scoops daily in 2 doses; max 6 pkts or scoops daily
>>*Oral pwdr:* 9 g pkts; 9 g equal 4 g *anhydrous cholestyramine resin* (60/pck); *Bulk can:* 378 g w. scoop
>
>**Questran®Light** initially 1 pkt or scoop daily; usual

Diarrhea: Chronic

maintenance 2-4 pkts or scoops daily in 2 doses
   Light: 5 g pkts; 5 g equals 4 g *anhydrous cholestyramine resin* (60/pck); *Bulk can:* 210 g w. scoop

Comment: Use *cholestyramine* only if diarrhea due to bile salt malabsorption.

▶*difenoxin/atropine* **(C)**
   Motofen® 2 tabs, then 1 tab after each loose stool or 1 tab q 3-4 hours prn; max 8 tab/day x 2 days
      Pediatric: <2 years: not recommended
      Tab: dif 1 mg/*atrop* 0.025 mg

▶*diphenoxylate/atropine* **(B)(V)(G)**
   Lomotil® 5-20 mg/day in divided doses
      Pediatric: <2 years: not recommended
      2-12 years: initially 0.3-0.4 mg/kg/day in 4 doses
      Tab: diphen 2.5 mg/*atrop* 0.025 mg; *Liq: diphen* 2.5 mg/*atrop* 0.025 mg per 5 ml (2 oz w. dropper)

▶*attapulgite* **(C)(G)**
   Donnagel® (OTC) 30 ml after each loose stool; max 7 doses/day
      Pediatric: <2 years: not recommended
      3-6 years: 7.5 ml after each loose stool
      Liq: 600 mg/15 ml (120, 240 ml)
   Donnagel®Chewable Tab 2 tabs after each loose stool; max 14 tabs/day
      Pediatric: <3 years: not recommended
      3-6 years: 1/2 tab after each stool; max 7 doses/day
      6-12 years: 1 tab after each loose stool; max 7 tabs/day

▶*loperamide* **(B)(OTC)(G)**
   Imodium® (OTC) 4-16 mg/day in divided doses
      Pediatric: <5 years: not recommended
      Cap: 2 mg
   Imodium®A-D (OTC) 4-16 mg/day in divided doses
      Pediatric: <2 years: not recommended
      2-5 years (24-47 lb): 1 mg up to tid x 2 days
      6-8 years (48-59 lb): 2 mg initially, then 1 mg after after each loose stool; max 4 mg/day x 2 days
      9-11 years (60-95 lb): 2 mg initially, then 1 mg after each loose stool; max 6 mg/day x 2 days
      Cplt: 2 mg; *Liq:* 1 mg/5 ml (2, 4 oz)

▶*loperamide/simethicone* **(B)(OTC)(G)**
   Imodium®Advanced 2 tabs chewed after loose stool, then 1 after the next loose stool; max 4 tabs/day

Diarrhea: Chronic

>*Pediatric:* 9-11 years: 1 tab chewed after loose stool, then 1/2 tab after next loose stool; max 3 tabs/day
>6-8 years: 1 tab chewed after loose stool, then 1/2 tab after next loose stool
>*Chew tab: loper* 2 mg/*simeth* 125 mg

Diarrhea: Traveler's

▶*ciprofloxacin* **(C)(G)** 500 mg bid x 3 days
>*Pediatric:* <18 years: not recommended
>**Cipro**® *Tab:* 100, 250, 500, 750 mg; *Oral susp:* 250, 500 mg/ 5 ml (100 ml; strawberry)

▶*rifaximen* **(C)** 200 mg tid x 3 days
>*Pediatric:* <12 years: not recommended
>**Xifaxin**® *Tab:* 200 mg

▶*trimethoprim/sulfamethoxazole* **(C)(G)** bid x 10 days
>*Pediatric: see page 597 for dose by weight*
>><2 months: not recommended
>>>2 months: 40 mg/kg/day of *sulfamethoxazole* in 2 doses bid x 10 days
>
>**Bactrim**®, **Septra**® 2 tabs bid x 10 days
>*Tab: trim* 80 mg/*sulfa* 400 mg*
>**Bactrim**®**DS, Septra**®**DS** 1 tab bid x 10 days
>*Tab: trim* 160 mg/*sulfa* 800 mg*
>**Bactrim**®**Pediatric Suspension, Septra**®**Pediatric Suspension** 20 ml bid x 10 days
>*Oral susp: trim* 40 mg/*sulfa* 200 mg per 5 ml (100 ml; cherry, alcohol 0.3%)

Comment: Trimethoprim/sulfamethoxazole is not recommended in pregnancy or lactation.

Digitalis Toxicity

Digoxin Binder
▶*digoxin immune fab (ovine)* **(B)** contents of one vial of **Digibind**® neutralizes 0.5 mg digoxin; dose based on amount of *digoxin* or *digitoxin* to be neutralized; see mfr literature
>*Pediatric:* see mfr literature
>**Digibind**® *Vial:* 38 mg

Diphtheria

Prophylaxis see ***Immunizations*** page 466
Post-exposure Prophylaxis for Non-immunized Persons
▶*erythromycin base* **(B)(G)** 500 mg qid x 14 days
       Pediatric: see page 588 for dose by weight
               <45 kg: 50 mg/kg/day in 4 doses x 14 days
               >45 kg: same as adult
   E-mycin® *Tab:* 250, 333 mg ent-coat
   Eryc® *Cap:* 250 mg ent-coat pellets
   Ery-Tab® *Tab:* 250, 333, 500 mg ent-coat
   PCE® *Tab:* 333, 500 mg
▶immunization series
see ***Immunizations: Childhood*** page 466
Post-exposure Prophylaxis for Immunized Persons
▶*Diphtheria* immunization booster

Diverticulitis

▶*amoxicillin* **(B)(G)** 500 mg q 8 hours or 875 mg q 12 hours x 7 days
   Amoxil® *Cap:* 250, 500 mg; *Tab:* 875*mg; *Chew tab:* 125, 200, 250, 400 mg (cherry-banana-peppermint, phenylalanine); *Oral susp:* 125, 250 mg/5 ml (80, 100, 150 ml; strawberry); 200, 400 mg/5 ml (50, 75, 100 ml; bubble gum); *Oral drops:* 50 mg/ml (30 ml; bubble gum)
   Trimox® *Cap:* 250, 500 mg; *Oral susp:* 125 mg/5 ml, 250 mg/5 ml (80, 100, 150 ml; raspberry-strawberry)
▶*amoxicillin/clavulanate* **(B)(G)** 500 mg tid or 875 mg bid x 7 days
   Augmentin® *Tab:* 250, 500, 875 mg; *Chew tab:* 125, 250 mg (lemon-lime), 200, 400 mg (cherry-banana, phenylalanine); *Oral susp:* 125 mg/5 ml (banana), 250 mg/5 ml (orange) (75, 100, 150 ml); 200, 400 mg/5 ml (50, 75, 100 ml; orange-raspberry, phenylalanine)
   Augmentin®ES-600 *Oral susp:* 600 mg/5 ml (50, 75, 100, 150 ml; orange-raspberry, phenylalanine)
   Augmentin®XR 2 tabs q 12 hours x 10 days
      Pediatric: <16 years: use other forms
      Tab: 1000 mg ext-rel
▶*ciprofloxacin* **(C)(G)** 500 mg bid x 7 days
   Cipro® *Tab:* 100, 250, 500, 750 mg; *Oral susp:* 250, 500 mg/

Diverticulitis

5 ml (100 ml; strawberry)
▶ *metronidazole* **(not for use in 1st; B in 2nd, 3rd)(G)** 250-500 mg q 8 hours or 750 mg q 12 hours x 7 days
  Flagyl®375 *Cap:* 375 mg
  Flagyl®ER *Tab:* 750 mg ext-rel
  Flagyl®, Protostat® *Tab:* 250*, 500*mg
Comment: Alcohol is contraindicated during treatment with oral *metronidazole* and for 72 hours after therapy due to a possible *disulfiram*-like reaction (nausea, vomiting, flushing, headache).
▶ *trimethoprim/sulfamethoxazole* **(C)(G)** bid x 7 days
  Bactrim®, Septra® 2 tabs bid x 7 days
    Tab: trim 80 mg/*sulfa* 400 mg*
  Bactrim®DS, Septra®DS 1 tab bid x 7 days
    Tab: trim 160 mg/*sulfa* 800 mg*
  Bactrim®Pediatric Suspension, Septra®Pediatric Suspension 20 ml bid x 7 days
    Oral susp: trim 40 mg/*sulfa* 200 mg per 5 ml (100 ml; cherry, alcohol 0.3%)
Comment: Trimethoprim/sulfamethoxazole is not recommended in pregnancy or lactation.

Diverticulosis

Bulk-Producing Agents
see **Constipation** *page 123*

Dry Eye Syndrome

Ophthalmic Immunomodulator/Anti-inflammatory
▶ *cyclosporine* **(C)** 1 drop q 12 hours
    Pediatric: <16 years: not recommended
  Restasis® *Ophth emul:* 0.05% (0.4 ml)
Comment: Contraindicated with active ocular infection. Allow at least 15 minutes between doses of artificial tears. May reinsert contact lenses after 15 minutes.

Ocular Lubricants
Comment: Remove contact lens prior to use.
▶ *dextran/hydroxypropyl methylcellulose* **(NR)** 1-2 drops prn
    Pediatric: same as adult
  Bion Tears® **(OTC)** *Ophth soln:* single-use containers (28/pck;

Dry Eye Syndrome

preservative-free)
▶*hydroxypropyl cellulose* **(NR)** 1/2 inch or 1 insert in each inferior cul-de-sac 1-2 times/day prn
    Pediatric: same as adult
  Lacrisert® *Ophth inserts:* 5 mg (60/pck; preservative-free)
  Hypotears®Ophthalmic Ointment (OTC) *Ophth oint:* 1% (3.5 g; preservative-free)

Comment: Place insert in the inferior cul-de-sac of the eye, beneath the base of the tarsus, not in apposition to the cornea nor beneath the eyelid at the level of the tarsal plate.

▶*hydroxypropyl methylcellulose* **(NR)** 1-2 drops prn
    Pediatric: same as adult
  GenTeal®Mild, GenTeal®Moderate (OTC) *Ophth soln:* (15 ml; perborate)
  GenTeal®Severe (OTC) *Ophth soln:* (15 ml; carbopol 980, perborate)

▶*petrolatum/mineral oil* **(NR)** apply 1/2 inch prn
    Pediatric: same as adult
  Hypotears®Ophthalmic Ointment (OTC) *Ophth oint:* 1% (3.5 g; benzalkonium chloride, alcohol 1%)
  Hypotears®PF Ophthalmic Ointment (OTC) *Ophth oint:* 1% (3.5 g; preservative-free, alcohol 1%)
  Lacri-Lube® **(OTC)** *Ophth oint:* 1% (3.5, 7 g)
  Lacri-Lube®NP **(OTC)** *Ophth oint:* 1% (0.7 g, 24/pck; preservative-free)

▶*petrolatum/lanolin/mineral oil* **(NR)** apply 1/4 inch prn
    Pediatric: same as adult
  Duratears Naturale® **(OTC)** *Ophth oint:* 3.5 g (preservative-free)

▶*polyethylene glycol/glycerin/hydroxypropyl methylcellulose* **(NR)** 1-2 drops prn.
    Pediatric: same as adult
  Visine®Tears (OTC) 1-2 drops prn
    Ophth soln: 1% (15, 30 ml)

▶*polyethylene glycol/propylene glycol* **(NR)** 1-2 drops prn.
    Pediatric: same as adult
  Systane® **(OTC)** 1-2 drops prn
    Ophth soln: (15 ml)

▶*polyvinyl alcohol* **(NR)** 1-2 drops prn
    Pediatric: same as adult
  Hypotears® **(OTC)** 1-2 drops prn
    Ophth soln: 1% (15, 30 ml)

Dry Eye Syndrome

Hypotears®PF (OTC) 1-2 drops q 3-4 hours prn
  Ophth soln: 1% (0.02 oz single-use containers, 30/pck; preservative-free)

Dyshidrosis

Topical Glucocorticosteroids *see page 483*
Comment: Intermediate to high potency indicated.

Dysfunctional Uterine Bleeding (DUB)

▶*medroxyprogesterone acetate* **(X)** 10 mg daily x 10-13 days
  Amen® *Tab:* 10 mg
  Cycrin®, Provera®, *Tab:* 2.5, 5, 10 mg
▶Oral contraceptives **(X)** with 35 mcg estrogen equivalent
see **Combined Oral Contraceptives** *page 471*
NSAIDs *see Pain page 305*
Oral Non-narcotic Analgesics *see Pain page 308*
Oral Narcotic Analgesics *see Pain page 308*

Dyslipidemia
(Hypercholesterolemia, Hyperlipidemia, Mixed Dyslipidemia)

Cholesterol Absorption Inhibitor
▶*ezetimibe* **(C)** 10 mg daily
    Pediatric: <10 years: not recommended
                >10 years: same as adult
  Zetia® *Tab:* 10 mg
Comment: Ezetimibe is contraindicated with concomitant statins in liver disease, persistent elevations in serum transaminase, pregnancy, and nursing mothers. Concomitant fibrates are not recommended. Potentiated by fenofibrate, gemfibrozil, and possibly cyclosporine. Separate dose of bile acid sequestrants required; take ezetimibe at least 2 hours before or 4 hours after.
HMG-CoA Reductase Inhibitors (Statins)
Comment: These agents decrease total cholesterol, LDL-C, TG, and apo B; Increase HDL-C. Before initiating and at 4-6 weeks, 3 months, and 6 months of therapy, check fasting lipid profile and LFTs. Side effects include myopathy and increased liver enzymes. A relative contraindication is concomitant use of cyclosporine, a macrolide antibiotic, various oral anti-fungal agents, and CYP-450 inhibitors. An absolute contraindication is active or chronic liver disease.

Dyslipidemia

▶*atorvastatin* **(X)** initially 10 mg daily; usual range 10-80 mg/day
    Pediatric: <10 years: not recommended
        >10 years (female post-menarche): same as adult
  Lipitor® *Tab:* 10, 20, 40, 80 mg

▶*fluvastatin* **(X)** initially 20-40 mg q HS; usual range 20-80 mg/day
    Pediatric: <18 years: not recommended
  Lescol® *Cap:* 20, 40 mg
  Lescol®**XL** *Tab:* 80 mg ext-rel

▶*lovastatin* **(X)**
  Mevacor® initially 20 mg daily at evening meal; may increase at 4 week intervals; max 80 mg/day in single or divided doses; if concomitant fibrates, niacin, or CrCl <30 ml/min, usual max 20 mg/day
    Pediatric: <10 years: not recommended
        10-17 years: initially 10-20 mg daily at evening meal; may increase at 4 week intervals; max 40 mg daily
    Tab: 10, 20, 40 mg
  Altoprev® initially 20 mg daily at evening meal; may increase at 4 week intervals; max 60 mg/day; if concomitant fibrates, or *niacin* >1 g/day, usual max 40 mg/day; if concomitant cyclosporine, *amiodorone*, or *verapamil*, or CrCl <30 ml/min, usual max 20 mg/day
    Pediatric: <20 years: not recommended
    Tab: 10, 20, 40, 60 mg ext-rel

▶*pravastatin* **(X)** initially 10-20 mg q HS; usual range 10-40 mg/day; may start at 40 mg/day
    Pediatric: <8 years: not recommended
        8-13 years: 20 mg daily
        14-18 years: 40 mg daily
  Pravachol® *Tab:* 10, 20, 40, 80 mg

▶*rosuvastatin* **(X)** initially 20 mg q PM; usual range 5-40 mg/day; adjust at 4 week intervals
    Pediatric: <10 years: not recommended
        >10 years (female post-menarche): same as adult
  Crestor® *Tab:* 5, 10, 20, 40 mg

▶*simvastatin* **(X)** initially 20 mg q PM; usual range 5-80 mg/day; adjust at 4 week intervals
    Pediatric: <10 years: not recommended
        >10 years (female post-menarche): same as adult
  Zocor® *Tab:* 5, 10, 20, 40, 80 mg

Dyslipidemia

Cholesterol Absorption Inhibitor/HMG-CoA Reductase Inhibitor Combination

▶*ezetimibe/simvastatin* **(X)**
    Pediatric: <10 years not recommended
    Tab: **Vytorin®10/10:** *ezetimibe* 10 mg/*simva* 10 mg
          Vytorin®10/20: *ezetimibe* 10 mg/*simva* 20 mg
          Vytorin®10/40: *ezetimibe* 10 mg/*simva* 40 mg
          Vytorin®10/80: *ezetimibe* 10 mg/*simva* 80 mg

Isobutyric Acid Derivatives and Fibrate

Comment: These agents decrease total cholesterol, LDL-C, and TG; increase HDL-C. They are indicated when the primary problem is very high TG level. Side effects include epigastric discomfort, dyspepsia, abdominal pain, cholelithiasis, myopathy, and neutropenia. Before initiating, and at 4-6 weeks, 3 months, and 6 months of therapy, check fasting CBC, lipid profile, LFT, and serum creatinine. Absolute contraindications include severe renal disease and severe hepatic disease.

Isobutyric Acid Derivatives

▶*clofibrate* **(C)** 2 g/day in divided doses
    Pediatric: not recommended
  Atromid-S® *Tab:* 500 mg
▶*gemfibrozil* **(C)(G)** 600 mg bid 30 minutes before AM and PM meal
    Pediatric: not recommended
  Lopid® *Tab:* 600*mg

Fibrates (Fibric Acid Derivatives)

▶*fenofibrate, micronized* **(C)** take with meals
    Pediatric: not recommended
  Antara® 43-130 mg daily; max 130 mg/day
    Cap: 43, 87, 130 mg
  TriCor® 54-160 mg daily; max 160 mg/day
    Tab: 54, 160 mg
  Lofibra® 67-200 mg daily; max 200 mg/day
    Tab: 67, 134, 200 mg

Nicotinic Acid Derivatives

Comment: These agents decrease total cholesterol, LDL, and TG; increase HD-C. Before initiating and at 4-6 weeks, 3 months, and 6 months of therapy, check fasting lipid profile, LFT, glucose, and uric acid. Side effects include hyperglycemia, upper GI distress, hyperuricemia, hepatotoxicity, and significant transient skin flushing. Take with food and take *aspirin* 300 mg 30 minutes before dose to decrease flushing. Relative contraindications include diabetes, hyperuricemia (gout), and PUD and absolute contraindications include severe gout and chronic liver disease.

▶*niacin* **(C)**
  Niaspan® 375 mg daily for first week, then 500 mg daily for second

Dyslipidemia

week, then 750 mg daily for third week, then 1 g daily for weeks 4-7; may increase by 500 mg q 4 weeks; usual range 1-2 g/day; max 2 g/day

    Pediatric: <21 years: not recommended

    Tab: 500, 750, 1000 mg ext-rel

Nicolar® initially 1 g tid; adjust in increments of 500 mg at 2-4 week intervals; max 6 g/day

    Pediatric: not recommended

    Tab: 500 mg

Slo-Niacin® one 250 or 500 mg tab q AM or HS or one-half 750 mg tab q AM or HS

    Pediatric: not recommended

    Tab: 250, 500, 750 mg cont-rel

Bile Acid Sequestrants

Comment: These agents decrease total cholesterol, LDL-C, and increase HDL-C, but have no effect on triglycerides. A relative contraindication is TG >200 mg/dL and an absolute contraindication is TG >400 mg/dL. Before initiating and at 4-6 weeks, 3 months, and 6 months of therapy, check fasting lipid profile. Side effects include sandy taste in mouth, abdominal gas, abdominal cramping, and constipation. These agents decrease the absorption of many other drugs.

▶*cholestyramine* **(C)**

    Pediatric: see mfr literature

    Questran®Powder for Oral Suspension initially 1 pkt or scoop daily; usual maintenance 2-4 pkts or scoops daily in 2 doses max 6 pkts or scoops daily

        Pwdr: 9 g pkts; 9 g equals 4 g anhydrous *cholestyramine* resin for reconstitution (60/pck); *Bulk can:* 378 g w. scoop

    Questran®Light initially 1 pkt or scoop daily; usual maintenance 2-4 pkts or scoops daily in 2 doses

        Light: 5 g pkts; 5 g equals 4 g anhydrous *cholestyramine* resin (60/pck): *Bulk can:* 210 g w. scoop

▶*colesevelam* **(B)**

    Pediatric: not recommended

  Monotherapy: 3 tabs bid or 6 tabs daily

  With an HMG-CoA Reductase Inhibitor: 4-6 tabs daily in a single dose or divided bid

    Welchol® *Tab:* 625 mg

▶*colestipol* **(C)**

    Pediatric: not recommended

    Colestid® 5-30 g daily or in divided doses

        Granules: unflavored: 5 g pkt; unflavored bulk: 300, 500 g

Dyslipidemia

w. scoop; flavored: 7.5 g pkt; flavored bulk: 450 g w. scoop

Colestid®Tab initially 2 g daily-bid; increase by 2 g daily-bid at 1-2 month intervals; usual maintenance 2-16 g/day

Tab: 1 g

Comment: Colestipol lowers LDL and total cholesterol.

Anti-lipid Combinations
Nicotinic acid derivative/HMG-CoA reductase inhibitor
▶ *niacin/lovastatin* **(X)**

Pediatric: <18 years: not recommended

Advicor® start at lowest niacin dose; may titrate niacin by no more than 500 mg/day every 4 weeks; max 2000/40 daily; concomitant cyclosporine or fibrate, max 1000/20 daily

Tab: **Advicor®500/20**: *niacin* 500 mg ext-rel/*lova* 20 mg
Advicor®750/20: *niacin* 750 mg ext-rel/*lova* 20 mg
Advicor®1000/20: *niacin* 1000 mg ext-rel/*lova* 20 mg

Anti-platelet/Anti-lipid Combinations
Salicylate/HMG-CoA Reductase Inhibitor (Statin) Combinations
▶ *aspirin, buffered/pravastatin* **(X)**

Pediatric: <10 years: not recommended
>10 years (female post-menarche): same as adult

Pravigard Pac® select according to desired daily aspirin dose and appropriate pravastatin starting dose; may increase pravastatin dose according to lipid values; max pravastatin 80 mg/day; refer to contraindications and precautions for aspirin and statin therapy

Tab: **Pravigard Pac®81/20**: *buf asa* 81 mg/*prava* 20 mg (30/pck)
Pravigard Pac®325/20: *buf asa* 325 mg/*prava* 20 mg (30/pck)
Pravigard Pac®325/40: *buf asa* 325 mg/*prava* 40 mg (30/pck)
Pravigard Pac®81/80: *buf asa* 81 mg/*prava* 80 mg (30/pck)
Pravigard Pac®325/80: *buf asa* 325 mg/*prava* 80 mg (30/pck)

Antihypertensive/Anti-lipid Combinations
Calcium Channel Blocker/HMG-CoA Reductase Inhibitor (Statin) Combinations
▶ *amlodipine/atorvastatin* **(X)**

Caduet® select according to blood pressure and lipid values; titrate amlodipine over 7-14 days; titrate atorvastatin according to monitored lipid values; max amlodipine 10 mg/day and max

atorvastatin 80 mg/day; refer to contraindications and precautions for CCB and statin therapy
> *Pediatric*: <10 years: not recommended
> >10 years (female post-menarche): same as adult

Tab: **Caduet®5/10**: *amlo* 5 mg/*ator* 10 mg
Caduet®5/20: *amlo* 5 mg/*ator* 20 mg
Caduet®5/40: *amlo* 5 mg/*ator* 40 mg
Caduet®5/80: *amlo* 5 mg/*ator* 80 mg
Caduet®10/10: *amlo* 10 mg/*ator* 10 mg
Caduet®10/20: *amlo* 10 mg/*ator* 20 mg
Caduet®10/40: *amlo* 10 mg/*ator* 40 mg
Caduet®10/80: *amlo* 10 mg/*ator* 80 mg

Dysmenorrhea: Primary

NSAIDs *see **Pain** page 305*
Oral Non-narcotic Analgesics *see **Pain** page 308*
Oral Narcotic Analgesics *see **Pain** page 308*
Benzeneacetic Acid Derivative
▶*diclofenac* **(B)** 50-100 mg once, then 50 tid
> *Pediatric:* <14 years: not recommended

Cataflam® *Tab:* 50 mg
Voltaren® 50-75 mg bid-qid; rarely
Tab: 25, 50, 75 mg e-c
Voltaren®-XR 100 mg qd; rarely, may use 100 mg bid
Tab: 100 mg ext rel

Comment: Diclofenac is contraindicated with *aspirin* allergy and late pregnancy.

Fenamate
▶*mefenamic acid* **(C)** 500 mg once, then 250 mg q 6 hours for up to 2-3 days; take with food
> *Pediatric:* <14 years: not recommended

Ponstel® *Cap:* 250 mg

Comment: Avoid *aspirin*.

COX-2 Inhibitor
Comment: Contraindicated with history of asthma, urticaria, and allergic-type reactions to sulfonamides, *aspirin*, or other NSAIDs.
▶*celecoxib* **(C; not for use in 3rd)** 400 mg x 1 dose, then 200 mg more on 1st day if needed, then 400 mg daily-bid; max 800 mg/day
> *Pediatric:* <18 years: not recommended

Celebrex® *Cap:* 100, 200 mg

Dysmenorrhea: Primary

Oral Contraceptives *see page 471*

Edema

Diuretics
Thiazide Diuretics
▶ *chlorthalidone* **(B)(G)** 12.5-200 mg daily
    Hygroton®, Hylidon®, Novothalidone®, Thalidone® *Tab:* 12.5, 25 mg
▶ *chlorothiazide* **(C)(G)** 0.5-1 g/day in single or divided doses; max 2 g/day
    Pediatric: <6 months: up to 15 mg/lb/day in 2 doses
               >6 months: 10 mg/lb/day in 2 doses
    Diuril® *Tab:* 250*, 500*mg; *Oral susp:* 250 mg/5 ml (237 ml)
▶ *hydrochlorothiazide* **(B)(G)**
    Pediatric: not recommended
    Esidrix® 25-100 mg daily
    Tab: 25, 50, 100 mg
    Hydrodiuril® initially 50-100 mg/day in single or divided doses; max 200 mg/day
    Tab: 25*, 50*mg
    Microzide® 12.5 mg daily; usual max 50 mg/day
    Cap: 12.5 mg
    Oretic® 25-50 mg bid; max 100 mg bid
    Tab: 25, 50 mg
▶ *hydroflumethiazide* **(B)** 50-100 mg/day
    Pediatric: not recommended
    Diucardin® *Tab:* 50 mg
▶ *methyclothiazide* **(B)** initially 2.5 mg daily; max 5 mg daily
    Pediatric: not recommended
    Enduron® *Tab:* 2.5, 5 mg
▶ *polythiazide* **(C)** 2-4 mg daily
    Pediatric: not recommended
    Renese® *Tab:* 1, 2, 4 mg

Potassium-Sparing Diuretics
▶ *amiloride* **(B)** initially 5 mg; may increase to 10 mg; max 20 mg
    Pediatric: not recommended
    Midamor® *Tab:* 5 mg
▶ *spironolactone* **(D)(G)** initially 50-100 mg in 1 or more doses; titrate at 2 week intervals

Edema

    Pediatric: not recommended
  Aldactone® *Tab:* 25, 50*, 100*mg
▶ *triamterene* **(B)** 100 mg bid; max 300 mg
    Pediatric: not recommended
  Dyrenium® *Cap:* 50, 100 mg

Loop Diuretics
▶ *bumetanide* **(C)(G)** 0.5-2 mg daily; may repeat at 4-5 hour intervals; max 10 mg/day
    Pediatric: <18 years: not recommended
  Bumex® *Tab:* 0.5*, 1*, 2*mg
▶ *ethacrynic acid* **(B)** initially 50-200 mg/day
    Pediatric: infants: not recommended
                >1 month: initially 25 mg/day; then adjust dose in 25 mg increments
  Edecrin® *Tab:* 25, 50 mg
▶ *furosemide* **(C)(G)** initially 40 mg bid
    Pediatric: not recommended
  Lasix® *Tab:* 20, 40*, 80 mg; *Oral soln:* 10 mg/ml (2, 4 oz w. dropper)
Comment: Furosemide is contraindicated with sulfa drug allergy.
▶ *torsemide* **(B)** 5 mg daily; may increase to 10 mg daily
    Pediatric: not recommended
  Demadex® *Tab:* 5*, 10*, 20*, 100*mg

Other Diuretics
▶ *indapamide* **(B)** initially 1.25 mg daily; may titrate dosage upward q 4 weeks if needed; max 5 mg/day
    Pediatric: not recommended
  Lozol® *Tab:* 1.25, 2.5 mg
Comment: Indapamide is contraindicated with sulfa drug allergy.
▶ *metolazone* **(B)**
    Pediatric: not recommended
  Mykrox® initially 0.5 mg q AM; max 1 mg/day
    Tab: 0.5 mg
  Zaroxolyn® 2.5- 5 mg daily
    Tab: 2.5, 5, 10 mg
Comment: Metolazone is contraindicated with sulfa drug allergy.

Diuretic Combinations
▶ *amiloride/hydrochlorothiazide* **(B)(G)** initially 1 tab daily; may increase to 2 tabs/day in single or divided doses
    Pediatric: not recommended
  Moduretic® *Tab: amil* 5 mg/*hydro* 50 mg*

Edema

▶*spironolactone/hydrochlorothiazide* **(D)(G)**
  Pediatric: not recommended
  Aldactazide®25 usual maintenance 50-100 mg in 1 or more doses
    Tab: spiro 25 mg/*hydro* 25 mg
  Aldactazide®50 usual maintenance 50-100 mg each in 1 or more doses
    Tab: spiro 50 mg/*hydro* 50 mg
▶*triamterene/hydrochlorothiazide* **(C)(G)**
  Pediatric: not recommended
  Dyazide® 1-2 caps daily
    Cap: triam 37.5 mg/*hydro* 25 mg
  Maxzide® 1 tab daily
    Tab: triam 75 mg/*hydro* 50 mg*
  Maxzide®-25 1-2 daily
    Pediatric: not recommended
    Tab: triam 37.5 mg/*hydro* 25 mg*

Emphysema

Inhaled Glucocorticosteroids *see Asthma page 58*
Parenteral Glucocorticosteroids *see page 389*
Oral Glucocorticosteroids *see page 387*
Inhaled Bronchodilators *see Asthma page 61*
Inhaled Non-selective Beta-Agonists *see Asthma page 61*
Expectorants *see page 529*
Antitussives *see page 530*

▶*isoproterenol* **(C)**
  Isuprel® acute: 1 inhalation, may repeat after 1 minute, max 5 inhalations/day; chronic: 1-2 inhalations q 3-4 hours
    Inhaler: 11.2 g (200 inh); 15 ml (300 inh)
  Isuprel®Inhaled Solution 5-15 inhalations of 1:200 or 3-7 inhalations of 1:100; may be repeated q 5-10 minutes if acute; max 5 treatments/day; chronic repeat q 3-4 hours
    Inhal soln: 1:200 (10, 60 ml); 1:100 (10 ml)
Oral Bronchodilators *see Asthma page 64*
Anticholinergics
▶*ipratropium* **(B)(G)**
  Atrovent® 2 inhalations qid; max 12 inhalations/day
    Inhaler: 14 g (200 inh)

Atrovent®Inhaled Solution 500 mcg by nebulizer tid-qid
Inhal soln: 0.02%; 500 mcg (2.5 ml)

Inhaled Bronchodilator/Anti-cholinergic Combination
▶*ipratropium/albuterol* **(C)** 2 inhalations qid; max 12 inhalations/day
Combivent® *Inhaler:* 14.7 g (200 inh)

Methylxanthines
see *Asthma* page 66

Methylxanthine/Expectorant Combinations
▶*dyphylline/guaifenesin* **(C)**
Lufyllin®GG 1 tab qid
Tab: dyph 200 mg/*guaif* 200 mg
Lufyllin®GG Elixir 30 ml qid
Elix: dyph 100 mg/*guaif* 100 mg per 15 ml (16 oz)

Other Methylxanthine Combination
▶*theophylline/potassium iodide/ephedrine/phenobarbital* **(X)(II)**
1 tab tid-qid prn; add an additional dose q HS as needed; dose may be increased to 1½ tab for severe attack
Pediatric: <6 years: not recommended
6-12 years: 1/2 tab tid
Quadrinal® *Tab: theo* 130 mg/*pot iod* 320 mg/*ephed* 24 mg/*phenol* 24 mg

---

Encopresis

Initial Bowel Evacuation
▶*mineral oil* **(C)** 1 oz x 1 day
▶Enemas 1-2 until clear x 2 days
▶*bisacodyl* **(B)**
Pediatric: <12 years: 1/2 suppository daily
Dulcolax® *Rectal supp:* 10 mg
▶*glycerin* suppository
Pediatric: <6 years: 1 pediatric suppository
>6 years: 1 adult suppository

Maintenance
▶*mineral oil* **(C)** 5-15 ml daily
▶*multivitamin* **(A)** 1 daily
see ***Vitamin & Mineral Supplements*** page 508

Endometriosis

NSAIDs see **Pain** page 305
Oral Non-narcotic Analgesics see **Pain** page 308
Oral Narcotic Analgesics see **Pain** page 308
Contraceptives see page 470
▶*medroxyprogesterone* **(X)** 30 mg daily
    Amen® *Tab:* 10 mg
    Cycrin®, **Provera**® *Tab:* 2.5, 5, 10 mg
▶*medroxyprogesterone acetate* injectable **(X)** 100-400 mg IM monthly
    Depo-Provera® Injectable: 300 mg/ml (2.5, 10 ml)
▶*norethidrone acetate* **(X)** initially 5 mg daily x 2 weeks; then increase by 2.5 mg/day every 2 weeks up to 15 mg/day maintenance dose; then continue for 6 to 9 months unless breakthrough bleeding is intolerable
    Aygestin® *Tab:* 5*mg

Gonadotropin Releasing Hormone Analogues
▶*goserelin (GnRH analogue)* implant **(X)** implant SC into upper abdominal wall; 1 SC implant q 28 days for up to 6 months; re-treatment not recommended
    Pediatric: <18 years: not recommended
    Zoladex® SC implant in syringe: 3.6 mg
▶*leuprolide acetate (GnRH analogue)* **(X)**
    Pediatric: <18 years: not recommended
    Lupron Depot®**3.75 mg** 3.75 mg SC monthly for up to 6 months; may repeat one 6-month cycle
        Syringe: 3.75 mg (single-dose depo susp for IM injection)
    Lupron Depot®**-3 Month** 22.5 mg IM q 3 months (84 days); max 2 injections
        Syringe: 22.5 mg (single-dose depo susp for IM injection)
Comment: Do not split doses.
▶*nafarelin acetate* **(X)** 1 spray (200 mcg) into one nostril q AM, then 1 spray (200 mcg) into the other nostril q PM x 6 months; if no response after 2 months, may increase to 2 sprays (400 mcg) bid
    Synarel® *Nasal spray:* 2 mg/ml (10 ml)
Comment: Start on 3rd or 4th day of menstrual period or after a negative pregnancy test.

Other Agents
▶*danazol* **(X)** initially 400 mg bid; gradual downward titration of dosage may be considered dependent upon patient response; mild cases may respond to 100-200 mg bid

Danocrine® *Cap:* 50, 100, 200 mg

Enuresis: Primary, Nocturnal

Vasopressin
▶*desmopressin acetate* **(B)**
    DDAVP® usual dosage 0.1-1.2 mg/day in 2-3 doses; 0.2 mg q HS prn for nocturnal enuresis
        Pediatric: <6 years: not recommended
                >6 years: 0.05 mg daily or q HS prn
    Tab: 0.1*, 0.2*mg
    DDAVP®Nasal Spray and **DDAVP®Rhinal Tube**
        Pediatric: <6 years: not recommended
                >6 years: 10 mcg or 0.1 ml of soln each nostril (20 mcg total dose) q HS prn; max 40 mcg total dose
    Nasal spray: 10 mcg/actuation (5 ml, 50 sprays); *Rhinal tube:* 0.1 mg/ml (2.5 ml)

Tricyclic Antidepressants
▶*imipramine* **(C)(G)**
    Pediatric: not recommended
    Tofranil® initially 75 mg daily (max 200 mg); adolescents Initially 30-40 mg daily (max 100 mg/day); if maintenance dose exceeds 75 mg daily, may switch to **Tofranil®PM** for divided or bedtime dose
    Tab: 10, 25, 50 mg
    Tofranil®PM initially 75 mg daily 1 hour before HS; max 200 mg
    Cap: 75, 100, 125, 150
    Tofranil®Injection 50 mg IM; lower dose for adolescents; switch to oral form as soon as possible
    Amp: 25 mg/2 ml (2 ml)

Epicondylitis

NSAIDs *see **Pain** page 305*
Oral Non-narcotic Analgesics *see **Pain** page 308*
Oral Narcotic Analgesics *see **Pain** page 308*
Topical Analgesics *see **Pain** page 308*
Parenteral Glucocorticosteroids *see page 389*
Oral Glucocorticosteroids *see page 387*

Epicondylitis

Topical Anesthetic *see page 383*
Topical Anesthetic/Steroid Combinations *see page 480*

Epididymitis

Comment: Treat x 4 weeks if underlying prostatitis present.
Primary Therapy
Age <35 years:
▶ *ceftriaxone* **(B)(G)** 250 mg IM x 1 dose
        Pediatric: <45 kg: 125 mg IM x 1 dose
                >45 kg: same as adult
   Rocephin® *Vial:* 250, 500 mg; 1, 2 g
▶ *doxycycline* **(D)(G)** 100 mg bid x 10 days
        Pediatric: see page 587 for dose by weight
                <8 years: not recommended
                >8 years, <100 lb: 2 mg/lb on first day in 2 doses,
                followed by 1 mg/lb/day in 1-2 doses x 10 days
                >8 years, >100 lb: same as adult
   Adoxa® *Tab:* 50, 100 mg ent-coat
   Doryx® *Cap:* 100 mg
   Monodox® *Cap:* 50, 100 mg
   Vibramycin® *Cap:* 50, 100 mg; *Syr:* 50 mg/5 ml (raspberry-apple, sulfites); *Oral susp:* 25 mg/5 ml (raspberry)
   Vibra-Tab® *Tab:* 100 mg film-coat
Comment: Doxycycline is contraindicated in pregnancy (discolors fetal tooth enamel).
▶ *ofloxacin* **(C)(G)** 300 mg bid x 10 day
        Pediatric: <18 years: not recommended
   Floxin® *Tab:* 200, 300, 400 mg
▶ *minocycline* **(D)(G)** 100 mg q 12 hours x 10 days
        Pediatric: <8 years: not recommended
                >8 years, <100 lb: 2 mg/lb on first day in 2 doses,
                followed by 1 mg/lb/ q 12 hours x 9 more days
                >8 years, >100 lb: same as adult
   Minocin® *Cap:* 100 mg ent-coat
Comment: Minocycline is contraindicated in pregnancy (discolors fetal tooth enamel).
▶ *tetracycline* **(D)(G)** 500 mg qid x 10 days
        Pediatric: <8 years: not recommended
                >8 years, <100 lb: 25-50 mg/kg/day in 2-4 doses

x 10 days
>8 years, >100 lb: same as adult

Achromycin®V *Cap:* 250, 500 mg

Sumycin® *Tab:* 250, 500 mg; *Cap:* 250, 500 mg; *Oral susp:* 125 mg/5 ml (100, 200 ml; fruit, sulfites)

Comment: Tetracycline is contraindicated in pregnancy (discolors fetal tooth enamel).

Age >35 years:

▶*ciprofloxacin* **(C)(G)** 500 mg bid x 10-14 days

Cipro® *Tab:* 100, 250, 500, 750 mg; *Oral susp:* 250, 500 mg/5 ml (100 ml; strawberry)

▶*norfloxacin* **(C)** 400 mg bid x 10-14 days

Pediatric: <18 years: not recommended

Noroxin® *Tab:* 400 mg

▶*ofloxacin* **(C)(G)** 300 mg bid x 12-14 days

Pediatric: <18 years: not recommended

Floxin® *Tab:* 200, 300, 400 mg

▶*trimethoprim/sulfamethoxazole* **(C)(G)** bid x 10 days

Pediatric: see page 597 for dose by weight
<2 months: not recommended
>2 months: 40 mg/kg/day of *sulfamethoxazole* in 2 doses bid x 10 days

Bactrim®, Septra® 2 tabs bid x 10-14 days
Tab: trim 80 mg/*sulfa* 400 mg*

Bactrim®DS, Septra®DS 1 tab bid x 10-14 days
Tab: trim 160 mg/*sulfa* 800 mg*

Bactrim®Pediatric Suspension, Septra®Pediatric Suspension 20 ml bid x 10-14 days
Oral susp: trim 40 mg/*sulfa* 200 mg per 5 ml (100 ml; cherry, alcohol 0.3%)

Comment: Trimethoprim/sulfamethoxazole is not recommended in pregnancy or lactation.

Erectile Dysfunction

Comment: Due to a degree of cardiac risk with sexual activity, consider cardiovascular status of patients before instituting therapeutic measures for erectile dysfunction.

Phosphodiesterase type 5 (PDE5) inhibitors

Comment: Oral PDE5 inhibitors (**Cialis®**, **Levitra®**, **Viagra®**) are contraindicated in patients taking nitrates. Caution with history of recent MI, stroke, life-

Erectile Dysfunction

threatening arrhythmia, hypotension, hypertension, cardiac failure, unstable angina, retinitis pigmentosa, CYP3A4 inhibitors (e.g., *cimetidine*, the "azoles," *erythromycin*, grapefruit juice), protease inhibitors (e.g., *ritonavir*), CYP3A4 inducers (e.g., *rifampin*, *carbamazepine*, *phenytoin*, *phenobarbital*), alcohol, antihypertensive agents. Side effects include headache, flushing, nasal congestion, rhinitis, dyspepsia, and diarrhea.

▶ *sildenafil citrate* **(B)** one dose 1 hour before sexual activity; usual initial dose 50 mg; may decrease to 25 mg or increase to max 100 mg/dose based on response; max one administration/day
  Viagra® *Tab:* 25, 50, 100 mg

▶ *tadalafil* **(B)** initially 10 mg prior to sexual activity at frequency of up to once daily; may decrease to 5 mg or increase to 20 mg based on response; max one administration/day
  Cialis® *Tab:* 5, 10, 20 mg

▶ *vardinafil* **(B)** initially 10 mg taken 60 min prior to sexual activity at frequency of up to once daily; may decrease to 5 mg or increase to 20 mg based on response; max one administration/day
  Levitra® *Tab:* 2.5, 5, 10, 20 mg

Prostaglandins (Urethral Suppository; Injection)

▶ *alprostadil* **(X)** *urethral suppository* initially 125 or 250 mcg inserted in the urethra after urination; adjust dose in stepwise manner on separate occasions; max two administrations/day
  Muse® *Urethral supp:* 125, 250, 500, 1000 mcg

Comment: Contraindicated with urethral stricture, balanitis, severe hypospadias and curvature, urethritis, predisposition to venous thrombosis, hyperviscosity syndrome. Extreme caution with anti-coagulant therapy (e.g., warfarin, heparin). Potential for hypotension and/or syncope.

▶ *alprostadil* **(X)** *injection* inject over 5-10 seconds into the dorsal lateral aspect of the proximal third of the penis; avoid visible veins; rotate injection sites and sides; if no initial response, may give next higher dose within 1 hour; if partial response, give next higher dose after 24 hours; max 60 mcg and 3 self-injections/week; allow at least 24 hours between doses; reduce dose if erection lasts >1 hour.
  Caverject® *Vial:* 5, 10, 20, 40 mcg/vial (pwdr for reconstitution w. diluent)
  Caverject®**Impulse** *Cartridge:* 10, 20 mcg (2 cartridge starter and refill pcks)
  Edex® *Vial:* 5, 10, 20, 40 mcg (6/pck); *Syringe:* 5, 10, 20, 40 mcg (4/pck); *Cartridge:* 10, 20, 40 mcg (2 cartridge starter and refill packs)

Comment: Determine dose of injectable prostaglandins in the office. Contraindicated with predisposition to priapism, penile angulation, cavernosal fibrosis,

Peyronie's disease, penile implant. Extreme caution with anti-coagulant therapy (e.g., *warfarin, heparin*).

Erysipelas

Comment: Most commonly due to GABHS.
Treatment of Choice
▶*penicillin v* **(B)** 250-500 mg q 6 hours x 10 days
    Pediatric: see page 594 for dose by weight
        25-50 mg/kg/day divided q 6 hours x 10 days
  Pen-Vee®K *Tab:* 250, 500 mg; *Oral soln:* 125 mg/5 ml (100, 200 ml); 250 mg/5 ml (100, 150, 200 ml)
  Veetids® *Tab:* 250, 500 mg; *Oral soln:* 125, 250 mg/5 ml (100, 200 ml)

Treatment if Penicillin Allergic
▶*erythromycin base* **(B)(G)** 250 mg q 6 hours x 10 days
    Pediatric: see page 588 for dose by weight
        30-40 mg/kg/day divided q 6 hours x 10 days
        >45 kg: same as adult
  E-Mycin® *Tab:* 250 mg ent-coat
  Eryc® *Cap:* 250 mg ent-coat
  Ery-Tab® *Tab:* 250, 333, 500 mg ent-coat
  PCE® *Tab:* 333, 500 mg

▶*erythromycin ethylsuccinate* **(B)(G)** 400 mg po qid x 7 days
    Pediatric: see page 589 for dose by weight
        30-50 mg/kg/day in 4 divided doses x 7 days; may double dose with severe infection; max 100 mg/kg/day
  Ery-Ped® *Oral susp:* 200 mg/5 ml (100, 200 ml; fruit); 400 mg/5 ml (60, 100, 200 ml; banana); *Oral drops:* 200, 400 mg/5 ml (50 ml; fruit); *Chew tab:* 200 mg wafer (fruit)
  E.E.S.® *Oral susp:* 200, 400 mg/5 ml (100 ml; fruit)
  E.E.S.®Granules *Oral susp:* 200 mg/5 ml (100, 200 ml; cherry)
  E.E.S.®400 Tablets *Tab:* 400 mg

Esophagitis

Antacids *see GERD page 177*
H$_2$ Antagonists *see GERD page 180*
Proton Pump Inhibitors *see GERD page 181*

Esophagitis

▶*sucralfate* **(B)(G)** 1 g qid for active ulcer; 1 g bid for maintenance
  Carafate® *Tab:* 1*g; *Oral susp:* 1 g/10 ml (14 oz)

Facial Hair, Excessive/Unwanted

Topical Hair Growth Retardant
▶*eflornithine* 13.9% cream **(C)** apply a thin layer to affected areas of face and under the chin bid a least 8 hours apart; rub in thoroughly; do not wash treated area for at least 4 hours following application
  Pediatric: not recommended
  Vaniqa® *Crm:* 13.9% (30, 60 g)
Comment: After **Vaniqa**® dries, may apply cosmetics or sunscreen. Hair removal techniques may be continued as needed.

Fecal Odor

▶*bismuth subgallate powder* **(B)(OTC)** 1-2 tabs tid with meals
  Devron® *Chew tab:* 200 mg; *Cap:* 200 mg
Comment: **Devron**® is an internal (oral) deodorant for control of odors from ileostomy or colostomy drainage or fecal incontinence.

Fever (Pyrexia)

▶*acetaminophen* **(B)(G)**
  Children's Tylenol® **(OTC)** 10-20 mg/kg q 4-6 hours prn
    Oral susp: 80 mg/tsp
      4-11 months (12-17 lb): 1/2 tsp q 4 hours prn
      12-23 months (18-23 lb): 3/4 tsp q 4 hours prn
      2-3 years (24-35 lb): 1 tsp q 4 hours prn
      4-5 years (36-47 lb): 1½ tsp q 4 hours prn
      6-8 years (48-59 lb): 2 tsp q 4 hours prn
      9-10 years (60-71 lb): 2½ tsp q 4 hours prn
      11 years (72-95 lb): 3 tsp q 4 hours prn
      All: max 5 doses/day
    Elix: 160 mg/5 ml (2, 4 oz)
    Chew tab: 80 mg
      2-3 years (24-35 lb): 2 tabs q 4 hours prn
      4-5 years (36-47 lb): 3 tabs q 4 hours prn
      6-8 years (48-59 lb): 4 tabs q 4 hours prn

Fever

        9-10 years (60-71 lb): 5 tabs q 4 hours prn
        11 years (72-95 lb): 6 tabs q 4 hours prn
        All: max 5 doses/day

Junior Strength:
        6-8 years: 2 tabs q 4 hours prn
        9-10 years: 2½ tabs q 4 hours prn
        11 years: 3 tabs q 4 hours prn
        12 years: 4 tabs q 4 hours prn
        All: max 5 doses/day

Chew tab: 160 mg
Junior cplt: 160 mg
Infant's Drops and Suspension: 80 mg/0.8 ml (1/2, 1 oz)
        <3 months: 0.4 ml q 4 hours prn
        4-11 months: 0.8 ml q 4 hours prn
        12-23 months: 1.2 ml q 4 hours prn
        2-3 years (24-35 lb): 1.6 ml q 4 hours prn
        4-5 years (36-47 lb): 2.4 ml q 4 hours prn
        All: max 5 doses/day

Extra Strength Tylenol® (OTC) 1 g q 4-6 hours prn; max 4 g/day
Pediatric: not recommended
Tab/Cplt/Gel tab/Gel cap: 500 mg
Liq: 500 mg/15 ml (8 oz)

FeverAll®Extra Strength Tylenol (OTC)
Pediatric: <3 months: not recommended
        3-36 months: 80 mg q 4 hours prn
        3-6 years: 120 mg q 4 hours prn
        >6 years: 325 mg q 4 hours prn
Rectal supp: 80, 120, 325 mg (6/box)

Maximum Strength Tylenol®Sore Throat (OTC) 500-1000 mg q 4-6 hours prn
Pediatric: not recommended
Liq: 1000 mg/30 ml (8 oz)

Tylenol® (OTC) 650 mg q 4-6 hours; max 4 g/day
Pediatric: <6 years: not recommended
        6-11 years: 325 mg q 4-6 hours prn; max 1.625 g/day

▶ *aspirin* **(D)(G)**
  Bayer® (OTC) 325-650 mg q 4 hours prn
  Pediatric: not recommended
  Tab/Cplt: 325 mg
  Children's Bayer® (OTC)

Fever

> *Pediatric:* 2-4 years (32-35 lb): 162 mg q 4 hours prn
> 4-6 years (36-45 lb): 243 mg q 4 hours prn
> 6-9 years (46-65 lb): 324 mg q 4 hours prn
> 9-11 years (66-76 lb): 324-405 mg q 4 hours prn
> 11-12 years (77-83 lb): 324-486 mg q 4 hours prn
> All: max 5 doses/day
>
> *Chew tab:* 81 mg
>
> **Extra Strength Bayer® (OTC)** 500 mg-1 g q 4-6 hours prn; max 4 g/day
>
> > *Pediatric:* not recommended
> > *Cplt:* 500 mg
>
> **Extended-Release Bayer® 8 Hour (OTC)** 650-1300 mg q 8 hours prn
>
> > *Pediatric:* not recommended
> > *Cplt:* 650 mg ext-rel

Comment: Aspirin-containing medications are contraindicated with history of allergic-type reaction to aspirin, children and adolescents with *Varicella* or other viral illness, and 3rd trimester pregnancy.

▶*aspirin/caffeine* **(D)(G)**

> **Anacin® (OTC)** 800 mg q 4 hours prn; max 4 g/day
>
> > *Pediatric:* <6 years: not recommended
> > 6-12 years: 400 mg q 4 hours prn; max 2 g/day
> > *Tab/Cplt:* 400 mg
>
> **Anacin® Maximum Strength (OTC)** 1 g tid-qid
>
> > *Pediatric:* not recommended
> > *Tab:* 500 mg

Comment: Aspirin-containing medications are contraindicated with history of allergic-type reaction to aspirin, children and adolescents with *Varicella* or other viral illness, and 3rd trimester pregnancy.

▶*aspirin/antacid* **(D)(G)**

> **Extra Strength Bayer®Plus (OTC)** 500 mg-1 g q 4-6 hours prn; usual max 4 g/day
>
> > *Pediatric:* not recommended
> > *Cplt:* 500 mg *aspirin* with *calcium carbonate*
>
> **Bufferin® (OTC)** 650 mg q 4 hours; max 3.9 mg/day
>
> > *Pediatric:* not recommended
> > *Tab:* 325 mg *aspirin* with *calcium carbonate, magnesium carbonate,* and *magnesium oxide*

Comment: Aspirin-containing medications are contraindicated with history of allergic-type reaction to aspirin, children and adolescents with *Varicella* or other viral illness, and 3rd trimester pregnancy.

▶*ibuprofen* **(B; not for use in 3rd)(G)**

Fever

Comment: Ibuprofen is contraindicated in children <6 months of age.

Children's Advil® (OTC), ElixSure®IB (OTC), Motrin® (OTC), PediaCare® (OTC), PediaProfen® (OTC)

Pediatric: 5-10 mg/kg q 6-8 hours; max 40 mg/kg/day
    <24 lb (<2 years): individualize
    24-35 lb (2-3 years): 5 ml q 6-8 hours prn
    36-47 lb (4-5 years): 7.5 ml q 6-8 hours prn
    48-59 lb (6-8 years): 10 ml or 2 tabs q 6-8 hours prn
    60-71 lb (9-10 years): 12.5 ml or 2 tabs q 6-8 hours prn
    72-95 lb (11 years): 15 ml or 3 tabs q 6-8 hours

Oral susp: 100 mg/5 ml (2, 4 oz; berry); *Junior tabs:* 100 mg

Children's Motrin®Drops (OTC), PediaCare®Drops (OTC)

Pediatric: <24 lb (<2 years): individualize
    24-35 lb (2-3 years): 2.5 ml q 6-8 hours prn

Oral drops: 50 mg/1.25 ml (15 ml; berry)

Children's Motrin®Chewables and Caplets (OTC)

Pediatric: 48-59 lb (6-8 years): 200 mg q 6-8 hours prn
    60-71 lb (9-10 years): 250 mg q 6-8 hours prn
    72-95 lb (11 years): 300 mg q 6-8 hours prn

Chew tab: 100*mg (citrus, phenylalanine)
Cplt: 100 mg

Motrin® (OTC) 400 mg q 6 hours prn

Pediatric: <6 months: not recommended
    >6 months, fever <102.5: 5 mg/kg q 6-8 hours prn
    >6 months, fever >102.5: 10 mg/kg q 6-8 hours prn
    All: max 40 mg/kg/day

Tab: 400 mg
Cplt: 100*mg
Chew tab: 50*, 100*mg (citrus, phenylalanine)
Oral susp: 100 mg/5 ml (4, 16 oz; berry)
Oral drops: 40 mg/ml (15 ml; berry)

Advil® (OTC), Motrin®IB (OTC), Nuprin® (OTC) 200-400 mg q 4-6 hours; max 1.2 g/day

Pediatric: not recommended
Tab, Cplt, Gel cap: 200 mg

▶ketoprofen **(B)(G)**
Pediatric: <16 years: not recommended

Actron® (OTC) 12.5-25 mg q 4-6 hours prn; max 75 mg/day

Tab/Cap: 12.5 mg

Fever

Orudis® 25-50 mg q 6-8 hours prn; max 300 mg/day
    Cap: 25, 50 mg
Orudis®KT (OTC) 12.5-25 mg q 4-6 hours prn; max 75 mg/day
    Tab: 12.5 mg; *Cplt:* 12.5 mg
Oruvail® 200 mg daily prn; max 200 mg/day
    Cap: 100, 150, 200 mg ext-rel

▶ *naproxen* **(B)(G)**
    Pediatric: <2 years: not recommended
                >2 years: 2.5-5 mg/kg bid-tid; max: 15 mg/kg/day
Aleve® (OTC) 400 mg x 1 dose; then 200 mg q 8-12 hours prn; max 10 days
    Tab/Cplt/Gel cap: 200 mg
Anaprox® 550 mg x 1 dose, then 550 mg q 12 hours or 275 mg q 6-8 hours; max 1.375 g first day and 1.1 g/day thereafter
    Tab: 275 mg
Anaprox®DS 1 tab bid
    Tab: 550 mg
EC-Naprosyn® 375 or 500 mg bid; may increase dose up to 1500 mg/day as tolerated
    Tab: 375, 500 mg del-rel
Naprelan® 1 g daily or 1.5 g daily for limited time; max 1 g/day thereafter
    Tab: 375, 500 mg
Naprosyn® initially 500 mg, then 500 mg q 12 hours or 250 mg q 6-8 hours prn; max 1.25 g first day and 1 g/day thereafter
    Tab: 250, 375, 500 mg; *Oral susp:* 125 mg/5 ml (473 ml; pineapple-orange)

Fibrocystic Breast Disease

▶ Contraceptives *see pages 470-478*
▶ *spironolactone* **(D)(G)** 10 mg bid pre-menstrually
    Aldactone® *Tab:* 25, 50*, 100*mg
▶ *vitamin E* **(A)** 400-600 IU daily
▶ *vitamin B6* **(A)** 50-100 mg daily
▶ *danazol* **(X)** 50-200 mg bid x 2-6 months
    Danocrine® *Cap:* 50, 100, 200 mg

Comment: Start on 3rd or 4th day of menstrual period or after a negative pregnancy test.

Fibromyalgia

NSAIDs see *Pain* page 305
Oral Non-narcotic Analgesics see *Pain* page 308
Oral Narcotic Analgesics see *Pain* page 308
Topical Analgesics see *Pain* page 308
Parenteral Glucocorticosteroids see page 389
Oral Glucocorticosteroids see page 387
Topical Anesthetic see page 383
Topical Anesthetic/Steroid Combinations see page 480
Other Agents
▶*amitriptyline* **(C)(G)** 20 mg q HS; increase gradually to 50 mg
    Pediatric: not recommended
  Amitryl®, Endep® *Tab:* 10, 25, 50, 75, 100, 150 mg
▶*cyclobenzaprine* **(B)(G)** 10 mg; usual range 20-40 mg/day in divided doses; max 60 mg/day x 2-3 weeks
    Pediatric: <15 years: not recommended
  Flexeril® *Tab:* 5, 10 mg
▶*fluazepam* **(X)(IV)(G)** 15 mg q HS, may increase to 30 mg
  Dalmane® *Cap:* 15, 30 mg
▶*trazodone* **(C)(G)** 50 mg q HS
  Desyrel® *Tab:* 50, 100, 150, 300 mg
▶*triazolam* **(X)(IV)** 0.125 mg q HS, may increase gradually to 0.5 mg
  Halcion® *Tab:* 0.125, 0.25*mg
▶*zolpidem* **(B)(IV)** 5 mg q HS, may increase to 10 mg
  Ambien® *Tab:* 5, 10 mg

Fifth Disease (Erythema Infectiosum)

Antipyretics see *Fever* page 168

Flatulence

▶*simethicone* **(C)(G)**
  Gas-X® (OTC) 2-4 tabs pc and HS prn
    Tab: 40, 80, 125 mg; *Cap:* 125 mg
  Mylicon® (OTC) 2-4 tabs pc and HS prn
    Tab: 40, 80, 125 mg; *Cap:* 125 mg
  Phazyme® Infant Oral Drops

Flatulence

> *Pediatric:* <2 years: 0.3 ml qid pc and HS prn
> 2-12 years: 0.6 ml qid pc and HS prn
> >12 years: 1.2 ml qid pc and HS prn
> *Oral drops:* 40 mg/0.6 ml (15, 30 ml w. calibrated dropper; orange, alcohol-free)

Phazyme®-95 1-2 tabs with each meal and HS prn
> *Tab:* 95 mg

Phazyme® Infant Oral Drops
> *Pediatric:* <2 years: 0.3 ml qid pc and HS prn
> 2-12 years: 0.6 ml qid pc and HS prn
> >12 years: 1.2 ml qid pc and HS prn
> *Oral drops:* 40 mg/0.6 ml (15, 30 ml w. calibrated dropper; orange, alcohol-free)

Maximum Strength Phazyme® 1-2 caps with each meal and HS prn
> *Cap:* 125 mg

▶*simethicone* **(NR)(G)**
Phazyme® Infant Oral Drops
> *Pediatric:* <2 years: 0.3 ml qid pc and HS prn
> 2-12 years: 0.6 ml qid pc and HS prn
> >12 years: 1.2 ml qid pc and HS prn
> *Oral drops:* 40 mg/0.6 ml (15, 30 ml w. calibrated dropper; orange, alcohol-free)

Fluoridation, Water, <0.6 ppm

▶*fluoride* **(NR)(G)**
Luride®
> *Pediatric:* Water fluoridation 0.3-0.6 ppm:
> <3 years: use drops
> 3-6 years: 0.25 mg daily
> 6-16 years: 0.5 mg daily
> Water fluoridation <0.3 ppm:
> <3 years: use drops
> 6 months-3 years: 0.25 mg daily
> 3-6 years: 0.5 mg daily
> 6-16 years: 1 mg daily
> *Chew tab:* 0.25, 0.5, 1 mg (sugar-free)

Luride® Drops
> *Pediatric:* Water fluoridation 0.3-0.6 ppm:

6 months-3 years: 0.25 ml daily
3-6 years: 0.5 ml daily
6-16 years: 1 ml daily
Water fluoridation <0.3 ppm:
6 months-3 years: 0.5 ml daily
3-6 years: 1 ml daily
6-16 years: 2 ml daily

Oral drops: 0.5 mg/ml (50 ml; sugar-free)

Combination Agents

▶*fluoride/vitamin A/vitamin D/vitamin C* **(NR)(G)**
Pediatric: Water fluoridation 0.3-0.6 ppm:
<3 years: not recommended
3-6 years: 0.25 mg fluoride/day
6-16 years: 0.5 mg fluoride/day
Water fluoridation <0.3 ppm:
<6 months: not recommended
6 months-3 years: 0.25 mg fluoride/day
3-6 years: 0.5 mg fluoride/day
6-16 years: 1 mg fluoride/day

Tri-Vi-Flor® Drops
Oral drops: fluoride 0.25 mg/*vit A* 1500 u/*vit D* 400 u/*vi C* 35 mg per ml (50 ml)
Oral drops: fluoride 0.5 mg/*vit A* 1500 u/*vit D* 400 u/*vit C* 35 mg per ml (50 ml)

▶*fluoride/vitamin A/vitamin D/vitamin C/iron* **(NR)**
Pediatric: Water fluoridation 0.3-0.6 ppm:
<3 years: not recommended
3-6 years: 0.25 mg fluoride/day
6-16 years: 0.5 mg fluoride/day
Water fluoridation <0.3 ppm:
<6 months: not recommended
6 months-3 years: 0.25 mg fluoride/day
3-6 years: 0.5 mg fluoride/day
6-16 years: 1 mg fluoride/day

Tri-Vi-Flor® w. Iron Drops
Oral drops: fluoride 0.25 mg/*vit A* 1500 u/*vit D* 400 u/*vit C* 35 mg/*iron* 10 mg per ml (50 ml)

Folliculitis Barbae

Topical Agents
▶ *benzoyl peroxide* **(B)** 5% daily after shaving
  Pediatric: same as adult
see Acne Vulgaris for benzoyl peroxide preparations page 31
▶ *clindamycin* **(B)** topical apply bid
  Pediatric: same as adult
  Cleocin®T *Pad:* 1% (60/pck; alcohol 50%); *Lotn:* 1% (60 ml); *Gel:* 1% (30, 60 g); *Soln w. applicator:* 1% (30, 60 ml; alcohol 50%)
▶ *hydrocortisone* 1% **(C)(G)** apply q HS
  Pediatric: same as adult
see Topical Glucocorticosteroids page 483
▶ *tazarotene* **(X)** apply daily at HS
  Pediatric: not recommended
  Avage®Cream *Crm:* 0.1% (30 g)
  Tazorac®Cream *Crm:* 0.05, 0.1% (15, 30, 60 g)
  Tazorac®Gel *Gel:* 0.05, 0.1% (30, 100 g)
▶ *tretinoin* **(C)** apply daily at HS
  Pediatric: <12 years: not recommended
  Avita® *Crm:* 0.025% (20, 45 g); *Gel:* 0.025% (20, 45 g)
  Renova® *Crm:* 0.02% (40 g); 0.05% (40, 60 g)
  Retin-A®Cream *Crm:* 0.025, 0.05, 0.1% (20, 45 g)
  Retin-A® Gel *Gel:* 0.01, 0.025% (15, 45 g; alcohol 90%)
  Retin-A®Liquid *Liq:* 0.05% (28 ml; alcohol 55%)
  Retin-A®Micro *Microspheres:* 0.04, 0.1% (20, 45 g)

Foreign Body: Esophagus

▶ *glucagon* **(B)** 0.02 mg/kg IV or IM with serial x-rays; max 1 mg
  Glucagon® (rDNA origin or beef/pork derived)
    Vial: 1 mg/ml w. diluent
Comment: Facilitates passage of foreign body from esophagus into stomach.

Foreign Body: Eye

▶ *proparacaine* **(NR)** 1-2 drops to anesthetize surface of eye; then flush with normal saline

Ophthaine® *Ophth soln:* 0.5% (15 ml)
Comment: Facilitates location and removal of foreign body.

Gastritis

Antacids *see GERD page 177*
H₂ Antagonists *see GERD page 180*

Gastroesophageal Reflux Disease (GERD)

Comment: Precipitators of reflux include narcotics, benzodiazepines, calcium antagonists, alcohol, nicotine, chocolate, and peppermint.

Antacids
Comment: Antacids with *aluminum hydroxide* may potentiate constipation. Antacids with *magnesium hydroxide* may potentiate diarrhea.

▶*aluminum hydroxide* **(C)**
    ALTernaGEL® (OTC) 5-10 ml between meals and HS prn; max 90 ml/day
        Pediatric: not recommended
        Liq: 500 mg/5 ml (5, 12 oz)
    Amphojel® (OTC) 10 ml 5-6 times/day between meals and HS prn; max 60 ml/day
        Pediatric: not recommended
        Oral susp: 320 mg/5 ml (12 oz)
    Amphojel®Tab (OTC) 600 mg 5-6 times/day between meals and HS prn; max 3.6 g/day
        Pediatric: not recommended
        Tab: 300, 600 mg

▶*aluminum hydroxide/magnesium hydroxide* **(C)(G)**
    Maalox® (OTC) 10-20 ml qid and HS prn
        Pediatric: not recommended
        Oral susp: alum 225 mg/*mag* 200 mg per 5 ml (5, 12, 26 oz; mint, lemon, cherry)
    Maalox®Therapeutic Concentrate (OTC) 10-20 ml qid pc and HS prn
        Pediatric: not recommended
        Oral susp: alum 600 mg/*mag* 300 mg per 5 ml (12 oz; mint)

▶*aluminum hydroxide/magnesium hydroxide/simethicone* **(C)(G)**

Maalox®Plus (OTC) 10-20 ml qid pc and HS prn
> *Pediatric:* not recommended
> *Tab: alum* 200 mg/*mag* 200 mg/*sim* 25 mg

Extra Strength Maalox®Plus (OTC) 10-20 ml qid pc and HS prn
> *Pediatric:* not recommended
> *Tab: alum* 350 mg/*mag* 350 mg/*sim* 30 mg
> *Oral susp: alum* 500 mg/*mag* 450 mg/*sim* 40 mg per 5 ml (5, 12, 26 oz)

Extra Strength Maalox®Plus Tab (OTC) 1-3 tabs qid pc and HS prn
> *Pediatric:* not recommended
> *Tab: alum* 350 mg/*mag* 350 mg/*sim* 30 mg

Mylanta® (OTC) 10-20 ml between meals and HS prn
> *Pediatric:* not recommended
> *Liq: alum* 200 mg/*mag* 200 mg/*sim* 20 mg per 5 ml (5, 12, 24 oz)

Mylanta®Double Strength (OTC) 10-20 ml between meals and HS prn
> *Pediatric:* not recommended
> *Liq: alum* 700 mg/*mag* 400 mg/*sim* 40 mg per 5 ml (5, 12, 24 oz)

▶ *aluminum hydroxide/magnesium carbonate* **(C)(G)**
Maalox®HRF (OTC) 10-20 ml qid pc and HS prn
> *Pediatric:* not recommended
> *Oral susp: alum* 280 mg/*mag* 350 mg per 10 ml (10 oz)

▶ *aluminum hydroxide/magnesium trisilicate* **(C)(G)**
Gaviscon® (OTC) 2-4 tabs chewed qid pc and HS prn
> *Pediatric:* not recommended
> *Tab: alum* 80 mg/*mag* 20 mg

Gaviscon®Liquid (OTC) 15-30 ml qid pc and HS prn
> *Pediatric:* not recommended
> *Liq: alum* 95 mg/*mag* 359 mg per 15 ml (6, 12 oz)

Gaviscon®Extra Strength (OTC) 2-4 tabs qid pc and HS prn
> *Pediatric:* not recommended
> *Tab: alum* 160 mg/*mag* 105 mg

Gaviscon®Extra Strength Liquid (OTC) 10-20 ml qid prn
> *Pediatric:* not recommended
> *Liq: alum* 508 mg/*mag* 475 mg per 10 ml (12 oz)

▶ *aluminum hydroxide/magnesium hydroxide/simethicone* **(C)(G)**
Maalox®Maximum Strength (OTC) 10-20 ml qid prn; max 60 ml/day

Gastroesophageal Reflux Disease

Pediatric: not recommended
Oral susp: alum 500 mg/*mag* 450 mg/*sim* 40 mg per 5 ml (5, 12, 26 oz; mint or cherry)

▶*calcium carbonate* **(C)(G)**
  Children's Mylanta®Tab (OTC)
    Pediatric: <2 years: not recommended
      2-5 years (24-47 lb): 1 tab as needed up to tid
      6-11 years (48-95 lb): 2 tabs as needed up to tid
    Tab: 400 mg
  Children's Mylanta® (OTC)
    Pediatric: <2 years: not recommended
      2-5 years (24-47 lb): 1 tab as needed up to tid
      6-11 years (48-95 lb): 2 tabs as needed up to tid
    Liq: 400 mg/5 ml (4 oz)
  Maalox®Tab (OTC) chew 2-4 tabs prn; max 12 tabs/day
    Pediatric: not recommended
    Chew tab: 600 mg (wild berry, lemon, or wintergreen, phenylalanine)
  Maalox®Maximum Strength Tab (OTC) 1-2 tabs prn; max 8 tabs/day
    Pediatric: not recommended
    Tab: 1 g (wild berry, lemon, or wintergreen, phenylalanine)
  Rolaids®Extra Strength (OTC) 1-2 tabs dissolved in mouth or chewed q 1 hour as needed; max 8 tabs/day
    Tab: 1000 mg
  Tums® (OTC) 1-2 tabs dissolved in mouth or chewed q 1 hour as needed; max 16 tabs/day
    Tab: 500 mg
  Tums®E-X 1-2 tabs dissolved in mouth or chewed q 1 hour as needed; max 16 tabs/day
    Tab: 750 mg

▶*calcium carbonate/magnesium hydroxide* **(C)**
  Mylanta®Tab (OTC) 2-4 tabs between meals and HS prn
    Pediatric: not recommended
    Tab: cal 350 mg/*mag* 150 mg
  Mylanta®DS Tab (OTC) 2-4 tabs between meals and HS prn
    Pediatric: not recommended
    Tab: cal 700 mg/*mag* 300 mg
  Rolaids®Sodium-Free (OTC) 1-2 tabs dissolved in mouth or chewed q 1 hour as needed
    Tab: cal 317 mg/*mag* 64 mg

Gastroesophageal Reflux Disease

▶ *calcium carbonate/magnesium carbonate* **(C)**
    Mylanta®Gel Caps (OTC) 2-4 caps as needed
        Gel cap: cal 550 mg/mag 125 mg
▶ *dihydroxyaluminum* **(NR)**
    Rolaids® **(OTC)** 1-2 tabs dissolved in mouth or chewed q 1 hour as needed; max 24 tabs/day
        Tab: 334 mg

H_2 Antagonists

▶ *cimetidine* **(B)(G)** 800 mg bid or 400 mg qid; max 12 weeks
        Pediatric: <16 years: not recommended
    Tagamet® *Tab:* 200, 300, 400*, 800*mg
    Tagamet®HB (OTC) 1 tab ac as prophylaxis or 1 tab bid as treatment
        Tab: 200 mg
    Tagamet®HB Oral Suspension (OTC) 1 tsp ac as prophylaxis or 1 tsp bid as treatment
        Oral susp: 200 mg/20 ml (12 oz)
    Tagamet®Liquid *Liq:* 300 mg/5 ml (mint-peach, alcohol 2.8%)
▶ *famotidine* **(B)** 20 mg bid; max 6 weeks
        Pediatric: 0.5 mg/kg/day q HS prn or in 2 doses; max 40 mg/day
    Maximum Strength Pepcid®AC (OTC) 1 tab ac
        Tab: 20 mg
    Pepcid® *Tab:* 20 mg **(OTC)**; *Tab:* 40 mg; *Oral susp:* 40 mg/5 ml (50 ml)
    Pepcid®AC (OTC) 1 tab ac; max 2 doses/day
        Tab/Rapid dissolving tab: 10 mg
    Pepcid®Complete (OTC) 1 tab ac; max 2 doses/day
        Tab: fam 10 mg/$CaCO_2$ 800 mg/mg hydroxide 165 mg
    Pepcid®RPD *Tab:* 20 mg rapid dissolving **(OTC)**; *Tab:* 40 mg rapid dissolving
▶ *nizatidine* **(B)(OTC)(G)** 150 mg bid
        Pediatric: not recommended
    Axid® *Cap:* 150, 300 mg
    Axid®AR 1 tab ac; max 150 mg/day
        Cap: 150 mg
▶ *ranitidine* **(B)**
        Pediatric: <1 month: not recommended
        1 month-16 years: 2-4 mg/kg/day in 2 divided doses; max 300 mg/day

Gastroesophageal Reflux Disease

> Duodenal/Gastric Ulcer: 2-4 mg/kg/day divided bid; max 300 mg/day
> Erosive Esophagitis: 5-10 mg/kg/day divided bid; max 300 mg/day

	20 lb, 9 kg	0.6 ml
	30 lb, 13.6 kg	0.9 ml
	40 lb, 18.2 kg	1.2 ml
	50 lb, 22.7 kg	1.5 ml
	60 lb, 27.3 kg	1.8 ml
	70 lb, 31.8 kg	2.1 ml

Zantac® 150 mg bid or 300 mg q HS
  Tab: 150, 300 mg
Zantac®75 (OTC) 1 tab ac
  Tab: 75 mg
Zantac®Efferdose dissolve 25 mg tab in 5 ml water and dissolve 150 mg tab in 6-8 oz water
  Efferdose: 25, 150 mg effervescent
Zantac®Syrup *Syr:* 15 mg/ml (peppermint, alcohol 7.5%)

▶ *ranitidine bismuth citrate* **(C)** 400 mg bid
  Pediatric: not recommended
  Tritec® *Tab:* 400 mg

Proton Pump Inhibitors

▶ *esomeprazole* **(B)** 20-40 mg daily; max 8 weeks
  Pediatric: not recommended
  Nexium® *Cap:* 20, 40 mg del-rel
▶ *lansoprazole* **(B)** 15-30 mg daily
  Pediatric: <12 years: not recommended
  Prevacid® *Cap:* 15, 30 mg ent-coat del-rel granules; may open and sprinkle; do not chew
  Prevacid®for Oral Suspension *Oral susp:* 15, 30 mg ent-coat del-rel granules/pkt; mix in 2 tblsp water and drink immediately; 30 pkt/box (strawberry)
  Prevacid®SoluTab *Tab:* 15, 30 mg orally disintegrating
▶ *omeprazole* **(C)(OTC)** 20 mg daily
  Pediatric: not recommended
  Prilosec® **(OTC)** *Cap:* 10, 20, 40 mg ent-coat del-rel granules (may open and sprinkle; do not chew)
▶ *pantoprazole* **(B)** 40 mg daily
  Pediatric: not recommended
  Protonix® *Tab:* 40 mg ent-coat del-rel
▶ *rabeprazole* **(B)(OTC)** 20 mg daily

Gastroesophageal Reflux Disease

    Pediatric: not recommended
  AcipHex® (OTC) *Tab:* 20 mg ent-coat del-rel
Promotility Agent
▶*metoclopramide* **(B)(G)** 5-15 mg qid 30 minutes ac and HS prn
    Pediatric: <18 years: not recommended
  Reglan® *Tab:* 5, 10*mg; *Syr:* 5 mg/5 ml
Comment: Metoclopropamide is contraindicated when stimulation of GI motility may be dangerous. Observe for tardive dyskinesia and Parkinsonism. Avoid concomitant drugs which may cause an extrapyramidal reaction (e.g., phenothiazines, *haloperidol*).

Giardiasis (*Giardia lamblia*)

▶*furazolidone* **(C)** 100 mg qid; max 7 days
    Pediatric: see page 591 for dose by weight
        <1 month: not recommended
        >1 month: 5 mg/kg/day in 4 doses; max 7 days
  Furoxone® *Tab:* 100 mg; *Liq:* 50 mg/15 ml (60 ml; 8 oz)
▶*metronidazole* **(not for use in 1st; B in 2nd, 3rd)** 250 mg tid x 5-10 days
    Pediatric: 35-50 mg/kg/day in 3 divided doses x 10 days
  Flagyl®375 *Cap:* 375 mg
  Flagyl®ER *Tab:* 750 mg ext-rel
  Flagyl®, Protostat® *Tab:* 250*, 500*mg
Comment: Alcohol is contraindicated during treatment with oral *metronidazole* and for 72 hours after therapy due to a possible *disulfiram*-like reaction (nausea, vomiting, flushing, headache).
▶*tinidazole* **(not for use in 1st; B in 2nd, 3rd)** 2 g in a single dose; take with food
    Pediatric: <3 years: not recommended
             >3 years: 50 mg/kg daily in a single dose; take with food; max 2 g
  Tindamax® *Tab:* 250*, 500*mg
▶*nitazoxanide* **(B)** dose by age q 12 hours x 3 days
    Pediatric: 12-47 months: 5 ml q 12 hours x 3 days
             4-11 years: 10 ml q 12 hours x 3 days
  Alinia® *Tab:* 500 mg; *Oral susp:* 100 mg/5 ml (60 ml)
Comment: **Alinia®** is intended for pediatric use only. Take with food.
▶*quinacrine* **(C)** 100 mg tid x 5-7 days

Pediatric: 2 mg/kg tid x 5 days; max 300 mg/day
Atabrine®

Gingivitis/Periodontitis

Anti-infective Oral Rinses
Comment: Treatments should be preceded by brushing and flossing the teeth. Avoid foods and liquids for 2-3 hours after a treatment.
▶ *chlorhexidine gluconate* **(B)** swish 15 ml undiluted for 30 seconds bid; do not swallow; do not rinse mouth after treatment.
    Peridex®, PerioGard® *Oral soln:* 0.12% (480 ml)

Glaucoma: Open Angle

Comment: Other ophthalmic medications should not be administered within 5-10 minutes of administering an ophthalmic anti-glaucoma medication. Contact lenses should be removed prior to instillation of anti-glaucoma medications and may be replaced 15 minutes later. Interactions with ophthalmic anti-glaucoma agents include MAOIs, CNS depressants, beta-blockers, tricyclic antidepressants, and hypoglycemics.

Ophthalmic Alpha-2 Agonists
Comment: Contraindicated with concomitant MAOI use. Cautious use with CNS depressants, beta-blockers (ocular and systemic), antihypertensives, cardiac glycosides, and tricyclic antidepressants.
▶ *apraclonidine* ophthalmic solution **(C)** 1-2 drops tid
    Iopidine® *Ophth soln:* 0.5% (5 ml; benzalkonium chloride)
▶ *brimonidine* ophthalmic solution **(B)** 1 drop q 8 hours
    Alphagan® *Ophth soln:* 0.2% (5, 10 ml; benzalkonium chloride)
    Alphagan®P *Ophth soln:* 0.15% (5, 10 ml; purite)

Ophthalmic Carbonic Anhydrase Inhibitors
Comment: Contraindicated in patients with sulfa allergy.
▶ *brinzolamide* ophthalmic suspension **(C)** 1 drop tid
    Azopt® *Ophth susp:* 1% (2.5, 5, 10 ml; benzalkonium chloride)
▶ *dorzolamide* ophthalmic solution **(C)** 1 drop tid
    Trusopt® *Ophth soln:* 2% (5, 10 ml; benzalkonium chloride)

Ophthalmic Cholinergics (Miotics)
▶ *carbachol/hydroxypropyl methylcellulose* ophthalmic solution **(C)** 2 drops daily-tid
    Isopto®Carbachol *Ophth soln: carb* 0.75% or 2.25%/*hydroxy* 1%

Glaucoma: Open Angle

(15 ml); *carb* 1.5% or 3%/*hydroxy* 1% (15, 30 ml; benzalkonium chloride)

▶*pilocarpine* **(C)(G)**

Ocusert®Pilo change ophthalmic insert once weekly
Ophth inserts: 20 mcg/hr (8/pck)

Pilocar®Ophthalmic Solution 1-2 drops 1-6 times/day
Ophth soln: 0.5, 1, 2, 3, 4, 6, 8% (15 ml)

Pilopine HS®Ophthalmic Gel apply 1/2 inch q HS or more frequently as needed
Gel: 4% (3.5 g)

▶*pilocarpine/hydroxypropyl methylcellulose* **(C)** 2 drops tid-qid or more frequently as needed

Isopto®Carpine *Ophth soln:* pilo 0.25, 0.5, 5, 8, 10%/*hydroxy* 5% (15 ml); *pilo* 1, 2, 3, 4, 6%/*hydrox* 5% (15, 30 ml; benzalkonium chloride)

Ophthalmic Cholinesterase Inhibitors

▶*demecarium bromide* ophthalmic solution **(X)** 1-2 drops q 12-48 hours

Humorsol® *Ophth soln:* 0.125, 0.25% (5 ml)

▶*echothiophate iodide* ophthalmic solution **(C)** initially 1 drop of 0.03% bid, then increase strength as needed

Phospholine®Iodide *Ophth soln:* 0.03, 0.06, 0.125, 0.25% (5 ml)

Ophthalmic Cardioselective Beta-Blockers

Comment: Generally contraindicated in severe COPD, history of or current bronchial asthma, sinus bradycardia, 2nd or 3rd degree AV block.

▶*betaxolol* ophthalmic solution **(C)** 1-2 drops bid

Betoptic® *Ophth soln:* 0.05% (2.5, 5, 10, 15 ml; benzalkonium chloride)

Betoptic®S *Ophth soln:* 0.25% (2.5, 5, 10, 15 ml; benzalkonium chloride)

Ophthalmic Non-cardioselective Beta-Blockers

Comment: Generally contraindicated in severe COPD, history of or current bronchial asthma, sinus bradycardia, 2nd or 3rd degree AV block.

▶*carteolol* ophthalmic solution **(C)** 1 drop bid

Ocupress® *Ophth soln:* 1% (5, 10 ml; benzalkonium chloride)

▶*levobunolol* **(C)** ophthalmic solution 0.25% 1-2 drops bid; 0.5% 1-2 drops daily-bid

Betagan® *Ophth soln:* 0.25% (5, 10 ml); 0.5% (2, 5, 10, 15 ml; benzalkonium chloride)

▶*metipranolol* ophthalmic solution **(C)** 1 drop bid

OptiPranolol® *Ophth soln:* 0.3% (5, 10 ml; benzalkonium

Glaucoma: Open Angle

chloride)
▶*timolol* ophthalmic solution and gel **(C)** 1 drop bid; max 1 drop 0.5% bid
   Timoptic® *Ophth soln:* 0.25, 0.5% (5, 10, 15 ml; benzalkonium chloride)
   Timoptic®Ocudose *Ophth soln:* 0.25, 0.5% (0.45 ml/dose, 60-dose; preservative-free)
   Timoptic®-XE *Ophth gel:* 0.25, 0.5% (2.5, 5 ml; preservative-free)
▶*timolol hemihydrate* ophthalmic solution **(C)** 1 drop bid
   Betimol® *Ophth soln:* 0.25, 0.5% (5, 10, 15 ml; benzalkonium chloride)

Ophthalmic Prostamide Analogue
▶*bimatropost* ophthalmic solution **C)** 1 drop q HS
   Lumigan® *Ophth soln:* 0.03% (2.5 ml; benzalkonium chloride)
▶*latanoprost* ophthalmic solution **(C)** 1 drop q HS
   Xalatan® *Ophth soln:* 0.005% (2.5 ml; benzalkonium chloride)
▶*travoprost* ophthalmic solution **(C)** 1 drop q HS
   Travatan® *Ophth soln:* 0.004% (2.5 ml; benzalkonium chloride)

Ophthalmic Sympathomimetics
Comment: Contraindicated in narrow-angle glaucoma. Use with caution in cardiovascular disease, hypertension, hyperthyroidism, diabetes, and asthma.
▶*dipivefrin* ophthalmic solution **(B)** 1 drop q 12 hours
   Propine® *Ophth soln:* 0.1% (5, 10, 15 ml; benzalkonium chloride)

Ophthalmic Carbonic Anhydrase Inhibitor/Non-cardioselective Beta-Blocker
▶*dorzolamine/timolol* ophthalmic solution **(C)** 1 drop bid
   Cosopt® *Ophth soln: dorz* 2%*/tim* 5% (5, 10 ml; benzalkonium chloride)

Ophthalmic Synthetic Docosanoid
▶*unoprostone isopropyl* ophthalmic solution **(C)** 1 drop bid
   Rescula® *Ophth soln:* 0.15% (5 ml; benzalkonium chloride)

Oral Carbonic Anhydrase Inhibitors
▶*acetazolamide* **(C)** 250-1000 mg in doses or 500 mg bid sust-rel tabs
   Diamox® *Tab:* 125*, 250*mg
   Diamox®Sequels *Tab:* 500 mg sust-rel
▶*dichlorphenamide* **(C)** initial dose 100-200 mg, followed by 100 mg q 12 hours until desired response; maintenance 25-50 mg daily-tid
   Daranide® *Tab:* 50 mg
▶*methazolamide* **(C)** 50-100 mg bid-tid
   Neptazne® *Tab:* 25, 50 mg
Comment: Administer ophthalmic osmotic and miotic agents concomitantly.

Gonorrhea

Comment: Empiric therapy requires concomitant treatment for chlamydia. Treat all sexual contacts.

Primary Therapy

▶*cefixime* **(B)(G)** 400 mg x 1 dose
        Pediatric: <6 months: not recommended
                6 months-12 years, <50 kg: 8 mg/kg/day in 1-2 doses x 10 days
                >12 years, >50 kg: same as adult
    Suprax®Oral Suspension *Oral susp:* 100 mg/5 ml (50, 75, 100 ml; strawberry)

▶*ceftriaxone* **(B)** 250 mg IM x 1 dose
        Pediatric: <45 kg: 125 mg IM x 1 dose or 50 mg/kg IM
                >45 kg: same as adult
    Rocephin® *Vial:* 250, 500 mg; 1, 2 g

Alternative Therapy

▶*azithromycin* **(B)** 2 g x 1 dose
        Pediatric: not recommended for treatment of gonorrhea in children
    Zithromax® *Tab:* 250, 500 mg; *Oral susp:* 100 mg/5 ml (15 ml); 200 mg/5 ml (15, 22.5, 30 ml); (cherry-vanilla-banana); *Pkt:* 1 g for reconstitution (cherry-banana)
    Zithromax®Tri-pak *Tab:* 3-500 mg tabs/pck
    Zithromax®Z-pak *Tab:* 6-250 mg tabs/pck
    Zmax® *Oral susp:* 2 g ext rel (cherry-banana)

▶*cefotaxime* 500 mg IM x 1 dose
    Claforan® *Vial:* 500 mg; 1, 2 g

▶*cefotetan* 1 g IM x 1 dose
        Pediatric: not recommended
    Cefotan® *Vial:* 1, 2 g

▶*cefoxitin* **(B)** 2 g IM x 1 dose
        Pediatric: <3 months: not recommended
    Mefoxin® *Vial:* 1, 2 g

plus
    probenecid **(B)(G)**
    Benemid® 1 g 30 minutes before cefoxitin
        Pediatric: <2 years: not recommended
                2-14 years: 25 mg/kg 30 minutes before cefoxitin
        Tab: 500*mg; *Cap:* 500 mg

Gonorrhea

▶*cefpodoxime proxetil* **(B)** 200 mg x 1 dose
        Pediatric: <2 months: not recommended
                      2 months-12 years: 10 mg/kg/day (max 400 mg/dose) or 5 mg/kg/day bid (max 200 mg/dose)
    Vantin® *Tab:* 100, 200 mg; *Oral susp:* 50, 100 mg/5 ml (50, 75, 100 mg; lemon-creme)

▶*ceftizoxime* **(B)** 1 g IM x 1 dose
        Pediatric: <6 months: not recommended
    Cefizox® *Vial:* 500 mg; 1, 2, 10 g

▶*cefuroxime axetil* **(B)(G)** 1000 mg x 1 dose
        Pediatric: 30 mg/kg/day in 2 doses x 10 days
    Ceftin® *Tab:* 125, 250, 500 mg; *Oral susp:* 125, 250 mg/5 ml (50, 100 ml; tutti-frutti)

▶*demeclocycline* **(X)** 600 mg initially, followed by 300 mg q 12 hours x 4 days (total 3 g)
        Pediatric: <8 years: not recommended
    Declomycin® *Tab:* 300 mg

▶*enoxacin* **(C)** 400 mg x 1 dose
        Pediatric: <18 years: not recommended
    Penetrex® *Tab:* 200, 400 mg

▶*imipramine* **(C)** 400 mg x 1 dose
        Pediatric: <18 years: not recommended
    Maxaquin® *Tab:* 400 mg

▶*norfloxacin* **(C)** 800 mg x 1 dose
        Pediatric: <18 years: not recommended
    Noroxin® *Tab:* 400 mg

▶*spectinomycin* **(B)** 2 g IM x 1 dose
        Pediatric: 40 mg/kg IM x 1 dose
    Trobicin® *Vial:* 2 g

▶*trovafloxacin* **(C)** 100 mg x 1 dose
        Pediatric: <18 years: not recommended
    Trovan® *Tab:* 100, 200 mg

Comment: Trovafloxacin is indicated only for life- or limb-threatening infection.

Combination Therapy

▶*trovafloxacin/azithromycin* **(C) Trovan®** 100 mg tab <u>plus</u> **Zithromax®** 1 g pkt together as a single one-time dose
        Pediatric: <18 years: not recommended
    Trovan®/Zithromax®Compliance Pak®
        Trovan®: *Tab:* 100 mg
        Zithromax®: *Pkt:* 1 g for reconstitution (cherry-banana)

Comment: Trovafloxacin is indicated only for life- or limb-threatening infection.

Gout

Acute Attack
NSAIDs *see Pain page 305*
Oral Non-narcotic Analgesics *see Pain page 308*
Oral Narcotic Analgesics *see Pain page 308*
Topical Analgesics *see Pain page 308*
Parenteral Glucocorticosteroids *see page 389*
Oral Glucocorticosteroids *see page 387*
Topical Anesthetic *see page 383*
Prophylaxis
▶*allopurinol* **(C)(G)** initially 100 mg daily; increase by 100 mg weekly; max 800 mg/day and 300 mg/dose; usual range for mild symptoms 200-300 mg/day; for severe symptoms 400-600 mg/day
  Zyloprim® *Tab:* 100*, 300*mg
▶*colchicine* **(C)(G)** 0.5-0.6 mg/day or every other day
    Tab: 0.5, 0.6 mg
▶*probenecid* **(B)(G)** 250 mg bid x 1 week; maintenance 500 mg bid
      Pediatric: <2 years: not recommended
               2-14 years: 25 mg/kg in 1 dose
  Benemid® *Tab:* 500*mg; *Cap:* 500 mg
Comment: Avoid concomitant use of *probenecid* and salicylates.
▶*probenecid/colchicine* **(C)** 1 tab daily x 1 week; may increase by 1 tab q 4 weeks within tolerance; usual maintenance 1 tab bid
  ColBenemid® *Tab: proben* 500 mg/*colch* 0.5 mg*
Comment: Avoid concomitant use of *probenecid* and *salicylate*.
▶*sulfinpyrazone* **(C)** initially 200-400 mg bid; may gradually increase to 800 mg bid
  Anturane® *Cap:* 100, 200 mg
Comment: Goal is serum uric acid <6.5 mg/dL.
Pseudogout
see Pseudogout page 356

Growth Failure

▶*mecasermin* (recombinant human insulin-like growth factor-1 [rhIGF-1])
  Increlex® **(B)** see mfr product literature
    Vial: 10 mg/ml (benzyl alcohol)
    Comment: **Increlex®** is indicated for growth failure in children with severe

Growth Failure

primary IGF-1 deficiency (primary IGFD) or in those with growth hormone (GH) gene deletion who have developed neutralizing antibodies to GH.

▶ *sermorelin acetate* (pituitary hormone)

Geref® (C) 30 mg/kg SC daily at HS; discontinue when epiphyses have fused

> *Vial:* 0.5, 1 mg lyophilized pwdr with 0.9% NaCl for reconstitution

▶ *somatropin* (rDNA origin)

Genotropin® (B) initially not more than 0.04 mg/kg/week divided into 6-7 doses; may increase at 4-8 week intervals; max 0.08 mg/kg/week divided into 6-7 doses

> *Pediatric:* usually 0.16-0.024 mg/kg/week divided into 6-7 doses
>
> *Intra-Mix Device:*
>> 1.5 mg (1.3 mg/ml after reconstitution)
>> 5.8 mg (5 mg/ml after reconstitution)
>> (2-chamber cartridge w. diluent)
>
> *Pen or Intra-Mix Device:*
>> 5.8 mg (5 mg/ml after reconstitution)
>> 13.8 mg (512 mg/ml after reconstitution)
>> (2 chamber cartridge w. diluent)

Genotropin®Miniquick (B) initially not more than 0.04 mg/kg/week divided into 6-7 doses; may increase at 4-8 week intervals; max 0.08 mg/kg/week divided into 6-7 doses

> *Pediatric:* usually 0.16-0.024 mg/kg/week divided into 6-7 doses
>
> *MiniQuick:* 0.2, 0.4, 0.6, 0.8, 1, 1.2, 1.4, 1.6, 1.8, 2 mg/0.25 ml (pwdr for SC injection after reconstitution) (2 chamber cartridge w. diluent)

Humatrope® (C)

> *Pediatric:* initially 0.18 mg/kg/week IM or SC divided into equal doses given either on 3 alternate days or 6 times per week; max 0.3 mg/kg/week
>
> *Vial:* 5 mg w. 5 ml diluent

Norditropin® (C)

> *Pediatric:* 0.024-0.034 mg/kg 6 to 7 times/week SC
>
> *Vial:* 4 mg (12 IU), 8 mg (24 IU); *Cartridge for inj:* 5, 10, 15 mg/1.5 ml

Nutropin® (C)

> *Pediatric:* 0.7 mg/kg/week SC in divided daily doses
>
> *Vial:* 5, 10 mg/vial w. diluent

Growth Failure

Nutropin®AQ (C)
>   <35 years: initially not more than 0.006 mg/kg SC daily; may increase to max 0.025 mg/kg SC daily
>   >35 years: initially not more than 0.006 mg/kg SC daily; may increase to max 0.0125 mg/kg SC daily
>   *Pediatric:* Prepubertal: up to 0.043 mg/kg SC daily
>   Pubertal: up to 0.1 mg/kg SC daily
>   Turner Syndrome: up to 0.0375 mg/kg/week divided into equal doses 3-7 times/week
>   *Vial:* 5 mg/ml (2 ml)

Nutropin®Depot 1.5 mg/kg SC monthly on same day each month; max 22.5 mg/inj; divide injection if >22.5 mg
>   *Pediatric:* same as adult
>   *Vial:* 13.5, 18, 22.5 mg/vial (pwdr for injection after reconstitution; single-use w. diluent and needle)

Saizen® (B)
>   *Pediatric:* 0.06 mg/kg IM or SC 3 times/week
>   *Vial:* 5 mg (pwdr for SC injection w. diluent)

▶*somatrem* **(C)**
Protropin®
>   *Pediatric:* 0.3 mg/kg/week IM or SC divided into daily doses
>   *Vial:* 5 mg (15 IU), 10 mg (30 IU)

Comment: Administer growth hormones by SC injection into thigh, buttocks, or abdomen. Rotate sites with each dose. Contraindicated in children with fused epiphyses or evidence of neoplasia.

Headache: Migraine

Ergotamine Agents
▶*dihydroxyergotamine mesylate* **(X)**
DHE 45® 1 mg SC, IM, or IV; may repeat at 1 hour intervals; max 3 mg/day SC or IM/day; max 2 mg IV/day; max 6 mg/week
>   *Pediatric:* not recommended
>   *Amp:* 1 mg/ml (1 ml)

Migranal® 1 spray in each nostril; may repeat 15 minutes later; max 6 sprays/day and 8 sprays/week
>   *Pediatric:* not recommended
>   *Nasal spray:* 4 mg/ml; 0.5 mg/spray (caffeine)

▶*ergotamine* **(X)(G)**
Ergomar® 1 tab SL at onset of attack, then q 30 minutes as

Headache: Migraine

needed; max 3 tabs/day and 5 tabs/week
>   *Tab:* 2 mg
▶ *ergotamine/caffeine* **(X)(G)**
Cafergot® 2 tabs at onset of attack; then 1 tab every 1/2 hour if needed; max 6/attack, 10/week
>   *Pediatric:* not recommended
>   *Tab:* ergot 1 mg/*caf* 100 mg

Cafergot®Suppository 1 suppository rectally at onset of headache; may repeat x 1 after 1 hour; max 2/attack, 5/week
>   *Rectal supp:* ergot 2 mg/*caf* 100 mg

Wigraine® 2 tabs at onset of headache, then 1 tab q 1/2 hour as needed; max 6/attack, 10/week
>   *Pediatric:* not recommended
>   *Tab:* ergot 1 mg/*caf* 100 mg

Wigraine®Suppository 1 supp at onset of headache, then repeat q 1hour as needed; max 3/attack <u>and</u> 5/week
>   *Pediatric:* not recommended
>   *Supp:* ergot 2 mg/*caf* 100 mg

5-HT Receptor Agonists (Abortive Agents)

Comment: Contraindications to 5-HT receptor agonists include cardiovascular disease, ischemic heart disease cerebral vascular syndromes, peripheral vascular disease, uncontrolled hypertension, hemiplegic or basilar migraine.

▶ *almotriptan* **(C)** 6.25 or 12.5 mg; may repeat once after 2 hours; max 2 doses/day
>   *Pediatric:* <18 years: not recommended
>   **Axert®** *Tab:* 6.25 mg

▶ *eletriptan* **(C)** 20 or 40 mg; may repeat once after 2 hours; max 80 mg/day
>   *Pediatric:* <18 years: not recommended
>   **Relpax®** *Tab:* 20, 40 mg

▶ *frovatriptan* **(C)** 2.5 mg with fluids; may repeat once after 2 hours; max 7.5 mg/day
>   *Pediatric:* <18 years: not recommended
>   **Frova®** *Tab:* 2.5 mg

▶ *naratriptan* **(C)** 1 or 2.5 mg with fluids; may repeat once after 4 hours; max 5 mg/day
>   *Pediatric:* <18 years: not recommended
>   **Amerge®** *Tab:* 1, 2.5 mg

▶ *rizatriptan* **(C)** initially 5 or 10 mg; may repeat in 2 hours if needed; max 30 mg/day
>   *Pediatric:* <18 years: not recommended

Headache: Migraine

Maxalt® *Tab:* 5, 10 mg
Maxalt®-MLT *MLT tab:* 5, 10 mg orally-disintegrating
▶*sumatriptan* **(C)**
    Pediatric: <18 years: not recommended
Imitrex®Injectable 6 mg SC; may repeat after 1 hour if needed; max 2 doses/day
    Prefilled syringe: 4, 6 mg/0.5 ml (2/pck with or without auto injector)
Imitrex®Tab 25-200 mg x 1 dose; may be repeated at intervals of at least 2 hours if needed; max 200 mg/day
    Tab: 25, 50, 100 mg rapid rel
Imitrex®Nasal Spray 5-20 mg intranasally; may repeat once after 2 hours if needed; max 40 mg/day
    Pediatric: <18 years: not recommended
    Nasal spray: 25, 20 mg/spray (single-dose)
▶*zolmitriptan* **(C)** initially 2.5 mg; may repeat after 2 hours if needed; max 10 mg/day
    Pediatric: <18 years: not recommended
Zomig® *Tab:* 2.5*, 5 mg
Zomig®Nasal Spray *Nasal spray:* 5 mg/spray (6/box)
Zomig®-ZMT *Tab:* 2.5, 5*mg orally-disintegrating (orange, phenylalanine)

Comment: Do not use *ergotamine/caffeine* and *sumatriptan* within 24 hours of each other.

Other Analgesics
▶*acetaminophen/aspirin/caffeine* **(D)(G)**

Comment: Aspirin-containing medications are contraindicated with history of allergic-type reaction to aspirin, children and adolescents with *Varicella* or other viral illness, and 3rd trimester pregnancy.

    Excedrin®Migraine (OTC) 2 tabs q 6 hours prn; max 8 tabs/day x 2 days
        Pediatric: not recommended
        Tab: acet 250 mg/*asp* 250 mg/*caf* 65 mg
▶*isometheptene mucate/dichloralphenazone/acetaminophen* **(C)(IV)**
    Midrin® 2 caps initially followed by one q 1 hour until relieved; max 5 caps/12 hours
        Pediatric: not recommended
        Cap: iso 65 mg/*dichlor* 100 mg/*acet* 325 mg

Prophylaxis
▶*topiramate* **(C)** initially 25 mg daily in the PM; then 25 mg bid; then 25 mg in the AM and 50 mg in the PM; then, 50 mg bid

Pediatric: not recommended
Topamax® *Tab:* 25, 50, 100, 200 mg
Topamax®Sprinkle Caps *Cap:* 15, 25, 50 mg

Beta-Blockers

▶*atenolol* **(D)(G)** initially 25 mg bid; max 150 mg/day in divided doses
Pediatric: not recommended
Tenormin® *Tab:* 25, 50, 100 mg

▶*metoprolol* **(C)(G)**
Pediatric: not recommended
Lopressor® initially 50 mg/day in divided doses; max 300 mg/day
Tab: 50*, 100*mg
Toprol®-XL initially 50-100 mg daily; increase at weekly intervals if needed; max 400 mg/day
Tab: 25*, 50*, 100*, 200*mg ext-rel

▶*nadolol* **(C)(G)** initially 20 mg daily; max 240 mg/day in divided doses
Pediatric: not recommended
Corgard® *Tab:* 20*, 40*, 80*, 120*, 160*mg

▶*propranolol* **(C)(G)**
Inderal® initially 10 mg bid; usual range 160-320 mg/day in divided doses
Pediatric: not recommended
Tab: 10*, 20*, 40*, 60*, 80*mg
Inderal®LA initially 80 mg daily in a single dose; increase q 3-7 days; usual range 120-160 mg/day; max 320 mg/day in a single dose
Pediatric: not recommended
Cap: 60, 80, 120, 160 mg sust-rel
InnoPran®XL initially 80 mg q HS; max 120 mg/day
Cap: 80, 120 mg ext-rel

▶*timolol* **(C)(G)** initially 5 mg bid; max 60 mg/day in divided doses
Pediatric: not recommended
Blocadren® *Tab:* 5, 10*, 20*mg

Calcium Antagonists

▶*diltiazem* **(C)(G)**
Cardizem® initially 30 mg qid; may increase gradually every 1 to 2 days; max 360 mg/day in divided doses
Pediatric: not recommended
Tab: 30, 60, 90, 120 mg
Cardizem®CD initially 120-180 mg daily; adjust at 1 to 2 week intervals; max 480 mg/day

Pediatric: not recommended
Cap: 120, 180, 240, 300, 360 mg ext-rel

Cardizem®LA initially 180-240 mg daily; titrate at 2 week intervals; max 540 mg/day
Pediatric: not recommended
Tab: 120, 180, 240, 300, 360, 420 mg ext-rel

Cardizem®SR initially 60-120 mg bid; adjust at 2 week intervals; max 360 mg/day
Pediatric: not recommended
Cap: 60, 90, 120 mg sust-rel

▶*nifedipine* **(C)(G)**
Pediatric: not recommended

Adalat® initially 10 mg tid; usual range 10-20 mg tid; max 180 mg/day
Cap: 10, 20 mg

Procardia® initially 10 mg tid; titrate over 7-14 days: max 30 mg/dose and 180 mg/day in divided doses
Cap: 10, 20 mg

Procardia®XL initially 30-60 mg daily; titrate over 7-14 days; max 90 mg/day in divided doses

▶*verapamil* **(C)(G)**
Pediatric: not recommended

Calan® 80-120 mg tid; increase daily or weekly if needed
Tab: 40, 80*, 120*mg

Covera®HS initially 180 mg q HS; titrate in steps to 240 mg; then to 360 mg; then to 480 mg if needed
Tab: 180, 240 mg ext-rel

Isoptin® initially 80-120 mg tid
Tab: 40, 80, 120 mg

Isoptin®SR initially 120-180 mg in the AM; may increase to 240 mg in the AM; then 180 mg q 12 hours or 240 mg in the AM and 120 mg in the PM, then 240 mg q 12 hours
Tab: 120, 180*, 240*mg sust-rel

TCA Antidepressants

▶*amitriptyline* **(C)** 10-20 mg q HS
Pediatric: not recommended
Amitryl®, **Endep®** *Tab:* 10, 25, 50, 75, 100, 150 mg

▶*doxepin* **(C)(G)** 10-200 mg q HS
Pediatric: not recommended
Adapin®, **Sinequan®** *Cap:* 10, 25, 50, 75, 100, 150 mg; *Oral conc:* 10 mg/ml (4 oz w. dropper)

▶*imipramine* **(C)(G)** 10-200 mg q HS
Tofranil® 25-50 mg; max 200 mg/day; if maintenance dose exceeds 75 mg daily, may switch to **Tofranil®PM**
Pediatric: <6 years: not recommended
6-12 years: initially 25 mg
>12 years: 50 mg
Max 2.5 mg/kg/day
Tab: 10, 25, 50 mg
Tofranil®PM initially 75 mg daily; max 200 mg
Pediatric: not recommended
Cap: 75, 100, 125, 150
Tofranil®Injection up to 50 mg IM; lower dose for adolescents; switch to oral form when possible
Pediatric: not recommended
Amp: 25 mg/2 ml (2 ml)
▶*nortriptyline* **(D)** 10-150 mg q HS
Pediatric: not recommended
Aventyl®, Pamelor® *Cap:* 10, 25, 50, 75 mg; *Oral soln:* 10 mg/5 ml (16 oz); *Cap:* 10, 25, 50, 75 mg; *Oral soln:* 10 mg/5 ml (16 oz)

SSRI Antidepressant
▶*fluoxetine* **(C)(G)**
Prozac® initially 20 mg daily; may increase after 1 week; doses >20 mg/day should be divided into AM and noon doses; max 80 mg/day
Pediatric: <8 years: not recommended
8-17 years: initially 10 or 20 mg/day; start lower weight children at 10 mg/day; if starting at 10 mg daily, may increase after 1 week to 20 mg daily
Tab: 10*mg; *Cap:* 10, 20, 40 mg; *Oral soln:* 20 mg/5 ml (4 oz; mint)
Prozac®Weekly following daily fluoxetine therapy at 20 mg/day for 13 weeks, may initiate **Prozac®Weekly** 7 days after the last 20 mg fluoxetine dose
Pediatric: not recommended
Cap: 90 mg ent-coat del-rel pellets

Other Agents
▶*divalproex sodium* **(D)**
Pediatric: <10 years: not recommended
>10 years: same as adult
Depakene® *Cap:* 250 mg; *Syr:* 250 mg/5 ml (16 oz)
Depakote® *Tab:* 125, 250 mg

Headache: Migraine

    Depakote®ER *Tab:* 250, 500 mg ext-rel
    Depakote®Sprinkle *Cap:* 125 mg
▶ *methysergide* **(C)** 4-8 mg daily in divided doses with food; max 8 mg/day; max 6 month treatment course; wean off over last 2-3 weeks of treatment course; separate treatment courses by 3-4 week drug-free interval
    Sansert® *Tab:* 2 mg

Headache: Tension (Muscle Contraction Headache)

NSAIDs *see **Pain** page 305*
Oral Non-narcotic Analgesics *see **Pain** page 308*
Oral Narcotic Analgesics *see **Pain** page 308*
Topical Analgesics *see **Pain** page 308*
Parenteral Glucocorticosteroids *see page 389*
Oral Glucocorticosteroids *see page 387*
Topical Anesthetic *see page 383*
Topical Anesthetic/Steroid Combinations *see page 480*
TCA Antidepressants
▶ *amitriptyline* **(C)(G)** 50-100 mg/day
    Pediatric: not recommended
    Amitryl®, Endep® *Tab:* 10, 25, 50, 75, 100, 150 mg
    ▶ *desipramine* **(C)(G)** 50-100 mg bid
        Pediatric: not recommended
    Norpramin® *Tab:* 10, 25, 50, 75, 100, 150 mg
▶ *imipramine* **(C)(G)**
    Pediatric: not recommended
    Tofranil® initially 75 mg daily (max 200 mg); adolescents Initially 30-40 mg daily (max 100 mg/day); if maintenance dose exceeds 75 mg daily, may switch to **Tofranil®PM** for divided or bedtime dose
        Tab: 10, 25, 50 mg
    Tofranil®PM initially 75 mg daily 1 hour before HS; max 200 mg
        Cap: 75, 100, 125, 150
    Tofranil®Injection 50 mg IM; lower dose for adolescents; switch to oral form as soon as possible
        Amp: 25 mg/2 ml (2 ml)
▶ *nortriptyline* **(D)(G)** 25-50 mg/day
    Pediatric: not recommended
    Pamelor® *Cap:* 10, 25, 50, 75 mg; *Oral soln:* 10 mg/5 ml (16 oz)

Analgesics

▶ *butalbital/acetaminophen* **(C)(II)(G)**
  Pediatric: <12 years: not recommended
  Axocet®, Bupap®, Dolgic® 1 tab q 4 hours prn; max 6 tabs/day
    Tab: but 50 mg/*acet* 650 mg
  Phrenilin®, Promicet® 1 tab q 4 hours prn; max 6 tabs/day
    Tab: but 50 mg/*acet* 325 mg
  Phrenilin®Forte 1 cap q 4 hours prn; max 6 caps/day
    Cap: but 50 mg/*acet* 650 mg
▶ *butalbital/acetaminophen/codeine/caffeine* **(C)(III)(G)**
  Fioricet®with Codeine 1-2 tabs at onset q 4 hours prn; max 6 tabs/day
    Pediatric: <12 years: not recommended
    Tab: but 50 mg/*acet* 325 mg/*cod* 30 mg/*caf* 40 mg
▶ *butalbital/aspirin/caffeine* **(C)(III)(G)**
  Fiorinal® 1-2 tabs q 4 hours prn; max 6 caps/day
    Cap: but 50 mg/*asa* 325 mg/*caf* 40 mg
▶ *butalbital/aspirin/codeine/caffeine* **(C)(III)(G)**
  Fiorinal®with Codeine 1-2 tabs q 4 hours prn; max 6 caps/day
    Cap: but 50 mg/*asp* 325 mg/*cod* 30 mg/*caf* 40 mg
▶ *butorphanol* **(C)(IV)(G)** initially 1 spray in 1 nostril; may repeat after 60-90 minutes if needed; may repeat again in 3-4 hours
  Pediatric: <18 years: not recommended
  Butorphanol®Nasal Spray *Nasal spray:* 10 mg/ml, 1 mg/actuation (2.5 ml)
  Stadol®NS *Nasal spray:* 10 mg/ml, 1 mg/actuation (2.5 ml)
▶ *tramadol* **(C)(G)** 50-100 mg q 4-6 hours prn
  Ultram® *Tab:* 50*mg
▶ *tramadol/acetaminophen* **(C)(G)** 2 tabs q 4-6 hours; max 8 tabs/day; max 5 days
  Pediatric: not recommended
  Ultracet® *Tab:* tram 37.5/*acet* 325 mg
Other Narcotic Analgesics and Combinations see *Pain* page 308

Helicobacter pylori Infection (*H. Pylori Bacterium*)

Helicobacter Pylori
Eradication Regimens

Comment: There are many H_2 receptor blocker-based and PPI-based treatment regimens suggested in the professional literature for the eradication of the *H. pylori* organism and subsequent ulcer healing. Generally,

Helicobacter pylori

regimens range from 10 to 14 days for eradication and 2 to 6 more weeks of continued gastric acid suppression. A 2-antibiotic combination may increase treatment effectiveness and decrease the likelihood of resistant strain emergence. Empirical treatment is not recommended. Diagnosis should be confirmed before treatment is started. Antibiotic choices include doxycycline, tetracycline, amoxicillin, amoxicillin/ clavulanate, clarithromycin, clindamycin, metronidazole. Follow-up visits are recommended at 2 weeks and 6 weeks to evaluate treatment outcomes.

Regimen 1: Helidac®Therapy *bismuth subsalicylate* 525 mg qid + *tetracycline* 500 mg qid + *metronidazole* 250 mg qid x 14 days
    bismuth subsalicylate **(B; D in 3rd)** *Chew tab:* 262.4 mg (112/pck); *tetracycline* **(D)** *Cap:* 500 mg (56/pck);
    metronidazole **(not for use in 1st; B in 2nd, 3rd)** *Tab:* 250 mg (56/pck)

Regimen 2: PrevPac® *amoxicillin* 500 mg 2 caps bid + *lansoprazole* 30 mg bid + *clarithromycin* 500 mg bid x 14 days (one pack per day);
    lansoprazole **(B)** *Cap:* 30 mg (2/pck); *amoxicillin* **(B)** *Cap:* 500 mg (4/pck); *clarithromycin* **(C)** *Tab:* 500 mg (2/pck)

Regimen 3: *omeprazole* 40 mg daily + *clarithromycin* 500 mg tid x 2 weeks; then continue *omeprazole* 10-40 mg daily x 6 more weeks

Regimen 4: *lansoprazole* 30 mg tid + *amoxicillin* 1 g tid x 10 days; then continue *lansoprazole* 15-30 mg daily x 6 more weeks

Regimen 5: *omeprazole* 40 mg daily + *amoxicillin* 1 g bid + *clarithromycin* 500 mg bid x 10 days; then continue *omeprazole* 10-40 mg daily x 6 more weeks

Regimen 6: *bismuth subsalicylate* 525 mg qid + *metronidazole* 250 mg qid + *tetracycline* 500 mg qid + H_2 receptor agonist x 2 weeks; then continue H_2 receptor agonist x 6 more weeks

Regimen 7: *bismuth subsalicylate* 525 mg qid + *metronidazole* 250 mg qid + *amoxicillin* 500 mg qid + H_2 receptor agonist x 2 weeks; then continue H_2 receptor agonist x 6 more weeks

Regimen 8: *ranitidine bismuth citrate* 400 mg bid + *clarithromycin* 500 mg bid x 2 weeks; then continue *ranitidine bismuth citrate* 400 mg bid x 2 more weeks

Regimen 9: *omeprazole* 20 mg or *lansoprazole* 30 mg q AM + *bismuth subsalicylate* 524 mg qid + *metronidazole* 500 mg tid + *tetracycline* 500 mg qid x 2 weeks; then continue *omeprazole* 20 mg or *lansoprazole* 30 mg q AM for 6 more weeks

Hemorrhoids

▶ *dibucaine* **(C)(G)** 1 applicatorful or suppository bid and after each stool; max 6 supp/day
  Pediatric: not recommended
  Nupercainal® (OTC) *Rectal oint:* 1% (30, 60 g); *Rectal supp:* 1% (12, 14/pck)

▶ *hydrocortisone* **(C)(G)**
  Pediatric: not recommended
  Anusol®-HC 1 suppository rectally bid-tid or 2 rectally bid x 2 weeks
    Rectal supp: 25 mg (12, 24/pck)
  Anusol®-HC Cream 2.5% apply bid-qid
    Rectal crm: 2.5% (30 g)
  Anusol®HC-1 (OTC) apply tid-qid; max 7 days
    Rectal crm: 1% (0.7 oz)
  Nupercainal® (OTC) apply tid-qid
    Rectal crm: 1% (30 g)
  Proctocort® 1 suppository rectally bid-tid or 2 bid x 2 weeks
    Rectal supp: 30 mg (12/pck)
  Proctocream®HC 2.5% apply rectally bid-qid
    Rectal crm: 2.5% (30 g)
  Proctofoam®HC 1% apply rectally tid-qid
    Rectal foam: 1% (14 applications/10 g)

▶ *petrolatum/mineral oil/shark liver oil/phenylephrine* **(C)(G)**
  Preparation H®Ointment (OTC) apply up to qid
    Rectal oint: 1, 2 oz

▶ *petrolatum/glycerin/shark liver oil/phenylephrine* **(C)(G)**
  Preparation H®Cream (OTC) apply up to qid
    Rectal crm: 0.9, 1.8 oz

▶ *phenylephrine/cocoa butter/shark liver oil* **(C)(G)**
  Preparation H®Suppositories (OTC) 1 rectally up to qid
    Rectal supp: phen 0.25%/cocoa 85.5%/shark 3% (12, 24, 45/pck)
    Rectal oint: phen 0.25%/petro 1.9%/mineral oil 14%/shark 3% (1, 2 oz)
    Rectal crm: phen 0.25%/petro 18%/gly 12%/shark 3% (0.9, 1.8 oz)

▶ *witch hazel*
  Tucks® (OTC) apply up to 6 times/day; leave on x 5-15 minutes
    Pad: 12, 40, 100/pck; *Gel:* 19.8 g

Hemorrhoids

▶ *lidocaine* 3% cream **(B)** apply bid-tid prn
    Pediatric: reduce dosage commensurate with age, body weight, and physical condition
    LidaMantle® *Crm:* 3% (1 oz)

Bulk-forming Agents, Stool Softeners, and Stimulant Laxatives
see Constipation page 123

Hepatitis A (HAV)

Comment: Schedule first immunization at least 2 weeks before expected exposure. Booster dose recommended 6-12 months later. Under 1 year administer in vastus lateralis; over 1 year administer in deltoid.

Prophylaxis (Hepatitis A)
▶ *hepatitis A vaccine, inactivated* **(C)**
    Havrix® 1440 El.U IM; repeat in 6-12 months
        Pediatric: <2 years: not recommended
                    2-18 years: 720 El.U IM; repeat in 6-12 months or 360 El.U IM; repeat in 1 month
    Vaqta® 25 U (1 ml) IM; repeat in 6 months
        Pediatric: <2 years: not recommended
                    2-18 years: 0.5 ml IM; repeat in 6-18 months
    Vial: 25 U/ml single-dose (preservative-free); *Prefilled syringe:* 25 U/ml, (0.5, 1 ml single-dose)

Prophylaxis (Hepatitis A and B Combination)
▶ *hepatitis A* inactivated/*hepatitis B* surface antigen (recombinant vaccine **(C)**
    Pediatric: <18 years: not recommended
    Twinrix® 1 ml IM in deltoid; repeat in 1 month and 6 months
    Vial (soln): hepatitis A inactivated 720 IU/*hepatitis B* surface antigen (recombinant) 20 mcg/ml (1, 10 ml); *Prefilled syringe: hepatitis A* inactivated 720 IU/*hepatitis B* surface antigen (recombinant) 20 mcg/ml

---

Hepatitis B (HBV)

Comment: Under 1 year administer in vastus lateralis; over 1 year administer in deltoid.

Prophylaxis (Hepatitis B)
▶ *hepatitis B* recombinant vaccine **(C)**
    Engerix-B®Adult 20 mcg (1 ml) IM; repeat in 1 and 6 months

Pediatric: infant-19 years: 10 mcg (1/2 ml) IM; repeat in 1 and 6 months
Vial: 20 mcg/ml single-dose (preservative-free, thimerosal); *Prefilled syringe*: 20 mcg/ml

Engerix-B®Pediatric/Adolescent
Pediatric: infant-19 years: 10 mcg IM; repeat in 1 and 6 months
Vial: 10 mcg/0.5 ml single-dose (preservative-free, thimerosal); *Prefilled syringe:* 10 mcg/0.5 ml

Recombivax HB®Adult 10 mcg (1 ml) IM in deltoid; repeat in 1 and 6 months
Vial: 10 mcg/ml single-dose; *Vial:* 10 mcg/3 ml multi-dose

Recombivax HB®Pediatric/Adolescent 5 mcg (0.5 ml) IM; repeat in 1 and 6 months
Pediatric: birth-19 years: 5 mcg (0.5 ml) IM; repeat in 1 and 6 months
>19 years: use adult formulation or 10 mcg (1 ml) pediatric/adolescent formulation
Vial: 5 mcg/0.5 ml single-dose

Prophylaxis (Hepatitis A and B Combination)

▶*hepatitis A inactivated/hepatitis B surface antigen (recombinant) vaccine* **(C)**
Pediatric: <18 years: not recommended
Twinrix® 1 ml IM in deltoid; repeat in 1 months and 6 months
Vial (soln): hepatitis A inactivated 720 IU/*hepatitis B* surface antigen (recombinant) 20 mcg/ml (1, 10 ml); *Prefilled syringe: hepatitis A* inactivated 720 IU/*hepatitis B* surface antigen (recombinant) 20 mcg/ml

Chronic HBV Infection Treatment
Nucleoside Analogues (Reverse Transcriptase Inhibitors & HBV Polymerase Inhibitors)

Comment: Nucleoside analogues are indicated for chronic hepatitis infection with viral replication and either elevated ALT/AST or histologically active disease.

▶*adefovir dipivoxil* **(C)** 10 mg daily
CrCl 20-49 mL/min: 10 mg q 48 hours
CrCl 10-19 mL/min: 10 mg q 72 hours
Pediatric: not recommended
Hepsera® *Tab:* 10 mg

▶*entecavir* **(C)** take on an empty stomach
Nucleoside naïve: 0.5 mg daily
Nucleoside naïve, CrCl 30-49 mL/min: 0.25 mg daily

Hepatitis B

Nucleoside naïve, CrCl 10-29 mL/min: 0.15 mg daily
Nucleoside naïve, CrCl <10 mL/min: 0.05 mg daily
Lamivudine-refractory: 1 mg daily
Lamivudine-refractory, renal impairment: see mfr literature
> *Pediatric:* <16 years: not recommended

Baraclude® *Tab:* 0.5, 1 mg; *Oral Soln* 0.05 mg/ml (orange, parabens)

▶ *lamivudine* **(C)** 100 mg daily
> *Pediatric:* not recommended

Epivir-HBV® *Tab:* 100 mg
Epivir-HBV® Oral Solution
> *Oral Soln:* 5 mg/ml (240 ml; strawberry-banana)

Interferon Alpha

▶ *interferon alfa-2b* **(C)** 5 million IU SC or IM daily or 10 million IU SC or IM 3 times/week x 16 weeks; reduce dose by half or interrupt dose if WBCs, granulocyte count, or platelet count decreases
> *Pediatric:* <1 year: not recommended
>> >1 year: 3 million IU/m^2 3 times/week x 1 week; then increase to 6 million IU/m^2 3 times/week to 16-24 weeks; max 10 million IU/dose; reduce dose by half or interrupt dose if WBCs, granulocyte count, or platelet count decreases

Intron A® *Vial (pwdr):* 5, 10, 18, 25, 50 million IU/vial (pwdr + diluent; single-dose) (benzoyl alcohol); *Vial (soln):* 3, 5, 10 million IU/vial (single-dose); *Multidose vials (soln):* 18, 25 million IU/vial soln; *Multidose pens (soln):* 3, 5, 10 million IU/0.2 ml (6 doses/pen)

Hepatitis C (HCV)

Chronic HCV Infection Treatment
Nucleoside Analogues (Reverse Transcriptase Inhibitors)

Comment: Nucleoside analogues are indicated for patients with compensated liver disease previously untreated with *alpha interferon* or who have relapsed after *alpha interferon* therapy. Primary toxicity is hemolytic anemia. Contraindicated in male partners of pregnant women; use 2 forms of contraception during therapy and for 6 months after discontinuation.

▶ *ribavirin* **(X)**
> *Interferon*-naive: treat for 24-48 weeks
> Relapse: treat for 24 weeks
>> >18 years (<75 kg): 400 mg in AM and 600 mg in PM
>> >18 years (>75 kg): 600 mg in AM and 600 mg in PM

Pediatric: not recommended
Copegus® *Tab:* 200 mg
Rebetol® *Tab:* 100 mg; *Cap:* 200*mg
Rebetol®Solution *Soln:* 40 mg/ml (120 ml)

Interferon Alpha

▶*interferon alfacon-1* **(C)**

Pediatric: <18 years: not recommended

Infergon® 9 mcg SC three times/week x 24 weeks, then 15 mcg SC 3 times/week x 6 months; allow at least 48 hours between doses

Vial (soln): 9, 15 mcg/vial soln (6-single dose/pck; preservative-free)

Wellferon® 3 million IU SC or IM 3 times/week x 18-24 months

Vial (soln): 3 million IU/ml (preservative-free)

Pediatric: <1 year: not recommended

>1 year: 3 million IU/m^2 3 times/week x 1 week; then increase to 6 million IU/m^2 3 times/week to 16-24 weeks; max 10 million IU/reduce dose by half or interrupt dose if WBCs, granulocyte count, or platelet count decreases

▶*interferon alfa-2b*

Intron A® *Vial (pwdr):* 5, 10, 18, 25, 50 million IU/vial (pwdr w. diluent; single-dose) (benzoyl alcohol); *Vial (soln):* 3, 5, 10 million IU/vial (single-dose); *Multidose vials (soln):* 18, 25 million IU/vial Soln; *Multidose pens (soln):* 3, 5, 10 million IU/0.2 ml (6 doses/pen)

▶*peginterferon alfa-2a* **(C)** administer 180 mcg SC once weekly (on the same day of the week); treat for 48 weeks; consider discontinuing if adequate response after 12-24 weeks

Pediatric: <18 years: not recommended

PEGasys® *Vial:* 180 mcg/ml (single-dose); *Monthly pck (vials):* 180 mcg/ml (1 ml, 4/pck)

▶*peginterferon alfa-2b* **(C)** administer SC once weekly (on the same day of the week); treat for 1 year; consider discontinuing if inadequate response after 24 weeks; initially:

37-45 kg: 40 mcg (100 mg/ml, 0.4 ml)
46-56 kg: 50 mcg (100 mg/ml, 0.5 ml)
57-72 kg: 64 mcg (160 mg/ml, 0.4 ml)
73-88 kg: 80 mcg (160 mg/ml, 0.5 ml)
89-106 kg: 96 mcg (240 mg/ml, 0.4 ml)
107-136 kg: 120 mcg (240 mg/ml, 0.5 ml)
137-160 kg: 150 mcg (300 mg/ml, 0.5 ml)

Pediatric: <18 years: not recommended

Hepatitis C

PEG-Intron® *Vial:* 50, 80, 120, 150 mcg/ml (single-dose)
PEG-Intron®Redipen *Pen:* 50, 80, 120, 150 mcg/ml (disposable pens)

Nucleoside Analogue (Reverse Transcriptase Inhibitor)/Interferon Combination

▶*ribavirin/interferon alfa-2b* **(X)**
<75 kg (>18 yrs): *ribavirin* 400 mg in AM and 600 mg in PM x 24 weeks

plus

interferon alfa-2b 3 million IU SC 3 times/week
>75 kg (>18 yrs): *ribavirin* 600 mg in AM and 600 mg in PM x 24 weeks

plus

interferon alfa-2b 3 million IU SC 3 times/week
Pediatric: <18 years: not recommended

Rebetron®Combination Therapy
Comb pack: rib 200*mg caps + *interf* 3 million IU per vial;
rib 200*mg caps + *interf* 18 million IU per vial or pen

Comment: **Rebetron®** is indicated for patients with compensated liver disease previously untreated with *alpha interferon* or who have relapsed after *alpha interferon* therapy. Contraindicated in male partners of pregnant women (the *ribavirin*, a nucleoside analogue, is pregnancy category X); use 2 forms of contraception during therapy and for 6 months after discontinuation.

Herpangina

Analgesics
▶*acetaminophen* **(B)** see ***Fever*** *page 168*
▶*tramadol* **(C)(G)** 50-100 mg q 4-6 hours prn
Pediatric: <16 years: not recommended
Ultram® *Tab:* 50*mg
▶*tramadol/acetaminophen* **(C)** 2 tabs q 4-6 hours; max 8 tabs/day; max 5 days
CrCl <30 ml/min: max 2 tabs q 12 hours; max 5 days
Pediatric: not recommended
Ultracet® *Tab: tram* 37.5 mg/*acet* 325 mg

Oral Narcotic Analgesics see ***Pain*** *page 308*

Topical Anesthetics
▶*lidocaine* viscous soln **(B)** 15 ml gargle or mouthwash; repeat after 3 hours; max 8 doses/day
Pediatric: <3 years: 1.25 ml apply to affected area with

cotton-tipped applicator; may repeat after 3 hours; max 8 doses/day
Xylocaine®2% Viscous Solution *Viscous soln:* 2% (20 ml, 100, 450 ml)

Antipyretics see *Fever* page 168

Herpes Genitalis (Herpes Simplex Virus Type II)

Primary Infection
▶*acyclovir* **(B)(G)** 400 mg tid x 7-10 days or 200 mg 5 times/day x 10 days or until clinically resolved
    Pediatric: see page 568 for dose by weight
        <2 years: not recommended
        >2 years, <40 kg: 20 mg/kg 5 times/day x 10 days or until clinically resolved
        >2 years, >40 kg: 800 mg 5 times/day x 10 days or until clinically resolved
    Zovirax® *Cap:* 200 mg; *Tab:* 400, 800 mg
    Zovirax®Oral Suspension *Oral susp:* 200 mg/5 ml (banana)
▶*acyclovir* **(B)(G)** cream apply q 3 hours 6 times/day x 7 days
    Pediatric: <2 years: not recommended
        >2 years: same as adult
    Zovirax®Cream *Crm:* 5% (3, 15 g); *Oint:* 5% (3, 15 g)
▶*famciclovir* **(B)** 250 mg tid x 7-10 days or until clinically resolved
    Pediatric: <18 years: not recommended
    Famvir® *Tab:* 125, 250, 500 mg
▶*valacyclovir* **(B)** 1 g bid x 10 days or until clinically resolved
    Pediatric: not recommended
    Valtrex® *Cplt:* 500, 1000 mg

Recurrent Episodes
cont-rel Initiate treatment of recurrent episodes within 1 day of onset of lesions.
▶*acyclovir* **(B)(G)** 200 mg 5 times/day x 5 days
    Pediatric: see page 568 for dose by weight
        <2 years: not recommended
        >2 years, <40 kg: 20 mg/kg 5 times/day x 5 days
        >2 years, >40 kg: 800 mg 5 times/day x 5 days
    Zovirax® *Cap:* 200 mg; *Tab:* 400, 800 mg
    Zovirax®Oral Suspension *Oral susp:* 200 mg/5 ml (banana)
▶*famciclovir* **(B)** 125 mg bid x 5 days
    Pediatric: <18 years: not recommended
    Famvir® *Tab:* 125, 250, 500 mg

Herpes Genitalis

▶*valacyclovir* **(B)** 500 mg bid x 3-5 days or until clinically resolved
    Pediatric: not recommended
  Valtrex® *Cplt:* 500, 1000 mg

Suppression Therapy
▶*acyclovir* **(B)(G)** 400 mg bid x 1 year
    Pediatric: see page 568 for dose by weight
        <2 years: not recommended
        >2 years, <40 kg: 20 mg/kg bid x 1 year
        >2 years, >40 kg: 400 mg bid x 1 year
  Zovirax® *Cap:* 200 mg; *Tab:* 400, 800 mg
  Zovirax®Oral Suspension *Oral susp:* 200 mg/5 ml (banana)
▶*famciclovir* **(B)** 250 mg bid x 1 year
    Pediatric: <18 years: not recommended
  Famvir® *Tab:* 125, 250, 500 mg
▶*valacyclovir* **(B)** 500 mg daily x 1 year (for < 9 recurrences/year)
or 1 g daily x 1 year (for >9 recurrences/year)
    Pediatric: not recommended
  Valtrex® *Cplt:* 500, 1000 mg

Herpes labialis
(Herpes Simplex Virus Type II, Cold Sore, Fever Blister)

Primary Infection
▶*acyclovir* **(B)** 200 mg 5 times/day x 7-10 days
    Pediatric: see page 568 for dose by weight
        <2 years: not recommended
        >2 years, <40 kg: 20 mg/kg 5 times/day x 7-10 days
        >2 years, >40 kg: 800 mg 5 times/day x 7-10 days
  Zovirax® *Cap:* 200 mg; *Tab:* 400, 800 mg
  Zovirax®Oral Suspension *Oral susp:* 200 mg/5 ml (banana)
▶*valacyclovir* **(B)** 2 g q 12 hours x 1 day
    Pediatric: not recommended
  Valtrex® *Cplt:* 500, 1000 mg

Suppression Therapy (for 6 or more outbreaks/year)
▶*acyclovir* **(B)(G)** 200 mg 2-5 times/day x 1 year
    Pediatric: see page 568 for dose by weight
        <2 years: not recommended
        >2 years, <40 kg: 20 mg/kg 2-5 times/day x 1 year
        >2 years, >40 kg: 200 mg 2-5 times/day x 1 year
  Zovirax® *Cap:* 200 mg; *Tab:* 400, 800 mg

Zovirax®Oral Suspension *Oral susp:* 200 mg/5 ml (banana)
Topical Therapy
▶*acyclovir* **(B)(G)** oint apply q 3 hours 6 times/day x 7 days
    Pediatric: <2 years: not recommended
             >2 years: same as adult
    Zovirax®Cream *Crm:* 5% (3, 15 g); *Oint:* 5% (3, 15 g)
▶*docosanol* **(B)** apply and gently rub in 5 times daily until healed
    Pediatric: not recommended
    Abreva® (OTC) *Crm:* 10% (2 g)
▶*penciclovir* **(B)** apply q 2 hours while awake x 4 days
    Pediatric: not recommended
    Denavir® *Crm:* 1% (2 g)

Herpes zoster (Shingles)

Oral Antivirals
▶*famciclovir* **(B)** 500 mg tid x 7 days
    Pediatric: <18 years: not recommended
    Famvir® *Tab:* 125, 250, 500 mg
▶*valacyclovir* **(B)** 1 g tid x 7 days
    Pediatric: not recommended
    Valtrex® *Cplt:* 500, 1000 mg
▶*acyclovir* **(B)(G)** 800 mg 5 times/day x 7-10 days
    Pediatric: see page 568 for dose by weight
             <2 years: not recommended
             >2 years, <40 kg: 20 mg/kg 5 times/day x 7-10 days
             >2 years, >40 kg: 800 mg 5 times/day x 7-10 days
    Zovirax® *Cap:* 200 mg; *Tab:* 400, 800 mg
    Zovirax®Oral Suspension *Oral susp:* 200 mg/5 ml (banana)
Prophylaxis against Secondary Infection
▶*silver sulfadiazine* **(B)** apply qid
    Pediatric: not recommended
    Silvadene® *Crm:* 1% (20, 50, 85, 400, 1000 g jar; 20 g tube)
Analgesics
▶*acetaminophen* **(B)** see ***Fever*** page 168
▶*aspirin* **(D)** see ***Fever*** page 169
Comment: Aspirin-containing medications are contraindicated with history of allergic-type reaction to aspirin, children and adolescents with *varicella* or other viral illness, and 3rd trimester pregnancy.
▶*tramadol* **(C)(G)** 50-100 mg q 4-6 hours prn
    Pediatric: <16 years: not recommended

Ultram® *Tab:* 50*mg
▶*tramadol/acetaminophen* **(C)(G)** 2 tabs q 4-6 hours; max 8 tabs/day; max 5 days
  CrCl <30 ml/min: max 2 tabs q 12 hours; max 5 days
    Pediatric: not recommended
  Ultracet® *Tab:* tram 37.5/acet 325 mg
Oral Narcotic Analgesics see *Pain* page 308
Post-herpetic Neuralgia see page 349
Secondary Infection Prophylaxis
▶*silver sulfadiazine* **(B)** apply qid
    Pediatric: not recommended
  Silvadene® *Crm:* 1% (20, 50, 85, 400, 1000 g/jar; 20 g tube)

Hiccups: Intractable

▶*chlorpromazine* **(C)** 25-50 mg tid-qid
    Pediatric: <6 months: not recommended
      >6 months: 0.25 mg/lb orally q 4-6 hours prn or
      0.5 mg/lb rectally q 6-8 hours prn
  Thorazine® *Tab:* 10, 25, 50, 100, 200 mg; *Spansule:* 30, 75, 150 mg sust-rel; *Syr:* 10 mg/5 ml (4 oz; orange custard); *Oral conc:* 30 mg/ml (4 oz); 100 mg/ml (2, 8 oz); *Supp:* 25, 100 mg

Hidradenitis Suppurativa

Oral Anti-infectives
▶*doxycycline* **(D)(G)** 100 mg bid x 7-14 days
    Pediatric: see page 587 for dose by weight
      <8 years: not recommended
      >8 years, <100 lb: 2 mg/lb on first day in 2 doses, followed by 1 mg/lb/day in 1-2 doses
      >8 years, >100 lb: same as adult
  Adoxa® *Tab:* 50, 100 mg ent-coat
  Doryx® *Cap:* 100 mg
  Monodox® *Cap:* 50, 100 mg
  Vibramycin® *Cap:* 50, 100 mg; *Syr:* 50 mg/5 ml (raspberry-apple, sulfites); *Oral susp:* 25 mg/5 ml (raspberry)
  Vibra-Tab® *Tab:* 100 mg film-coat
Comment: Doxycycline is contraindicated in pregnancy (discolors fetal tooth

enamel).
▶ *erythromycin base* **(B)(G)** 1-1.5 g daily x 7-14 days
> *Pediatric: see page 588 for dose by weight*
> <45 kg: 30-50 mg in 2-4 doses x 7-14 days
> >45 kg: same as adult

E-Mycin® *Tab:* 250; 333 mg ent-coat
Eryc® *Cap:* 250 mg ent-coat
Ery-Tab® *Tab:* 250, 333, 500 mg ent-coat
PCE® *Tab:* 333, 500 mg

▶ *minocycline* **(D)** 100 mg bid x 7-14 days
> *Pediatric:* <8 years: not recommended
> >8 years: same as adult

Dynacin® *Cap:* 50, 100 mg
Minocin® *Cap:* 50, 100 mg; *Oral susp:* 50 mg/5 ml (2 oz; custard, sulfites, alcohol 5%)

Comment: Minocycline is contraindicated in pregnancy (discolors fetal tooth enamel).

▶ *tetracycline* **(D)(G)** 250 mg qid or 500 mg tid x 7-14 days
> *Pediatric: see page 595 for dose by weight*
> <8 years: not recommended
> >8 years, <100 lb: 25-50 mg/kg/day in 2-4 doses x 7-14 days
> >8 years, >100 lb: same as adult

Achromycin®**V** *Cap:* 250, 500 mg
Sumycin® *Tab:* 250, 500 mg; *Cap:* 250, 500 mg; *Oral susp:* 125 mg/5 ml (100, 200 ml; fruit, sulfites)

Comment: Tetracycline is contraindicated in pregnancy (discolors fetal tooth enamel).

Topical Anti-infectives
▶ *clindamycin* **(B)** topical apply bid x 7-14 days
Cleocin®**T** *Pad:* 1% (60/pck; alcohol 50%); *Lotn:* 1% (60 ml); *Gel:* 1% (30, 60 g); *Soln w. applicator:* 1% (30, 60 ml; alcohol 50%)

Hookworm (*Uncinariasis*)

Anthelmintics
▶ *albendazole* **(C)** 400 mg as a single dose; may repeat in 3 weeks
> *Pediatric:* <2 years: 200 mg daily x 3 days; may repeat in 3 weeks
> 2-12 years: 400 mg daily x 3 days; may repeat in 3

Hookworm

weeks
    Albenza® *Tab:* 200 mg
▶ *mebendazole* **(C)(G)** 100 mg AM and PM x 3 consecutive days or 500 mg as a single dose; may repeat in 2-3 weeks if needed
    Pediatric: same as adult (chew or crush and mix with food)
    Vermox® *Chew tab:* 100 mg
▶ *pyrantel pamoate* **(C)** 11 mg/kg x 1 dose; max 1 g/dose
    Pediatric: 25-37 lb: 1/2 tsp x 1 dose
              38-62 lb: 1 tsp x 1 dose
              63-87 lb: 1½ tsp x 1 dose
              88-112 lb: 2 tsp x 1 dose
              113-137 lb: 2½ tsp x 1 dose
              138-162 lb: 3 tsp x 1 dose
              163-187 lb: 3½ tsp x 1 dose
              >187 lb: 4 tsp x 1 dose
    Antiminth® **(OTC)** *Cap:* 180 mg; *Liq:* 50 mg/ml (30 ml); 144 mg/ml (30 ml); *Oral susp:* 50 mg/ml (60 ml)
    Pin-X® **(OTC)** *Cap:* 180 mg; *Liq:* 50 mg/ml (30 ml); 144 mg/ml (30 ml); *Oral susp:* 50 mg/ml (30 ml)
▶ *thiabendazole* **(C)** treat bid x 7 days
    Pediatric: same as adult
              <30 lb: consult mfr literature
              >30 lb 2 doses/day with meals
              30-50 lbs: 250 mg bid with meals
              >50 lb: 10 mg/lb/dose bid with meals; max 3g/day
    Mintezol® *Chew tab:* 500*mg (orange); *Oral susp:* 500 mg/5 ml (120 ml; orange)
Comment: Thiabendazole is not for prophylaxis. May impair mental alertness.

Human Immunodeficiency Virus (HIV)

*see **Anti-HIV Drugs** page 503*
Appetite Stimulants
▶ *dronabinol* (cannabinoid) **(B)(III)** initially 2.5 mg bid before lunch and dinner; may reduce to 2.5 mg q HS or increase to 2.5 mg before lunch and 5 mg before dinner; max 20 mg/day in divided doses
    Pediatric: not recommended
    Marinol® *Cap:* 2.5, 5, 10 mg (sesame oil)
▶ *megestrol* **(X)** (progestin)
    Pediatric: not recommended
    Megace® initially 800 mg/day; maintenance usually 400-800

mg/day
>   *Tab:* 20*, 40* mg
> **Megace®ES** 625 mg/day
>   *Oral susp (concentrate):* 125 mg/ml; 625 mg/5 ml (5 oz; lemon-lime)
> **Megace®Oral Suspension** initially 800 mg/day; maintenance usually 400-800 mg/day
>   *Oral susp:* 40 mg/ml (8 oz; lemon-lime)

Hyperhidrosis (Perspiration, Excessive)

▶ *aluminum chloride* **(NR)** 20% solution apply q HS; wash treated area the following morning; after 1-2 treatments, may reduce frequency to 1-2 x/week
   Drysol® *Soln:* 35, 60 ml (alcohol 93%)
cont-rel Apply to clean dry skin (e.g., underarms). Do not apply to broken, irritated, or recently shaved skin.

Hyperhomocysteinemia

Comment: Elevated homocysteine is associated with cognitive impairment, vascular dementia, and dementia of the Alzheimer's type.
Homocystein-lowering Nutritional Supplement
▶ *L-methylfolate/riboflavin/pyridoxine/cyanocobalamin* **(NR)** 1-2 tabs daily
   Cerefolin® *Tab:* L-meth 5.635 mg/*ribo* 5 mg/*pyr* 50 mg/*cyan* 1 mg per tab

Hyperphosphatemia

Phosphate Binders
Comment: Monitor for development of hypercalcemia. Normal serum PO_4^- is 2.5-4.5 mg/dL and normal serum calcium is 8.5-10.5 mg/dL.
▶ *calcium acetate* **(C)** initially 2 tabs or caps with each meal; then titrate gradually to keep serum phosphate is <6 mg/dL; usual maintenance is 3-4 tabs or caps with each meal
   Pediatric: not recommended
   PhosLo® *Tab:* 667 mg; *Cap:* 667 mg
▶ *lanthanumcarbonate* **(C)** initially 750 mg to 1.5 g per day in divided

doses; take with meals; titrate at 2-3 week intervals in increments of 750 mg/day based on serum phosphate; usual range 1.5-3 g/day; usual max 3750 mg/day
> *Pediatric:* not recommended
> **Fosrenol®** *Chew tab:* 250, 500, 750 mg; 1 g

▶ *sevelamer* **(C)** initially 800 to 1600 mg with each meal; titrate by 1 tab at 2 week intervals to maintain serum phosphate ≤5.5 mg/dL
> *Pediatric:* not recommended
> **Renagel®** *Tab:* 400, 800 mg

Hyperpigmentation

Comment: De-pigmenting agents may be used for hyperpigmented skin conditions including chloasma, melasma, freckles, senile lentigenes. Limit treatments to small areas at one time. Sunscreen ≥30 SPF recommended.

▶ *hydroquinone* **(C)(G)** apply sparingly to affected area and rub in bid
> **Eldoquin®** *Crm:* 2% (30 g; sulfites)
> **Eldoquin®Forte** *Crm:* 4% (30 g; sulfites)
> **Lustra®** *Crm:* 4% (1, 2 oz; sulfites)
> **Lustra®AF** *Crm:* 4% (1, 2 oz; sunscreen, sulfites)

▶ *monobenzone* **(C)** apply sparingly to affected area and rub in bid-tid; depigmentation occurs in 1-4 months
> **Benoquin®** *Crm:* 20% (1.25 oz)

▶ *tazarotene* **(X)(G)** apply daily at HS
> *Pediatric:* not recommended
> **Avage®Cream** *Crm:* 0.1% (30 g)
> **Tazorac®Cream** *Crm:* 0.05, 0.1% (15, 30, 60 g)
> **Tazorac®Gel** *Gel:* 0.05, 0.1% (30, 100 g)

▶ *tretinoin* **(C)** apply daily at HS
> *Pediatric:* <12 years: not recommended
> **Avita®** *Crm/Gel:* 0.025% (20, 45 g)
> **Renova®** *Crm:* 0.02% (40 g); 0.05% (40, 60 g)
> **Retin-A®Cream** *Crm:* 0.025, 0.05, 0.1% (20, 45 g)
> **Retin-A®Gel** *Gel:* 0.01, 0.025% (15, 45 g; alcohol 90%)
> **Retin-A®Liquid** *Liq:* 0.05% (28 ml; alcohol 55%)
> **Retin-A®Micro** *Microspheres:* 0.04, 0.1% (20, 45 g)

Combination Agents

▶ *hydroquinone/fluocinolone/tretinoin* **(C)**
apply sparingly to affected area and rub in daily at HS
> *Pediatric:* not recommended
> **Tri-Luma®** *Crm:* hydro 4%/fluo 0.01%/tretin 0.05% (30 g;

parabens, sulfites)
- ▶*hydroquinone/padimate O/oxybenzone/octyl methoxycinnamate* **(C)** apply sparingly to affected area and rub in bid
    Pediatric: <12 years: not recommended
    Glyquin® *Crm:* 4% (1 oz jar)
- ▶*hydroquinone/ethyldihydroxypropyl PABA/dioxybenzone/ oxybenzone* **(C)** apply sparingly to affected area and rub in bid; max 2 months
    Pediatric: not recommended
    Solaquin® *Crm:* hydro 2%/PABA 5%/dioxy 3%/oxy 2% (1oz; sulfites)
- ▶*hydroquinone/padimate/dioxybenzone/oxybenzone* **(C)** apply sparingly to affected area and rub in bid; max 2 months
    Pediatric: not recommended
    Solaquin®Forte *Crm:* hydro 4%/pad 0.5%/dioxy 3%/oxy 2% (1oz; sunscreen, sulfites)
- ▶*hydroquinone/padimate/dioxybenzone* **(C)** apply sparingly to affected area and rub in bid; max 2 months
    Pediatric: not recommended
    Solaquin®Forte Gel *Gel:* hydro 4%/pad 0.5%/dioxy 3% (1 oz; alcohol, sulfites)

Hypertension: Primary

see ***JNC-VII Recommendations*** *page 462*
Beta-Blockers, Cardioselective
Comment: Cardioselective beta-blockers are less likely to cause bronchospasm, peripheral vasoconstriction, or hypoglycemia than non-cardioselective beta-blockers.
- ▶*acebutolol* **(B)(G)** initially 400 mg in 1-2 doses; usual range 200-800 mg/day; max 1.2 g/day in 2 doses
    Pediatric: not recommended
    Sectral® *Cap:* 200, 400 mg
- ▶*atenolol* **(D)(G)** initially 50 mg daily; may increase after 1-2 weeks to 100 mg daily; max 100 mg/day
    Pediatric: not recommended
    Tenormin® *Tab:* 25, 50, 100 mg
- ▶*betaxolol* **(C)** initially 10 mg daily; may increase to 20 mg/day after 7-14 days; usual max 20 mg/day
    Pediatric: not recommended

Hypertension: Primary

Kerlone® *Tab:* 10*, 20 mg
▶ *bisoprolol* **(C)** 5 mg daily; max 20 mg daily
    Pediatric: not recommended
  Zebeta® *Tab:* 5, 10 mg
▶ *metoprolol* **(C)(G)**
    Pediatric: not recommended
  Lopressor® initially 100 mg/day in 1-2 doses; increase if needed weekly; usual range 100-450 mg/day
    Tab: 50*, 100*mg
  Toprol®-XL initially 50-100 mg daily; increase at weekly intervals if needed; max 400 mg/day
    Tab: 25*, 50*, 100*, 200*mg ext-rel

Beta-Blockers, Non-cardioselective
Comment: Non-cardioselective beta-blockers are more likely to cause bronchospasm, peripheral vasoconstriction, and/or hypoglycemia than cardioselective beta-blockers.

▶ *nadolol* **(C)(G)** initially 40 mg daily; usual maintenance 40-80 mg daily; max 320 mg/day
    Pediatric: not recommended
  Corgard® *Tab:* 20*, 40*, 80*, 120*, 160*mg
▶ *penbutolol* **(C)** 20 mg daily
    Pediatric: not recommended
  Levatol® *Tab:* 20*mg
▶ *pindolol* **(B)(G)** initially 5 mg bid; may increase after 3-4 weeks in 10 mg increments; max 60 mg/day
    Pediatric: not recommended
  Visken® *Tab:* 5, 10 mg
▶ *propranolol* **(C)(G)**
  Inderal® initially 40 mg bid; usual maintenance 120-240 mg/day; max 640 mg/day
    Pediatric: initially 1 mg/kg/day; usual range 2-4 mg/kg/day in 2 doses; max 16 mg/kg/day
    Tab: 10*, 20*, 40*, 60*, 80*mg
  Inderal®LA initially 80 mg daily in a single dose; increase q 3-7 days; usual range 120-160 mg/day; max 320 mg/day in a single dose
    Pediatric: not recommended
    Cap: 60, 80, 120, 160 mg sust-rel
  InnoPran®XL initially 80 mg q HS; max 120 mg/day
    Cap: 80, 120 mg ext-rel
▶ *timolol* **(C)(G)** initially 10 mg bid, increase weekly if needed; usual

maintenance 20-40 mg/day; max 60 mg/day in 2 doses
> *Pediatric:* not recommended
>
> **Blocadren®** *Tab:* 5, 10*, 20*mg

Beta-Blocker, Non-cardioselective/Alpha-1 Blockers

▶*carvedilol* **(C)**
> **Coreg®** initially 6.25 mg bid; may increase at 1-2 week intervals to 12.5 mg bid; max 25 mg bid
> *Pediatric:* <18 years: not recommended
> *Tab:* 3.125, 6.25, 12.5, 25 mg

▶*carteolol* **(C)**
> **Cartrol®** initially 2.5 mg daily, gradually increase to 5 or 10 mg daily; usual maintenance 2.5-5 mg daily
> *Pediatric:* not recommended
> *Tab:* 2.5, 5 mg

▶*labetalol* **(C)(G)** initially 100 mg bid; increase after 2-3 days if needed; usual maintenance 200-400 mg bid; max 2.4 g/day
> *Pediatric:* not recommended
>
> **Normodyne®** *Tab:* 100*, 200*, 300 mg
> **Trandate®** *Tab:* 100*, 200*, 300*mg

Diuretics

Thiazide Diuretics

▶*chlorthalidone* **(B)(G)** 12.5-200 mg daily
> **Hygroton®** *Tab:* 12.5, 25 mg
> **Hylidon®** *Tab:* 12.5, 25 mg
> **Novothalidone®** *Tab:* 12.5, 25 mg
> **Thalidone®** *Tab:* 12.5, 25 mg

▶*chlorothiazide* **(C)(G)** 0.5-1 g/day in single or divided doses; max 2 g/day
> *Pediatric:* <6 months: up to 15 mg/lb/day in 2 doses
> >6 months: 10 mg/lb/day in 2 doses
>
> **Diuril®** *Tab:* 250*, 500*mg; *Oral susp:* 250 mg/5 ml (237 ml)

▶*hydrochlorothiazide* **(B)(G)**
> *Pediatric:* not recommended
>
> **Esidrix®** 25-100 mg daily
> *Tab:* 25, 50, 100 mg
> **Hydrodiuril®** initially 50-100 mg/day in single or divided doses; max 200 mg/day
> *Tab:* 25*, 50*mg
> **Microzide®** 12.5 mg daily; usual max 50 mg/day
> *Cap:* 12.5 mg
> **Oretic®** 25-50 mg bid; max 100 mg bid

Hypertension: Primary

    Tab: 25, 50 mg
▶*hydroflumethiazide* **(B)** 50-100 mg/day
    Pediatric: not recommended
   Diucardin® *Tab:* 50 mg
▶*methyclothiazide* **(B)** initially 2.5 mg daily; max 10 mg daily
    Pediatric: not recommended
   Enduron® *Tab:* 2.5, 5 mg
▶*polythiazide* **(C)** 2-4 mg daily
    Pediatric: not recommended
   Renese® *Tab:* 1, 2, 4 mg

Potassium-Sparing Diuretics

▶*amiloride* **(B)** initially 5 mg; may increase to 10 mg; max 20 mg
    Pediatric: not recommended
   Midamor® *Tab:* 5 mg
▶*spironolactone* **(D)(G)** initially 50-100 mg in 1 or more doses; titrate at 2 week intervals
    Pediatric: not recommended
   Aldactone® *Tab:* 25, 50*, 100*mg
▶*triamterene* **(B)** 100 mg bid; max 300 mg
    Pediatric: not recommended
  Dyrenium®
    Cap: 50, 100 mg

Loop Diuretics

▶*bumetanide* **(C)(G)** 0.5-2 mg daily; may repeat at 4-5 hour intervals; max 10 mg/day
    Pediatric: <18 years: not recommended
   Bumex® *Tab:* 0.5*, 1*, 2*mg
▶*ethacrynic acid* **(B)** initially 50-200 mg/day
    Pediatric: infant: not recommended
                >1 month: initially 25 mg/day; then adjust dose in 25 mg increments
   Edecrin® *Tab:* 25, 50 mg
▶*furosemide* **(C)(G)** initially 40 mg bid
    Pediatric: not recommended
   Lasix® *Tab:* 20, 40*, 80 mg; *Oral Soln:* 10 mg/ml (2, 4 oz w. dropper)
Comment: Furosemide is contraindicated with sulfa drug allergy.
▶*torsemide* **(B)** 5 mg daily; may increase to 10 mg daily
    Pediatric: not recommended
   Demadex® *Tab:* 5*, 10*, 20*, 100*mg

Other Diuretics

Hypertension: Primary

▶*indapamide* **(B)** initially 1.25 mg daily; may titrate dosage upward q 4 weeks if needed; max 5 mg/day
    Lozol® *Tab:* 1.25, 2.5 mg
Comment: Indapamide is contraindicated with sulfa drug allergy.

▶*metolazone* **(B)**
    Pediatric: not recommended
    Mykrox® initially 0.5 mg q AM; max 1 mg/day
        Tab: 0.5 mg
    Zaroxolyn® 2.5- 5 mg daily
        Tab: 2.5, 5, 10 mg
Comment: Metolazone is contraindicated with sulfa drug allergy.

Diuretic Combinations

▶*amiloride/hydrochlorothiazide* **(B)(G)** initially 1 tab daily; may increase to 2 tabs/day in single or divided doses
    Pediatric: not recommended
    Moduretic® *Tab: amil* 5 mg/*hydro* 50 mg*

▶*deserpidine/methylclothiazide* **(C)** titrate methylchlothiazide 2.5-10 mg daily
    Pediatric: not recommended
    Tab: **Enduronyl®0.25/5**: *deser* 0.25 mg/*methylclo* 5mg*
            Enduronyl®0.5/5: *deser* 0.5 mg/*methylclo* 5mg*

▶*spironolactone/hydrochlorothiazide* **(D)(G)**
    Pediatric: not recommended
    Aldactazide®25 usual maintenance 50-100 mg in 1 or more doses
        Tab: spiro 25 mg/*hydro* 25 mg
    Aldactazide®50 usual maintenance 50-100 mg in 1 or more doses
        Tab: spiro 50 mg/*hydro* 50 mg

▶*triamterene/hydrochlorothiazide* **(C)(G)**
    Pediatric: not recommended
    Dyazide® 1-2 caps daily
        Cap: triam 37.5 mg/*hydro* 25 mg
    Maxzide® 1 tab daily
        Tab: triam 75 mg/*hydro* 50 mg*
    Maxzide®-25 1-2 daily
        Pediatric: not recommended
        Tab: triam 37.5 mg/*hydro* 25 mg*

ACE Inhibitors

▶*benazepril* **(C; D in 2nd, 3rd)(G)** initially 10 mg daily; usual maintenance
20-40 mg/day in 1-2 doses; usual max 80 mg/day
    Pediatric: not recommended

Hypertension: Primary

Lotensin® *Tab:* 5, 10, 20, 40 mg
▶*captopril* **(C; D in 2nd, 3rd)(G)** initially 25 mg bid-tid; after 1-2 weeks increase to 50 mg bid-tid
　　　Pediatric: not recommended
Capoten® *Tab:* 12.5*, 25*, 50*, 100*mg
▶*enalapril* **(C; D in 2nd, 3rd)(G)** initially 2.5 mg/day; max 40 mg/day; usual range 10-40 mg in 1-2 doses
　　　Pediatric: not recommended
Vasotec® *Tab:* 2.5*, 5*, 10, 20 mg
▶*fosinopril* **(C; D in 2nd, 3rd)** initially 10 mg daily; usual maintenance 20-40 mg/day in single or divided doses; max 80 mg/day
　　　Pediatric: <6 years, <50 kg: not recommended
　　　　　　　　6-12 years, >50 kg: 5-10 mg daily
Monopril® *Tab:* 10*, 20, 40 mg
▶*lisinopril* **(C; D in 2nd, 3rd)** initially 10 mg daily; usual range 20-40 mg/day
　　　Pediatric: not recommended
Prinivil® *Tab:* 2.5, 5*, 10, 20, 40 mg
Zestril® *Tab:* 2.5, 5, 10, 20, 40 mg
▶*moexipril* **(C; D in 2nd, 3rd)** initially 7.5 mg daily; usual range 15-30 mg/day in 1-2 doses; max 30 mg/day
　　　Pediatric: not recommended
Univasc® *Tab:* 7.5*, 15*mg
▶*perindopril* **(C; D in 2nd, 3rd)** 2-8 mg daily-bid; max 16 mg/day
　　　Pediatric: not recommended
Aceon® *Tab:* 2*, 4*, 8*mg
▶*quinapril* **(C; D in 2nd, 3rd)** initially 10 mg daily; usual maintenance 20-80 mg daily in 1-2 doses
　　　Pediatric: not recommended
Accupril® *Tab:* 5*, 10, 20, 40 mg
▶*ramipril* **(C; D in 2nd, 3rd)** initially 2.5 mg bid; usual maintenance 2.5-20 mg in 1-2 doses
　　　Pediatric: not recommended
Altace® *Cap:* 1.25, 2.5, 5, 10 mg
▶*trandolapril* **(C; D in 2nd, 3rd)** initially 1-2 mg daily; adjust at 1 week intervals; usual range 2-4 mg in 1-2 doses; max 8 mg/day
　　　Pediatric: not recommended
Mavik® *Tab:* 1, 2, 4 mg

Angiotensin II Receptor Antagonists
▶*candesartan* **(C; D in 2nd, 3rd)** initially 16 mg daily; range 8-32 mg in 1-2 doses

Hypertension: Prima

    Pediatric: not recommended
  Atacand® *Tab:* 4, 8, 16, 32 mg

▶*eprosartan* **(C; D in 2nd, 3rd)** initially 400 mg bid or 600 mg daily; max 800 mg/day
    Pediatric: not recommended
  Teveten® *Tab:* 400*, 600 mg

▶*irbesartan* **(C; D in 2nd, 3rd)** initially 150 mg daily; titrate up to 300 mg
    Pediatric: not recommended
  Avapro® *Tab:* 75, 150, 300 mg

▶*losartan* **(C; D in 2nd, 3rd)** initially 50 mg daily; max 100 mg/day
    Pediatric: not recommended
  Cozaar® *Tab:* 25, 50 mg

▶*olmesartan medoxomil* **(C; D in 2nd, 3rd)** initially 20 mg daily; after 2 weeks, may increase to 40 mg daily
    Pediatric: not recommended
  Benicar® *Tab:* 5, 20, 40 mg

▶*telmisartan* **(C; D in 2nd, 3rd)** initially 40 mg daily; usual dose 20-80 mg
    Pediatric: not recommended
  Micardis® *Tab:* 40, 80 mg

▶*valsartan* **(C; D in 2nd, 3rd)** initially 80 mg daily; may increase to 160 or 320 mg daily after 2-4 weeks; usual range 80-320 mg/day
    Pediatric: not recommended
  Diovan® *Tab:* 80, 160, 320 mg

Calcium Channel Blockers
Benzothiazepines
▶*diltiazem* **(C)(G)**
  Cardizem® initially 30 mg qid; may increase gradually every 1 to 2 days; max 360 mg/day in divided doses
    Pediatric: not recommended
    Tab: 30, 60, 90, 120 mg
  Cardizem®CD initially 120-180 mg daily; adjust at 1 to 2 week intervals; max 480 mg/day
    Pediatric: not recommended
    Cap: 120, 180, 240, 300, 360 mg ext-rel
  Cardizem®LA initially 180-240 mg daily; titrate at 2 week intervals; max 540 mg/day
    Pediatric: not recommended
    Tab: 120, 180, 240, 300, 360, 420 mg ext-rel
  Cardizem®SR initially 60-120 mg bid; adjust at 2 week intervals;

max 360 mg/day
> *Pediatric:* not recommended
> *Cap:* 60, 90, 120 mg sust-rel

Dilacor®XR initially 180 or 240 mg in AM; usual range 180-480 mg/day; max 540 mg/day
> *Pediatric:* not recommended
> *Cap:* 120, 180, 240 mg ext-rel

Tiazac® initially 120-240 mg daily; adjust at 2 week intervals; usual max 540 mg/day
> *Pediatric:* not recommended
> *Cap:* 120, 180, 240, 300, 360, 420 mg ext-rel

▶ *diltiazem maleate* **(C)** initially 120-180 mg daily; adjust at 2 week intervals; usual range 120-480 mg daily
> *Pediatric:* not recommended

Tiamate® *Cap:* 120, 180, 240 mg ext-rel

Dihydropyridines

▶ *amlodipine* **(C)** initially 5 mg daily; max 10 mg/day
> *Pediatric:* not recommended

Norvasc® *Tab:* 2.5, 5, 10 mg

▶ *felodipine* **(C)** initially 5 mg daily; usual range 2.5-10 mg daily; adjust at 2 week intervals; max 10 mg/day
> *Pediatric:* not recommended

Plendil® *Tab:* 2.5, 5, 10 mg ext-rel

▶ *isradipine* **(C)**
> *Pediatric:* not recommended

DynaCirc® initially 2.5 mg bid; adjust in increments of 5 mg/day at 2-4 week intervals; max 20 mg/day
> *Cap:* 2.5, 5 mg

DynaCirc®CR initially 5 mg daily; adjust in increments of 5 mg/day
at 2-4 week intervals; max 20 mg/day
> *Tab:* 5, 10 mg cont-rel

▶ *nicardipine* **(C)(G)**
> *Pediatric:* <18 years: not recommended

Cardene® initially 20 mg tid; adjust at intervals of at least 3 days; max 120 mg/day
> *Cap:* 20, 30 mg

Cardene®SR 30-60 mg bid
> *Cap:* 30, 45, 60 mg sust-rel

▶ *nifedipine* **(C)(G)**
Adalat® initially 10 mg tid; usual range 10-20 mg tid; max 180

Hypertension: Primary

mg/day
    Cap: 10, 20 mg
Procardia® initially 10 mg tid; titrate over 7-14 days: max 30 mg/dose and 180 mg/day in divided doses
    Cap: 10, 20 mg
Procardia®**XL** initially 30-60 mg daily; titrate over 7-14 days; max dose 90 mg/day
    Tab: 30, 60, 90 mg ext-rel

▶*nisoldipine* **(C)**
    Sular® initially 20 mg daily; may increase by 10 mg weekly; usual maintenance 20-40 mg/day; max 60 mg/day
        Pediatric: not recommended
        Tab: 10, 20, 30, 40 mg ext-rel

Diphenylalkylamines

▶*verapamil* **(C)(G)**
        Pediatric: not recommended
    Calan® 80-120 mg tid; increase daily or weekly if needed
        Tab: 40, 80*, 120*mg
    Covera®**HS** initially 180 mg q HS; titrate in steps to 240 mg; then to 360 mg; then to 480 mg if needed
        Tab: 180, 240 mg ext-rel
    Isoptin® initially 80-120 mg tid
        Tab: 40, 80, 120 mg
    Isoptin®**SR** initially 120-180 mg in the AM; may increase to 240 mg in the AM; then 180 mg q 12 hours or 240 mg in the AM and 120 mg in the PM, then 240 mg q 12 hours
        Tab: 120, 180*, 240*mg sust-rel
    Verelan® initially 240 mg daily; adjust in 120 mg increments; max 480 mg/day
        Cap: 120, 180, 240, 360 mg sust-rel
    Verelan®**PM** initially 200 mg q HS, may titrate upwards to 300 mg, then 400 mg if needed
        Cap: 100, 200, 300 mg ext-rel

Alpha-1 Antagonists

Comment: Educate the patient regarding potential side effects of hypotension when taking an alpha-1 antagonist, especially with first dose. Start at lowest dose and titrate upward.

▶*doxazosin* **(C)(G)** initially 1 mg daily at HS; increase dose slowly every 2 weeks if needed; max dose 16 mg/day
    Pediatric: not recommended
    Cardura® *Tab:* 1*, 2*, 4*, 8*mg

Hypertension: Primary

Cardura®XL *Tab:* 4, 8 mg

▶*prazosin* **(C)(G)** first dose at HS, 1 mg bid-tid; increase dose slowly; usual range 6-15 mg/day in divided doses; max 20-40 mg/day
> *Pediatric:* not recommended

Minipress® *Cap:* 1, 2, 5 mg

▶*terazosin* **(C)** 1 mg q HS, then increase dose slowly; usual range 1-5 mg q HS; max 20 mg/day
> *Pediatric:* not recommended

Hytrin® *Cap:* 1, 2, 5, 10 mg

Central Alpha-Agonists

▶*clonidine* **(C)**
> *Pediatric:* <12 years: not recommended

Catapres® initially 0.1 mg bid; usual range 0.2-0.6 mg/day in divided doses; max 2.4 mg/day
> *Tab:* 0.1*, 0.2*, 0.3*mg

Catapres®-TTS initially 0.1 mg patch weekly; increase after 1-2 weeks if needed; max 0.6 mg/day
> *Patch:* 0.1, 0.2 mg (12/box); 0.3 mg (4/box)

▶*guanabenz* **(C)(G)** initially 4 mg bid; may increase by 4-8 mg/day every 1-2 weeks; max 32 mg/day
> *Pediatric:* not recommended

Wytensin® *Tab:* 4, 8 mg

▶*guanfacine* **(B)(G)** initially 1 mg/day q HS; may increase to 2 mg/day q HS; usual max 3 mg/day
> *Pediatric:* not recommended

Tenex® *Tab:* 1, 2 mg

▶*methyldopa* **(B)(G)** initially 250 mg bid-tid; titrate at 2 day intervals; usual maintenance 500 mg-2 g/day; max 3 g/day
> *Pediatric:* initially 10 mg/kg/day in 2-4 doses; max 65 mg/kg/day or 3 g/day, whichever is less

Aldomet® *Tab:* 125, 250, 500 mg; *Oral susp:* 250 mg/5 ml (473 ml)

Aldosterone Receptor Blocker

▶*eplerenone* **(B)** initially 25-50 mg daily; may increase to 50 mg bid; max 100 mg/day
> *Pediatric:* not recommended

Inspra® *Tab:* 25, 50 mg

Comment: Contraindicated with concomitant potent CYP3A4 inhibitors. Risk of hyperkalemia with concomitant ACE-I or ARB. Monitor serum potassium at baseline, 1 week, and 1 month. Caution with serum Cr >2 mg/dL (male) or >1.8 mg/dL (female) and/or CrCl < 50 ml/min, and DM with proteinuria.

Peripheral Adrenergic Blocker

Hypertension: Primary

▶*guanethidine* **(C)** initially 10 mg daily; may adjust dose at 5-7 day intervals; usual range 25-50 mg/day
> *Pediatric:* not recommended

Ismelin® *Tab:* 10, 25 mg

Other Agents

▶*hydralazine* **(C)(G)** initially 10 mg qid x 2-4 days; then increase to 25 mg qid for remainder of 1st week; then increase to 50 mg qid; max 300 mg/day
> *Pediatric:* initially 0.75 mg/kg/day in 4 doses; increase gradually over 3-4 weeks; max 7.5 mg/kg/day or 2000 mg/day

Apresoline® *Tab:* 10, 25, 50, 100 mg

▶*minoxidil* **(C)** initially 5 mg daily; may increase at 3 day intervals to 10 mg/day, then 20 mg/day, then 40 mg/day; usual range 10-40 mg/day; max 100 mg/day
> *Pediatric:* initially 0.2 mg/kg daily; may increase in 50-100% increments every 3 days; usual range 0.25-1 g/kg/day; max 50 mg/day

Loniten® *Tab:* 2.5*, 10*mg

Combination Agents

ACEI/Diuretic Combinations

▶*benazepril/hydrochlorothiazide* **(C; D in 2nd, 3rd)**
Lotensin®HCT titrate individual components
> *Pediatric:* not recommended
> *Tab:* **Lotensin®HCT 5/6.25**: *benaz* 5 mg/*hydro* 6.25 mg*
> **Lotensin®HCT 10/12.25**: *benaz* 10 mg/*hydro* 12.25 mg*
> **Lotensin®HCT 20/12.25**: *benaz* 20 mg/*hydro* 12.25 mg*
> **Lotensin®HCT 20/25**: *benaz* 20 mg/*hydro* 25 mg*

▶*captopril/hydrochlorothiazide* **(C; D in 2nd, 3rd)(G)**
> *Pediatric:* not recommended

Capozide® initially one 25/25 tab daily; adjust at 6 week intervals; max 150 mg *captopril* and 50 mg *hydrochlorothiazide* per day
> *Tab:* **Capozide®25/15**: *capt* 25 mg/*hydro* 15 mg*
> **Capozide®25/25**: *capt* 25 mg/*hydro* 25 mg*
> **Capozide®50/15**: *capt* 50 mg/*hydro* 15 mg*
> **Capozide®50/25**: *capt* 50 mg/*hydro* 25 mg*

▶*enalapril/hydrochlorothiazide* **(C; D in 2nd, 3rd)**
> *Pediatric:* not recommended

Vaseretic® initially 5/12.5 or 10/25 daily; then adjust at 2-3 week intervals; max 20 mg enalapril/day

Hypertension: Primary

> *Tab:* **Vaseretic®5/12.5**: *enal* 5 mg/*hydro* 12.5 mg
> **Vaseretic®10/25**: *enal* 10 mg/*hydro* 25 mg

▶ *lisinopril/hydrochlorothiazide* **(C; D in 2nd, 3rd)**
  Pediatric: not recommended
  Prinzide® usual maintenance 1-2 tabs of 10/12.5 or 20/12.5 daily or 1 tab of 20/25 daily
> *Tab:* **Prinzide®10/12.5**: *lis* 10 mg/*hydro* 12.5 mg
> **Prinzide®20/12.5**: *lis* 20 mg/*hydro* 12.5 mg
> **Prinzide®20/25**: *lis* 20 mg/*hydro* 25 mg

  Zestoretic® initially 10/12.5 or 20/12.5 daily; then adjust every 2-3 weeks as needed
> *Tab:* **Zestoretic®10/12.5**: *lis* 10 mg/*hydro* 12.5 mg
> **Zestoretic®20/12.5**: *lis* 20 mg/*hydro* 12.5 mg
> **Zestoretic®20/25**: *lis* 20 mg/*hydro* 25 mg

▶ *moexipril/hydrochlorothiazide* **(C; D in 2nd, 3rd)**
  Pediatric: not recommended
  Uniretic® 1 tab daily; adjust at 2-3 week intervals; usual max 30 mg moexipril/50 mg *hydrochlorothiazide* per day
> *Tab:* **Uniretic®7.5/12.5**: *moex* 7.5 mg/*hydro* 12.5mg*
> **Uniretic®15/12.5**: *moex* 15 mg/*hydro* 12.5 mg*
> **Uniretic®15/25**: *moex* 15 mg/*hydro* 25 mg*

▶ *quinapril/hydrochlorothiazide* **(C; D in 2nd, 3rd)**
  Pediatric: not recommended
  Accuretic® initially 10/12.5 or 20/12.5 daily; then adjust every 2-3 weeks as needed
> *Tab:* **Accuretic®10/12.5**: *quin* 10 mg/*hydro* 12.5mg*
> **Accuretic®20/12.5**: *quin* 20 mg/*hydro* 12.5 mg*
> **Accuretic®20/25**: *quin* 20 mg/*hydro* 25 mg*

Angiotensin II Receptor Antagonist/Diuretic Combinations

▶ *candesartan/hydrochlorothiazide* **(C; D in 2nd, 3rd)**
  Pediatric: not recommended
  Atacand®HCT initially one 16/12.5 mg tab daily; may increase to one 32/12.5 mg tab daily
> *Tab:* **Atacand®16/12.5**: *can* 16 mg/*hydro* 12.5 mg
> **Atacand®32/12.5**: *can* 32 mg/hydro 12.5 mg

▶ *eprosartan/ hydrochlorothiazide* **(C; D in 2nd, 3rd)** initially one 600/12.5 tab daily; may increase to one 600/25 tab daily max 800 mg/day
  Pediatric: not recommended
  Teveten®HCT
> *Tab:* **Teveten®HCT 600/12.5**: *epro* 600 mg/*hydro* 12.5 mg

Hypertension: Primary

Teveten®HCT 600/25: *epro* 600 mg/*hydro* 25 mg

▶*irbesartan/hydrochlorothiazide* **(C; D in 2nd, 3rd)**
> *Pediatric:* not recommended

Avalide® initially one 150/12.5 mg tab daily; may increase to one 300/12.5 mg tab/day
> *Tab:* **Avalide®150/12.5**: *irb* 150 mg/*hydro* 12.5 mg
> **Avalide®300/12.5**: *irb* 300 mg/*hydro* 12.5 mg

▶*losartan/hydrochlorothiazide* **(C; D in 2nd, 3rd)**
> *Pediatric:* not recommended

Hyzaar® initially one 50/12.5 mg tab daily; may increase to two 50/12.5 mg or one 100/25 mg tabs after 3 weeks if needed; max 100 mg *losartan*/day
> *Tab:* **Hyzaar®50/12.5**: *los* 50 mg/*hydro* 12.5 mg
> **Hyzaar®100/25**: *los* 100 mg/*hydro* 25 mg

▶*olmisartan medoxomil/hydrochlorothiazide* **(C; D in 2nd, 3rd)**
> *Pediatric:* not recommended

Benicar®HCT initially one 20/12.5 tab daily; may increase at 2-4 week intervals; max one 40/25 tab daily
> *Tab:* **Benicar®HCT 20/12.5**: *olmi* 20 mg/*hydro* 12.5 mg
> **Benicar®HCT 40/12.5**: *olmi* 40 mg/*hydro* 12.5 mg
> **Benicar®HCT 40/25**: *olmi* 40 mg/*hydro* 25 mg

▶*telmisartan/hydrochlorothiazide* **(C; D in 2nd, 3rd)**

Micardis®HCT one 40 mg/12.5 mg tab daily; adjust at 3-4 week intervals; usual max 160 mg/25 mg per day
> *Pediatric:* not recommended
> *Tab:* **Micardis®HCT 40/12.5**: *tel* 80 mg/*hydro* 12.5 mg
> **Micardis®HCT 80/12.5**: *tel* 160 mg/*hydro* 12.5 mg
> **Micardis®HCT 80/25**: *tel* 80 mg/*hydro* 12.5 mg

▶*valsartan/hydrochlorothiazide* **(C; D in 2nd, 3rd)**

Diovan®HCT one 80 mg/12.5 mg tab daily; adjust at 3-4 week intervals; usual max 160 mg/25 mg per day
> *Pediatric:* not recommended
> *Tab:* **Diovan®HCT 80/12.5**: *val* 80 mg/*hydro* 12.5 mg
> **Diovan®HCT 160/12.5**: *val* 160 mg/*hydro* 12.5 mg
> **Diovan®HCT 160/25**: *val* 160 mg/*hydro* 25 mg

Central Alpha-Agonist/Diuretic Combinations

▶*clonidine/chlorthalidone* **(C)**

Combipres® 1 tab daily-bid
> *Pediatric:* not recommended
> *Tab:* **Combipres®0.1**: *clon* 0.1 mg/*chlorthal* 15 mg*
> **Combipres®0.2**: *clon* 0.2 mg/*chlorthal* 15 mg*

Hypertension: Primary

Combipres®0.3: *clon* 0.3 mg/*chlorthal* 15 mg*

▶*methyldopa/chlorothiazide* **(C)**
    Pediatric: not recommended
  Aldoclor® initially 250 mg daily-tid, then gradually titrate as needed
    Pediatric: not recommended
    Tab: *meth* 250 mg/*chlor* 250 mg

▶*methyldopa/hydrochlorothiazide* **(C)(G)**
  Aldoril® initially **Aldoril®15** bid-tid or **Aldoril®25** bid
    Pediatric: not recommended
    Tab: **Aldoril®15**: *meth* 250 mg/*hydro* 15 mg
          Aldoril®25: *meth* 250 mg/*hydro* 25 mg
          Aldoril®D30: *meth* 500 mg/*hydro* 30 mg
          Aldoril®D50: *meth* 500 mg/*hydro* 50 mg

Beta-Blocker, Cardioselective/Diuretic Combinations

▶*atenolol/chlorthalidone* **(D)(G)**
    Pediatric: not recommended
  Tenoretic® initially one 50 mg tab daily; may increase to one 100 mg tab daily
    Tab: **Tenoretic®50**: *aten* 50 mg/*chlorthal* 25 mg*
          Tenoretic®100: *aten* 100 mg/*chlorthal* 25 mg*

▶*bisoprolol/hydrochlorothiazide* **(C)**
    Pediatric: not recommended
  Ziac® initially one 2.5/6.25 mg tab daily; adjust at 14 day intervals; max two 10/6.25 mg tabs daily
    Tab: **Ziac®2.5**: *bis* 2.5 mg/*hydro* 6.25 mg
          Ziac®5: *bis* 5 mg/*hydro* 6.25
          Ziac®10: *bis* 10 mg/*hydro* 6.25

▶*metoprolol/hydrochlorothiazide* **(C)**
    Pediatric: not recommended
  Lopressor®HCT titrate individual components
    Tab: **Lopressor®HCT 50/25**: *met* 50 mg/*hydro* 25mg*
          Lopressor®HCT 100/25: *met* 100 mg/*hydro* 25mg*
          Lopressor®HCT 100/50: *met* 100 mg/*hydro* 50mg*

Beta-Blocker, Non-cardioselective/Diuretic Combinations

▶*nadolol/bendroflumethiazide* **(C)**
  Corzide® titrate individual components
    Pediatric: not recommended
    Tab: **Corzide®40/5**: *nad* 40 mg/*bend* 5mg*
          Corzide®80/5: *nad* 80 mg/*bend* 5mg*

Hypertension: Primary

▶ *propranolol/hydrochlorothiazide* **(C)(G)**
    Pediatric: not recommended
  Inderide® titrate individual components
    Tab: **Inderide®40/25**: *pro* 40 mg/*hydro* 25 mg*
        Inderide®80/25: *pro* 80 mg/*hydro* 25 mg*
  Inderide®LA titrate individual components
    Cap: **Inderide®LA 80/50**: *pro* 80 mg/*hydro* 50 mg sust-rel
        Inderide®LA 120/50: *pro* 120 mg/*hydro* 50 mg sust-rel
        Inderide®LA 160/50: *pro* 160 mg/*hydro* 50 mg sust-rel

▶ *timolol/hydrochlorothiazide* **(C)**
    Pediatric: not recommended
  Timolide® usual maintenance 2 tabs/day in 1-2 doses
    Tab: tim 10 mg/*hydro* 25 mg

Alpha-1 Antagonist/Diuretic Combinations

▶ *prazosin/polythiazide* **(C)**
    Pediatric: not recommended
  Minizide® titrate individual components
    Cap: **Minizide®1**: *praz* 1 mg/*poly* 0.5 mg
        Minizide®2: *praz* 2 mg/*poly* 0.5 mg
        Minizide®5: *praz* 5 mg/*poly* 0.5 mg

Peripheral Adrenergic Blocker/Diuretic Combination

▶ *guanethidine/hydrochlorothiazide* **(C)**
  Esmil® titrate individual components
    Pediatric: not recommended
    Tab: **Esmil 10/25**: *guan* 1 mg/*hydro* 25 mg

ACEI/Calcium Agonist Combinations

▶ *amlodipine/benazepril* **(C; D in 2nd, 3rd)**
    Pediatric: not recommended
  Lotrel® titrate individual components
    Cap: **Lotrel®2.5/10**: *amlo* 2.5 mg/*benaz* 10 mg
        Lotrel®5/10: *amlo* 5 mg/*benaz* 10 mg
        Lotrel®5/20: *amlo* 5 mg/*benaz* 20 mg
        Lotrel®10/20: *amlo* 10 mg/*benaz* 20 mg
        Lotrel®5/40: *amlo* 5 mg/*benaz* 40 mg
        Lotrel®10/40: *amlo* 10 mg/*benaz* 40 mg

▶ *enalapril/diltiazem* **(C; D in 2nd, 3rd)**
    Pediatric: not recommended
  Teczem® titrate individual components
    Tab: enal 5 mg/*dil* 180 mg ext-rel

▶ *enalapril/felodipine* **(C; D in 2nd, 3rd)** initially 1 tab daily; after 1-2 weeks may increase to 2 tabs/day

      Pediatric: <18 years: not recommended
  Lexxel® titrate individual components
      Tab: **Lexxel®5/2.5**: *enal* 5 mg/*felo* 2.5 mg ext-rel
           Lexxel®5/5: *enal* 5 mg/*felo* 5 mg ext-rel

▶*trandolapril/verapamil* **(C; D in 2nd, 3rd)**
      Pediatric: not recommended
  Tarka® titrate individual components
      Tab: **Tarka®1/240**: *tran* 1 mg/*ver* 240 mg ext-rel
           Tarka®2/180: *tran* 1 mg/*ver* 240 mg ext-rel
           Tarka®2/240: *tran* 2 mg/*ver* 240 mg ext-rel
           Tarka®4/240: *tran* 4 mg/*ver* 240 mg ext-rel

Other Combination Agents

▶*clonidine/chlorthalidone* **(C)**
      Pediatric: not recommended
  Clorpres® initially one 0.1/15 mg tab daily; may increase to 0.3/15 mg tab bid as needed
      Tab: **Clorpres®0.1/15**: *clon* 0.1 mg/*chlorthal* 15 mg
           Clorpres®0.2/15: *clon* 0.2 mg/*chlorthal* 15 mg
           Clorpres®0.3/15: *clon* 0.3 mg/*chlorthal* 15 mg

▶*hydralazine/hydrochlorothiazide* **(C)**
      Pediatric: not recommended
  Apresazide® 1 cap bid
      Cap: **Apresazide®25/25**: *hydral* 25 mg/*hydro* 25 mg
           Apresazide®50/50: *hydral* 50 mg/*hydro* 50 mg

▶*reserpine/chlorothiazide* **(C)** one 25/12.5 mg tab daily-bid or one 50/0.125 mg tab daily
      Pediatric: not recommended
  Diupres®
      Tab: **Diupres®25**: *reser* 25 mg/*chlor* 0.125 mg
           Diupres®50: *reser* 50 mg/*chlor* 0.125 mg
  Hydropres®
      Tab: **Hydropres®25**: *reser* 25 mg/*chlor* 0.125 mg
           Hydropres®50: *reser* 50 mg/*chlor* 0.125 mg

▶*reserpine/hydroflumethiazide* **(C)** one 1.25/25 tab daily-bid or one 1.25/50 tab daily
      Pediatric: not recommended
  Salutensin®
      Tab: **Salutensin®1.25/25**: *enal* 1.25 mg/*hydroflu* 25 mg
           Salutensin®1.25/50: *enal* 1.25 mg/*hydroflu* 50 mg

Anti-hypertensive/Anti-lipid Combinations
  Calcium Channel Blocker/HMG-CoA Reductase Inhibitor (Statin)

Combinations

▶*amlodipine/atorvastatin* **(X)**
> *Pediatric*: <10 years: not recommended
> >10 years (female post-menarche): same as adult

Caduet® select according to blood pressure and lipid values; titrate *amlodipine* over 7-14 days; titrate *atorvastatin* according to monitored lipid values; max *amlodipine* 10 mg/day and max *atorvastatin* 80 mg/day; refer to contraindications and precautions for CCB and statin therapy

> *Tab:* **Caduet®5/10**: *amlo* 5 mg/*ator* 10 mg
> **Caduet®5/20**: *amlo* 5 mg/*ator* 20 mg
> **Caduet®5/40**: *amlo* 5 mg/*ator* 40 mg
> **Caduet®5/80**: *amlo* 5 mg/*ator* 80 mg
> **Caduet®10/10**: *amlo* 10 mg/*ator* 10 mg
> **Caduet®10/20**: *amlo* 10 mg/*ator* 20 mg
> **Caduet®10/40**: *amlo* 10 mg/*ator* 40 mg
> **Caduet®10/80**: *amlo* 10 mg/*ator* 80 mg

Hyperthyroidism

▶*methimazole* **(D)** initially 15-60 mg/day in 3 divided doses; maintenance 5-15 mg/day
> *Pediatric:* initially 0.4 mg/kg/day in 3 divided doses;
> maintenance 0.2 mg/kg/day or 1/2 initial dose

Tapazole® *Tab:* 5*, 10*mg

Comment: Methimazole potentiates anticoagulants. Contraindicated in nursing mothers.

▶*propylthiouracil (PTU)* **(D)(G)**
Propyl-Thyracil® initially 100-900 mg/day in 3 doses;
> maintenance usually 50-600 mg/day in 2 doses
> *Pediatric:* 6-10 years: initially 50-150 mg/day or 5-7 mg/
> kg/day in 3 doses
> >10 years: initially 150-300 mg/day or 5-7 mg/
> kg/day in 3 doses
> Maintenance: 0.2 mg/kg/day or 1/2-2/3 of initial dose

Comment: Preferred agent in pregnancy. Side effects include dermatitis, nausea, agranulocytosis, and hypothyroidism. Should be taken regularly for 2 years. Do not discontinue abruptly.

▶*propranolol* **(C)(G)** 40-240 mg daily
> *Pediatric*: not recommended

Hyperthyroidism

Inderal® *Tab:* 10*, 20*, 40*, 60*, 80*mg
Inderal®**LA** initially 80 mg daily in a single dose; increase q 3-7 days; usual range 120-160 mg/day; max 320 mg/day in a single dose
   Cap: 60, 80, 120, 160 mg sust-rel
InnoPran®**XL** initially 80 mg q HS; max 120 mg/day
   Cap: 80, 120 mg ext-rel

Hypertriglyceridemia

Isobutyric Acid Derivative
▶*gemfibrozil* **(C)(G)**
   Pediatric: not recommended
   Lopid® 600 mg bid 30 minutes before AM and PM meals
      Tab: 600*mg
Fibrates (Fibric Acid Derivatives)
▶*fenofibrate, micronized* **(C)** take with meals
   Pediatric: not recommended
   Antara® 43-130 mg daily; max 130 mg/day
      Cap: 43, 87, 130 mg
   TriCor® 54-160 mg daily; max 160 mg/day
      Tab: 54, 160 mg
   Lofibra® 67-200 mg daily; max 200 mg/day
      Tab: 67, 134, 200 mg
Nicotinic Acid Derivatives
Comment: Contraindicated in liver disease. Decrease total cholesterol, LDL-C, and TG; increase HDL-C. Before initiating and at 4-6 weeks, 3 months, and 6 months of therapy, check fasting lipid profile, LFT, glucose, and uric acid. Significant side effect of transient skin flushing. Take with food and take *aspirin* 300 mg 30 minutes before dose to decrease flushing.
▶*niacin* **(C)**
   Niaspan® 375 mg daily for first week, then 500 mg daily for second week, then 750 mg daily for third week, then 1 g daily for weeks 4-7; may increase by 500 mg q 4 weeks; usual range 1-3 g/day
      Tab: 500, 750, 1000 mg ext-rel
   Nicolar® initially 1 g tid; adjust in increments of 500 mg at 2-4 week intervals; max 6 g/day
      Tab: 500 mg
   Slo-Niacin® one 250 or 500 mg tab q AM or HS or one-half 750 mg tab q AM or HS
      Tab: 250, 500, 750 mg cont-rele

Hypertriglyceridemia

HMG-CoA Reductase Inhibitors

▶ *atorvastatin* **(X)** initially 10 mg daily; usual range 10-80 mg daily
        Pediatric: <10 years: not recommended
                 >10 years (female post-menarche): same as adult
    Lipitor® *Tab:* 10, 20, 40, 80 mg

▶ *fluvastatin* **(X)** initially 20-40 mg q HS; usual range 20-80 mg/day
        Pediatric: <18 years: not recommended
    Lescol® *Cap:* 20, 40 mg
    Lescol®XL *Tab:* 80 mg ext-rel

▶ *lovastatin* **(X)** initially 20 mg daily at evening meal; may increase at 4 week intervals; max 80 mg/day in single or divided doses
    If concomitant fibrates, *niacin*, or CrCl <30 ml/min: usual max 20 mg/day
        Pediatric: <10 years: not recommended
                 10-17 years: initially 10-20 mg daily at evening meal; may increase at 4 week intervals; max 40 mg daily
                 >17 years: same as adult
                 If concomitant fibrates, niacin, or CrCl <30 ml/min: usual max 20 mg/day
    Mevacor® *Tab:* 10, 20, 40 mg

▶ *pravastatin* **(X)** initially 10-20 mg q HS; usual range 10-40 mg/day; may start at 40 mg/day
        Pediatric: <8 years: not recommended
                 8-13 years: 20 mg daily
                 14-18 years: 40 mg daily
    Pravachol® *Tab:* 10, 20, 40, 80 mg

▶ *simvastatin* **(X)** initially 20 mg q PM; usual range 5-80 mg/day; adjust at 4 week intervals
        Pediatric: <20 years: not recommended
    Zocor® *Tab:* 5, 10, 20, 40, 80 mg

Nicotinic acid derivative/HMG-CoA reductase inhibitor Combination

▶ *niacin/lovastatin* **(X)**
        Pediatric: <18 years: not recommended
    Tab: **Advicor®500 mg/20 mg**: *niacin* 500 mg ext-rel/*lova* 20 mg
            Advicor®750 mg/20 mg: *niacin* 750 mg ext-rel/*lova* 20 mg
            Advicor®1000 mg/20 mg: *niacin* 1000 mg ext-rel/*lova* 20 mg

Hypocalcemia

Comment: Hypocalcemia resulting in metabolic bone disease may be secondary to hyperparathyroidism, pseudoparathyroidism, and chronic renal disease. Normal serum Ca^{++} range is approximately 8.5-12 mg/dL. Signs and symptoms of hypocalcemia include confusion, increased neuromuscular excitability, muscle spasms, paresthesias, hyperphosphatemia, positive Chvostek's sign, and positive Trousseau's sign. Signs and symptoms of hypercalcemia include fatigue, lethargy, decreased concentration and attention span, frank psychosis, anorexia, nausea, vomiting, constipation, bradycardia, heart block, shortened QT interval.

Calcium supplements

Comment: Take calcium supplements after meals to avoid gastric upset. Dosages of calcium over 2000 mg/day have not been shown to have any additional benefit. Calcium decreases *tetracycline* absorption. Calcium absorption is decreased by corticosteroids.

▶ *calcitonin-salmon* **(C)**
  Calcimar® 100 IU/day SC or IM
    Vial: 200 IU/ml (2 ml)
  Miacalcin® 200 units intranasally daily; alternate nostrils each day
    Nasal spray: 14 dose (2 ml)
  Miacalcin®Injection 100 units/day SC or IM
    Vial: 2 ml

▶ *calcium carbonate* **(C)(OTC)(G)**
  Rolaids® chew 2 tabs bid; max 14 tabs/day
    Tab: calcium carbonate: 550 mg
  Rolaids®Extra Strength chew 2 tabs bid; max 8 tabs/day
    Tab: 1000 mg
  Tums® chew 2 tabs bid; max 16 tabs/day
    Tab: 500 mg
  Tums®Extra Strength chew 2 tabs bid; max 10 tabs/day
    Tab: 750 mg
  Tums®Ultra chew 2 tabs bid; max 8 tabs/day
    Tab: 1000 mg
  Os-Cal®500 (OTC) 1-2 tab bid-tid
    Tab: elemental calcium carbonate 500 mg

▶ *calcium carbonate/vitamin D* **(C)(G)**
  Os-Cal®250+D (OTC) 1-2 tab tid
    Tab: elemental calcium carbonate 250 mg/*vit D* 125 IU
  Os-Cal®500+D (OTC) 1-2 tab bid-tid
    Tab: elemental calcium carbonate 500 mg/*vit D* 125 IU
  Viactiv® (OTC) 1 tab tid

Chew tab: elemental calcium 500 mg/*vit D* 100 IU/*Vit K* 40 mEq

▶ *calcium citrate*
    Citracal® (OTC) 1-2 tabs bid
        Tab: elemental calcium citrate 200 mg

▶ *calcium citrate/vitamin D* **(C)(G)**
    Citracal®+D (OTC) 1-2 cplts bid
        Cplt: elemental calcium citrate 315 mg/*vit D* 200 IU
    Citracal®250+D (OTC) 1-2 tabs bid
        Tab: elemental calcium citrate 250 mg/*vit D* 62.3 IU

Vitamin D Analog

Comment: Concurrent vitamin D supplementation is contraindicated for patients taking *calcitrol* or *doxecalciferol* due to the risk of vitamin D toxicity.

▶ *calcitrol* **(C)**
    Pre-dialysis: initially 0.25 mcg daily; may increase to 0.5 mcg daily
    Dialysis: initially 0.25 mcg daily; may increase by 0.25 mcg/day at 4-8 week intervals; usual maintenance 0.5-1 mcg/day
    Hypoparathyroidism: initially 0.25 mcg q AM; may increase by 0.25 mcg/day at 4-8 week intervals; usual maintenance 0.5-2 mcg/day
        Pediatric:
            Predialysis: <3 years: 10-15 ng/kg/day
                        >3 years: initially 0.25 mcg daily; may increase to 0.5 mcg/day
            Dialysis: not recommended
            Hypoparathyroidism: initially 0.25 mcg daily; may increase by 0.25 mcg/day at 2-4 week intervals; usual maintenance (1-5 years) 0.25-0.75 mcg/day, (>6 years) 0.5-2 mcg/day
    Rocaltrol® *Cap:* 0.25, 0.5 mcg
    Rocaltrol®Solution *Soln:* 1 mcg/ml (15 ml, single-use dispensers)

▶ *doxecalciferol* **(C)** initially 0.25 mcg q AM; may increase by 0.25 mcg/day at 4-8 week intervals; usual maintenance 0.5-2 mcg/day
        Pediatric: initially 0.25 mcg daily; may increase by 0.25 mcg 0.25 mcg/day at 2-4 week intervals; usual maintenance (1-5 years) 0.25-0.75 mcg/day, (>6 years) 0.5-2 mcg/day
    Hectorol® *Cap:* 0.25, 0.5 mcg

Hypokalemia

Comment: Normal serum K⁺ range is approximately 3.5-5.5 mEq/L. Signs and symptoms of hypokalemia include neuromuscular weakness, muscle twitching and cramping, hyporeflexia, postural hypotension, anorexia, nausea and vomiting, depressed ST segment, flattened T wave, and cardiac tachyarrhythmias. Signs and symptoms of hyperkalemia include peaked T waves, elevated ST segment, and widened QRS complexes.

Prophylaxis:

Comment: Usual dose range 8-10 mEq/day.

Treatment of Hypokalemia: Non-emergency (K⁺ < 2.5 mEq/L)
cont-rel Usual dose range 40-120 mEq/day in divided doses. Solutions are preferred; potentially serious GI side effects may occur with tablet formulations or when taken on an empty stomach.

Potassium Supplements

▶*potassium* **(C)(G)**
  Pediatric: not recommended

  K-Dur® (as chloride) *Tab:* 10, 20* mEq sust-rel

  K-Lor®for Oral Solution (as chloride) *Pkts for reconstitution:* 20 mEq/pkt (fruit)

  Klor-Con®/25 (as chloride) *Pkts for reconstitution:* 25 mEq/pkt

  Klor-Con®/EF 25 (as bicarbonate) *Pkts for reconstitution:* 25 mEq/pkt

  Klor-Con®Extended-Release (as chloride) *Tab:* 8, 10 mEq sust-rel

  Klor-Con®M (as chloride) *Tab:* 10, 20 mEq sust-rel

  Klor-Con®Powder 20 mEq (as chloride) *Pkts for reconstitution:* 20 mEq/pkt (30/carton; fruit)

  Klorvess® (as bicarbonate and citrate) *Tab:* 20 mEq effervescent for solution; *Granules:* 20 mEq/pkt effervescent for solution; *Oral liq:* 20 mEq/15 ml (16 oz)

  Klotrix® (as chloride) *Tab:* 10 mEq sust-rel

  K-Lyte® (as bicarbonate and citrate) *Tab:* 25 mEq effervescent for solution (lime and orange)

  K-Lyte®/CL (as chloride) *Tab:* 25 mEq effervescent for solution (citrus and fruit)

  K-Lyte®/CL 50 (as chloride) *Tab:* 50 mEq effervescent for solution (citrus and fruit)

  K-Lyte®/DS (as bicarbonate and citrate) *Tab:* 50 mEq effervescent for solution (lime and orange)

  K-Tab® (as chloride) *Tab:* 10 mEq sust-rel

  Micro-K® (as chloride) *Cap:* 8, 10 mEq sust-rel

Rum-K® (as chloride) *Oral conc:* 20 mEq/10 ml
Slow-K® (as chloride) *Cap:* 8 mEq sust-rel
K-Norm® (as chloride) *Tab:* 10 mEq ext-rel

Hypomagnesemia

Comment: Normal serum Mg^{++} range is approximately 1.2-2.6 mEq/L. Signs and symptoms of hypomagnesemia include confusion, disorientation, hallucinations, hyper-reflexia, tetany, convulsions, tachyarrhythmia, positive Chvostek's sign, and positive Trousseau's sign. Signs and symptoms of hypermagnesemia include drowsiness, lethargy, muscle weakness, hypoactive reflexes, slurred speech, bradycardia, hypotension, convulsions, and cardiac arrhythmias.

Magnesium Supplements
▶*magnesium* **(B)**
    Slow-Mag® 2 tabs daily
        Tab: 64 mg (as chloride)/110 mg (as carbonate)
▶*magnesium oxide* **(B)**
    Mag-Ox 400® 1-2 tabs daily
        Tab: 400 mg

Hypoparathyroidism

Vitamin D Analog
cont-rel Concurrent vitamin D supplementation is contraindicated for patients taking *calcitrol* or *doxecalciferol* due to the risk of vitamin D toxicity.
▶*calcitrol* **(C)** initially 0.25 mcg q AM; may increase by 0.25 mcg/day at 4-8 week intervals; usual maintenance 0.5-2 mcg/day
    Pediatric: initially 0.25 mcg daily; may increase by 0.25 mcg 0.25 mcg/day at 2-4 week intervals; usual maintenance (1-5 years) 0.25-0.75 mcg/day, (>6 years) 0.5-2 mcg/day
    Rocaltrol® *Cap:* 0.25, 0.5 mcg
    Rocaltrol® Solution *Soln:* 1 mcg/ml (15 ml, single-use dispensers)
▶*doxecalciferol* **(C)** initially 0.25 mcg q AM; may increase by 0.25 mcg/day at 4-8 week intervals; usual maintenance 0.5-2 mcg/day
    Pediatric: initially 0.25 mcg daily; may increase by 0.25 mcg 0.25 mcg/day at 2-4 week intervals; usual maintenance (1-5 years) 0.25-0.75 mcg/day, (>6 years) 0.5-2 mcg/day
    Hectorol® *Cap:* 0.25, 0.5 mcg

Hypotension: Orthostatic

Alpha-1 Agonist
▶ *midodrine* **(C)** 10 mg tid; last dose before 6:00 pm to prevent supine hypertension
      Pediatric: not recommended
    ProAmatine® *Tab:* 2.5*, 5*, 10*mg

Hypothyroidism

Comment: Take thyroid replacement hormone in the morning on an empty stomach. For the elderly, start thyroid hormone replacement at 25 mcg/day. Target TSH is 0.4-5.5 mIU/L; target T_4 is 4.5-12.5 mcg%. Signs and symptoms of thyroid toxicity include tachycardia, palpitations, nervousness, chest pain, heat intolerance, and weight loss.

Oral Thyroid Hormone Supplements

T_3

▶ *liothyronine* **(A)** initially 25 mcg daily; may increase by 25 mcg every 1-2 weeks as needed; usual maintenance 25-75 mcg/day
      Pediatric: initially 5 mcg/day; may increase by 5 mcg/day every 3-4 days
          Cretinism: maintenance dose:
              <1 years: 20 mcg/day
              1-3 years: 50 mcg/day
              >3 years: same as adult
    Cytomel® *Tab:* 5, 25, 50 mcg

T_4

▶ *levothyroxine* **(A)**
    Levoxyl® initially 25-100 mcg/day; increase by 25 mcg/day q 2-3 weeks as needed; maintenance 100-200 mcg/day
      Pediatric: <6 months: 8-10 mcg/kg/day
              6 months-1 year: 6-8 mcg/kg/day
              1-5 years: 5-6 mcg/kg/day
              6-12 years: 4-5 mcg/kg/day
      Tab: 25*, 50* (dye-free), 75*, 88*, 100*, 112*, 125*, 137*, 150*, 175*, 200*, 300*mcg

Hypothyroidism

Synthroid® initially 50 mcg/day; increase by 25 mcg/day q 2-3 weeks as needed; max 300 mcg/day
Pediatric: <6 months: 8-10 mcg/kg/day
6 months-1 year: 6-8 mcg/kg/day
1-5 years: 5-6 mcg/kg/day
6-12 years: 4-5 mcg/kg/day
Tab: 25*, 50* (dye-free), 75*, 88*, 100*, 112*, 125*, 137*, 150*, 175*, 200*, 300*mcg

Unithroid® initially 50 mcg/day; increase by 25 mcg/day q 2-3 weeks as needed; max 300 mcg/day
Pediatric: 0-3 months: 10-15 mcg/kg/day
3-6 months: 8-10 mcg/kg/day
6-12 months: 6-8 mcg/kg/day
1-5 years: 5-6 mcg/kg/day
6-12 years: 4-5 mcg/kg/day
>12 years: 2-3 mcg/kg/day
Growth and Puberty Complete: same as adult
Tab: 25*, 50* (dye-free), 75*, 88*, 100*, 112*, 125*, 150*, 175*, 200*, 300*mcg

T_3/ T_4 Combination

▶ *liothyronine/levothyroxine* **(A)** initially 15-30 mg/day; increase by 15/day q 2-3 weeks to target goal; usual maintenance 60-120 mg/day
Pediatric: <6 months: 4.6-6 mcg/kg/day
6 months-1 year: 3.6-4.8 mcg/kg/day
1-5 years: 3-3.6 mcg/kg/day
6-12 years: 2.4-3 mcg/kg/day
>12 years: 1.2-1.8
Growth and Puberty Complete: same as adult

Armour®Thyroid Tab *Tab:* per grain: T_3 9 mcg/T_4 38 mcg: 1/4 , 1/2, 1, 1½, 2, 3*, 4*, 5* gr; 15, 30, 60, 90, 120, 180*, 240*, 300*mg

Thyrolar®
Tab: per grain: T_3 12.5 mcg/ T_4 50 mcg: 1/4, 1/5, 1, 2, 3 gr

Parenteral Thyroid Hormone Supplement

▶*levothyroxine sodium* **(A)** 1/2 oral dose by IV or IM and titrate
Myxedema Coma: 200-500 mcg IV x 1 dose; may administer 100-300 mcg (or more) IV on second day if needed; then 50-100 mcg IV daily; switch to oral form as soon as possible
Pediatric: not recommended

Hypothyroidism

T₄ *Inj:* 200, 500 mcg (pwdr for IM or IV administration after reconstitution)

Impetigo Contagiosa (Indian Fire)

Comment: The most common infectious organisms are *Staphylococcus aureus* and *Streptococcus pyogenes*.

Topical Anti-infectives
▶*mupirocin* **(B)(G)** apply to lesions bid
  Pediatric: same as adult
  Bactroban® *Oint:* 2% (22 g); *Crm:* 2% (15, 30 g)
  Centany® *Oint:* 2% (15, 30 g)

Oral Anti-infectives
▶*amoxicillin* **(B)(G)** 500-875 mg bid or 250-500 mg tid x 10 days
  Pediatric: see page 569 for dose by weight
    <40 kg (88 lb): 20-40 mg/kg/day in 3 doses x 10 days or 25-45 mg/kg/day in 2 doses x 10 days
    >40 kg: same as adult
  Amoxil® *Cap:* 250, 500 mg; *Tab:* 875*mg; *Chew tab:* 125, 200, 250, 400 mg (cherry-banana-peppermint, phenylalanine);
  Oral susp: 125, 250 mg/5 ml (80, 100, 150 ml; strawberry); 200, 400 mg/5 ml (50, 75, 100 ml; bubble gum); *Oral drops:* 50 mg/ml (30 ml; bubble gum)
  Trimox® *Cap:* 250, 500 mg; *Oral susp:* 125, 250 mg/5 ml (80, 100, 150 ml; raspberry-strawberry)
▶*amoxicillin/clavulanate* **(B)(G)** 500 mg tid or 875 mg bid x 10 days
  Pediatric: see pages 571-572 for dose by weight
    40-45 mg/kg/day divided tid x 10 days or
    90 mg/kg/day divided bid x 10 days
  Augmentin® *Tab:* 250, 500, 875 mg; *Chew tab:* 125, 250 mg (lemon-lime), 200, 400 mg (cherry-banana, phenylalanine); *Oral susp:* 125 mg/5 ml (banana), 250 mg/5 ml (orange) (75, 100, 150 ml); 200, 400 mg/5 ml (50, 75, 100 ml; orange-raspberry, phenylalanine)
  Augmentin®**ES-600** *Oral susp:* 600 mg/5 ml (50, 75, 100, 150 ml; orange-raspberry, phenylalanine)
  Augmentin®**XR** 2 tabs q 12 hours x 10 days
    Pediatric: <16 years: use other forms
    Tab: 1000 mg ext-rel

Impetigo Contagiosa

▶ *azithromycin* **(B)** 500 mg x 1 dose on day 1, then 250 mg daily on days 2-5 or 500 mg daily x 3 days or 2 g in a single dose
> *Pediatric:* not recommended for bronchitis in children

Zithromax® *Tab:* 250, 500 mg; *Oral susp:* 100 mg/5 ml (15 ml); 200 mg/5 ml (15, 22.5, 30 ml); (cherry-vanilla-banana); *Pkt:* 1 g for reconstitution (cherry-banana)
Zithromax®**Tri-pak** *Tab:* 3-500 mg tabs/pck
Zithromax®**Z-pak** *Tab:* 6-250 mg tabs/pck
Zmax® *Oral susp:* 2 g ext rel (cherry-banana)

▶ *cefaclor* **(B)(G)**
Ceclor® 250 mg tid x 7 days
> *Pediatric: see page 575 for dose by weight*
> 20-40 mg/kg/day in 3 doses x 10 days
> *Pulvule:* 250, 500 mg; *Oral susp:* 125, 250 mg/5 ml (75, 150 ml); 187, 375 mg/5 ml (50, 100 ml) (strawberry)

Ceclor®**CD** 500 mg q 12 hours x 7 days
> *Pediatric:* <16 years: not recommended
> *Tab:* 375, 500 mg ext-rel

Ceclor®**CDpak** 500 mg q 12 hours x 7 days
> *Pediatric:* <16 years: not recommended
> *Tab:* 500 mg (14 tabs/CDpak)

Raniclor® 500 mg q 12 hours x 7 days
> *Pediatric:* 20-40 mg/kg/day in 3 doses x 10 days
> *Chew tab:* 125, 187, 250, 375 mg

▶ *cefadroxil* **(B)** 1-2 g in 1-2 doses x 10 days
> *Pediatric: see page 576 for dose by weight*
> 30 mg/kg/day in 2 doses x 10 days

Duricef® *Cap:* 500 mg; *Tab:* 1 g; *Oral susp:* 250 mg/5 ml (100 ml); 500 mg/5 ml (75, 100 ml) (orange-pineapple)

▶ *cefpodoxime proxetil* **(B)** 200 mg bid x 10 days
> *Pediatric: see page 578 for dose by weight*
> <2 months: not recommended
> 2 months-12 years: 10 mg/kg/day (max 400 mg/dose) or 5 mg/kg/day bid (max 200 mg/dose) x 10 days

Vantin® *Tab:* 100, 200 mg; *Oral susp:* 50, 100 mg/5 ml (50, 75, 100 ml; lemon-creme)

▶ *cefprozil* **(B)** 500 mg bid x 10 days
> *Pediatric: see page 579 for dose by weight*
> <6 months: not recommended
> 6 months-12 years:

Impetigo Contagiosa

Cefzil® *Tab:* 250, 500 mg; *Oral susp:* 125, 250 mg/5 ml (50, 75, 100 ml; bubble gum, phenylalanine)

▶*cefuroxime axetil* **(B)(G)** 250-500 mg bid x 10 days
Pediatric: see page 581 for dose by weight
15 mg/kg bid x 10 days

Ceftin® *Tab:* 125, 250, 500 mg; *Oral susp:* 125, 250 mg/5 ml (50, 100 ml; tutti-frutti)

▶*cephalexin* **(B)(G)** 250-500 mg qid or 500 mg bid x 10 days
Pediatric: see page 582 for dose by weight
25-50 mg/kg/day in 4 doses x 10 days

Keflex® *Cap:* 250, 500, 750 mg; *Oral susp:* 125, 250 mg/5 ml (100, 200 ml)
Keftab® *Tab:* 500 mg
Keftab®K-pak *Tab:* 20-500 mg tabs/K-pak

▶*cephradine* **(B)** 250 mg q 6 hours or 500 mg q 12 hours; max 4 g/day
Pediatric: see page 583 for dose by weight
<9 months: not recommended
>9 months: 25-50 mg/kg/day divided q 6-12 hours; max 4 g/day

Velosef® *Cap:* 250, 500 mg; *Oral susp:* 125, 250 mg/5 ml (100, 200 ml)

▶*clarithromycin* **(C)(G)** 500 mg or 500 mg ext-rel daily x 7 days
Pediatric: see page 584 for dose by weight
<6 months: not recommended
>6 months: 7.5 mg/kg bid x 7 days

Biaxin® *Tab:* 250, 500 mg
Biaxin®Oral Suspension *Oral susp:* 125, 250 mg/5 ml (50, 100 ml; fruit-punch)
Biaxin®XL *Tab:* 500 mg ext-rel

▶*dicloxacillin* **(B)(G)** 500 mg q 6 hours x 10 days
Pediatric: see page 586 for dose by weight
12.5-25 mg/kg/day in 4 doses x 10 days

Dynapen® *Cap:* 125, 250, 500 mg; *Oral susp:* 62.5 mg/5 ml (80, 100, 200 ml)

▶*erythromycin base* **(B)(G)** 250 mg qid, or 333 mg tid, or 500 mg bid x 7-10 days
Pediatric: see page 588 for dose by weight
<45 kg: 30-50 mg in 2-4 doses x 7-10 days
>45 kg: same as adult

E-mycin® *Tab:* 250, 333 mg ent-coat
Eryc® *Cap:* 250 mg ent-coat pellets

Ery-Tab® *Tab:* 250, 333, 500 mg ent-coat
PCE® *Tab:* 333, 500 mg

▶*loracarbef* **(B)** 200 mg bid x 10 days
    Pediatric: see page 593 for dose by weight
        15 mg/kg/day in 2 doses x 10 days
    Pediatric: 30 mg/kg/day in 2 doses x 7 days
Lorabid® *Pulvule:* 200, 400 mg; *Oral susp:* 100 mg/5 ml (50, 100 ml); 200 mg/5 ml (50, 75, 100 ml) (strawberry bubble gum)

▶*penicillin G (benzathine)* **(B)** 1.2 million units IM x 1 dose
    Pediatric: <60 lb: 300,000-600,000 units IM x 1 dose
        >60 lb: 900,000 units x 1 dose
Bicillin®L-A *Cartridge-needle unit:* 600,000 units (1 ml); 1.2 million units (2 ml)

▶*penicillin G (benzathine/procaine)* **(B)(G)** 2.4 million units IM x 1 dose
    Pediatric: <30 lb: 600,000 units IM x 1 dose
        30-60 lb: 900,000-1.2 million units IM x 1 dose
Bicillin®C-R *Cartridge-needle unit:* 600,000 units (1 ml); 1.2 million units (2 ml); 2.4 million units (4 ml)

▶*penicillin v* **(B)** 250-500 mg q 6 hours x 10 days
    Pediatric: see page 594 for dose by weight
        50 mg/kg/day in 4 doses x 3 days
        >12 years: same as adult
Pen-Vee®K *Tab:* 250, 500 mg; *Oral soln:* 125 mg/5 ml (100, 200 ml); 250 mg/5 ml (100, 150, 200 ml)
Veetids® *Tab:* 250, 500 mg; *Oral soln:* 125, 250 mg/5 ml (100, 200 ml)

Incontinence: Urinary
Overactive Bladder/Stress Incontinence/Urge Incontinence

▶*estrogen* replacement **(X)** see **Menopause** page 270

▶*imipramine* **(C)(G)**
    Pediatric\: not recommended
Tofranil® initially 75 mg daily (max 200 mg); adolescents
Initially 30-40 mg daily (max 100 mg/day); if maintenance dose exceeds 75 mg daily, may switch to **Tofranil®PM** for divided or bedtime dose
    Tab: 10, 25, 50 mg
Tofranil®PM initially 75 mg daily 1 hour before HS; max 200 mg

Incontinence: Urinary

        Cap: 75, 100, 125, 150
▶ *pseudoephedrine* **(C)(G)** 30-60 mg tid
    Sudafed® **(OTC)** *Tab:* 30 mg; *Liq:* 15 mg/5 ml (1, 4 oz)

Urge Incontinence
▶ *darifenacin* **(C)**
       Pediatric: not recommended
    Enablex® 7.5-15 mg daily with liquid; max 15 mg/day
       Tab: 7.5, 15 mg ext-rel
▶ *dicyclomine* **(B)(G)** 10-20 mg qid
       Pediatric: not recommended
    Bentyl® *Tab:* 20 mg; *Cap:* 10 mg; *Syr:* 10 mg/5 ml (16 oz)
▶ *flavoxate* **(B)** 100-200 mg tid-qid
       Pediatric: not recommended
    Urispas® *Tab:* 100 mg
▶ *hyoscyamine* **(C)(G)**
    Cystospaz® 1-2 tabs qid
       Tab: 0.15 mg
    IB-Stat® 1 oral spray q 12 hours
       Oral spray: 0.125 mg/ml
    Levbid® 1-2 tabs q 12 hours prn; max 4 tabs/day
       Pediatric: <12 years: not recommended
       Tab: 0.375*mg ext-rel
    Levsin® 1-2 tabs q 4 hours prn; max 12 tabs/day
       Pediatric: <6 years: not recommended
               6-12 years: 1 tab q 4 hours prn
       Tab: 0.125*mg
    Levsin®Drops 1-2 ml q 4 hours prn; max 60 ml/day
       Pediatric:
           3.4 kg: 4 drops q 4 hours prn; max 24 drops/day
           5 kg: 5 drops q 4 hours prn; max 30 drops/day
           7 kg: 6 drops q 4 hours prn; max 36 drops/day
           10 kg: 8 drops q 4 hours prn; max 40 drops/day
       Oral drops: 0.125 mg/ml (15 ml; orange, alcohol 5%)
    Levsin®Elixir 5-10 ml q 4 hours prn
       Pediatric:
           <10 kg: use drops
           10-19 kg: 1.25 ml q 4 hours prn
           20-39 kg: 2.5 ml q 4 hours prn
           40-49 kg: 3.75 ml q 4 hours prn
           >50 kg: 5 ml q 4 hours prn
       Elix: 0.125 mg/5 ml (16 oz; orange, alcohol 20%)

Incontinence: Urinary

Levsinex®SL 1-2 tabs q 4 hours SL or po; max 12 tabs/day
> *Pediatric:* 2-12 years: ½-1 tab q 4 hours; max 6 tabs/day
> *Tab:* 0.125 mg sublingual

Levsinex®Timecaps 1-2 caps q 12 hours; may adjust to 1 cap q 8 hours
> *Pediatric:* 2-12 years: 1 cap q 12 hours; max 2 caps/day
> *Cap:* 0.375 mg time-rel

NuLev® dissolve 1-2 tabs on tongue, with or without water, q 4 hours prn; max 12 tabs/day
> *Pediatric:* <2 years: not recommended
> 2-12 years: dissolve ½-1 tab on tongue, with or without water, q 4 hours prn; max 6 tabs/day
> *Tab:* 0.125 mg orally-disintegrating (mint, phenylalanine)

Symax®SL 1-2 tabs SL q 4 hours prn
> *Pediatric:* <2 years: not recommended
> 2-12 years: ½-1 tab SL q 4 hours prn
> *SL tab:* 0.125 mg sublingual

Symax®SR 1 tab q 12 hours prn
> *Pediatric:* <12 years: not recommended
> *SL tab:* 0.375 mg

▶ *oxybutynin chloride* **(B)**
Ditropan® 5 mg bid-tid; max 20 mg/day
> *Pediatric:* <5 years: not recommended
> 5-12 years: 5 mg bid; max 15 mg/day
> *Tab:* 5*mg; *Syr:* 5 mg/5 ml

Ditropan®XL initially 5 mg daily; may increase weekly in 5 mg increments as needed; max 30 mg/day
> *Tab:* 5, 10, 15 mg ext-rel

Oxytrol®Transdermal Patch apply patch to clean dry area of the abdomen, hip, or buttock; one patch twice weekly; rotate sites
> *Pediatric:* not recommended
> *Transdermal patch:* 3.9 mg/day

▶ *propantheline* **(C)** 15-30 mg tid
> *Pediatric:* not recommended
Pro-Banthine® *Tab:* 7.5, 15 mg

▶ *solifenacin* **(C)** 5-10 mg daily
> *Pediatric:* not recommended
VESIcare® *Tab:* 5, 10 mg

▶ *tolterodine tartrate* **(C)**
> *Pediatric:* not recommended
Detrol® 2 mg bid; may decrease to 1 mg bid

Incontinence: Urinary

    Tab: 1, 2 mg
  Detrol®XL 2-4 mg daily
    Cap: 2, 4 mg ext-rel

Vasopressin
▶*desmopressin acetate* **(B)(G)**
  DDAVP® usual dosage 0.1-1.2 mg/day in 2-3 doses; 0.2 mg q HS prn for nocturnal enuresis
    Pediatric: <6 years: not recommended
             >6 years: 0.5 mg daily or q HS prn
    Tab: 0.1*, 0.2*mg
  DDAVP®Nasal Spray and **DDAVP®Rhinal Tube**
    Pediatric: <6 years: not recommended
             >6 years: 10 mcg or 0.1 ml of soln each nostril (20 mcg total dose) q HS prn; max 40 mcg total dose
    Nasal spray: 10 mcg/actuation (5 ml, 50 sprays); *Rhinal tube:* 0.1 mg/ml (2.5 ml)

Overflow Incontinence/Atonic Bladder
▶*bethanechol* **(C)** 10-30 mg tid
  Urecholine® *Tab:* 5, 10, 25, 50 mg

Overflow Incontinence/Prostatic Enlargement
Alpha-1 Blockers
Comment: Educate the patient regarding the potential side effect of hypotension when taking an alpha-1 blocker, especially with first dose. Start at lowest dose and titrate upward.
▶*terazosin* **(C)** initially 1 mg q HS; titrate to 10 mg q HS; max 20 mg/day
  Hytrin® *Cap:* 1, 2, 5, 10 mg
▶*doxazosin* **(C)** initially 1 mg q HS; may double dose every 1-2 weeks; max 8 mg/day
  Cardura® *Tab:* 1*, 2*, 4*, 8*mg
  Cardura®XL *Tab:* 4, 8 mg
▶*prazosin* **(C)(G)** 1-15 mg q HS; max 15 mg/day
  Minipress® *Tab:* 1, 2, 5 mg
▶*tamsulosin* **(C)** initially 0.4 mg daily; may increase to 0.8 mg daily after 2-4 weeks if needed
  Flomax® *Cap:* 0.4 mg

5-Alpha Reductase Inhibitor
▶*finasteride* **(X)** 5 mg daily
  Proscar® *Tab:* 5 mg

Influenza (Flu)

Comment: Flu vaccine is contraindicated with allergy to egg or chicken proteins, egg products, and/or allergy to latex, active infection, acute respiratory disease, active neurological disorder; history of Guillain-Barre syndrome. Have epinephrine 1:1000 on hand. Flu vaccine is contraindicated for children under 18 years-of-age who are taking aspirin and/or an aspirin-containing product due to the risk of developing Reye's syndrome. Under 1 year-of-age, administer flu vaccine in the vastus lateralis. Over 1 year-of-age, administer flu vaccine in the deltoid. Flu vaccine formulations change annually. Administer flu vaccine one month before flu season. The influenza vaccine reduces hospitalization by about 70% and mortality by about 80% in the elderly.

Prophylaxis (Nasal Spray)

▶*trivalen, live atteunuated influenza* vaccine, types A and B **(C)** 1 spray each nostril; >50 years not recommended

    Pediatric: <5 years: not recommended
        Never vaccinated with **FluMist**®: 5-8 years: 2 doses 46-74 days apart
        Previously vaccinated with **FluMist**®: 5-8 years: same as adult

  FluMist®**Nasal Spray** 0.5 ml IM annually
    Nasal spray: 0.5 ml (0.25 ml/spray; 10/box; preservative-free)

Prophylaxis (Injectable)

▶*trivalent inactivated influenza subviron vaccine, types A and B* **(C)**

  Flushield® 0.5 ml IM annually
    Pediatric: <6 months: not recommended
        Never vaccinated: <9 years: 2 doses at least 4 weeks apart
        9-12 years: same as adult
        Previously vaccinated: 6-35 months: 0.25 ml IM x 1 dose
        3-8 years: same as adult

  Fluzone® 0.5 ml IM annually
    Vial: 5 ml (thimerosal)

  Fluzone®**Preservative-Free: Adult Dose** 0.5 ml IM annually
    Pediatric: <6 months: not recommended
        Not previously vaccinated: 6 months-8 years: 0.25 ml IM; repeat in 1 month
        Previously vaccinated: 6-35 months: 0.25 ml IM x 1 dose
        >3 years: same as adult
    Prefilled syringe: 0.5 ml (10/box; preservative-free; trace thimerosal)

Influenza

Fluzone®Preservative-Free: Pediatric Dose
Pediatric: <6 months: not recommended
Not previously vaccinated: 6 months-8 years: 0.25 ml IM; repeat in 1 month
Previously vaccinated: 6-35 months: 0.25 ml IM x 1 dose
>3 years: 0.5 ml IM (use **Fluzone®for Adult**)
Prefilled syringe: 0.5 ml (10/box; preservative-free; trace thimerosal)

Prophylaxis and Treatment
Neuraminidase Inhibitors
Comment: Effective for influenza type A and B. Indicated for treatment of uncomplicated acute illness in patients who have been symptomatic for no more than 2 days; therefore, start within 2 days of symptom onset or exposure. Indicated for influenza prophylaxis in patients >13 years.

▶*oseltamivir* **(C)**
Treatment: 75 mg bid x 5 days
Pediatric: <1 year: not recommended
1-13 years: <15 kg: 30 ml bid x 5 days; 15-23 kg: 45 mg bid x 5 days; 23-40 kg: 60 mg bid x 5 days
>40 kg: same as adult
Prophylaxis: 75 mg daily for at least 7 days and up to 6 weeks
Pediatric: <13 years: not recommended
Tamiflu® *Cap:* 75 mg; *Oral susp:* 12 mg/ml (100 ml; tutti-frutti)
cont-rel **Tamiflu®** is effective for influenza type A and B.

▶*zanamivir* **(C)** 2 inhalations (10 mg) bid x 5 days
Pediatric: <7 years: not recommended
>7 years: same as adult
Relenza®Inhaler *Inhaler:* 5 mg/inh blister; 4 blisters/Rotadisk (5 Rotadisks/box w. 1 inhaler)
Comment: Use caution with asthma and COPD.
50 mg/5 ml (2, 8 oz; raspberry)
Antipyretics *see Fever page 168*

Insect Bite/Sting

Topical Anesthetic
▶*lidocaine* 3% cream **(B)** apply bid-tid prn
Pediatric: reduce dosage commensurate with age, body weight and physical condition
LidaMantle® *Crm:* 3% (1 oz)
Oral 1st Generation Antihistamines *see page 525*

Oral 2nd Generation Antihistamines *see page 527*
Topical Antihistamine/Glucocorticosteroid
▶*chlorcyclizine/hydrocortisone* **(C)** apply 2-5 times/day
    Mantadil® *Crm: chlor 2%/hydro 0.5% (15 g)*
Topical Glucocorticosteroids *see page 483*
Parenteral Glucocorticosteroids *see page 389*
Oral Glucocorticosteroids *see page 387*
Other Agents
▶*epinephrine* **(C)(G)** 1:1000 0.3-0.5 ml SC
    Pediatric: 0.01 ml/kg SC
Tetanus prophylaxis
▶*tetanus toxoid* vaccine **(C)(G)** 0.5 cc IM x 1 dose if previously immunized
    Vial: 5 Lf units/0.5 ml (0.5, 5 ml); *Prefilled syringe:* 5 Lf units/0.5 ml (0.5 ml)

For patients not previously immunized see **Tetanus page 397**

Insomnia

Melatonin Receptor Agonist
▶*ramelteon* **(C)(IV)** 8 mg within 30 minutes of bedtime; delayed effect if taken with a meal
    Pediatric: not recommended
  Rozerem® *Tab:* 8 mg

Nonbenzodiazepines
▶*zaleplon* **(C)(IV)** (imidazopyridine) 5-10 mg at HS or after going to bed if unable to sleep; do not take if unable to sleep for at least 4 hours before required to be active again; max 20 mg/day x 1 month; delayed effect if taken with a meal
    Pediatric: not recommended
  Sonata® *Cap:* 5, 10 mg (tartrazine)

▶*zolpidem* **(B)(IV)(G)** (pyrazolopyrimidine) 5-10 mg or 6.25-12.5 ext-rel
q HS prn; max 12.5 mg/day x 1 month; do not take if unable to sleep for at least 8 hours before required to be active again; delayed effect if taken with a meal
    Pediatric: <18 years: not recommended
  Ambien® *Tab:* 5, 10 mg
  Ambien®**CR** *Tab:* 6.25, 12.5 mg ext-rel

▶*eszopiclone* **(C)(IV)** (pyrrolopyrazine) 1-3 mg; max 3 mg/day x 1

Insomnia

month; do not take if unable to sleep for at least 8 hours before required to be active again; delayed effect if taken with a meal
> *Pediatric:* <18 years: not recommended

Lunesta® *Tab:* 1, 2, 3 mg

Benzodiazepines

▶ *estazolam* **(X)(IV)(G)** initially 1 mg q HS prn; may increase to 2 mg q HS
> *Pediatric:* <18 years: not recommended

ProSom® *Tab:* 1*, 2*mg

▶ *flurazepam* **(X)(IV)(G)** 30 mg q HS prn
> *Pediatric:* <15 years: not recommended

Dalmane® *Cap:* 15, 30 mg

▶ *quazepam* **(X)(IV)** initially 15 mg q HS prn; may reduce to 7.5 mg after 1-2 days
> *Pediatric:* not recommended

Doral® *Tab:* 7.5, 15 mg

▶ *temazepam* **(X)(IV)(G)** 7.5-30 mg q HS prn; max 1 month
> *Pediatric:* <18 years: not recommended

Restoril® *Cap:* 7.5, 15, 30 mg

▶ *triazolam* **(X)(IV)** 0.125-0.25 mg q HS prn; max 0.5 mg q HS x 1 month
> *Pediatric:* <18 years: not recommended

Halcion® *Tab:* 0.125, 0.25*mg

Barbiturates

▶ *pentobarbital* **(D)(II)(G)**

Nembutal® 100 mg q HS prn
> *Cap:* 50, 100 mg

Nembutal®Suppository 120 or 200 mg suppository rectally q HS prn
> *Pediatric:* 2 months-1 year (10-20 lb): 30 mg supp
> 1-4 years (21-40 lb): 30 or 60 mg supp
> 5-12 years (41-80 lb): 60 mg supp
> 12-14 years (81-110 lb): 60 or 120 mg supp

Rectal supp: 30, 60, 120, 200 mg

Non-barbiturate

▶ *ethchlorvynol* **(C)**
> *Pediatric:* not recommended

Placidyl® usually 500 mg q HS prn; 200 mg q HS for early awakening; max 1000 mg as a single bedtime dose
> *Cap:* 200, 500, 750 mg

Oral 1st generation Antihistamines *see page 525*
Combination Analgesic/1st Generation Antihistamines
▶ *acetaminophen/diphenhydramine* **(B)**
    Excedrin®PM (OTC) 2 tabs q HS prn
        Pediatric: <12 years: not recommended
        Tab/Geltab: acet 500 mg/*diphen* 38 mg
    Tylenol®PM (OTC) 2 caps q HS prn
        Pediatric: <12 years: not recommended
        Tab/Cap/Gel cap: acet 500 mg/*diphen* 25 mg
Tricyclic Antidepressants *see **Depression** page 133*

Interstitial Cystitis

Comment: Avoid peppers and spicy food, citrus, vinegar, caffeine (e.g., coffee, tea, colas) alcohol, carbonated beverages, and other GU tract irritants.
Management of Pain and Urinary Urgency
▶*flavoxate* **(B)** 100-200 mg tid-qid
        Pediatric: <12 years: not recommended
    Urispas® *Tab:* 100 mg
▶*hyoscyamine* **(C)(G)**
    Cystospaz® 1-2 tabs qid
        Tab: 0.15 mg
    IB-Stat® 1 oral spray q 12 hours
        Oral spray: 0.125 mg/ml
    Levbid® 1-2 tabs q 12 hours prn; max 4 tabs/day
        Pediatric: <12 years: not recommended
        Tab: 0.375*mg ext-rel
    Levsin® 1-2 tabs q 4 hours prn; max 12 tabs/day
        Pediatric: <6 years: not recommended
                6-12 years: 1 tab q 4 hours prn
        Tab: 0.125*mg
    Levsin®Drops 1-2 ml q 4 hours prn; max 60 ml/day
        Pediatric:
                3.4 kg: 4 drops q 4 hours prn; max 24 drops/day
                5 kg: 5 drops q 4 hours prn; max 30 drops/day
                7 kg: 6 drops q 4 hours prn; max 36 drops/day
                10 kg: 8 drops q 4 hours prn; max 40 drops/day
        Oral drops: 0.125 mg/ml (15 ml; orange, alcohol 5%)
    Levsin®Elixir 5-10 ml q 4 hours prn
        Pediatric: <10 kg: use drops
                10-19 kg: 1.25 ml q 4 hours prn

Interstitial Cystitis

> 20-39 kg: 2.5 ml q 4 hours prn
> 40-49 kg: 3.75 ml q 4 hours prn
> >50 kg: 5 ml q 4 hours prn

Elix: 0.125 mg/5 ml (16 oz; orange, alcohol 20%)

Levsinex®SL 1-2 tabs q 4 hours SL or po; max 12 tabs/day
> *Pediatric:* 2-12 years: ½-1 tab q 4 hours; max 6 tabs/day
> *SL tab:* 0.125 mg

Levsinex®Timecaps 1-2 caps q 12 hours; may adjust to 1 cap q 8 hours
> *Pediatric:* 2-12 years: 1 cap q 12 hours; max 2 caps/day
> *Cap:* 0.375 mg time-rel

NuLev® dissolve 1-2 tabs on tongue, with or without water, q 4 hours prn; max 12 tabs/day
> *Pediatric:* <2 years: not recommended
> 2-12 years: dissolve ½-1 tab on tongue, with or without water, q 4 hours prn; max 6 tabs/day
> *Tab:* 0.125 mg orally-disintegrating (mint, phenylalanine)

Symax®SL 1-2 tabs sublingually q 4 hours prn; max 12 tabs/day
> *Pediatric:* <2 years: not recommended
> 2-12 years: ½-1 tab SL q 4 hours prn
> *SL tab:* 0.125 mg

Symax®SR 1-2 tabs q 12 hours prn; max 4 tabs/day
> *Pediatric:* <12 years: not recommended
> *Tab:* 0.375 mg sust-rel

▶ *methenamine/phenyl salicylate/methylene blue/benzoic acid/atropine sulfate/hyoscyamine* **(C)(G)** 2 tabs qid
> *Pediatric:* <6 years: not recommended
> **Urised®** *Tab:* meth 40.8 mg/*phenyl sa* 18.1 mg/*meth blue* 5.4 mg/*benz acid* 4.5 mg/*atro sul* 0.03 mg/*hyoscy* 0.03 mg

Comment: **Urised®** imparts a blue-green color to urine which may stain fabrics.

▶ *oxybutynin chloride* **(B)**
> **Ditropan®** 5 mg bid-tid; max 20 mg/day
> *Pediatric:* <5 years: not recommended
> 5-12 years: 5 mg bid; max 15 mg/day
> *Tab:* 5*mg; *Syr:* 5 mg/5 ml

> **Ditropan®XL** initially 5 mg daily; may increase weekly in 5 mg increments as needed; max 30 mg/day
> *Tab:* 5, 10, 15 mg ext-rel

▶ *pentosan* **(B)** 100 mg tid; re-evaluate at 3 and 6 months
> *Pediatric:* <16 years: not recommended

Elmiron® *Cap:* 100 mg
▶*phenazopyridine* **(B)(G)** 190-200 mg tid; max 2 days
　　　Pediatric: not recommended
　　Azo Standard® (OTC) *Tab:* 95 mg
　　Prodium® (OTC) *Tab:* 95 mg
　　Pyridium® *Tab:* 100, 200 mg ent-coat
　　Uristat® (OTC) *Tab:* 95 mg
　　Urogesic® *Tab:* 100, 200 mg
Comment: Phenazopyridine imparts an orange-red color to urine which may stain fabrics.
▶*propantheline* **(C)** 15-30 mg tid
　　Pro-Banthine® *Tab:* 7.5, 15 mg
▶*tolterodine tartrate* **(C)** 2 mg bid; may decrease to 1 mg bid
　　Detrol® 2 mg bid; may decrease to 1 mg bid
　　　Tab: 1, 2 mg
　　Detrol®XL 2-4 mg daily
　　　Cap: 2, 4 mg ext-rel

Anticholinergic/Sedative Combination
▶*chlordiazepoxide/clidinium* **(D)(IV)** 1-2 caps ac and HS; max 8 caps/day
　　　Pediatric: not recommended
　　Librax® *Cap:* chlor 5 mg/clid 2.5 mg

Tricyclic Antidepressants
▶*amitriptyline* **(C)(G)** 25-50 mg q HS
　　　Pediatric: not recommended
　　Amitryl®, **Endep®** *Tab:* 10, 25, 50, 75, 100, 150 mg
▶*imipramine* **(C)(G)**
　　　Pediatric: not recommended
　　Tofranil® initially 75 mg daily (max 200 mg); adolescents initially 30-40 mg daily (max 100 mg/day); if maintenance dose exceeds 75 mg daily, may switch to **Tofranil®PM** for divided or bedtime dose
　　　Tab: 10, 25, 50 mg
　　Tofranil®PM initially 75 mg daily 1 hour before HS; max 200 mg
　　　Cap: 75, 100, 125, 150
　　Tofranil®Injection 50 mg IM; lower dose for adolescents; switch to oral form as soon as possible
　　　Amp: 25 mg/2 ml (2 ml)

Intertrigo

Comment: Intertrigo is an irritation and rash secondary to adjacent skin surfaces rubbing together. Treatment is dependent upon symptoms and presence of infection.
Topical Glucocorticosteroids *see page 483*
Topical Anti-fungals *see Tinea Corporis page 399*
Topical Anti-infectives *see Skin Infection: Bacterial page 384*

Iritis: Acute

▶*loteprednol etabonate* (**C**) 1-2 drops qid; may increase to 1 drop hourly as needed
    Pediatric: not recommended
    Lotemax®Ophthalmic Solution *Ophth soln:* 0.3% (2.5, 5, 10, 15 ml)

▶*prednisone acetate* (**C**) 1 drop q 1 hour x 24-48 hours, then 1 drop q 2 hours while awake x 24-48 hours, then 1 drop bid-qid until resolved
    Pediatric: not recommended
    Pred Forte® *Ophth soln:* 1% (1, 5, 10, 15 ml)

Iron Overload

Iron Chelating Agent
▶*deferasirox* (**C**) (tridentate ligand) initially 20 mg/kg/day; titrate; may increase 5-10 mg/kg q 3-6 months based on serum ferritin trends; max 30 mg/kg/day
    Pediatric: <2 years: not recommended
    Exjade® *Tab for oral soln:* 125, 250, 500 mg

Comment: For the treatment of chronic iron overload due to blood transfusions (transfusional hemosiderosis). Monitor serum ferritin monthly. Consider interrupting therapy if serum ferritin falls below 500 mcg/L. Take **Exjade®** on an empty stomach. Completely disperse tablet(s) in 3.5 oz liquid if dose is <1 g or 7 oz liquid if >1 g.

Irritable Bowel Syndrome

Bulk-Producing Agents *see Constipation page 123*

Irritable Bowel Syndrome

Constipating Agents

▶ *difenoxin/atropine* **(C)** 2 tabs, then 1 tab after each loose stool or 1 tab q 3-4 hours as needed; max 8 tab/day x 2 days
    Pediatric: <12 years: not recommended
  Motofen® *Tab:* difen 1 mg/*atro* 0.025 mg

▶ *diphenoxylate/atropine* **(C)(G)** 2 tabs or 10 ml qid
    Pediatric: <2 years: not recommended
                2-12 years: initially 0.3-0.4 mg/kg/day in 4 doses
  Lomotil® *Tab:* difen 2.5 mg/*atro* 0.025 mg; *Liq:* difen 2.5 mg/*atro* 0.025 mg per 5 ml (2 oz)

▶ *loperamide* **(B)(G)**
  Imodium® **(OTC)** 4 mg initially, then 2 mg after each loose stool; max 16 mg/day
    Pediatric: <5 years: not recommended
    Cap: 2 mg

  Imodium®A-D (OTC) 4 mg initially, then 2 mg after each loose stool; usual max 8 mg/day x 2 days
    Pediatric: <2 years: not recommended
                2-5 years (24-47 lb): 1 mg up to tid x 2 days
                 6-8 years (48-59 lb): 2 mg initially, then 1 mg after each loose stool; max 4 mg/day x 2 days
                 9-11 years (60-95 lb): 2 mg initially, then 1 mg after each loose stool; max 6 mg/day x 2 days
    Cplt: 2 mg; *Liq:* 1 mg/5 ml (2, 4 oz)

▶ *loperamide/simethicone* **(B)(G)**
  Imodium®Advanced (OTC) 2 tabs chewed after loose stool, then 1 after the next loose stool; max 4 tabs/day
    Pediatric: 6-8 years: 1 tab chewed after loose stool, then 1/2 after next loose stool; max 2 tabs/day
                 9-11 years: 1 tab chewed after loose stool, then 1/2 after next loose stool; max 3 tabs/day
    Chew tab: lop 2 mg/*sim* 125 mg

Antispasmodic/Anticholinergic Combination

▶ *dicyclomine* **(B)(G)** initially 20 mg bid-qid; may increase to 40 mg qid po; usual IM dose 80 mg/day divided qid; do not use IM route for more than 1-2 days
    Pediatric: not recommended
  Bentyl® *Tab:* 20 mg; *Cap:* 10 mg; *Syr:* 10 mg/5 ml (16 oz); *Vial:* 10 mg/ml (10 ml); *Amp:* 10 mg/ml (2 ml)

▶ *methscopolomine bromide* **(B)** 1 tab q 6 hours prn
    Pediatric: not recommended

Irritable Bowel Syndrome

    Pamine® *Tab:* 2.5 mg
    Pamine®Forte *Tab:* 5 mg
Anticholinergics
▶*hyoscyamine* **(C)(G)**
    Cystospaz® 1-2 tabs qid
        Tab: 0.15 mg
    IB-Stat® 1 oral spray q 12 hours
        Oral spray: 0.125 mg/ml
    Levbid® 1-2 tabs q 12 hours prn; max 4 tabs/day
        Pediatric: <12 years: not recommended
        Tab: 0.375*mg ext-rel
    Levsin® 1-2 tabs q 4 hours prn; max 12 tabs/day
        Pediatric: <6 years: not recommended
                6-12 years: 1 tab q 4 hours prn
        Tab: 0.125*mg
    Levsin®Drops 1-2 ml q 4 hours prn; max 60 ml/day
        Pediatric:
            3.4 kg: 4 drops q 4 hours prn; max 24 drops/day
            5 kg: 5 drops q 4 hours prn; max 30 drops/day
            7 kg: 6 drops q 4 hours prn; max 36 drops/day
            10 kg: 8 drops q 4 hours prn; max 40 drops/day
        Oral drops: 0.125 mg/ml (15 ml; orange, alcohol 5%)
    Levsin®Elixir 5-10 ml q 4 hours prn
        Pediatric: <10 kg: use drops
                10-19 kg: 1.25 ml q 4 hours prn
                20-39 kg: 2.5 ml q 4 hours prn
                40-49 kg: 3.75 ml q 4 hours prn
                >50 kg: 5 ml q 4 hours prn
        Elix: 0.125 mg/5 ml (orange, alcohol 20%)
    Levsinex®SL 1-2 tabs q 4 hours SL or po; max 12 tabs/day
        Pediatric: 2-12 years: ½-1 tab q 4 hours; max 6 tabs/day
        Tab: 0.125 mg sublingual
    Levsinex®Timecaps 1-2 caps q 12 hours; may adjust to 1 cap q 8 hours
        Pediatric: 2-12 years: 1 cap q 12 hours; max 2 caps/day
        Cap: 0.375 mg time-rel
    NuLev® dissolve 1-2 tabs on tongue, with or without water, q 4 hours prn; max 12 tabs/day
        Pediatric: <2 years: not recommended
                2-12 years: dissolve ½-1 tab on tongue, with or without water, q 4 hours prn; max 6 tabs/day

Tab: 0.125 mg orally-disintegrating (mint, phenylalanine)

Symax®SL 1-2 tabs SL q 4 hours prn
   Pediatric: <2 years: not recommended
   2-12 years: ½-1 tab SL q 4 hours prn
   SL tab: 0.125 mg

Symax®SR 1 tab q 12 hours prn
   Pediatric: <12 years: not recommended
   SL tab: 0.375 mg

▶ *simethicone* **(C)(G)** 0.3 ml qid pc and HS
   Mylicon®Drops (OTC) *Oral drops:* 40 mg/0.6 ml (30 ml)

▶ *phenobarbital/hyoscyamine/atropine/scopolamine* **(C)(IV)(G)**
   Donnatal® 1-2 tabs ac and HS
       Pediatric: not recommended
       Tab: pheno 16.2 mg/*hyo* 0.1037 mg/*atro* 0.0194 mg/*scop* 0.0065 mg

   Donnatal®Elixir 1-2 tsp ac and HS
       Pediatric: 10 lb: 0.5 ml q 4 hours or 0.75 ml q 6 hours
                    20 lb: 1 ml q 4 hours or 1.5 ml q 6 hours
                    30 lb: 1.5 ml q 4 hours or 2 ml q 6 hours
                    50 lb: 1/2 tsp q 4 hours or 3/4 tsp q 6 hours
                    75 lb: 3/4 tsp q 4 hours or 1 tsp q 6 hours
                    100 lb: 1 tsp q 4 hours or 1½ tsp q 6 hours
       Elix: pheno 16.2 mg/*hyo* 0.1037 mg/*atro* 0.0194 mg/*scop* 0.0065 mg per 5 ml (4, 16 oz)

   Donnatal®Extentabs 1 tab q 12 hours
       Pediatric: not recommended
       Tab: pheno 48.6 mg/*hyo* 0.3111 mg/*atro* 0.0582 mg/*scop* 0.0195 mg ext-rel

Anticholinergic/Sedative Combination
▶ *chlordiazepoxide/clidinium* **(D)(IV)** 1-2 caps ac and HS: max 8 caps/day
   Pediatric: not recommended
   Librax® *Cap: chlor* 5 mg/*clid* 2.5 mg

Tricyclic Antidepressants
▶ *amitriptyline* **(C)(G)** 25-50 mg q HS
   Pediatric: not recommended
   Amitryl®, Endep® *Tab:* 10, 25, 50, 75, 100, 150 mg

▶ *imipramine* **(C)(G)** 25-50 mg tid
   Pediatric: not recommended
   Tofranil® initially 75 mg daily (max 200 mg); adolescents initially 30-40 mg daily (max 100 mg/day); if maintenance dose

exceeds 75 mg daily, may switch to **Tofranil®PM** for divided or bedtime dose
  Tab: 10, 25, 50 mg
Tofranil®PM initially 75 mg daily 1 hour before HS; max 200 mg
  Cap: 75, 100, 125, 150
Tofranil®Injection 50 mg IM; lower dose for adolescents; switch to oral form as soon as possible
  Amp: 25 mg/2 ml (2 ml)

Keratitis/Keratoconjunctivitis: Herpes Simplex

▶*idoxuridine* **(C)** instill 1 drop q 1 hour during day and every other hour at night or 1 drop every minute for 5 minutes and repeat q 4 hours during day and night
  Herplex® *Ophth soln:* 0.1% (15 ml)
▶*trifluridine* **(C)** instill 1 drop q 2 hours while awake (max 9 drops/day) until reepithelialization; then 1 drop q 4 hours x 7 more days (at least 5 drops/day); max 21 days
    Pediatric: <6 years: not recommended
           >6 years: same as adult
  Viroptic® *Ophth soln:* 1% (7.5 ml; thimerosal)
▶*vidarabine* **(C)** apply 1/2 inch in lower conjunctival sac 5 times/day q 3 hours until reepithelialization occurs, then bid x 7 more days
    Pediatric: <2 years: not recommended
  Vira-A® *Ophth oint:* 3% (3.5 g)

Keratitis/Keratoconjunctivitis: Vernal

Ophthalmic Mast Cell Stabilizers
Comment: Contact lens wear is contraindicated
▶*cromolyn sodium* **(B)** 1-2 drops 4-6 times/day
    Pediatric: <4 years: not recommended
           >4 years: same as adult
  Crolom®, Opticrom® *Ophth soln:* 4% (10 ml; benzalkonium chloride)
▶*iodoxamide tromethamine* **(B)** 1-2 drops qid; max 3 months
    Pediatric: <2 years: not recommended
           >2 years: same as adult
  Alomide® *Ophth susp:* 0.1% (10 ml)

Labyrinthitis

▶*meclizine* **(B)** 25 mg tid
    Pediatric: not recommended
  Antivert® *Tab:* 12.5, 25, 50*mg
  Bonine® (OTC) *Cap:* 15, 25, 30 mg; *Tab:* 12.5, 25, 50 mg; *Chew tab/Film-coated tab:* 25 mg
  Dramamine®II (OTC) *Tab:* 25*mg
▶*promethazine* **(C)(G)** 25 mg tid
    Pediatric: <2 years: not recommended
             >2 years: 0.5 mg/lb or 6.25-25 mg tid
  Phenergan® *Tab:* 12.5*, 25*, 50 mg; *Plain syr:* 6.25 mg/5 ml; *Fortis syr:* 25 mg/5 ml; *Rectal supp:* 12.5, 25, 50 mg
▶*scopolamine* **(C)**
  Transderm Scop® 1 patch behind ear at least 4 hours before travel; each patch is effective for 3 days
    Transdermal patch: 1.5 mg (4/box)

Lactose Intolerance

▶*lactase* enzyme
    Pediatric: same as adult
  Lactaid®Drops (OTC) 5-7 drops to each quart of milk and shake gently; may increase to 10-15 drops if needed; usual max 18,000 u/dose
    Oral drops: 1250 U/5 gtts (7 ml w. dropper)
  Lactaid®Extra Strength (OTC) 2 caps with first bite of dairy food; max 4 caps/dose
    Cap: 4500 FCC units
  Lactaid®Original (OTC) 3 caps with first bite of dairy food; max 6 caps/dose
    Cap: 3000 FCC units
  Lactaid®Ultra (OTC) 1 cap with first bite of dairy food; max 2 caps/dose
    Chew tab: 9000 FCC units (vanilla-twist)

Larva Migrans: Cutaneous or Visceral

▶*thiabendazole* **(C)**

Larva Migrans

Cutaneous Larva Migrans: treat x 2 days
Visceral Larva Migrans: treat x 7 days
> *Pediatric:* same as adult
>> <30 lb: consult mfr literature
>> >30 lb: 2 doses/day with meals
>> 30-50 lbs: 250 mg bid with meals
>> 30-50 lbs: 250 mg bid with meals
>> >50 lb: 10 mg/lb/dose bid with meals; max 3g/day

Mintezol® *Chew tab:* 500*mg (orange); *Oral susp:* 500 mg/5 ml (120 ml; orange)

Comment: Thiabendazole is not for prophylaxis.

Lead Poisoning

Comment: Chelation therapy for lead poisoning requires maintenance of adequate hydration, close monitoring of renal and hepatic function, and monitoring for neutropenia; discontinue therapy at first sign of toxicity. Contraindicated with severe renal disease or anuria.

Chelating Agents

▶*deferoxaminemesylate* **(C)** initially 1 g IM, followed by 500 mg IM every 4 hours x 2 doses; then repeat every 4-12 hours if needed; max 6 g/day
> *Pediatric:* <3 months: not recommended
>> >3 months: same as adult

Desferal® *Vial:* 250 mg/ml after reconstitution (500 mg)

▶*edetate calcium disodium (EDTA)* **(B)** administer IM or IV; use IM route of administration for children and overt lead encephalopathy
> *Pediatric:* same as adult

Serum lead level: 20-70 mcg/dL: 1 g/m^2 per day
> IV: infuse over 8-12 hours
> IM: divided doses q 8-12 hours
> Treat for 5 days; then stop for 2-4 days; may repeat if serum lead level is >70 mcg/dL

Calcium Disodium Versenate® *Amp:* 200 mg/ml (5 ml)

▶*succimer* **(C)** may swallow caps whole or put contents onto a small amount of soft food or a spoon and swallow, followed by a fruit drink
> *Pediatric:* <12 months: not recommended
>> >12 months: same as adult

Serum lead level: >45 mcg/dL: initially 10 mg/kg (or 350 mg/m^2) every 8 hours for 5 days; then reduce frequency to every 12 hours for 14 more days; allow at least 14 days between courses

unless serum lead levels indicate a need for more prompt treatment; treatment for more than 3 consecutive weeks not recommended
Chemet® *Cap:* 100 mg

Leg Cramps: Nocturnal Recumbency

▶*quinine sulfate* **(C)(G)** 1 tab or cap q HS
    Pediatric: <16 years: not recommended
    Tab: 260 mg; *Cap:* 260, 300, 325 mg
  Qualaquin® *Cap:* 324 mg

Lentigines: Benign, Senile

Comment: Wash affected area with a soap-free cleanser; pat dry and wait 20 to 30 minutes; then apply sparingly to affected area; use only once daily in PM. Avoid eyes, ears, nostrils, mouth, and healthy skin. Avoid sun exposure. Cautious use of concomitant astringents, alcohol-based products, sulfur-containing products, salicylic acid-containing products, soap, and other topical agents.

Topical Retinoids
▶*tazarotene* **(X)** apply daily at HS
    Pediatric: not recommended
  Avage®**Cream** *Crm:* 0.1% (30 g)
  Tazorac®**Cream** *Crm:* 0.05, 0.1% (15, 30, 60 g)
  Tazorac®**Gel** *Gel:* 0.05, 0.1% (30, 100 g)
▶*tretinoin* **(C)** apply daily at HS
    Pediatric: <12 years: not recommended
    >12 years: same as adult
  Avita® *Crm:* 0.025% (20, 45 g); *Gel:* 0.025% (20, 45 g)
  Renova® *Crm:* 0.02% (40 g); 0.05% (40, 60 g)
  Retin-A®**Cream** *Crm:* 0.025, 0.05, 0.1% (20, 45 g)
  Retin-A®**Gel** *Gel:* 0.01, 0.025% (15, 45 g; alcohol 90%)
  Retin-A®**Liquid** *Liq:* 0.05% (28 ml; alcohol 55%)
  Retin-A®**Micro** *Microspheres:* 0.04, 0.1% (20, 45 g)

Listeriosis

▶*erythromycin base* **(B)(G)** 500 mg qid x 10 days
    Pediatric: see page 588 for dose by weight

Listeriosis

> <45 kg: 30-40 mg/kg/day in 4 doses x 10 days
> >45 kg: same as adult

E-mycin® *Tab:* 250, 333 mg ent-coat
Eryc® *Cap:* 250 mg ent-coat
Ery-Tab® *Tab:* 250, 333, 500 mg ent-coat
PCE® *Tab:* 333, 500 mg

▶*erythromycin ethylsuccinate* **(B)(G)** 400 mg po qid x 7 days
> *Pediatric: see page 589 for dose by weight*
>
> 30-50 mg/kg/day in 4 divided doses x 7 days; may double dose with severe infection; max 100 mg/kg/day

Ery-Ped® *Oral susp:* 200 mg/5 ml (100, 200 ml; fruit); 400 mg/5 ml (60, 100, 200 ml; banana); *Oral drops:* 200, 400 mg/5 ml (50 ml; fruit); *Chew tab:* 200 mg wafer (fruit)
E.E.S.® *Oral susp:* 200, 400 mg/5 ml (100 ml; fruit)
E.E.S.®Granules *Oral susp:* 200 mg/5 ml (100, 200 ml; cherry)
E.E.S.®400 Tablets *Tab:* 400 mg

Low Back Strain

NSAIDs *see **Pain** page 305*
Oral Non-narcotic Analgesics *see **Pain** page 308*
Oral Narcotic Analgesics *see **Pain** page 308*
Topical Analgesics *see **Pain** page 308*
Parenteral Glucocorticosteroids *see page 389*
Oral Glucocorticosteroids *see page 387*
Topical Anesthetic *see page 383*
Topical Anesthetic/Steroid Combinations *see page 480*

Lyme Disease

Stage 1
▶*amoxicillin* **(B)(G)** 500-875 mg bid or 250-500 mg tid x 10 days
> *Pediatric: see page 569 for dose by weight*
>
> <40 kg (88 lb): 20-40 mg/kg/day in 3 doses x 10 days or 25-45 mg/kg/day in 2 doses x 10 days
> >40 kg: same as adult

Amoxil® *Cap:* 250, 500 mg; *Tab:* 875*mg; *Chew tab:* 125, 200, 250, 400 mg (cherry-banana-peppermint, phenylalanine);

Lyme Disease

Oral susp: 125, 250 mg/5 ml (80, 100, 150 ml; strawberry); 200, 400 mg/5 ml (50, 75, 100 ml; bubble gum); *Oral drops:* 50 mg/ml (30 ml; bubble gum)

Trimox® *Cap:* 250, 500 mg; *Oral susp:* 125, 250 mg/5 ml (80, 100, 150 ml; raspberry-strawberry)

▶ *cefuroxime axetil* **(B)(G)** 500 mg bid x 20 days

    Pediatric: <3 months: not recommended
              >3 months: 15 mg/kg bid x 20 days

Ceftin® *Tab:* 125, 250, 500 mg; *Oral susp:* 125, 250 mg/5 ml (50, 100 ml; tutti-frutti)

▶ *clarithromycin* **(C)(G)** 500 mg bid or 500 mg ext-rel daily x 14-21 days

    Pediatric: see page 584 for dose by weight
              <6 months: not recommended
              >6 months: 7.5 mg/kg bid x 7 days

Biaxin® *Tab:* 250, 500 mg

Biaxin®**Oral Suspension** *Oral susp:* 125, 250 mg/5 ml (50, 100 ml; fruit-punch)

Biaxin®**XL** *Tab:* 500 mg ext-rel

▶ *doxycycline* **(D)(G)** 100 mg bid x 14-21 days

    Pediatric: see page 587 for dose by weight
              <8 years: not recommended
              >8 years, <100 lb: 2 mg/lb on first day in 2 doses, followed by 1 mg/lb/day in 1-2 doses
              >8 years, >100 lb: same as adult

Adoxa® *Tab:* 50, 100 mg ent-coat

Doryx® *Cap:* 100 mg

Monodox® *Cap:* 50, 100 mg

Vibramycin® *Cap:* 50, 100 mg; *Syr:* 50 mg/5 ml (raspberry-apple, sulfites); *Oral susp:* 25 mg/5 ml (raspberry)

Vibra-Tab® *Tab:* 100 mg film-coat

Comment: Doxycycline is contraindicated in pregnancy (discolors fetal tooth enamel).

(D)(G) 200 mg on first day; then 100 mg q 12 hours x 9 more days

    Pediatric: <8 years: not recommended
              >8 years, <100 lb: 2 mg/lb on first day in 2 doses, followed by 1 mg/lb/ q 12 hours x 9 more days
               >8 years, >100 lb: same as adult

Minocin® *Cap:* 100 mg ent-coat

Comment: Minocycline is contraindicated in pregnancy (discolors fetal tooth

Lyme Disease

▶*tetracycline* **(D)(G)** 250-500 mg qid ac x 21 days
> *Pediatric: see page 595 for dose by weight*
>> <8 years: not recommended
>> >8 years, <100 lb: 25-50 mg/kg/day in 2-4 doses x 7 days
>> >8 years, >100 lb: same as adult

Achromycin®V *Cap:* 250, 500 mg

Sumycin® *Tab:* 250, 500 mg; *Cap:* 250, 500 mg; *Oral susp:* 125 mg/5 ml (100, 200 ml; fruit, sulfites)

Comment: Tetracycline is contraindicated in pregnancy (discolors fetal tooth enamel).

Lymphadenitis

Comment: Therapy should continue for no less than 5 days after resolution of symptoms.

▶*amoxicillin/clavulanate* **(B)(G)** 500 mg tid or 875 mg bid x 10 days
> *Pediatric: see pages 571-572 for dose by weight*
>> 40-45 mg/kg/day divided tid x 10 days or
>> 90 mg/kg/day divided bid x 10 days

Augmentin® *Tab:* 250, 500, 875 mg; *Chew tab:* 125, 250 mg (lemon-lime), 200, 400 mg (cherry-banana, phenylalanine); *Oral susp:* 125 mg/5 ml (banana), 250 mg/5 ml (orange) (75, 100, 150 ml); 200, 400 mg/5 ml (50, 75, 100 ml; orange-raspberry, phenylalanine)

Augmentin®ES-600 *Oral susp:* 600 mg/5 ml (50, 75, 100, 150 ml; orange-raspberry, phenylalanine)

Augmentin®XR 2 tabs q 12 hours x 10 days
> *Pediatric:* <16 years: use other forms
> *Tab:* 1000 mg ext-rel

▶*cephalexin* **(B)(G)** 500 mg bid x 10 days
> *Pediatric: see page 582 for dose by weight*
>> 25-50 mg/kg/day in 4 doses x 10 days

Keflex® *Cap:* 250, 500, 750 mg; *Oral susp:* 125, 250 mg/5 ml (100, 200 ml)

Keftab® *Tab:* 500 mg

Keftab®K-pak *Tab:* 20-500 mg tabs/K-pak

▶*dicloxacillin* **(B)** 500 mg qid x 10 days
> *Pediatric: see page 586 for dose by weight*
>> 12.5-25 mg/kg/day in 4 doses x 10 days

Dynapen® *Cap:* 125, 250, 500 mg; *Oral susp:* 62.5 mg/5 ml (80, 100, 200 ml)

Lymphogranuloma Venereum

Comment: Treat all sexual contacts.
▶ *doxycycline* **(D)(G)** 100 mg bid x 21 days
    Pediatric: see page 587 for dose by weight
        <8 years: not recommended
        >8 years, <100 lb: 2 mg/lb on first day in 2 doses, followed by 1 mg/lb/day in 1-2 doses x 21 days
        >8 years, >100 lb: same as adult
  Adoxa® *Tab:* 50, 100 mg ent-coat
  Doryx® *Cap:* 100 mg
  Monodox® *Cap:* 50, 100 mg
  Vibramycin® *Cap:* 50, 100 mg; *Syr:* 50 mg/5 ml (raspberry-apple, sulfites); *Oral susp:* 25 mg/5 ml (raspberry)
  Vibra-Tab® *Tab:* 100 mg film-coat

Comment: Doxycycline is contraindicated in pregnancy (discolors fetal tooth enamel).

▶ *erythromycin base* **(B)(G)** 500 mg qid x 21 days
    Pediatric: see page 588 for dose by weight
        <45 kg: 30-40 mg/kg/day in 4 doses x 21 days
        >45 kg: same as adult
  E-mycin® *Tab:* 250, 333 mg ent-coat
  Eryc® *Cap:* 250 mg ent-coat
  Ery-Tab® *Tab:* 250, 333, 500 mg ent-coat
  PCE® *Tab:* 333, 500 mg

▶ *minocycline* **(D)(G)** 200 mg bid x 21 days
    Pediatric: <8 years: not recommended
        >8 years, <100 lb: 2 mg/lb on first day in 2 doses, followed by 1 mg/lb/ q 12 hours x 9 more days
        >8 years, >100 lb: same as adult
  Minocin® *Cap:* 100 mg ent-coat

Comment: Minocycline is contraindicated in pregnancy (discolors fetal tooth enamel).

▶ *tetracycline* **(D)** 500 mg qid x 21 days
    Pediatric: see page 595 for dose by weight
        <8 years: not recommended
        >8 years, <100 lb: 25-50 mg/kg/day in 2-4 doses x 7 days

>8 years, >100 lb: same as adult
Achromycin®V *Cap:* 250, 500 mg
Sumycin® *Tab:* 250, 500 mg; *Cap:* 250, 500 mg; *Oral susp:* 125 mg/5 ml (100, 200 ml; fruit, sulfites)

Comment: Tetracycline is contraindicated in pregnancy (discolors fetal tooth enamel).

Malaria (*P. falciparum, P. vivax malaria*)

▶*doxycycline* **(D)(G)** 100 mg daily; initiate 1 to 2 days prior to travel; Take during travel; continue for 4 weeks after leaving the endemic area
    Pediatric: see page 587 for dose by weight
        <8 years: not recommended
        >8 years, <100 lb: 1 mg/lb/day prior to travel; take during travel; continue for 4 weeks after leaving the endemic area
        >8 years, >100 lb: same as adult
Adoxa® *Tab:* 50, 100 mg ent-coat
Doryx® *Cap:* 100 mg
Monodox® *Cap:* 50, 100 mg
Vibramycin® *Cap:* 50, 100 mg; *Syr:* 50 mg/5 ml (raspberry-apple, sulfites); *Oral susp:* 25 mg/5 ml (raspberry)
Vibra-Tab® *Tab:* 100 mg film-coat

Comment: Doxycycline is contraindicated in pregnancy (discolors fetal tooth enamel).

▶*minocycline* **(D)(G)** 100 mg daily; initiate 1 to 2 days prior to travel; Take during travel; continue for 4 weeks after leaving the endemic area
    Pediatric: <8 years: not recommended
        >8 years, <100 lb: 2 mg/lb on first day in 2 doses, followed by 1 mg/lb/ q 12 hours x 9 more days
        >8 years, >100 lb: same as adult
Minocin® *Cap:* 100 mg ent-coat

Comment: Minocycline is contraindicated in pregnancy (discolors fetal tooth enamel).

▶*tetracycline* **(D)** 250 mg daily; initiate 1 to 2 days prior to travel; Take during travel; continue for 4 weeks after leaving the endemic area
    Pediatric: see page 595 for dose by weight
        <8 years: not recommended
        >8 years, <100 lb: 25-50 mg/kg/day in 4 doses x 10 days

Malaria

>8 years, >100 lb: same as adult

Achromycin®V *Cap:* 250, 500 mg

Sumycin® *Tab:* 250, 500 mg; *Cap:* 250, 500 mg; *Oral susp:* 125 mg/5 ml (100, 200 ml; fruit, sulfites)

Comment: *Tetracycline* is contraindicated in pregnancy (discolors fetal tooth enamel).

Anti-malarials

▶*quinine sulfate* **(C)(G)** 1 tab or cap every 8 hours x 7 days

    Pediatric: <16 years: not recommended

    Tab: 260 mg; *Cap:* 260, 300, 325 mg

Qualaquin® *Cap:* 324 mg

Comment: **Qualaquin®** is indicated in the treatment of uncomplicated *P. falciparum* malaria (including chloroquine-resistant strains).

▶*atovaquone/proquanil* **(C)** take as a single dose with food or a milky drink at the same time each day; repeat dose if vomited within 1 hour

    Prophylaxis: 1 tab daily starting 1-2 days before entering endemic area, during stay, and for 7 days after return

    Treatment (Acute, Uncomplicated): 4 tabs daily x 3 days

        Pediatric: <5 kg: not recommended

        5-40 kg: see dose below

    Prophylaxis: daily dose starting 1-2 days before entering endemic area, during stay, and for 7 days after return:

        Pediatric: 5-20 kg: 1 ped tab

            21-30 kg: 2 ped tabs

            31-40 kg: 3 ped tabs

            >40 kg: same as adult

    Treatment (Acute, Uncomplicated): daily dose x 3 days

        Pediatric: 5-8 kg: 2 ped tabs

            9-10 kg: 3 ped tabs

            11-20 kg: 1 adult tab

            21-30 kg: 2 adult tabs

            31-40 kg: 3 adult tabs

            >40 kg: same as adult

Malarone® *Tab: atov* 250 mg/*proq* 100 mg

Malarone®Pediatric *Tab: atov* 62.5 mg/*proq* 25 mg

Comment: *Atovaquone* is antagonized by *tetracycline* and *metoclopramide*. Concomitant *rifampin* is not recommended. May elevate LFTs.

▶*chloroquine* **(C)(G)**

    Prophylaxis: 500 mg once weekly (on the same day of each week); start 2 weeks prior to exposure, continue while in the endemic area, and continue 4 weeks after departure

Treatment: initially 1 g; then 500 mg 6 hours, 24 hours, and 48

Malaria

hours after initial dose or initially 200-250 mg IM; may repeat in 6 hours; max 1 g in first 24 hours; continue to 1.875 g in 3 days

> *Pediatric:* Suppression: 8.35 mg/kg (max 500 mg) weekly (on the same day of each week)
> Treatment: initially 16.7 mg/kg (max 1 g); then 8.35 mg/kg (max 500 mg) 6 hours, 24 hours, and 48 hours after initial dose or initially 6.25 mg/kg IM; may repeat in 6 hours; max 12.5 mg/kg/day

Aralen® *Tab:* 500 mg; *Amp:* 50 mg/ml (5 ml)

▶ *hydroxychloroquine* **(C)(G)**

Prophylaxis: 400 mg once weekly (on the same day of each week); start 2 weeks prior to exposure, continue while in the endemic area, and continue 4 weeks after departure

Treatment: initially 800 mg; then 400 mg 6 hours, 24 hours, and 48 hours after initial dose

> *Pediatric:* Suppression: 6.45 mg/kg (max 400 mg) weekly (on the same day of each week) beginning 2 weeks prior to arrival, continuing while in endemic area, and continuing 4 weeks after departure
> Treatment: initially 12.9 mg/kg (max 800 mg); then 6.45 mg/kg (max 400 mg) 6 hours, 24 hours, and 48 hours after initial dose

Plaquenil® *Tab:* 200 mg

▶ *mefloquine* **(C)**

Prophylaxis: 250 mg once weekly (on the same day of each week); start 1 week prior to exposure, continue while in the endemic area, and continue for 4 weeks after departure

Treatment: 1250 mg as a single dose

> *Pediatric:* <6 months: not recommended
> Prophylaxis: >6 months: 3-5 mg/kg (max 250 mg) weekly (on the same day of each week); start 1 weeks prior to exposure, continue while in the endemic area, and continue for 4 weeks after departure
> Treatment: >6 months: 25-50 mg/kg as a single dose; max 250 mg

Lariam® *Tab:* 250*mg

Comment: Mefloquine is contraindicated with active or recent history of depression, generalized anxiety disorder, psychosis, schizophrenia or any other psychiatric disorder or history of convulsions.

Mastitis (Breast Abscess)

Anti-infectives
▶ *amoxicillin/clavulanate* **(B)(G)** 500 mg tid or 875 mg bid x 10 days
> *Pediatric: see pages 571-572 for dose by weight*
>> 40-45 mg/kg/day divided tid x 10 days or
>> 90 mg/kg/day divided bid x 10 days

Augmentin® *Tab:* 250, 500, 875 mg; *Chew tab:* 125, 250 mg (lemon-lime), 200, 400 mg (cherry-banana, phenylalanine); *Oral susp:* 125 mg/5 ml (banana), 250 mg/5 ml (orange) (75, 100, 150 ml); 200, 400 mg/5 ml (50, 75, 100 ml; orange-raspberry, phenylalanine)

Augmentin®**ES-600** *Oral susp:* 600 mg/5 ml (50, 75, 100, 150 ml; orange-raspberry, phenylalanine)

Augmentin®**XR** 2 tabs q 12 hours x 10 days
> *Pediatric:* <16 years: use other forms
> *Tab:* 1000 mg ext-rel

▶ *cefaclor* **(B)**
Ceclor® 250 mg tid x 7 days
> *Pediatric: see page 575 for dose by weight*
>> 20-40 mg/kg/day in 3 doses x 10 days
> *Pulvule:* 250, 500 mg; *Oral susp:* 125, 250 mg/5 ml (75, 150 ml); 187, 375 mg/5 ml (50, 100 ml) (strawberry)

Ceclor®**CD** 500 mg q 12 hours x 7 days
> *Pediatric:* <16 years: not recommended
> *Tab:* 375, 500 mg ext-rel

Ceclor®**CDpak** 500 mg q 12 hours x 7 days
> *Pediatric:* <16 years: not recommended
> *Tab:* 500 mg (14 tabs/CDpak)

Raniclor® 500 mg q 12 hours x 7 days
> *Pediatric:* 20-40 mg/kg/day in 3 doses x 10 days
> *Chew tab:* 125, 187, 250, 375 mg

▶ *ceftriaxone* **(B)(G)** 1-2 grams IM daily continued 2 days after signs of infection have disappeared; max 4 g/day
> *Pediatric:* 50 mg/kg IM daily continued 2 days after signs of infection have disappeared

Rocephin® *Vial:* 250, 500 mg; 1, 2 g

▶ *cephalexin* **(B)(G)** 500 mg bid x 10 days
> *Pediatric: see page 582 for dose by weight*
>> 25-50 mg/kg/day in 4 doses x 10 days

Keflex® *Cap:* 250, 500, 750 mg; *Oral susp:* 125, 250 mg/5 ml

Mastitis

    (100, 200 ml)
    Keftab® *Tab:* 500 mg
    Keftab®K-pak *Tab:* 20-500 mg tabs/K-pak
▶ *clindamycin* **(B)** 300 mg tid x 10 days
    Pediatric: not recommended
    Cleocin® *Cap:* 75 (tartrazine), 150 (tartrazine), 300 mg
    Cleocin®Pediatric Granules *Oral susp:* 75 mg/5 ml (100 ml; cherry)
▶ *erythromycin base* **(B)(G)** 250-500 mg qid x 10 days
    Pediatric: see page 588 for dose by weight
        <45 kg: 30-40 mg/kg/day in 4 doses x 10 days
        >45 kg: same as adult
    E-mycin® *Tab:* 250, 333 mg ent-coat
    Eryc® *Cap:* 250 mg ent-coat
    Ery-Tab® *Tab:* 250, 333, 500 mg ent-coat
    PCE® *Tab:* 333, 500 mg

Meniere's Disease

▶ *diazepam* **(D)(IV)(G)** initially 1-2.5 mg tid-qid; may increase gradually
    Pediatric: <6 months: not recommended
        >6 months: same as adult
    Valium® *Tab:* 2*, 5*, 10*mg
▶ *dimenhydrinate* **(B)** 50 mg q 4-6 hours
    Pediatric: <2 years: not recommended
        2-6 years: 12.5-25 mg q 6-8 hours; max 75 mg/day
        6-11 years: 25-50 mg q 6-8 hours; max 150 mg/day
    Dramamine® (OTC) *Tab:* 50*mg; *Chew tab:* 50 mg phenylalanine, tartrazine)
    Liq: 12.5 mg/5 ml (4 oz)
▶ *diphenhydramine* **(B)(OTC)(G)** 25-50 mg q 6-8 hours; max 100 mg/day
    Pediatric: <2 years: not recommended
        2-6 years: 6.25 mg q 4-6 hours; max 37.5 mg/day
        6-12 years: 12.5-25 mg q 4-6 hours; max 150 mg/day
    Benadryl® (OTC) *Chew tab:* 12.5 mg (grape, phenylalanine); *Liq:* 12.5 mg/5 ml (4, 8 oz); *Cap:* 25 mg; *Tab:* 25 mg; *Dye-free Softgel:* 25 mg; *Dye-free liq:* 12.5 mg/5 ml (4, 8 oz)
▶ *meclizine* **(B)(G)** 25-100/day in divided doses
    Pediatric: not recommended

Antivert® *Tab:* 12.5, 25, 50*mg
Amp: 50 mg/ml (1 ml); *Vial:* 50 mg/ml (1 ml single-use); 50 mg/ml (10 ml multidose)
Bonine® **(OTC)** *Cap:* 15, 25, 30 mg; *Tab:* 12.5, 25, 50 mg; *Chew tab/Film-coat tab:* 25 mg
Dramamine®II 25 mg bid; max 50 mg/day
Tab: 25*mg

▶*promethazine* **(C)** 12.5-25 q 4-6 hours po or rectally
Pediatric: <2 years: not recommended
>2 years: 0.5 mg/lb or 6.25-25 mg q 4-6 hours po or rectally
Phenergan® *Tab:* 12.5*, 25*, 50 mg; *Plain syr:* 6.25 mg/5 ml; *Fortis syr:* 25 mg/5 ml; *Rectal supp:* 12.5, 25, 50 mg

▶*scopolamine* **(C)**
Pediatric: not recommended
Transderm Scop® 1 patch behind ear; each patch is effective for 3 days
Patch: 1.5 mg (4/box)

Meningitis (*Neisseria meningitides*)

Prophylaxis
Comment: Have epinephrine 1:1000 readily available.

▶*neisseria meningitidis polysacaccharides* **(C)** 0.5 ml SC x 1 dose; if at high risk, may revaccinate after 3-5 years; age >55 years contact mfr
Pediatric: <2 years: contact mfr
>2 years: same as adult; if at high risk, may revaccinate children first vaccinated <4 years of age after 2-3 years
Menactra (A/C/Y/W-135®)
Vial (single-dose): 4 mcg each of group A, C, Y, and W-135 per 0.5 ml (pwdr for SC inj after reconstitution; preservative-free diluent); *Vial (multidose):* 4 mcg each of group A, C, Y, and W-130 per 0.5 ml (pwdr for SC inj after reconstitution (5 doses/vial; preservative-free)
Comment: Latex allergy is a contraindication to **Menactra®**.

▶*neisseria meningitidis polysacaccharides* **(C)** 0.5 ml SC x 1 dose; if at high risk, may revaccinate after 3-5 years
Pediatric: <2 years: not recommended (except >3 months of age as short-term protection against group A)
>2 years: same as adult; if at high risk, may

Meningitis

revaccinate children first vaccinated <4 years of age after 2-3 years (older children after 3-5 years)

Menomune-A/C/Y/W-135®
Vial (single-dose): 50 mcg each of group A, C, Y, and W-135 per 0.5 ml (pwdr for SC inj after reconstitution; preservative-free diluent); *Vial (multidose):* 50 mcg each of group A, C, Y, and W-130 per 0.5 ml (pwdr for SC inj after reconstitution (10 doses/vial: thimerosal diluent)

Comment: Use precaution with latex allergy.

Menopause

Comment: Estrogen replacement lowers LDL and raises HDL. *Estrogen* replacement is indicated for osteoporosis prevention. Exogenous *estrogen* administration increases risk for endometrial cancer, MI, stroke, invasive breast cancer, pulmonary embolism, and DVT. *Estrogen* replacement is contraindicated in known or suspected pregnancy, known or suspected cancer of the breast, known or suspected *estrogen*-dependent neoplasia, undiagnosed genital bleeding, and active thrombophlebitis or thromboembolic disorders. Use HRT with caution in patients with cardiovascular or peripheral vascular disease.

Vaginal Rings

▶ *estradiol, acetate* **(X)**

Femring®Vaginal Ring insert high into vagina; replace every 90 days
  Vag ring: 0.05, 0.1 mg/24 hours (1/pck)

▶ *estradiol, micronized* **(X)**

Estring®Vaginal Ring insert high into vagina; replace every 90 days
  Vag ring: 7.5 mcg/24 hours (1/pck)

Regimens for Patients with an Intact Uterus

Vaginal Preparations (with Uterus)

Comment: Vaginal preparations provide relief from vaginal and urinary symptoms only (i.e., atrophic vaginitis, dyspareunia, dysuria, and urinary frequency).

▶ *estradiol, micronized* **(X)**

Estrace®Vaginal Cream 2-4 g daily x 1-2 weeks, then gradually reduced to 1/2 initial dose x 1-2 weeks, then maintenance dose of 1 g 1-3 times/week
  Vag crm: 0.01% (12, 42.5 g with calib applicator)

▶ *estrogen, conjugated equine* **(X)**

Premarin®Vaginal Cream 0.5-2 g/day intravaginally; cyclically

(3 weeks on, 1 week off)
> *Vag crm:* 1.5 oz w. applicator marked in 1/2 g increments to max of 2 g

Transdermal Systems (with Uterus)
Comment: Alternate sites. Do not apply patches on or near breasts.

▶ *estradiol* **(X)**

Climara® initially 0.025 mg/day patch once/week to trunk (3 weeks on and 1 week off)
> *Transdermal patch:* 0.025, 0.0375, 0.05, 0.075, 0.1 mg/day (4/pck)

Esclim® apply twice weekly x 3 weeks, then 1 week off; use with an oral progestin to prevent endometrial hyperplasia
> *Transdermal patch:* 0.025, 0.0375, 0.05, 0.075, 0.1 mg/day (8, 48/pck)

Vivelle® initially one 0.0375 mg/day patch twice weekly to trunk area; use with an oral progestin to prevent endometrial hyperplasia
> *Transdermal patch:* 0.025, 0.0375, 0.05, 0.075, 0.1 mg/day (8, 48/pck)

Vivelle®-Dot initially one 0.05 mg/day patch twice weekly to lower abdomen, below the waist; use with an oral progestin to prevent endometrial hyperplasia
> *Transdermal patch:* 0.025, 0.0375, 0.05, 0.075, 0.1 mg/day (8, 24/pck)

▶ *estradiol/ levonorgestrel* **(X)** apply 1 patch weekly to lower abdomen; avoid waistline; alternate sites

Climara®Pro *Transdermal patch:* 0.045 mg/*levo* 0.015 mg per day (4/pck)

▶ *estradiol/norethindrone* **(X)**

CombiPatch® apply twice weekly or q 3-4 days
> *Transdermal patch:* 9 cm^2: *est* 0.05 mg/*noreth* 0.14 mg; 16 cm^2: *est* 0.05 mg/*noreth* 0.25 mg

Comment: May cause irregular bleeding in first 6 months of therapy, but usually decreases over time (often to amenorrhea).

Oral Agents (with Uterus)
▶ *estradiol* **(X)(G)**

Estrace® 1-2 mg daily cyclically (3 weeks on and 1 week off)
> *Tab:* 0.5, 1, 2*mg (tartrazine)

▶ *estradiol/norethindrone* **(X)** 1 tab daily

Activella® *Tab:* estra 1 mg/*noreth* 0.5 mg
FemHRT®1/5 *Tab:* est 5 mcg/*noreth* 1 mg

Menopause

▶ *estradiol/norgestimate* **(X)** one-1mg estradiol tab daily x 3 days, then 1-*estradiol* 1 mg/*norgestimate* 0.09 mg tab daily x 3 days; repeat this pattern continuously
    Ortho-Prefest® *Tab:* estra 1 mg/norgest 0.09 mg (30/blister pck)

▶ *estrogen, conjugated/medroxyprogesterone* **(X)**
    Prempro® 1 tab daily
        Tab: **Prempro®0.3/1.5**: *conj est* 0.3 mg/*medroxy* 1.5 mg
                Prempro®0.45/1.5: *conj est* 0.45 mg/*medroxy* 1.5 mg
                Prempro®0.625/2.5: *conj est* 0.625 mg/*medroxy* 2.5 mg
                Prempro®0.625/5: *conj est* 0.625 mg/*medroxy* 5 mg
    Premphase® 0.625 *estrogen* on days 1-14, then 0.625 mg *estrogen*/ 5 mg *medroxyprogesterone* on days 15-28
        Tab (in dial dispenser): conj est 0.625 mg (14 maroon tabs) + medroxy 5 mg (14 blue tabs)

▶ *estrogen, esterified (plant derived)* **(X)**
    Menest® 0.3-2.5 mg daily cyclically, 3 weeks on and 1 week off (with progestins in the latter part of the cycle to prevent endometrial hyperplasia)
        Tab: 0.3, 0.625, 1.25, 2.5 mg

▶ *estrogen, esterified/methyltestosterone* **(X)**
    Estratest® 1 tab daily cyclically, 3 weeks on and 1 week off
        Tab: ester est 1.25 mg/*meth* 2.5 mg
    Estratest®HS 1-2 tabs daily cyclically, 3 weeks on and 1 week off
        Tab: ester est 0.625 mg/*meth* 1.25 mg
    Syntest®D.S. 1-2 tabs daily cyclically, 3 weeks on and 1 week off
        Tab: ester est 1.25 mg/*meth* 2.5 mg
    Syntest®H.S. 1 tab daily cyclically, 3 weeks on and 1 week off
        Tab: ester est 0.625 mg/*meth* 1.25 mg

▶ *ethinyl estradiol* **(X)** 0.02-0.05 mg q 1-2 days cyclically, 3 weeks on and 1 week off (with progestins in the latter part of the cycle to prevent endometrial hyperplasia)
    Estinyl® *Tab:* 0.02 (tartrazine), 0.05 mg

▶ *estropipate, piperazine estrone sulfate* **(X)(G)**
    Ogen® 0.625-1.25 mg daily cyclically (3 weeks on and 1 week off)
        Tab: 0.625, 1.25, 2.5 mg
    Ortho-Est® 0.75-6 mg daily cyclically (3 weeks on and 1 week off)
        Tab: 0.625, 1.25 mg

▶ *medroxyprogesterone* **(X)** 5-10 mg daily for 12 sequential days of each 28-day cycle to prevent endometrial hyperplasia in the post-menopausal women with an intact uterus receiving conjugated estrogens

Amen® *Tab:* 10 mg
Cycrin®, **Provera**® *Tab:* 2.5, 5, 10 mg
▶ *norethidrone acetate* **(X)** 2.5-10 mg daily x 5-10 days during second half of menstrual cycle
Aygestin® *Tab:* 5*mg
▶ *progesterone, micronized* **(X)**
Prometrium® 200 mg daily in the PM for 12 sequential days of Each 28-day cycle to prevent endometrial hyperplasia in the post-menopausal woman with an intact uterus receiving conjugated estrogens
Cap: 100, 200 mg (peanut oil)

Regimens for Patients without Uterus
Oral Agents (without Uterus)
▶ *estradiol* **(X)(G)**
Estrace® 1-2 mg daily
Tab: 0.5*, 1*, 2*mg (tartrazine)
▶ *estrogen, conjugated (equine)* **(X)**
Premarin® 1 tab daily
Tab: 0.3, 0.45, 0.625, 0.9, 1.25, 2.5 mg
▶ *estrogen, conjugated (synthetic)* **(X)** 1 tab daily; may titrate up to max 1.25 mg/day
Cenestin® *Tab:* 0.3, 0.625, 0.9, 1.25 mg
Enjuvia® *Tab:* 0.3, 0.45, 0.625 mg
▶ *estrogen, esterified (plant derived)* **(X)** 1 tab daily
Estratab® *Tab:* 0.3, 0.625, 2.5 mg
Menest® *Tab:* 0.3, 0.625, 1.25, 2.5 mg
▶ *ethinyl estradiol* **(X)** 0.02-0.05 mg q 1-2 days
Estinyl® *Tab:* 0.02 (tartrazine), 0.05 mg

Topical Agents (without Uterus)
▶ *estradiol* **(X)**
Estrasorb® apply 3.48 g (2 pouches) every morning; apply one pouch to each leg from the upper thigh to the calf; rub in for 3 minutes; rub excess on hands onto buttocks
Emul: 0.025 mg/day/pouch (2.5 mg/g; 1.74 g/pouch)
EstroGel® apply 1.25 g (one compression) to one arm from wrist to shoulder once daily at the same time each day
Gel: 0.06 % per compression (93 g)

Transdermal Systems (without Uterus)
Cont rel. Alternate sites. Do not apply patches on or near breasts.
▶ *estradiol* **(X)**
Alora® initially 0.05 mg/day apply patch twice weekly to lower

Menopause

abdomen, upper quadrant of buttocks or outer aspect of hip
> *Transdermal patch:* 0.025, 0.05, 0.075, 0.1 mg/day (8, 24/pck)

Climara® initially 0.025 mg/day patch once/week to trunk
> *Transdermal patch:* 0.025, 0.0375, 0.05, 0.075, 0.1 mg/day (4, 8, 24/pck)

Esclim® initially 0.025 mg/day apply patch twice weekly to buttocks, femoral triangle, or upper arm
> *Transdermal patch:* 0.025, 0.0375, 0.05, 0.075, 0.1 mg/day (8/pck)

Estraderm® initially apply one 0.05 mg/day patch twice weekly to trunk
> *Transdermal patch:* 0.05, 0.1 mg/day (8, 24/pck)

Menostar® apply one patch weekly to lower abdomen, below the waist; avoid the breasts; alternate sites
> *Transdermal patch:* 14 mcg/day (4/pck)

Vivelle® initially one 0.0375 mg/day patch twice weekly to trunk area; adjust after one month of therapy
> *Transdermal patch:* 0.025, 0.0375, 0.05, 0.075, 0.1 mg/day (8, 48/pck)

Vivelle®-Dot initially apply one 0.05 mg/day patch twice weekly to lower abdomen, below the waist; adjust after one month of therapy
> *Transdermal patch:* 0.025, 0.0375, 0.05, 0.075, 0.1 mg/day (8, 24/pck)

Comment: The *estrogens* in **Alora®**, **Climara®**, **Estraderm®**, and **Vivelle-Dot®** are plant-derived.

Mitral Valve Prolapse

▶ *propranolol* **(C)(G)**
Inderal® 10-30 mg tid-qid
> *Tab:* 10*, 20*, 40*, 60*, 80*mg

Inderal®LA initially 80 mg daily in a single dose; increase q 3-7 days; usual range 120-160 mg/day; max 320 mg/day in a single dose
> *Cap:* 60, 80, 120, 160 mg sust-rel

InnoPran®XL initially 80 mg q HS; max 120 mg/day
> *Cap:* 80, 120 mg ext-rel

Mononucleosis (Mono)

Analgesics
▶ *acetaminophen* **(B)** see ***Fever*** *page 168*
Oral Narcotic Analgesics see ***Pain*** *page 308*
Parenteral Glucocorticosteroids *see page 389*
Oral Glucocorticosteroids *see page 387*
▶ *prednisone* **(C)** initially 40-80 mg/day, then taper off over 5-7 days

Motion Sickness

▶ *dimenhydrinate* **(B)(OTC)** 50-100 mg q 4-6 hours; start ½-1 hour before travel; max 400 mg/day
    Dramamine®
        Pediatric: <2 years: not recommended
            2-6 years: 12.5-25 mg; max 75 mg/day; start ½-1 hour before travel; may repeat q 6-8 hours
            6-11 years: 25-50 mg; max 150 mg/day; start ½-1 hour before travel; may repeat q 6-8 hours
        Tab: 50*mg; *Chew tab:* 50 mg (phenylalanine, tartrazine); *Liq:* 12.5 mg/5 ml (4 oz)
▶ *meclizine* **(B)(G)** 25-50 mg 1 hour before travel; may repeat q 24 hours as needed; max 50 mg/day
        Pediatric: not recommended
    Antivert® *Tab:* 12.5, 25, 50*mg
    Bonine® (OTC) *Cap:* 15, 25, 50 mg; *Tab:* 12.5, 25, 50 mg; *Chew tab/Film-coat tab:* 25 mg
    Dramamine®II (OTC) *Tab:* 25 mg
▶ *prochlorperazine* **(C)(G)**
    Compazine® 5-10 mg q 4 hours as needed
        Pediatric: not recommended
        Tab: 5 mg; *Syr:* 5 mg/5 ml (4 oz; fruit); *Rectal supp:* 2.5, 5, 25 mg
    Compazine®Spansule 15 mg q AM or 10 mg q 12 hours
        Spansules: 10, 15 mg sust-rel
▶ *promethazine* **(C)(G)** 25 mg 30-60 minutes before travel; may repeat in 8-12 hours
        Pediatric: <2 years: not recommended
            >2 years: 12.5-25 mg 30-60 minutes before travel; may repeat in 8-12 hours

Phenergan® *Tab:* 12.5*, 25*, 50 mg; *Plain syr:* 6.25 mg/5 ml; *Fortis syr:* 25 mg/5 ml; *Rectal supp:* 12.5, 25, 50 mg

▶ *scopolamine* **(C)**

Scopace® 0.4-0.8 mg 1 hour before travel; may repeat in 8 hours
Pediatric: not recommended
Tab: 0.4 mg

Transderm Scop® 1 patch behind ear at least 4 hours before travel; each patch is effective for 3 days
Pediatric: not recommended
Transdermal patch: 1.5 mg (4/box)

Multiple Sclerosis

Immunomodulators

Comment: The role of immunomodulators in the treatment of MS is to slow progression of physical disability and to decrease frequency of clinical exacerbations.

▶ *glatiramer acetate* **(B)**
Pediatric: <18 years: not recommended

Copaxone® 20 mg SC daily
Prefilled syringe: 20 mg/ml (mannitol, preservative-free)

▶ *interferon beta-1a* **(C)**
Pediatric: <18 years: not recommended

Avonex® 30 mcg IM weekly
Vial: 33 mcg/vial pwdr for reconstitution (single-dose w. diluent, 4 vials/kit; albumin [human], preservative-free)

Rebif® initially 8.8 mcg SC 3x/week (at least 48 hours apart and preferably in the late afternoon or evening); increase over 4 weeks to usual dose 44 mcg 3x/week
Prefilled syringe: 22 mcg/0.5 ml (12/box); 44 mcg/0/5 ml (1, 3, 12/box) (albumin [human], preservative-free)

▶ *interferon beta-1b* **(C)** 0.25 mg (8 million IU) SC qod
Pediatric: not recommended

Betaseron®
Vial: 0.3 mg/vial pwdr for reconstitution (single-dose w. diluent) (albumin [human])

Mumps (Infectious Parotitis)

Prophylaxis

▶ *Measles, mumps, rubella, live, attenuated, neomycin vaccine* **(C)**
   MMR II 25 mcg SC (preservative-free)
Comment: Contraindications: hypersensitivity to *neomycin* or eggs, primary or acquired immune deficiency, immunosuppressant therapy, bone marrow or lymphatic malignancy, and pregnancy (within 3 months after vaccination).
see ***Immunizations: Childhood*** *page 466*
Parenteral Glucocorticosteroids *see page 389*
Oral Glucocorticosteroids *see page 387*
Antipyretics *see* ***Fever*** *page 168*

Muscle Strain

NSAIDs *see* ***Pain*** *page 305*
Oral Non-narcotic Analgesics *see* ***Pain*** *page 308*
Oral Narcotic Analgesics *see* ***Pain*** *page 308*
Topical Analgesics *see* ***Pain*** *page 308*
Parenteral Glucocorticosteroids *see page 389*
Oral Glucocorticosteroids *see page 387*
Topical Anesthetic *see page 383*
Topical Anesthetic/Steroid Combinations *see page 480*
Skeletal Muscle Relaxants
Comment: Usual length of treatment for acute injury is approximately 5 days.
▶*baclofen* **(C)** 5 mg tid; titrate up by 5 mg every 3 days to 20 mg tid; max 80 mg/day
   Pediatric: not recommended
   Atrofen®, Lioresal® *Tab:* 10*, 20*mg
Comment: Baclofen is indicated for chronic spasticity associated with multiple sclerosis and spinal cord injury or disease. Potential for seizures or hallucinations on abrupt withdrawal.
▶*carisoprodol* **(C)(G)** 1 tab tid-qid
   Pediatric: not recommended
   Soma® *Tab:* 350 mg
▶*chlorzoxazone* **(NR)(G)** 1 caplet qid; max 750 mg qid
   Pediatric: not recommended
   Parafon Forte®DSC *Cplt:* 500*mg
▶*cyclobenzaprine* **(B)(G)** 10 mg tid; usual range 20-40 mg/day in divided doses; max 60 mg/day x 2-3 weeks
   Pediatric: <15 years: not recommended
   Flexeril® *Tab:* 5, 10 mg

Muscle Strain

▶*dantrolene* **(C)** 25md daily x 7 days; then 25 mg tid x 7 days; then 50 mg tid x 7 days; max 100 mg qid
> *Pediatric:* 0.5 mg/kg daily x 7 days; then 0.5 mg/kg tid x 7 days; then 1 mg/kg tid x 7 days; then 2 mg/kg tid; max 100 mg qid

Dantrium® *Tab:* 25, 50, 100 mg

Comment: Dantrolene is indicated for chronic spasticity associated with multiple sclerosis and spinal cord injury or disease.

▶*diazepam* **(C)(IV)** 2-10 mg bid-qid; may increase gradually
> *Pediatric:* <6 months: not recommended
> >6 months: initially 1-2.5 mg bid-qid; may increase gradually

Valium® *Tab:* 2, 5, 10 mg

▶*metaxalone* **(B)** 2 tabs tid-qid
> *Pediatric:* not recommended

Skelaxin® *Tab:* 400*, 800*mg

▶*methocarbamol* **(C)(G)** initially 1.5 g qid x 2-3 days; maintenance 4 g daily in divided doses
> *Pediatric:* <16 years: not recommended

Robaxin® *Tab:* 500 mg
Robaxin®**-750** *Tab:* 750 mg
Robaxin®**Injection** 10 ml IM or IV; max 30 ml/day; max 3 days; max 5 ml/gluteal injection q 8 hours; max IV rate 3 ml/min
> *Vial:* 100 mg/ml (10 ml)

▶*orphenadrine* **(C)** 1 tab bid
> *Pediatric:* not recommended

Banflex® *Tab:* 100 mg
Norflex® *Tab:* 100 mg sust-rel

▶*tizanidine* **(C)** 1-4 mg q 6-8 hours; max 36 mg/day
> *Pediatric:* not recommended

Zanaflex® *Tab:* 2*, 4**mg; *Cap:* 2, 4, 6 mg

Skeletal Muscle Relaxant/NSAID Combinations

Comment: Aspirin-containing medications are contraindicated with history of allergic-type reaction to aspirin, children and adolescents with *Varicella* or other viral illness, and 3rd trimester pregnancy.

▶*carisoprodol/aspirin* **(C)(III)(G)** 1-2 tabs qid
> *Pediatric:* not recommended

Soma®**Compound** *Tab: caris* 200 mg/*asa* 325 mg (sulfites)

▶*methocarbamol/aspirin* **(D)** 2 tabs qid (or 3 tabs qid x 1-3 days for severe conditions)

Robaxisal® *Tab: methocarb* 400 mg/*asa* 325 mg
▶ *meprobamate/aspirin* **(D)(IV)** 1-2 tabs tid-qid
    Pediatric: not recommended
Equagesic® *Tab: mepro* 200 mg/*asa* 325*mg

Skeletal Muscle Relaxant/NSAID/Caffeine Combinations
▶ *orphenadrine/aspirin/caffeine* **(D)**
    Pediatric: not recommended
Norgesic® 1-2 tabs tid-qid
    Tab: orphen 25 mg/*asa* 385 mg/*caf* 30 mg
Norgesic®Forte ½-1 tab tid-qid; max 4 tabs/day
    Tab: orphen 50 mg/*asa* 770 mg/*caf* 60*mg

Skeletal Muscle Relaxant/NSAID/Codeine Combinations
▶ *carisoprodol/aspirin/codeine* **(C; D in 3rd)(III)**
    Pediatric: not recommended
Soma®Compound w. Codeine 1-2 tabs qid
    Tab: caris 200 mg/*asa* 325 mg/*cod* 16 mg (sulfites)

Narcolepsy

Antinarcoleptic Agent
▶ *modafinil* **(C)(IV)** 100-200 mg q AM; max 400 mg/day
    Pediatric: <16 years: not recommended
Provigil® *Tab:* 100, 200*mg

Comment: **Provigil®** also promotes wakefulness in patients with shift work sleep disorder and excessive sleepiness due to obstructive sleep apnea/hypopnea syndrome.

Stimulants
▶ *dextroamphetamine sulfate* **(C)(II)(G)** initially start with 10 mg daily; increase by 10 mg at weekly intervals if needed; may switch to daily dose with sust-rel spansules when titrated
    Pediatric: <3 years: not recommended
        3-5 years: 2.5 mg daily; may increase by 2.5 mg daily at weekly intervals if needed
        6-12 years: initially 5 mg daily-bid; may increase by 5 mg/day at weekly intervals; usual max 40 mg/day
        >12 years: initially 10 mg daily; may increase by 10 mg/day at weekly intervals; max 40 mg/day
Dexedrine® *Tab:* 5*mg (tartrazine)
Dexedrine®Spansule *Cap:* 5, 10, 15 mg sust-rel
Dextrostat® *Tab:* 5, 10 mg (tartrazine)

Narcolepsy

▶ *dextroamphetamine saccharate/dextroamphetamine sulfate/ amphetamine aspartate/amphetamine sulfate* **(C)(II)**

Adderall® initially 10 mg daily; may increase weekly by 10 mg/day; usual max 60 mg/day in 2-3 divided doses; first dose on awakening and then q 4-6 hours prn

Pediatric: <6 years: not indicated
6-12 years: initially 5 mg daily; may increase weekly by 5 mg/day; usual max 40 mg/day in 2-3 divided doses

Tab: 5**mg: 1.25 mg of each drug
7.5**mg: 1.875 mg of each drug
10**mg: 2.5 mg of each drug
12.5**mg: 3.125 mg of each drug
15**mg: 3.75 mg of each drug 20 mg: 5 mg of each drug
20**mg: 5 mg of each drug
30**mg: 7.5 mg of each drug
(all double-scored)

Adderall®XR not recommended for adult

Pediatric: <6 years: not recommended
6-12 years: initially 10 mg daily in the AM; may increase by 10 mg weekly; max 30 mg/day
13-17 years: initially 10 mg daily; may increase to 20 mg/day after 1 week; max 30 mg/day

Cap: 5 mg: 1.25 mg of each drug ext-rel
10 mg: 2.5 mg of each drug ext-rel
15 mg: 3.75 mg of each drug ext-rel
20 mg: 5 mg of each drug ext-rel
25 mg: 6.25 mg of each drug ext-rel
30 mg: 7.5 mg of each drug ext-rel
Do not chew; may sprinkle on apple sauce

Comment: **Adderall®** is also indicated to improve wakefulness in patients with shift-work sleep disorder and excessive sleepiness due to obstructive sleep apnea/ hypopnea syndrome.

▶ *dexmethylphenidate* **(C)(II)**

Focalin®

Pediatric: <6 years: not recommended
>6 years: initially 2.5 mg bid; allow at least 4 hours between doses; may increase at 1 week intervals; max 20 mg/day

Tab: 2.5, 5, 10*mg (dye-free)

▶ *methamphetamine* **(C)(II)(G)**

Desoxyn®Granumets
> *Pediatric:* <6 years: not recommended
> >6 years: initially 5 mg daily-bid; may increase by 5 mg/day at weekly intervals; usual effective dose 20-25 mg/day
>
> *Tab:* 5, 10, 15 mg sust-rel

▶ *methylphenidate* (regular-acting) **(C)(II)(G)**
> **Methylin®, Methylin®Chewable, Methylin®Oral Solution** usual dose 20-30 mg/day in 2 or 3 divided doses 30-45 minutes before a meal; may increase to 60 mg/day
> > *Pediatric:* <6 years: not recommended
> > >6 years: initially 5 mg twice daily before breakfast and lunch; may increase 5-10 mg/week; max 60 mg/day
> >
> > *Tab:* 5, 10*, 20*mg; *Chew tab:* 2.5, 5, 10 mg (grape, phenylalanine); *Oral soln:* 5, 10 mg/5 ml; grape)
>
> **Ritalin®** 10-60 mg/day in 2-3 divided doses 30-45 minutes ac; max 60 mg/day
> > *Pediatric:* <6 years: not recommended
> > >6 years: initially 5 mg bid ac (before breakfast and lunch); may gradually increase by 5-10 mg at weekly intervals as needed; max 60 mg/day
> >
> > *Tab:* 5, 10*, 20*mg

▶ *methylphenidate* (long-acting) **(C)(II)**
> **Concerta®** initially 18 mg q AM; may increase in 18 mg increments as needed; max 54 mg/day
> > *Tab:* 18, 27, 36, 54 mg sust-rel
>
> **Metadate®CD** 1 cap daily in the AM
> > *Pediatric:* <6 years: not recommended
> > >6 years: initially 20 mg daily; may gradually increase by 20 mg/day at weekly intervals as needed; max 60 mg/day
> >
> > *Cap:* 10, 20, 30 mg immed- and ext-rel beads (dye-free)

Comment: May sprinkle on food, but do not crush or chew.
> **Metadate®ER** 1 tab daily in the AM
> > *Pediatric:* <6 years: not recommended
> > >6 years: use in place of regular-acting *methylphenidate* when the 8-hour dose of Metadate®-ER corresponds to the titrated 8-hour dose of regular-acting *methylphenidate*
> >
> > *Tab:* 10, 20 mg ext-rel (dye-free)

Narcolepsy

Methylin®ER usual dose 20-30 mg/day in 2 or 3 divided doses 30-45 minutes before a meal; may increase to 60 mg/day
> *Pediatric:* <6 years: not recommended
>> >6 years: initially 5 mg twice daily before breakfast and lunch; may increase by 5-10 mg/week; max 60 mg/day
>
> *Tab:* 10, 20 mg ext-rel

Ritalin®LA 1 cap daily in the AM
> *Pediatric:* <6 years: not recommended
>> >6 years: use in place of regular-acting *methylphenidate* when the 8-hour dose of **Ritalin®LA** corresponds to the titrated 8-hour dose of regular-acting *meethylphenidate*; max 60 mg/day
>
> *Cap:* 10, 20, 30, 40 mg ext-rel (immed- and ext-rel beads)

Ritalin®SR 1 cap daily in the AM
> *Pediatric:* <6 years: not recommended
>> >6 years: use in place of regular-acting *methylphenidate* when the 8-hour dose of Ritalin®SR corresponds to the titrated 8-hour dose of regular-acting *meethylphenidate*; max 60 mg/day
>
> *Tab:* 20 mg sust-rel (dye-free)

▶*methylphenidate* (transdermal patch) **(C)(II)(G)** 1 patch daily in the AM
> *Pediatric:* <6 years: not recommended
>> >6 years: initially 10 mg patch daily in the AM; may Increase by 5-10 mg/week; max 60 mg/day
>
> *Transdermal patch:* 10, 15, 20, 30 mg

▶*pemoline* **(B)(IV)** 18.75-112.5 mg/day; usually start with 37.5 mg in AM; increase weekly by 18.75 mg/day if needed; max 112.5 g/day
> *Pediatric:* <6 years: not recommended
>> >6 years: same as adult

Cylert®
> *Tab:* 18.75*, 37.5*, 75*mg

Cylert®Chewable *Chew tab:* 37.5*mg

Comment: Monitor baseline serum ALT and repeat every 2 weeks thereafter.

Nausea/Vomiting

Prophylaxis (for Prevention of Motion Sickness and Post-op Nausea and Vomiting)

Anti-cholinergic Agents
▶*scopolamine* **(C)**
   Scopace® 0.4-0.8 mg 1 hour before travel; may repeat in 8 hours
      Pediatric: not recommended
      Tab: 0.4 mg
   Transderm Scop® 1 patch behind ear at least 4 hours before travel; each patch is effective for 3 days
      Pediatric: not recommended
      Transdermal patch: 1.5 mg (4/box)

Mild Nausea
▶*phosphorolated carbohydrate* solution **(C)(G)** 1-2 tblsp q 15 minutes until nausea subsides; max 5 doses/day
      Pediatric: 1-2 tsp q 15 minutes until nausea subsides; max 5 doses/day
   Emetrol® (OTC)
      Soln: dextrose 1.87 g/fructose 1.87 g/phosphoric acid 21.5 mg per 5 ml (4, 8, 16 oz)

Cannabinoid
▶*dronabinol* **(C)(III)** initially 5 mg/m^2 1 to 3 hours before chemotherapy; then q 2-4 hours prn; max 4-6 doses/day, 15 mg/m^2
   Marinol® *Cap:* 2.5, 5, 10 mg (sesame seed oil)
▶*nabilone* **(C)(II)** 1-2 mg bid; max 6 mg/day in 3 divided doses; initially 1-3 hours before chemotherapy; may give 1-2 mg the night before chemo; may continue 48 hours after each chemo cycle
   Cesamet® *Cap:* 1 mg (sesame seed oil)

Antihistamines
▶*diphenhydramine* **(C)(G)** 10-50 mg IV or deep IM q 6-8 hours prn; max 400 mg/day
      Pediatric: 5 mg/kg/day in 4 divided doses; max 300 mg/day
   Benadryl® *Vial:* 50 mg/ml (1 ml single-use); 50 mg/ml (10 ml multidose); *Amp:* 50 mg/ml (1 ml); *Prefilled syringe:* 50 mg/ml (1 ml)
▶*meclizine* **(C)(G)**
   Travel: 25-50 mg 1 hour prior to travel; repeat every 24 hours
   Vertigo of vestibular origin: 25-100 mg/day in divided doses
      Pediatric: 5 mg/kg/day in 4 divided doses; max 300 mg/day
   Antivert® *Tab:* 12.5, 25, 50*mg; *Amp:* 50 mg/ml (1 ml)
      Vial: 50 mg/ml (1 ml single-use); 50 mg/ml (10 ml multidose)

Moderate to Severe Nausea
Phenothiazines
▶*chlorpromazine* **(C)(G)** 10-25 mg po q 4 hours prn or 50-100 mg

Nausea/Vomiting

rectally q 6-8 hours prn
> *Pediatric:* <6 months: not recommended
> >6 months: 0.25 mg/lb orally q 4-6 hours prn or 0.5 mg/lb rectally q 6-8 hours prn

Thorazine® *Tab:* 10, 25, 50, 100, 200 mg; *Spansule:* 30, 75, 150 mg sust-rel; *Syr:* 10 mg/5 ml (4 oz; orange custard); *Conc:* 30 mg/ml (4 oz); 100 mg/ml (2, 8 oz); *Supp:* 25, 100 mg

▶*perphenazine* **(C)** 5 mg IM (may repeat in 6 hours) or 8-16 mg/day po in divided doses; max 15 mg/day IM; max 24 mg/day po
> *Pediatric:* not recommended

Trilafon® *Tab:* 2, 4, 8, 16 mg; *Oral conc:* 16 mg/ 5 ml (118 ml); *Amp:* 5 mg/ml (1 ml)

▶*prochlorperazine* **(C)(G)** 5-10 mg tid-qid prn; usual max 40 mg/day
Compazine®
> *Pediatric:* <2 years or 20 lb: not recommended
> > 20-29 lb: 2.5 mg daily-bid prn; max 7.5 mg/day
> > 30-39 lb: 2.5 mg bid-tid prn; max 10 mg/day
> > 40-85 lb: 2.5 mg tid or 5 mg bid prn; max 15 mg/day
>
> *Tab:* 5, 10 mg; *Syr:* 5 mg/5 ml (4 oz; fruit)

Compazine®Suppository 25 mg rectally bid prn; usual max 50 mg/day
> *Pediatric:* <2 years or 20 lb: not recommended
> > 20-29 lb: 2.5 mg daily-bid prn; max 7.5 mg/day
> > 30-39 lb: 2.5 mg bid-tid prn; max 10 mg/day
> > 40-85 lb: 2.5 mg tid or 5 mg bid prn; max 15 mg/day
>
> *Rectal supp:* 2.5, 5, 25 mg

Compazine®Injectable 5-10 mg tid-qid prn
> *Pediatric:* <2 years or 20 lb: not recommended
> >2 years or 20 lb: 0.06 mg/kg x 1 dose
>
> *Vial:* 5 mg/ml (2, 10 ml)

Compazine®Spansule 15 mg q AM prn or 10 mg q 12 hours prn usual max 40 mg/day
> *Pediatric:* not recommended
> *Spansule:* 10, 15 mg sust-rel

▶*promethazine* **(C)(G)** 25 mg po or rectally q 4-6 hours prn
> *Pediatric:* <2 years: not recommended
> >2 years: 0.5 mg/lb or 6.25-25 mg q 4-6 hours prn

Phenergan® *Tab:* 12.5*, 25*, 50 mg; *Plain syr:* 6.25 mg/5 ml; *Fortis syr:* 25 mg/5 ml; *Rectal supp:* 12.5, 25, 50 mg

▶*thiethylperazine* **(X)** 10-30 mg tid
> *Pediatric:* not recommended

Torecan® *Tab:* 10 mg
  Amp: 10 mg/2 ml (2 ml)

Substance P/Neurokinin 1 Receptor Antagonist

▶*aprepitant* **(B)** administer with corticosteroid and 5-HT-3 receptor antagonist
  Day 1 of chemotherapy cycle: 125 mg 1 hour prior to chemotherapy
  Day 2 & 3: 80 mg in the morning
  Pediatric: not recommended
  Emend® *Cap:* 80, 125 mg (1x 25 mg, 2x 80 mg tri-fold pck)

5-HT-3 Receptor Antagonists

Comment: The selective 5-HT-3 receptor antagonists indicated for prevention of nausea and vomiting associated with highly emetogenic chemotherapy.

▶*dolasetron* **(B)** administer 100 mg IV over 30 seconds, 30 min prior to administration of chemotherapy or 2 hours before surgery; max 100 mg/dose
  Pediatric: <2 years: not recommended
    2-16 years: 1.8 mg/kg
  Anzimet® *Tab:* 50, 100 mg; *Amp:* 12.5 mg/0.625 ml; *Prefilled carpuject syringe:* 12.5 mg (0.625 ml); *Vial:* 100 mg/5 ml (single-use)
    Vial: 500 mg/25 ml (multidose)

▶*granisetron* **(B)** administer IV over 30 seconds, 30 min prior to administration of chemotherapy; max 1 dose/week
  Pediatric: <2 years: not recommended
    >2 years: 10 mcg/kg
  Kytril® *Tab:* 1 mg; *Oral soln:* 2 mg/10 ml (30 ml; orange); *Vial:* 1 mg/ml (1 ml single-dose; preservative-free); 1 mg/ml (4 ml multidose; benzyl alcohol)

▶*ondansetron* **(C)(G)**
  Oral Forms:
    Highly emetogenic chemotherapy:
      24 mg x 1 dose 30 min prior to start of single-day chemotherapy
    Moderately emetogenic chemotherapy:
      8 mg q 8 hours x 2 doses beginning 30 minutes prior to start of chemotherapy; then 8 mg q 12 hours x 1-2 days following
  Pediatric:
    <4 years: not recommended
    4-11 years, moderately emetogenic chemotherapy:
      4 mg q 4 hours x 3 doses beginning 30 min prior to start;

Nausea/Vomiting

       then 4 mg q 8 hours x 1-2 days following
    Zofran® *Tab:* 4, 8, 24 mg
    Zofran®ODT *Tab:* 4, 8 mg orally-disintegrating (strawberry, phenylalanine)
    Zofran®Oral Solution *Oral soln:* 4 mg/5 ml (50 ml; strawberry, phenylalanine); *Parenteral form:* see mfr literature
    Zofran®Injection *Vial:* 2 mg/ml (2 ml single-dose); 2 mg/ml (20 ml multidose); 32 mg/50 ml (50 ml multidose)

▶ *palonosetron* **(B)** administer IV over 30 seconds, 30 min prior to administration of chemotherapy; max 1 dose/week
    Pediatric: <18 years: not recommended
    Aloxi® *Vial (single-use):* 0.025 mg/5 ml (mannitol)

Anti-dopaminergic (Promotility Agent)

▶ *metoclopramide* **(B)** 10 mg 30 minutes before each meal and at HS for 2-8 weeks
    Reglan® *Tab:* 5, 10*mg

Comment: Metoclopropamide is contraindicated when stimulation of GI motility may be dangerous. Observe for tardive dyskinesia and Parkinsonism. Avoid concomitant drugs which may cause an extrapyramidal reaction (e.g., phenothiazines, *haloperidol*).

Nerve Agent Poisoning

▶ *atropine sulfate* **(NR)(G)** 2 mg IM
    Pediatric: 15-40 lb: 0.5 mg IM
               40-90 lb: 1 mg IM
               >90 lb: same as adult
    Atropen® *Pen (single-use):* 0.5, 1, 2 mg (0.5 ml)

Obesity

Comment: Target BMI is 27-30 (≤27 preferred).

Lipase Inhibitor

▶ *orlistat* **(B)** 1 cap tid one hour before or during each main meal containing fat
    Pediatric: <12 years: not recommended
    Xenical® *Cap:* 120 mg

Comment: For use when BMI >30 kg/m² or BMI >27 kg/m² in the presence of other risk factors (i.e., HTN, DM, dyslipidemia).

Anorexigenics

Sympathomimetics

Comment: Side effects include hypertension, tachycardia, restlessness, insomnia, and dry mouth.

▶*benzphetamine* **(X)(III)** initially 25-50 mg daily in the mid-morning or mid-afternoon; may increase to bid-tid as needed
    Pediatric: not recommended
  Didrex® *Tab:* 50*mg

▶*diethylpropion* **(B)(IV)(G)** 25 mg tid 1 hour ac and mid-evening for night hunger if necessary or 75 mg Dospan daily mid-morning
    Pediatric: <16 years: not recommended
  Tenuate® *Tab:* 25 mg
  Tenuate®Dospan *Dospan tab:* 75 mg sust-rel

▶*methamphetamine* **(C)(II)** 10-15 mg q AM
    Pediatric: <12 years: not recommended
  Desoxyn® *Tab:* 5, 10, 15 mg sust-rel

▶*phendimetrazine* **(C)(III)**
    Pediatric: <12 years: not recommended
  Bontril®PDM 35 mg bid-tid 1 hour ac; may reduce to 17.5 mg (1/2 tab)/dose; max 210 mg/day in 3 evenly divided doses
    Tab: 35*mg
  Bontril®Slow-Release 105 mg in the AM 30-60 minutes before breakfast
    Cap: 105 mg slow-rel

▶*phentermine* **(C)(IV)(G)**
    Pediatric: <16 years: not recommended
  Adipex-P® 1 cap before breakfast or ½-1 tab before breakfast or 1/2 tab bid ac
    Cap: 37.5 mg; *Tab:* 37.5*mg
  Fastin® 1 cap before breakfast
    Cap: 30 mg
  Ionamin® 1 cap before breakfast or 10-14 hours prior to HS
    Cap: 15, 30 mg
  Pro-Fast® 1 cap before breakfast
    Cap: 18.75 mg
  Pro-Fast®SA 1 tab tid ac
    Tab: 8 mg
  Pro-Fast®SR 1 cap before breakfast
    Cap: 37.5 mg

Comment: Contraindicated within 14 days of taking an MAOI.

Mixed Neurotransmitter Reuptake Inhibitor

▶*sibutramine* **(C)(IV)** 5-10 mg daily; may increase to 15 mg daily after

Obesity

4 weeks
> *Pediatric:* <16 years: not recommended

Meridia® *Cap:* 5, 10, 15 mg

Comment: Use with caution with serotonergic agents.

Obsessive-Compulsive Disorder (OCD)

Selective Serotonin Reuptake Inhibitors (SSRIs)

▶*fluoxetine* **(C)(G)**
Prozac® initially 20 mg daily; may increase after 1 week; doses >20 mg/day should be divided into AM and noon doses; max 80 mg/day
> *Pediatric:* <8 years: not recommended
> 8-17 years: initially 10 or 20 mg/day; start lower weight children at 10 mg/day; if starting at 10 mg daily, may increase after 1 week to 20 mg daily

Tab: 10*mg; *Cap:* 10, 20, 40 mg; *Oral soln:* 20 mg/5 ml (4 oz; mint)

Prozac®Weekly following daily fluoxetine therapy at 20 mg/day for 13 weeks, may initiate **Prozac®Weekly** 7 days after the last 20 mg *fluoxetine* dose
> *Pediatric:* not recommended

Cap: 90 mg ent-coat del-rel pellets

▶*fluvoxamine* **(C)** initially 50 mg q HS; adjust in 50 mg increments at 4-7 day intervals; range 100-300 mg/day; over 100 mg/day, divide into 2 doses giving the larger dose at HS
> *Pediatric:* <8 years: not recommended
> 8-17 years: initially 25 mg q HS; adjust in 25 mg increments q 4-7 days; usual range 50-200 mg/day; over 50 mg/day, divide into 2 doses giving the larger dose at HS

Luvox® *Tab:* 25, 50*, 100*mg

▶*paroxetine maleate* **(D)(G)**
> *Pediatric:* not recommended

Paxil® initially 20 mg daily in AM; may increase by 10 mg/day at weekly intervals as needed; max 60 mg/day

Tab: 10*, 20*, 30, 40 mg

Paxil®CR initially 25 mg daily in AM; may increase by 12.5 mg at weekly intervals as needed; max 62.5 mg/day

Tab: 12.5, 25, 37.5 mg cont-rel ent-coat

Paxil®Suspension initially 20 mg daily in AM; may increase by 10 mg/day at weekly intervals as needed; max 60 mg/day
> *Oral susp:* 10 mg/5 ml (250 ml; orange)

▶*sertraline* **(C)** initially 50 mg daily; increase at 1 week intervals if needed; max 200 mg daily
> *Pediatric:* <6 years: not recommended
> 6-12 years: initially 25 mg daily; max 200 mg/day
> 13-17 years: initially 50 mg daily; max 200 mg/day

Zoloft® *Tab:* 15*, 50*, 100*mg; *Oral conc:* 20 mg per ml (60 ml, [dilute just before administering in 4 oz water, ginger ale, lemon-lime soda, lemonade, or orange juice]; alcohol 12%)

Tricyclic Antidepressant

▶*clomipramine* **(C)(G)** initially 25 mg daily in divided doses; gradually increase to 100 mg during first 2 weeks; max 250 mg/day; total maintenance dose may be given at HS
> *Pediatric:* <10 years: not recommended
> >10 years: initially 25 mg daily in divided doses; gradually increase; max 3 mg/kg or 100 mg, whichever is smaller

Anafranil® *Cap:* 25, 50, 75 mg

▶*imipramine* **(C)(G)**
Tofranil® initially 75 mg/day; max 200 mg/day
> *Pediatric:* adolescents initially 30-40 mg/day; max 100 mg/day
> *Tab:* 10, 25, 50 mg

Tofranil®PM initially 75 mg/day; max 200 mg/day
> *Pediatric:* not recommended
> *Cap:* 75, 100, 125, 150 mg

Onychomycosis (Fungal Nail)

Oral Agents

▶*griseofulvin, microsize* **(C)(G)** 1 g daily for at least 4 months for finger-nails and at least 6 months for toenails
> *Pediatric:* see page 592 for dose by weight
> 5 mg/lb/day

Grifulvin®V *Tab:* 250, 500 mg; *Oral susp:* 125 mg/5 ml (120 ml; alcohol 0.02%)

▶*griseofulvin, ultramicrosize* **(C)** 750 mg in 1 or more doses for at least 4 months for fingernails and at least 6 months for toenails

Onychomycosis

>Pediatric: <2 years: not recommended
>2 years: 3.3 mg/lb in 1 or more doses

Fulvicin®P/G *Tab:* 125, 165, 250, 330 mg
Grisactin® *Tab:* 250, 330 mg
Grisactin®Ultra *Cap:* 250 mg
Gris-PEG® *Tab:* 125, 250 mg

▶*itraconazole* **(C)(G)** 200 mg daily x 12 consecutive weeks for toenails; 200 mg bid x 1 week, off 3 weeks, then 200 mg bid x 1 additional week for fingernails

>*Pediatric:* not recommended

Sporanox® *Cap:* 100 mg; *Soln:* 10 mg/ml (150 ml; cherry-caramel); **Pulse Pack®**: 100 mg caps (7/pck)

▶*terbinafine* **(B)(G)** 250 mg daily x 6 weeks for fingernails; 250 mg daily x 12 weeks for toenails

>*Pediatric:* not recommended

Lamisil® *Tab:* 250 mg

Topical Agent

▶*ciclopirox* **(B)** apply evenly to entire onycholytic nail and surrounding 5 mm of skin daily, preferably at HS or 8 hours before washing; apply to nailbed, hyponychium, and under surface of nail plate when it is free of the nailbed; apply over previous coats, then remove with alcohol once per week; treat for up to 48 weeks.

>*Pediatric:* not recommended

Penlac®Nail Lacquer *Topical soln (nail lacquer):* 8% (3.3 ml)

Comment: File and trim nail while nail is free from drug. Remove unattached infected nail as frequently as monthly. For use with mild to moderate onychomycosis of the fingernails and toenails, without lunula involvement due to *Trichophyton rubrum* immunocompetent patients as part of a comprehensive treatment program. For use on nails and adjacent skin only.

Ophthalmia Neonatorum: Chlamydial

Prophylaxis

▶*erythromycin* ophthalmic ointment 0.5-1 cm ribbon into lower conjunctival sac of each eye x 1 application

Ilotycin®Ophthalmic Ointment *Ophth oint:* 5 mg/g (1/8 oz)

Treatment

▶*erythromycin ethylsuccinate* **(B)(G)** 50 mg/kg/day in 4 doses for at least 14 days

>*Pediatric:* see page 589 for dose by weight
>30-50 mg/kg/day in 4 divided doses x 7 days; may

double dose with severe infection; max 100 mg/kg/day for at least 14 days

Ery-Ped® *Oral susp:* 200 mg/5 ml (100, 200 ml; fruit); 400 mg/5 ml (60, 100, 200 ml; banana); *Oral drops:* 200, 400 mg/5 ml (50 ml; fruit); *Chew tab:* 200 mg wafer (fruit)

E.E.S.® *Oral susp:* 200, 400 mg/5 ml (100 ml; fruit)

E.E.S.®Granules *Oral susp:* 200 mg/5 ml (100, 200 ml; cherry)

Ophthalmia Neonatorum: Gonococcal

Prophylaxis

▶ *erythromycin* ophthalmic ointment **(G)** 0.5-1 cm ribbon into lower conjunctival sac of each eye x 1 application

Ilotycin®Ophthalmic Ointment *Ophth oint:* 5 mg/g (1/8 oz)

▶ *silver nitrate* 1% aqueous solution **(G)** 2 drops x 1 application

Ophth soln: 1% (single-dose wax ampule)

▶ *tetracycline* 1% ophthalmic ointment **(G)** x 1 application

Ophth oint: 1%, 10 mg/g (3.5 g)

Treatment

▶ *ceftriaxone* **(B)(G)**

Pediatric: 25-50 mg/kg IM x 1 dose; max 125 mg/dose

Rocephin® *Vial:* 250, 500 mg; 1, 2 g

Opioid Dependence
Opioid Withdrawal Syndrome

Narcotic Analgesic

▶ *methadone* **(C)**

Narcotic Detoxification: 15-40 mg daily in decreasing doses not to exceed 21 days

Narcotic Maintenance: (>21 days; see mfr literature)

Pediatric: not recommended

Dolophine® *Tab:* 5, 10 mg; *Dispersible tab:* 40 mg (dissolve in 120 ml orange juice or other citrus drink); *Oral conc:* 5, 10 mg/5 ml; 10 mg/10 ml

Comment: Methadone maintenance is allowed only by approved providers with strict state and federal regulations.

Opioid Antagonist

▶ *naltrexone* **(C)** 50 mg daily

ReVia® *Tab:* 50 mg

Opioid Dependence

Opioid Partial Agonist-Antagonist
▶*buprenorphine* **(C)** 8 mg in a single dose on day 1; then 16 mg in a single dose on day 2; target dose is 16 mg/day in a single dose
  Pediatric: <16 years: not recommended
 Subutex® dissolve under tongue; do not swallow whole
  SL tab: 2, 8 mg

Opioid Partial Agonist-Antagonist/Opioid Antagonist
▶*buprenorphine/naloxone* **(C)** adjust in 2-4 mg of buprenorphine/day in a single dose; usual range is 4-24 mg/day in a single dose; target dose is 16 mg/day in a single dose
  Pediatric: <16 years: not recommended
 Suboxone®2/0.5 SL Tab dissolve under tongue; do not swallow whole
  SL tab: bupre 2 mg/*nalox* 0.5 mg per tab (lemon-lime)
 Suboxone®8/2 SL Tab dissolve under tongue; do not swallow whole
  SL tab: bupre 8 mg/*nalox* 2 mg per tab (lemon-lime)
Comment: **Sobutex®** and **Suboxone®** maintenance is allowed only by approved providers with strict state and federal regulations.

Opioid Overdose

Opioid Antagonists
▶*nalmefene* **(B)** initially 0.25 mcg/kg IV/IM/SC, then incremental doses of 0.25 mcg/kg at 2-5 minute intervals; cumulative max 1 mcg/kg; if opioid dependency suspected use 0.1 mg/70 kg initially and then proceed as usual if no response in 2 minutes
  Pediatric: not recommended
 Revex® *Amp:* 100 mcg/1 ml (1 ml); 1 mg/ml (2 ml)
▶*naloxone* **(B)** 0.4-2 mg IV/IM/SC; repeat in 2-3 minutes if no response
  Pediatric: 0.01 mg/kg initially, repeat in 2-3 minutes at 0.1 mg/kg if response inadequate
 Narcan® *Vial:* 0.4, ml, 1 mg/ml (10 ml); *Prefilled syringe:* 0.4 mg/ml (1 ml), 1 mg/ml (2 ml); *Amp:* 0.4 mg/ml (1 ml), 1 mg/ml (2 ml) (parabens-free)

Osgood-Schlatter Disease

NSAIDs *see Pain page 305*

Oral Non-narcotic Analgesics *see **Pain** page 308*
Oral Narcotic Analgesics *see **Pain** page 308*
Topical Analgesics *see **Pain** page 308*
Parenteral Glucocorticosteroids *see page 389*
Oral Glucocorticosteroids *see page 387*
Topical Anesthetic *see page 614*
Topical Anesthetic/Steroid Combinations *see page 480*

Osteoarthritis

NSAIDs *see **Pain** page 305*
Oral Non-narcotic Analgesics *see **Pain** page 308*
Oral Narcotic Analgesics *see **Pain** page 308*
Topical Analgesics *see **Pain** page 308*
Parenteral Glucocorticosteroids *see page 389*
Oral Glucocorticosteroids *see page 387*
Topical Anesthetic *see page 383*
Topical Anesthetic/Steroid Combinations *see page 480*
COX-2 Inhibitor
Comment: Contraindicated with history of asthma, urticaria, and allergic-type reactions to *aspirin*, other NSAIDs, and sulfonamides.
▶*celecoxib* **(C; not for use in 3rd)** 100-400 mg daily-bid; max 800 mg/day
    Pediatric: <18 years: not recommended
  Celebrex® *Cap:* 100, 200 mg
Intra-articular Injection
▶*sodium hyaluronate* **(B)** 20 mg by intra-articular injection weekly x 5 weeks; proceed with *lidocaine* or other anesthetic; remove joint effusion prior to injection
    Pediatric: not recommended
  Hyalgan® *Vial:* 20 mg (2 ml); *Prefilled syringe:* 20 mg (2 ml)

Osteoporosis

Comment: Indications for bone density screening include:
    Post-menopausal women not receiving HRT, maternal history of hip fracture, personal history of fragility fracture, presence of high serum markers of bone resorption, smoker, height >67 inches, weight <125 lbs, taking a steroid, GnRH agonist, or anti-seizure drug, immobilization, hyperthyroidism, post-transplantation, malabsorption syndrome,

Osteoporosis

hyperparathyroidism, prolactinemia. The mnemonic "**ABONE**" [**A**ge >65, **B**ulk (weight <140 lbs at menopause), and **N**ever **E**strogens (for more than 6 months)], represent other indications for bone density screening.

Foods high in calcium include almonds, broccoli, baked beans, salmon, sardines, buttermilk, turnip greens, collard greens, spinach, pumpkin, rhubarb, and bran.

Calcium Supplements

Comment: Take calcium supplements after meals to avoid gastric upset. Dosages of calcium over 2000 mg/day have not been shown to have any additional benefit. Calcium decreases *tetracycline* absorption. Calcium absorption is decreased by corticosteroids.

▶ *calcitonin-salmon* **(C)**
    Calcimar® 100 IU daily SC or IM
        Vial: 200 IU/ml (2 ml)
    Fortical® 200 IU intranasally daily; alternate nostrils each day
        Nasal spray: 30 doses (3.7 ml)
    Miacalcin® 200 IU intranasally daily; alternate nostrils each day
        Nasal spray: 14 doses (2 ml)
    Miacalcin®Injection 100 units/day SC or IM
        Vial: 2 ml

Comment: Supplement diet with calcium (1 g/day) and vitamin D (400 IU/day).

▶ *calcium carbonate* **(C)(OTC)(G)**
    Rolaids® chew 2 tabs bid; max 14 tabs/day
        Chew tab: 550 mg
    Rolaids®Extra Strength chew 2 tabs bid; max 8 tabs/day
        Chew tab: 1000 mg
    Tums® chew 2 tabs bid; max 16 tabs/day
        Chew tab: 500 mg
    Tums®Extra Strength chew 2 tabs bid; max 10 tabs/day
        Chew tab: 750 mg
    Tums®Ultra chew 2 tabs bid; max 8 tabs/day
        Chew tab: 1000 mg
    Os-Cal®500 (OTC) 1-2 tab bid-tid
        Chew tab: elemental calcium carbonate 500 mg

▶ *calcium carbonate/vitamin D* **(C)(G)**
    Os-Cal®250+D (OTC) 1-2 tab tid
        Tab: elemental calcium carbonate 250 mg/*vit D* 125 IU
    Os-Cal®500+D (OTC) 1-2 tab bid-tid
        Tab: elemental calcium carbonate 500 mg/*vit D* 125 IU
    Viactiv® (OTC) 1 tab tid
        Chew tab: elemental calcium 500 mg/*vit D* 100 IU/
        vitamin K 40 mcg

▶ *calcium citrate* **(C)(G)**

Osteoporosis

Citracal® (OTC) 1-2 tabs bid
Tab: elemental calcium citrate 200 mg

▶*calcium citrate/vitamin D* **(C)(G)**

Citracal®+D (OTC) 1-2 cplt bid
Cplt: elemental calcium citrate 315 mg/vit D 200 IU

Citracal®250+D (OTC) 1-2 tabs bid
Tab: elemental calcium citrate 250 mg/vit D 62.3 IU

Vitamin D Analog

Comment: Concurrent vitamin D supplementation is contraindicated for patients taking *calcitrol* or *doxecalciferol* due to the risk of vitamin D toxicity.

▶*calcitrol* **(C)**

Pre-dialysis: initially 0.25 mcg daily; may increase to 0.5 mcg daily

Dialysis: initially 0.25 mcg daily; may increase by 0.25 mcg/day at 4-8 week intervals; usual maintenance 0.5-1 mcg/day

Hypoparathyroidism: initially 0.25 mcg q AM; may increase by 0.25 mcg/day at 4-8 week intervals; usual maintenance 0.5-2 mcg/day

Pediatric:

Pre-dialysis: <3 years: 10-15 ng/kg/day
>3 years: initially 0.25 mcg daily; may increase to 0.5 mcg/day

Dialysis: not recommended

Hypoparathyroidism: initially 0.25 mcg daily; may increase by 0.25 mcg/day at 2-4 week intervals; usual maintenance (1-5 years) 0.25-0.75 mcg/day, (>6 years) 0.5-2 mcg/day

Rocaltrol® *Cap:* 0.25, 0.5 mcg

Rocaltrol®Solution *Soln:* 1 mcg/ml (15 ml, single-use dispensers)

▶*doxecalciferol* **(C)** initially 0.25 mcg q AM; may increase by 0.25 mcg/day at 4-8 week intervals; usual maintenance 0.5-2 mcg/day

Pediatric: initially 0.25 mcg daily; may increase by 0.25 mcg 0.25 mcg/day at 2-4 week intervals; usual maintenance (1-5 years) 0.25-0.75 mcg/day, (>6 years) 0.5-2 mcg/day

Hectorol® *Cap:* 0.25, 0.5 mcg

Calcium Modifiers (Biphosphates)

Comment: Calcium modifiers should be swallowed whole in the AM with 6-8 oz of plain water 30 minutes before first meal, beverage, or other medications of the day. Monitor serum alkaline phosphatase.

▶*alendronate* **(C)**

Prevention: 5 mg daily or 35 mg weekly

Treatment: 10 mg daily or 70 mg weekly

Pediatric: not recommended

Osteoporosis

      Fosamax® *Tab:* 5, 10, 35, 40, 70 mg
▶*ibadronate* **(C)**
    Pediatric: not recommended
      Boniva® *Tab:* 2.5 mg
▶*risedronate* **(C)** 5 mg daily or 35 mg once weekly
    Pediatric: not recommended
      Actonel® *Tab:* 5, 30, 35 mg
▶*risedronat/calcium* **(C)** 1-5 mg *risedronate* tab weekly and 1-500 mg calcium tab on days 2-7 weekly
      Actonel®with Calcium® *Tab:* risedronate 5 mg <u>and</u> *Tab:* calcium 500 mg (4 *risedronate* tabs + 30 *calcium* tabs/pck)

Selective Estrogen Receptor Modulator
▶*raloxifene* **(X)** 60 mg daily
      Evista® *Tab:* 60 mg
Comment: Contraindicated in women who have history of, or current, venous thrombotic event.

Human Parathyroid Hormone
Comment: Calcium modifiers should be swallowed whole in the AM with 6-8 oz of plain water 30 minutes before first meal, beverage, or other medications of the day. Monitor serum alkaline phosphatase.
▶*teriparatide* **(C)** 20 mcg SC daily in the thigh or abdomen; may treat for up to 2 years
    Pediatric: not recommended
      Forteo®Multidose Pen *Multidose pen:* 250 mcg/ml (3 ml)
Comment: **Forteo®** is indicated for the treatment of post-menopausal osteoporosis in women who are at high risk for fracture and to increase bone mass in men with primary or hypogonadal osteoporosis who are at high risk for fracture.

Estrogen Supplements see ***Menopause*** *page 270*

Otitis Externa

Otic Anti-infective
▶*chloroxylenol/pramoxine* **(C)** otic 4-5 drops tid x 5-10 days
    Pediatric: <1 year: not recommended
               1-12 years: 5 drops bid x 10 days
      PramOtic® *Otic drops: chlorox/pramox* (5 ml w. dropper)
▶*ofloxacin* **(C)** otic 10 drops bid x 10 days
    Pediatric: <1 year: not recommended
               1-12 years: 5 drops bid x 10 days
      Floxin®Otic *Otic soln:* 0.3% (5 ml w. dropper)
Comment: May be used with PE tubes and perforated tympanic membrane.

Otitis Externa

Otic Anti-infective-/Corticosteroid Combinations

▶ *chloroxylenol/pramoxine/hydrocortisone* **(C)** otic drops 4 drops tid-qid x 5-10 days
        Pediatric: 3 drops tid-qid x 5-10 days
    Cortic®Otic Solution *Otic soln:* 10 ml
    Cortane®B Aqueous *Otic soln: chlo* 1 mg/*pram* 10 mg/*hydro* 10 mg per ml (10 ml w. dropper)
    Zoto-HC® *Otic soln: chlo* 1 mg/*pram* 10 mg/*hydro* 10 mg per ml (10 ml w. dropper)

▶ *ciprofloxacin/hydrocortisone* **(C)** otic susp 3 drops bid x 7 days
        Pediatric: <1 year: not recommended
                   >1 year: same as adult
    Cipro®HC Otic *Otic susp: cipro* 0.2%/*hydro* 1% (10 ml w. dropper)

▶ *colistin/neomycin/hydrocortisone/thonzonium* **(C)** otic susp 5 drops tid-qid x 5-10 days
        Pediatric: 4 drops tid-qid x 5-10 days
    Coly-Mycin S® *Otic susp:* 5, 10 ml
    Cortisporin®-TC Otic *Otic susp: colis* 3 mg/*neo* 3.3 mg/*hydro* 10 mg/*thon* 0.5 mg per ml (10 ml w. dropper)

▶ *polymyxin B/neomycin/hydrocortisone* **(C)** 4 drops tid-qid; max 10 days
        Pediatric: 3 drops tid-qid; max 10 days
    Cortisporin®Otic Suspension *Otic susp: poly B* 10,000 u/*neo* 3.5 mg/*hydro* 10 mg per 5 ml (10 ml w. dropper)
    Cortisporin®Otic Solution
        Otic soln: poly B 10000 u/*neo* 3.5 mg/*hydro* 10 mg per 5 ml (10 ml w. dropper)
    Lazersporin® *Otic soln:* 10 ml w. dropper
    PediOtic® *Otic susp: poly B* 10000 u/*neo* 3.5 mg/*hydro* 10 mg per 5 ml (10 ml w. dropper)

▶ *polymyxin B/neomycin/hydrocortisone/surfactant* **(C)** 4 drops tid-qid
        Pediatric: 3 drops tid-qid; max 10 days
    Cortisporin®-TC *Otic susp:* 10 ml w. dropper

Otic Astringents

▶ *acetic acid 2% in aluminum sulfate* **(C)** 4-6 drops in ear q 2-3 hours
        Pediatric: same as adult
    Domeboro®Otic *Otic soln:* 60 ml w. dropper

▶ *acetic acid/propylene glycol/benzethonium chloride/sodium acetate* **(C)** 3-5 drops q 4-6 hours

Pediatric: same as adult
Vosol® *Otic soln: acet* 2% (15, 30 ml)
▶*acetic acid/propylene glycol/hydrocortisone/benzethonium chloride/ sodium acetate* **(C)** 3-5 drops q 4-6 hours
Pediatric: same as adult
Vosol®HC *Otic soln: acet* 2%/*hydro* 1% (10 ml)

Otic Anesthetic/Analgesic Combinations
▶*antipyrine/benzocaine/glycerine* **(C)** fill ear canal and insert cotton plug; may repeat q 1-2 hours as needed
Pediatric: same as adult
A/B Otic® *Otic soln:* 15 ml w. dropper
Auralgan®Otic *Otic soln:* 10 ml w. dropper
Auroto® *Otic soln:* 15 ml w. dropper
Benzotic® *Otic soln:* 15 ml w. dropper
▶*benzocaine* **(C)**
Americaine®Otic 4-5 drops q 1-2 hours
Pediatric: <1 year: not recommended
>1 year: same as adult
Otic drops: 20% (15 ml dropper-top bottle)

Systemic Anti-infectives
Comment: Used for severe disease or with culture.
▶*amoxicillin/clavulanate* **(B)** 500 mg tid or 875 mg bid x 10 days
Pediatric: see pages 571-572 for dose by weight
40-45 mg/kg/day divided tid x 10 days or
90 mg/kg/day divided bid x 10 days
Augmentin® *Tab:* 250, 500, 875 mg; *Chew tab:* 125 mg (lemon-lime), 200 mg (cherry-banana, phenylalanine), 250 mg (lemon-lime), 400 mg (cherry-banana, phenylalanine); *Oral susp:* 125 mg/5 ml (banana), 250 mg/5 ml (orange) (75, 100, 150 ml); 200 mg/5 ml, 400 mg/5 ml (50, 75, 100 ml; orange-raspberry, phenylalanine)
Augmentin®ES-600 *Oral susp:* 600 mg/5 ml (50, 75, 100, 150 ml; orange-raspberry, phenylalanine)
Augmentin®XR 2 tabs q 12 hours x 10 days
Pediatric: <16 years: use other forms
Tab: 1000 mg ext-rel
▶*cefaclor* **(B)**
Ceclor® 500 mg tid x 10 days
Pediatric: see page 575 for dose by weight
20-40 mg/kg/day in 3 doses x 10 days
Pulvule: 250, 500 mg; *Oral susp:* 125, 250 mg/5 ml (75, 150 ml); 187, 375 mg/5 ml (50, 100 ml) (strawberry)

Ceclor®CD 500 mg q 12 hours x 7 days
   Pediatric: <16 years: not recommended
   Tab: 375, 500 mg ext-rel
Ceclor®CDpak 500 mg q 12 hours x 7 days
   Pediatric: <16 years: not recommended
   Tab: 500 mg (14 tabs/CDpak)
Raniclor® 500 mg q 12 hours x 7 days
   Pediatric: 20-40 mg/kg/day in 3 doses x 10 days
   Chew tab: 125, 187, 250, 375 mg
▶*dicloxacillin* **(B)** 500 mg qid x 7-10 days
   Pediatric: see page 586 for dose by weight
      12.5-25 mg/kg/day in 4 doses x 7-10 days
   Dynapen® *Cap:* 125, 250, 500 mg; *Oral susp:* 62.5 mg/5 ml (80, 100, 200 ml)
▶*trimethoprim/sulfamethoxazole* **(C)(G)**
   Pediatric: see page 597 for dose by weight
      <2 months: not recommended
      >2 months: 40 mg/kg/day of *sulfamethoxazole*
      in 2 doses bid x 10 days
Bactrim®, Septra® 2 tabs bid x 10 days
   Tab: trim 80 mg/*sulfa* 400 mg*
Bactrim®DS, Septra®DS 1 tab bid x 10 days
   Tab: trim 160 mg/*sulfa* 800 mg*
Bactrim®Pediatric Suspension, Septra®Pediatric Suspension
20 ml bid x 10 days
   Oral susp: trim 40 mg/*sulfa* 200 mg per 5 ml (100 ml; cherry, alcohol 0.3%)
Comment: Trimethoprim/sulfamethoxazole is not recommended in pregnancy or lactation.

Otitis Media: Acute

Systemic Anti-infectives
▶*amoxicillin* **(B)(G)** 500-875 mg bid or 250-500 mg tid x 10 days
   Pediatric: see page 569 for dose by weight
      <40 kg (88 lb): 20-40 mg/kg/day in 3 doses x 10
      days or 25-45 mg/kg/day in 2 doses x 10 days
   Amoxil® *Cap:* 250, 500 mg; *Tab:* 875*mg; *Chew tab:* 125, 200, 250, 400 mg (cherry-banana-peppermint, phenylalanine); *Oral susp:*

Otitis Media: Acute

125, 250 mg/5 ml (80, 100, 150 ml; strawberry); 200, 400 mg/5 ml (50, 75, 100 ml; bubble gum); *Oral drops:* 50 mg/ml (30 ml; bubble gum)

Trimox® *Cap:* 250, 500 mg; *Oral susp:* 125, 250 mg/5 ml (80, 100, 150 ml; raspberry-strawberry)

▶*amoxicillin/clavulanate* **(B)(G)** 500 mg tid or 875 mg bid x 10 days
   Pediatric: see pages 571-572 for dose by weight
       40-45 mg/kg/day divided tid x 10 days or
       90 mg/kg/day divided bid x 10 days

Augmentin® *Tab:* 250, 500, 875 mg; *Chew tab:* 125 mg (lemon-lime), 200 mg (cherry-banana, phenylalanine), 250 mg (lemon-lime), 400 mg (cherry-banana, phenylalanine); *Oral susp:* 125 mg/5 ml (banana), 250 mg/5 ml (orange) (75, 100, 150 ml); 200 mg/5 ml, 400 mg/5 ml (50, 75, 100 ml; orange-raspberry, phenylalanine)

Augmentin®**ES-600** *Oral susp:* 600 mg/5 ml (50, 75, 100, 150 ml; orange-raspberry, phenylalanine)

Augmentin®**XR** 2 tabs q 12 hours x 10 days
   Pediatric: <16 years: use other forms
   Tab: 1000 mg ext-rel

▶*ampicillin* **(B)** 250-500 mg qid x 10 days
   Pediatric: 50 mg/kg IM 30 minutes before procedure
   Omnipen®, **Principen**® *Cap:* 250, 500 mg; *Oral susp:* 125, 250 mg/5 ml (100, 150, 200 ml; fruit)

▶*azithromycin* **(B)(G)** 500 mg x 1 dose on day 1, then 250 mg daily on days 2-5 or 500 mg daily x 3 days or **Zmax**® 2 g in a single dose
   Pediatric: see page 573 for dose by weight
       12 mg/kg/day x 5 days; max 500 mg/day

Zithromax® *Tab:* 250, 500 mg; *Oral susp:* 100 mg/5 ml (15 ml); 200 mg/5 ml (15, 22.5, 30 ml); (cherry-vanilla-banana); *Pkt:* 1 g for reconstitution (cherry-banana)

Zithromax®**Tri-pak** *Tab:* 3-500 mg tabs/pck
Zithromax®**Z-pak** *Tab:* 6-250 mg tabs/pck
Zmax® *Oral susp:* 2 g ext rel (cherry-banana)

▶*cefaclor* **(B)(G)**
   Ceclor® 250 mg tid or 375 mg bid x 10 days
       Pediatric: see page 575 for dose by weight
           20-40 mg/kg/day in 3 doses x 10 days
       Pulvule: 250, 500 mg; *Oral susp:* 125, 250 mg/5 ml (75, 150 ml); 187, 375 mg/5 ml (50, 100 ml) (strawberry)
   Ceclor®**CD** 500 mg q 12 hours x 7 days
       Pediatric: <16 years: not recommended

Tab: 375, 500 mg ext-rel

Ceclor®CDpak 500 mg q 12 hours x 7 days
Pediatric: <16 years: not recommended
Tab: 500 mg (14 tabs/CDpak)

Raniclor® 500 mg q 12 hours x 7 days

▶*cefdinir* **(B)** 300 mg bid or 600 mg daily x 5-10 days
Pediatric: see page 574 for dose by weight
<6 months: not recommended
6 months-12 years: 14 mg/kg/day in 1-2 doses x 10 days

Omnicef® *Cap:* 300 mg; *Oral susp:* 125 mg/5 ml (60, 100 ml; strawberry)

▶*cefixime* **(B)**
Pediatric: see page 577 for dose by weight
<6 months: not recommended
6 months-12 years, <50 kg: 8 mg/kg/day in 1-2 doses x 10 days
>12 years, >50 kg: same as adult

Suprax®Oral Suspension *Oral susp:* 100 mg/5 ml (50, 75, 100 ml; strawberry)

▶*cefpodoxime proxetil* **(B)** 100 mg bid x 5 days
Pediatric: see page 578 for dose by weight
<2 months: not recommended
2 months-12 years: 10 mg/kg/day (max 400 mg/dose) or 5 mg/kg/day bid (max 200 mg/dose) x 5 days

Vantin® *Tab:* 100, 200 mg; *Oral susp:* 50, 100 mg/5 ml (50, 75, 100 ml; lemon-creme)

▶*cefprozil* **(B)** 250-500 mg bid or 500 mg daily x 10 days
Pediatric: see page 579 for dose by weight
2-12 years: 7.5 mg/kg bid x 10 days

Cefzil® *Tab:* 250, 500 mg; *Oral susp:* 125, 250 mg/5 ml (50, 75, 100 ml; bubble gum, phenylalanine)

▶*ceftibuten* **(B)** 400 mg daily x 10 days
Pediatric: see page 580 for dose by weight
9 mg/kg daily x 10 days; max 400 mg/day

Cedax® *Cap:* 400 mg; *Oral susp:* 90 mg/5 ml (30, 60, 90, 120 ml); 180 mg/5 ml (30, 60, 120 ml; cherry)

▶*ceftriaxone* **(B)** 1-2 g IM x 1 dose; max 4 g
Pediatric: 50 mg/kg IM x 1 dose

Otitis Media: Acute

    Rocephin® *Vial:* 250, 500 mg; 1, 2 g
▶*cefuroxime axetil* **(B)(G)** 250-500 mg bid x 10 days
      Pediatric: see page 581 for dose by weight
          15 mg/kg bid x 10 days
   Ceftin® *Tab:* 125, 250, 500 mg; *Oral susp:* 125, 250 mg/5 ml (50, 100 ml; tutti-frutti)
▶*cephalexin* **(B)(G)** 250 mg qid x 10 days
      Pediatric: see page 582 for dose by weight
          25-50 mg/kg/day in 4 doses x 10 days
   Keflex® *Cap:* 250, 500, 750 mg; *Oral susp:* 125, 250 mg/5 ml (100, 200 ml)
   Keftab® *Tab:* 500 mg
   Keftab®**K-pak** *Tab:* 20-500 mg tabs/pck
▶*cephradine* **(B)** 500 mg q 6-12 hours or 1 g q 12 hours; max 4 g/day
      Pediatric: see page 583 for dose by weight
          <9 months: not recommended
          >9 months: 25-50 mg/kg/day divided q 6-12 hours; max 4 g/day
   Velosef® *Cap:* 250, 500 mg; *Oral susp:* 125, 250 mg/5 ml (100, 200 ml)
▶*clarithromycin* **(C)(G)** 500 mg bid or 500 mg ext-rel daily
      Pediatric: see page 584 for dose by weight
          <6 months: not recommended
          >6 months: 7.5 mg/kg bid x 7 days
   Biaxin® *Tab:* 250, 500 mg
   Biaxin®**Oral Suspension** *Oral susp:* 125, 250 mg/5 ml (50, 100 ml; fruit-punch)
   Biaxin®**XL** *Tab:* 500 mg ext-rel
▶*erythromycin/sulfisoxazole* **(C)(G)**
      Pediatric: <2 months: not recommended
          >2 months: 50 mg/kg/day in 3 doses x 10 days
   Eryzole® *Oral susp: eryth* 200 mg/*sulf* 600 mg per 5 ml (100, 150, 200, 250 ml)
   Pediazole® *Oral susp: eryth* 200 mg/*sulf* 600 mg per 5 ml (100, 150, 200 ml; strawberry-banana)
▶*loracarbef* **(B)** 400 mg bid x 10 days
      Pediatric: see page 593 for dose by weight
          30 mg/kg/day in 2 doses x 7 days
   Lorabid® *Pulvule:* 200, 400 mg; *Oral susp:* 100 mg/5 ml (50, 100 ml); 200 mg/5 ml (50, 75, 100 ml) (strawberry bubble gum)

Otitis Media: Acute

▶*trimethoprim/sulfamethoxazole* **(C)(G)**
    Pediatric: see page 597 for dose by weight
        <2 months: not recommended
        >2 months: 40 mg/kg/day of *sulfamethoxazole*
        in 2 doses bid x 10 days
  Bactrim®, Septra® 2 tabs bid x 10 days
    Tab: trim 80 mg/*sulfa* 400 mg*
  Bactrim®DS, Septra®DS 1 tab bid x 10 days
    Tab: trim 160 mg/*sulfa* 800 mg*
  Bactrim®Pediatric Suspension, Septra®Pediatric Suspension
  20 ml bid x 10 days
    Oral susp: trim 40 mg/*sulfa* 200 mg per 5 ml (100 ml; cherry, alcohol 0.3%)

Comment: Trimethoprim/sulfamethoxazole is not recommended in pregnancy or lactation.

Otic Anti-infectives
▶*ofloxacin* **(C)** otic 10 drops bid x 14 days
    Pediatric: <6 months: not recommended
               6 months-12 years: 5 drops bid x 14 days
  Floxin®Otic *Otic soln:* 0.3% (5, 10 ml w. dropper)

Comment: May be used with patients with perforated tympanic membrane or tympanostomy tubes.

Otic Anti-infective-/Corticosteroid Combinations
Comment: Neomycin may cause ototoxicity.
▶*chloroxylenol/pramoxine/hydrocortisone* **(C)** otic drops 4 drops tid-qid x 5-10 days
    Pediatric: 3 drops tid-qid x 5-10 days
  Cortic®Ear Drops, Cortane®Ear Drops, Zoto-HC® *Otic drops:* 10 ml
▶*ciprofloxacin/hydrocortisone* **(C)** otic susp 3 drops bid x 7 days
    Pediatric: <1 year: not recommended
               >1 year: same as adult
  Cipro®HC *Otic susp: cipro* 0.3%/*dexa* 0.1% (10 ml)
▶*colistin/neomycin/hydrocortisone/thonzonium* **(C)** otic susp 5 drops tid-qid x 5-10 days
    Pediatric: 4 drops tid-qid x 5-10 days
  Coly-Mycin S® *Otic susp:* 5, 10 ml
▶*polymyxin B/neomycin/hydrocortisone* **(C)** 4 drops tid-qid; max 10 days
    Pediatric: 3 drops tid-qid; max 10 days
  Cortisporin® *Otic susp:* 10 ml w. dropper; *Otic soln:* 10 ml w.

Otitis Media: Acute

    dropper
    Lazersporin® *Otic soln:* 10 ml w. dropper
    PediOtic® *Otic susp:* 7.5 ml w. dropper
▶ *polymyxin B/neomycin/hydrocortisone/surfactant* **(C)** 4 drops tid-qid
    Pediatric: 3 drops tid-qid; max 10 days
    Cortisporin®-TC *Otic susp:* 10 ml w. dropper
▶ *ciprofloxacin/hydrocortisone* **(C)** otic susp 3 drops bid x 7 days
    Pediatric: <1 year: not recommended
            >1 year: same as adult

Otic Anesthetic/Analgesic Combinations

▶ *antipyrine/benzocaine/glycerine* **(C)** fill ear canal and insert cotton plug; may repeat q 1-2 hours as needed
    Pediatric: same as adult
    A/B Otic® *Otic soln:* 15 ml w. dropper
    Auralgan®Otic *Otic soln:* 10 ml w. dropper
    Auroto® *Otic soln:* 15 ml w. dropper
    Benzotic® *Otic soln:* 15 ml w. dropper
▶ *benzocaine* **(C)**
    Americaine®Otic 4-5 drops q 1-2 hours
    Pediatric: <1 year: not recommended
            >1 year: same as adult
    Otic drops: 20% (15 ml dropper-top bottle)

Otitis Media: Serous

Anti-infectives *see **Otitis Media: Acute** page 299*
Oral 1st Generation Antihistamines *see page 525*
Oral Decongestants *see page 528*
Oral Antihistamine/Decongestant Combinations *see page 531*
Oral Glucocorticosteroids *see page 387*

Paget's Disease: Bone

Comment: Calcium decreases *tetracycline* absorption. Calcium absorption is decreased by corticosteroids. Calcium absorption is decreased by foods such as rhubarb, spinach, and bran.

Calcium Modifiers
Comment: Calcium modifiers should be swallowed whole in the AM with 6-8 oz of plain water 30 minutes before first meal, beverage, or other medications of the day. Monitor serum alkaline phosphatase.

▶ *alendronate* **(C)** 40 mg daily x 6 months; then check serum alkaline phosphatase; may retreat
Fosamax® *Tab:* 5, 10, 35, 40, 70 mg
▶ *etidronate* **(C)** 5-10 mg/kg/day for <6 months or 11-20 mg/kg/day for <3 months; a 90-day drug-free period should follow completion of therapy, and then retreatment considered
Didronel® *Tab:* 200, 400*mg
▶ *risedronate* **(C)** 30 mg daily x 2 months; may re-treat after a 2-month post-treatment evaluation period
Actonel® *Tab:* 5, 30, 35 mg
▶ *tiludronate disodium* **(C)**
Skelid® 400 mg daily with 6-8 ounces plain water only for 3 months
Tab: 200 mg; *Oral soln:* 10 ml w. dropper

Comment: **Skelid**® is indicated in patients whose serum alkaline phosphatase is 2 times the upper limit of normal, who are symptomatic, or who are at risk for complications.

Pain

Antidepressants see **Depression** *page 132*
Skeletal Muscle Relaxants see **Muscle Strain** *page 277*
NSAIDs
▶ *diclofenac* **(B)**
  Pediatric: not recommended
  Cataflam® 50-100 mg once, then 50 tid; max 150 mg/day
    Tab: 50 mg
  Voltaren® 50-75 mg bid-qid; rarely
    Tab: 25, 50, 75 mg e-c
  Voltaren®**-XR** 100 mg qd; rarely, may use 100 mg bid
    Tab: 100 mg ext rel

Comment: Diclofenac is contraindicated with *aspirin* allergy and late pregnancy.
▶ *diflunisal* **(C)** initially 250-500 mg bid, then 500 mg q 8 hours if needed; max 1500 mg/day
  Pediatric: not recommended
  Dolobid® *Tab:* 250, 500 mg
▶ *etodolac* **(C)(G)**
  Pediatric: not recommended
  Lodine® 200-400 mg q 6-8 hours; max 1200 mg/day
    Cap: 200, 300 mg; *Tab:* 400, 500 mg

Pain

> **Lodine®XL** 400-1000 mg daily
>   *Tab:* 400, 500, 600 mg ext-rel

▶ *fenoprofen* **(B; D in 3rd)** 200 mg q 4-6 hours; max 3200 mg/day
>   *Pediatric:* not recommended
>   **Nalfon®** *Pulvule:* 200, 300 mg; *Tab:* 600 mg

▶ *flurbiprofen* **(B; D in 3rd)(G)** 200-300 mg/day in 2-4 divided doses; max single dose 100 mg
>   *Pediatric:* not recommended
>   **Ansaid®** *Tab:* 50, 100 mg

▶ *ibuprofen* **(B; not for use in 3rd)(G)** 200-400 mg q 4-6 hours prn; max 1.2 g/day
>   *Pediatric: see* **Fever** *page 168*
>   **Advil®** **(OTC)** *Tab:* 200 mg
>   **ElixSure®IB** **(OTC)** *Chew tab:* 100 mg
>   **Motrin®IB** **(OTC)** *Cplt:* 100*mg; *Chew tab:* 50*, 100*mg (citrus, phenylalanine) *Oral susp:* 100 mg/5 ml (4, 16 oz; berry); *Oral drops:* 40 mg/ml (15 ml; berry)
>   **Nuprin®** **(OTC)** *Tab/Cplt/Gel cap:* 200 mg

▶ *ketoprofen* **(B)(G)**
>   *Pediatric:* <16 years: not recommended
>   **Actron®** **(OTC)** 12.5-25 mg q 4-6 hours; max 75 mg/day
>   *Tab:* 12.5 mg; *Cap:* 12.5 mg
>   **Orudis®** 25-50 mg q 6-8 hours; max 300 mg/day
>   *Cap:* 25, 50 mg
>   **Orudis®KT** **(OTC)** 12.5-25 mg q 4-6 hours; max 75 mg/day
>   *Tab:* 12.5 mg; *Cplt:* 12.5 mg
>   **Oruvail®** 200 mg daily; max 200 mg/day
>   *Cap:* 100, 150, 200 mg ext-rel

▶ *ketorolac tromethamine* **(C)** 30-60 mg IM x 1 dose, then 10 mg q 6 hours po x 5 days; max 60 mg IM; max 10 mg/day po; max 5 days; may omit IM or IV dose
>   *Pediatric:* <2 years: not recommended
>   2-16 years (IM/IV): 1 mg/kg IM; max 30 mg IM x 1 dose or 0.5 mg/kg IV; max 15 mg IV x 1 dose; po not recommended
>   **Toradol®IM/IV** *Vial:* 15 mg/ml (1 ml); 30 mg/ml (1, 2 ml); 60 mg/ml (2 ml, 10/box) (alcohol); *Tubex:* 15 mg/ml (1 ml); 30 mg/ml (1, 2 ml); 60 mg/ml (2 ml, 10/box) (alcohol)
>   **Toradol®Oral** *Tab:* 10 mg

Comment: Use *ketorolac* tabs only as continuation therapy; max 5 days combined parenteral and oral therapy.

Pain

▶*naproxen sodium* **(B)(G)**
    Pediatric: <2 years: not recommended
                >2 years: 2.5-5 mg/kg bid-tid; max 15 mg/kg/day; use oral suspension
  Aleve® (OTC) 440 mg x 1 dose; then 220 mg q 8-12 hours; max 10 days
    Tab/Cplt/Gel cap: 220 mg
  Anaprox® 550 mg x 1 dose, then 550 mg q 12 hours or 275 mg q 6-8 hours; max 1.375 g first day and 1.1 g/day thereafter
    Tab: 275 mg
  Anaprox®DS 1 tab bid
    Tab: 550*mg
  EC-Naprosyn® 375 or 500 mg bid; may increase dose up to 1500 mg/day as tolerated
    Tab: 375, 500*mg del-rel
  Naprelan® 1 g daily or 1.5 g daily for limited time; max 1 g/day thereafter
    Tab: 375, 500 mg cont-rel
  Naprosyn® initially 500 mg; then 500 mg q 12 hours or 250 mg q 6-8 hours; max 1.25 g first day and 1 g/day thereafter
    Tab: 250, 375, 500 mg
  Naprosyn®Suspension initially 500 mg; then 500 mg q 12 hours or 250 mg q 6-8 hours; max 1.25 g first day and 1 g/day thereafter
    Oral susp: 125 mg/5 ml (473 ml; pineapple-orange)

▶*piroxicam* **(C)**
    Pediatric: not recommended
  Feldene® 20 mg daily or 10 mg bid; max 20 mg/day
    Cap: 10, 20 mg

▶*salicylate* **(C)** 1 g tid or 1500 mg bid; max 3 g/day
    Pediatric: not recommended
  Disalcid® 20 mg daily or 10 mg bid; max 20 mg/day
    Tab: 500*, 750*mg; *Cap:* 500 mg

Comment: Aspirin-containing medications are contraindicated with history of allergic-type reaction to aspirin, children and adolescents with *Varicella* or other viral illness, and 3rd trimester pregnancy.

▶*salicylate (as choline magnesium trisalicylate)* **(C)** 1-1.5 mg bid
    Pediatric: <12 kg: not recommended
                12-37 kg: 50 mg/kg/day in 2 doses
                >37 kg: 2.25 g/day in 2 doses
  Trilisate® *Tab:* 500*, 750*mg; 1*g

Pain

Trilisate®Liquid *Liq:* 500 mg/5 ml (cherry-cordial)
Comment: Aspirin-containing medications are contraindicated with history of allergic-type reaction to aspirin, children and adolescents with *Varicella* or other viral illness, and 3rd trimester pregnancy.

▶*sulindac* **(C; D in 2nd, 3rd)(G)** 200 mg bid x 7 days; max 400 mg/day
    Pediatric: not recommended
  Clinoril® *Tab:* 150, 200*mg

Topical Analgesics

▶*capsaicin* cream **(NR)** apply tid-qid prn
    Pediatric: <2 years: not recommended
             >2 years: apply sparingly tid-qid prn
  Axsain® *Crm:* 0.075% (1, 2 oz)
  Capin® *Lotn:* 0.025, 0.075% (59 ml)
  Capzasin®-P (OTC) *Crm:* 0.025% (1.5 oz); *Lotn:* 0.025% (2 oz)
  Capzasin®-HP (OTC) *Crm:* 0.075% (1.5 oz); *Lotn:* 0.075% (2 oz)
  Dolorac® *Crm:* 0.025% (28 g)
  DoubleCap® (OTC) *Crm:* 0.05% (2 oz)
  R-Gel® *Gel:* 0.025% (15, 30 g)
  Zostrix® (OTC) *Crm:* 0.025% (0.7, 1.5, 3 oz)
  Zostrix®HP (OTC) *Emol crm:* 0.075% (1, 2 oz)

▶*trolamine salicylate*
  Mobisyl® apply tid-qid
    Crm: 10%

Oral Non-narcotic Analgesics

▶*tramadol* **(C)(G)** 50-100 mg q 4-6 hours prn; max 400 mg/day
  Ultram® *Tab:* 50*mg
    Pediatric: <16 years: not recommended
  Ultram® ER *Tab:* 100, 200, 300 mg ext-rel
    Pediatric: <18 years: not recommended

▶*tramadol/acetaminophen* **(C)(G)** 2 tabs q 4-6 hours; max 8 tabs/day; max 5 days
  CrCl <30 ml/min: max 2 tabs q 12 hours; max 5 days
    Pediatric: not recommended
  Ultracet® *Tab:* tram 37.5/acet 325 mg

Oral Narcotic Analgesics

Comment: For reversal of opioid effects *see **Opioid Overdose** page 292*
▶*codeine sulfate* **(C)(III)(G)** 15-60 q 4-6 hours prn; max 60 mg/day
  Tab: 15, 30, 60 mg

Oral Narcotic Analgesic Combinations

Comment: For reversal of opioid effects *see **Opioid Overdose** page 292*

Pain

▶ *butalbital/acetaminophen* **(C)(G)** 1 tab q 4 hours prn; max 6/day
  Pediatric: <12 years: not recommended
  Cephadyn®, **Promacet®** *Tab: but* 50 mg/*acet* 650 mg
▶ *butalbital/acetaminophen/caffeine* **(C)(G)** 1-2 caps or tabs q 4 hours prn; max 6/day
  Esgic® *Tab: but* 50 mg/*acet* 325 mg/*caf* 40 mg; *Cap: but* 50 mg/*acet* 325 mg/*caf* 40 mg
  Esgic®Plus *Tab: but* 50 mg/*acet* 500 mg/*caf* 40 mg; *Cap: but* 50 mg/*acet* 500 mg/*caf* 40 mg
  Zebutal® *Cap: but* 50 mg/*acet* 500 mg/*caf* 40 mg
▶ *codeine/acetaminophen* **(C)(III)(G)** 15-60 mg of *codeine* q 4 hours prn; max 360 mg of *codeine*/day
  Phenaphen®#3 *Cap: cod* 30 mg/*acet* 300 mg
  Phenaphen®#4 *Cap: cod* 60 mg/*acet* 300 mg
  Tylenol®#1 *Tab: cod* 7.5 mg/*acet* 300 mg (sulfites)
  Tylenol®#2 *Tab: cod* 15 mg/*acet* 300 mg (sulfites)
  Tylenol®#3 *Tab: cod* 30 mg/*acet* 300 mg (sulfites)
  Tylenol®#4 *Tab: cod* 60 mg/*acet* 300 mg (sulfites)
  Tylenol®with Codeine Elixir (C)(V)
    Pediatric: 1 mg of *codeine*/kg/dose q 4-6 hours prn; max 60 mg of *codeine*/dose
      <3 years: not recommended
      3-6 years: 5 ml tid-qid
      7-12 years: 10 ml tid-qid
    Elix: cod 12 mg/*acet* 120 mg per 5 ml (cherry, alcohol 7%)
▶ *dihydrocodeine/acetaminophen/caffeine* **(C)(III)(G)**
    Pediatric: not recommended
  Panlor®DC 1-2 caps q 4-6 hours prn; max 10 caps/day
    Cap: dihydro 16 mg/*acet* 356.4 mg/*caf* 30 mg
  Panlor®SS 1 tab q 4 hours prn; max 5 tabs/day
    Tab: dihydro 32 mg/*acet* 712.8 mg/*caf* 60*mg
▶ *dihydrocodeine/aspirin/caffeine* **(D)(III)(G)** 1-2 caps q 4 hours prn
    Pediatric: not recommended
  Synalgos-DC® *Cap: dihydro* 16 mg/*asa* 356.4 mg/*caf* 30 mg
▶ *fentanyl citrate* transmucosal unit **(C)(II)**
    Pediatric: <16 years: not recommended
  Actiq® dissolve 1 lozenge in mouth; may repeat in 15 minutes; max 2 doses; max 4 units/day caps q 4 hours prn
    Loz: 0.2, 0.4, 0.6, 0.8, 1.2, 1.6 mg

Pain

▶*hydrocodone bitartate/acetaminophen* **(C)(III)(G)**
  Pediatric: not recommended
  Anexsia®5/500 1-2 tabs q 4-6 hours prn; max 8 tabs/day
    Tab: hydro 5 mg/*acet* 500 mg
  Anexsia®7.5/650 1 tab q 4-6 hours prn; max 6 tabs/day
    Tab: hydro 7.5 mg/*acet* 650 mg
  Hydrocet® 1-2 caps q 4-6 hours prn; max 8 caps/day
    Cap: hydro 5 mg/*acet* 500 mg
  Lorcet® 1-2 caps q 4-6 hours prn; max 8 caps/day
    Cap: hydro 5 mg/*acet* 500 mg
  Lorcet®10/650 1 tab q 4-6 hours prn; max 6 tabs/day
    Tab: hydro 10 mg/*acet* 650 mg
  Lorcet®-HD 1 cap q 4-6 hours prn; max 6 tabs/day
    Cap: hydro 5 mg/*acet* 500 mg
  Lorcet®Plus 1 tab q 4-6 hours prn; max 6 tabs/day
    Tab: hydro 7.5 mg/*acet* 650 mg
  Lortab®2.5/500 1-2 tabs q 4-6 hours prn; max 8 tabs/day
    Tab: hydro 2.5 mg/*acet* 500*mg
  Lortab®5/500 1-2 tabs q 4-6 hours prn; max 8 tabs/day
    Tab: hydro 5 mg/*acet* 500*mg
  Lortab®7.5/500 1 tab q 4-6 hours prn; max 6 tabs/day
    Tab: hydro 7.5 mg/*acet* 500*mg
  Lortab®10/500 1 tab q 4-6 hours prn; max 6 tabs/day
    Tab: hydro 10 mg/*acet* 500*mg
  Lortab®Elixir 3 tsp q 4-6 hours prn; max 18 tsp/day
    Liq: hydro 7.5 mg/*acet* 500 mg per 15 ml (tropical fruit punch, alcohol 7%)
  Maxidone® 1 tab q 4-6 hours prn; max 5 tabs/day
    Tab: hydro 10 mg/*acet* 750*mg
  Norco®5/325 1 tab q 4-6 hours prn; max 8 tabs/day
    Tab: hydro 5 mg/*acet* 325*mg
  Norco®7.5/325 1 tab q 4-6 hours prn; max 6 tabs/day
    Tab: hydro 7.5 mg/*acet* 325*mg
  Norco®10/325 1 tab q 4-6 hours prn; max 6 tabs/day
    Tab: hydro 10 mg/*acet* 325*mg
  Vicodin® 1 tab q 4-6 hours prn; max 8 tabs/day
    Tab: hydro 5 mg/*acet* 500*mg
  Vicodin®ES 1 tab q 4-6 hours prn; max 5 tabs/day
    Tab: hydro 7.5 mg/*acet* 750*mg
  Vicodin®HP 1 tab q 4-6 hours prn; max 6 tabs/day
    Tab: hydro 10 mg/*acet* 660*mg

Pain

Zydone®5/400 1-2 caps q 4-6 hours prn; max 8 caps/day
Cap: hydro 5 mg/*acet* 400 mg
Zydone®7.5/400 1-2 caps q 4-6 hours prn; max 8 caps/day
Cap: hydro 7.5 mg/*acet* 400 mg
Zydone®10/400 1-2 caps q 4-6 hours prn; max 6 caps/day
Cap: hydro 10 mg/*acet* 400 mg

▶*hydrocodone/ibuprofen* **(C; not for use in 3rd)(III)(G)**
Pediatric: not recommended
Reprexain® 1 tab q 4-6 hours prn; max 5 tabs/day
Tab: hydro 5 mg/*ibup* 200 mg
Vicoprofen® 1 tab q 4-6 hours prn; max 5 tabs/day
Tab: hydro 7.5 mg/*ibup* 200 mg

▶*hydromorphone* **(C)(II)(G)**
Pediatric: not recommended
Dilaudid® initially 2-4 mg q 4-6 hours prn
Tab: 2, 4, 8 mg (sulfites)
Dilaudid®Oral Liquid 2.5-10 mg q 3-6 hours prn
Liq: 5 mg/5 ml (sulfites)
Dilaudid®Rectal Suppository 2.5-10 mg q 6-8 hours prn
Rectal supp: 3 mg
Dilaudid®Injection initially 1-2 mg SC or IM q 4-6 hours prn
Amp: 1, 2, 4 mg/ml (1 ml)
Dilaudid®-HP Injection initially 1-2 mg SC or IM q 4-6 hours prn
Amp: 10 mg/ml (1 ml)

▶*meperidine* **(C; D in 2nd, 3rd)(II)(G)** 50-150 mg q 3-4 hours prn
Pediatric: 0.5-0.8 mg/lb q 3-4 hours prn; max adult dose
Demerol® *Tab:* 50, 100 mg; *Syr:* 50 mg/5 ml (banana, alcohol-free)

▶*meperidine/promethazine* **(C; D in 2nd, 3rd)(II)(G)**
Pediatric: not recommended
Mepergan® 1-2 tsp q 3-4 hours prn
Syr: mep 25 mg/*prom* 25 mg per ml
Mepergan®Fortis 1-2 tsp q 4-6 hours prn
Tab: mep 50 mg/*prom* 25 mg

▶*methadone* **(C)(II)** 2.5-10 mg PO, SC, or IM q 3-4 hours prn
Pediatric: not recommended
Dolophine® *Tab:* 5, 10 mg; *Dispersible tab:* 40 mg (dissolve in 120 ml orange juice or other citrus drink); *Oral conc:* 5, 10 mg/5 ml; 10 mg/10 ml; *Inj:* 10 mg/ml

Comment: Methadone maintenance is allowed only by approved treatment programs with strict state and federal regulations.

Pain

▶ *morphine sulfate* **(C)(II)(G)**
   Pediatric: not recommended
   MSIR® 5-30 mg q 4 hours prn
      Tab: 15*, 30*mg; *Cap:* 15, 30 mg
   MSIR®Oral Solution
      Oral soln: 10, 20 mg/5 ml (120 ml)
   MSIR®Oral Solution Concentrate
      Oral conc: 20 mg/ml (30, 120 ml w. dropper)
   Roxanol®Oral Solution 10-30 mg q 4 hours prn
      Oral soln: 20 mg/ml (1, 4, 8 oz)
   Roxanol®Rescudose
      Oral soln: 10 mg/2.5 ml (25 single-dose)
▶ *morphine sulfate*, immed- and sust-rel **(C)(II)(G)** dosage dependent upon previous opioid dosages; see product literature for conversion guidelines; not for as needed (prn) use; may sprinkle beads (in caps) on applesauce; however, do not crush, chew, or dissolve
   Pediatric: <18 years: not recommended
   Avinza® 1 cap q 24 hours
      Cap: 30, 60, 90, 120 mg immed- and ext-rel
   Kadian® 1 cap every 12-24 hours
      Cap: 20, 30, 50, 60, 100 mg sust-rel
   MS Contin® 1 tab every 24 hours
      Tab: 15, 30, 60, 100, 200 mg sust-release
   Oramorph®SR *Tab:* 15, 30, 60, 100 mg sust-rel
▶ *nalbuphine* **(B)(G)** 10 mg/70 kg IM, SC, or IV q 3-6 hours prn
   Pediatric: <18 years: not recommended
   Nubain® *Amp:* 10, 20 mg/ml (1 ml; sulfite-free, parabens-free)
▶ *oxycodone* **(B)(II)(G)** 5-15 mg q 4-6 hours prn
   Pediatric: not recommended
   OxyIR® 1 cap q 6 hours prn
      Cap: 5 mg
   Percolone® 1 tab q 6 hours prn
      Tab: 5 mg
   Roxycodone® 1 tab q 6 hours prn
      Tab: 5, 15*, 30*mg; *Soln:* 5 mg/ml
   Roxycodone®Intensol
      Soln: 20 mg/ml
▶ *oxycodone*, cont-rel **(B)(II)(G)** dosage dependent upon previous opioid dosages; see product literature for conversion guidelines
   Pediatric: not recommended

Pain

OxyContin® dose q 12 hours
  Tab: 10, 20, 40, 80 mg cont-rel
OxyFast® dose q 6 hours
  Oral conc: 20 mg/ml (30 ml w. dropper)

▶*oxycodone/acetaminophen* **(C)(II)(G)**
  Pediatric: not recommended
  Percocet®2.5/325 1-2 tabs q 4-6 hours prn; max 4 g *acetaminophen*/day
    Tab: oxy 2.5 mg/*acet* 325 mg
  Percocet®5/325 1-2 tabs q 4-6 hours prn; max 4 g *acetaminophen*/day
    Tab: oxy 5 mg/*acet* 325 mg
  Percocet®7.5/325 1-2 tabs q 4-6 hours prn; max 4 g *acetaminophen*/day
    Tab: oxy 7.5 mg/*acet* 325 mg
  Percocet®10/325 1-2 tabs q 4-6 hours prn; max 4 g *acetaminophen*/day
    Tab: oxy 10 mg/*acet* 325 mg
  Percocet®7.5/500 1 tab q 4-6 hours prn; max 4 g *acetaminophen*/day
    Tab: oxy 7.5 mg/*acet* 500 mg
  Percocet®10/650 1 tab q 4-6 hours prn; max 4 g *acetaminophen*/day
    Tab: oxy 10 mg/*acet* 650 mg
  Roxicet®5/325 1 tab/tsp q 6 hours prn
    Tab: oxy 5 mg/*acet* 325 mg
    Oral soln: oxy 5 mg/*acet* 325 mg per 5 ml
  Roxicet®5/500 1 caplet q 6 hours prn
    Cplt: oxy 5 mg/*acet* 500 mg
  Roxicet®Oral Solution 1 caplet q 6 hours prn
    Oral soln: oxy 5 mg/*acet* 325 mg per 5 ml
  Tylox® 1 cap q 6 hours prn
    Cap: oxy 5 mg/*acet* 500 mg

▶*oxycodone/ibuprophen* **(C)(II)(G)**
  Pediatric: not recommended
  Combunox® 1 tab q 6 hours prn
    Tab: oxy 5 mg/*ibu* 400*mg

▶*oxycodone hydrochloride/oxycodone terephthelate/aspirin* **(D)(II)(G)**
  Pediatric: not recommended
  Percodan® 1 tab q 6 hours prn
    Tab: oxy hydro 4.5 mg/*oxy tere* 0.38 mg/*asa* 325*mg
  Percodan®-Demi 1-2 tabs q 6 hours prn

Pain

       Pediatric: 6-12 years: 1/4 tab q 6 hours prn
                     12-18 years: 1/2 tab q 6 hours prn
       Tab: oxy hydro 2.25 mg/*oxy tere* 0.19 mg/*asa* 325 mg
    Roxiprin® 1-2 tabs q 6 hours prn
       Tab: oxy hydro 4.25 mg/*oxy tere* 0.38 mg/*asa* 325 mg

▶*oxymorphone* 1 supp q 4-6 hours prn
    Numorphan® *Rectal supp:* 5 mg
Comment: Store in refrigerator in original package.
    Opana® 1 tab q 4-6 hours prn
       Tab: 5, 10 mg
    Opana®ER 1 tab q 12 hours prn
       Tab: 5, 10, 20, 40 mg ext rel

▶*pentazocine/acetaminophen* **(C)(IV)** 1 caplet q 4 hours prn; max 6/day
       Pediatric: not recommended
    Talacen® *Cplt: pent* 25 mg/*acet* 650*mg (sulfites)

▶*pentazocine/aspirin* **(D)(IV)** 2 cplts tid-qid prn
       Pediatric: not recommended
    Talwin®Compound *Cplt: pent* 12.5 mg/*asa* 325 mg

▶*pentazocine/naloxone* **(C)(IV)** 1 tab q 3-4 hours prn
       Pediatric: not recommended
    Talwin®NX *Tab: pent* 50 mg/*nal* 0.5*mg

▶*pentazocine lactate* **(C)(IV)** 30 mg IM, SC, or IV q 3-4 hours; max 360 mg/day
       Pediatric: <1 year: not recommended
                   >1 year: 0.5 mg/kg IM
    Talwin®Injectable *Amp: pent* 30 mg/ml (1, 1.5, 2 ml)

▶*propoxyphene napsylate* **(C)(IV)(G)**
       Pediatric: not recommended
    Darvon® 1 cap q 4 hours prn; max 390 mg/day
       Cap: 65 mg
    Darvon®-N 1 tab q 4 hours prn; max 600 mg/day
       Tab: 100 mg

▶ *propoxyphene napsylate/acetaminophen* **(C)(IV)(G)**
       Pediatric: not recommended
    Balacet®325 1 tab q 4 hours prn; max 6 tabs/day
       Tab: prop 100 mg/*acet* 325 mg
    Darvocet®-A500 one tab q 4 hours prn; max 6 tabs/day
       Tab: prop 100 mg/*acet* 500 mg
    Darvocet®-N 50 2 tabs q 4 hours prn; max 12 tabs/day
       Tab: prop 50 mg/*acet* 325 mg
    Darvocet®-N 100 1 tab q 4 hours prn; max 6 tabs/day

Pain

> *Tab: prop* 100 mg/*acet* 650 mg

Wygesic® 1 tab q 4 hours prn; max 390 mg *propoxyphene*/day
> *Tab: prop* 65 mg/*acet* 650 mg

▶*propoxyphene napsylate/aspirin/caffeine* **(D)(IV)(G)** max 390 mg *propox nap*/day
> *Pediatric:* not recommended

Darvon®Compound-32 1 cap q 4 hours prn; max 12/day
> *Cap: prop* 32 mg/*asa* 389 mg/*caf* 32.4 mg

Darvon®Compound-65 1 cap q 4 hours prn; max 6/day
> *Cap: prop* 65 mg/*asa* 389 mg/*caf* 32.4 mg

Transdermal Opioid

Comment: For chronic severe pain.

▶*fentanyl* transdermal system **(C)(II)** apply to clean, dry, non-irritated, intact, skin; hold in place for 30 seconds; start at lowest dose and titrate upward; opioid-naive, change patch every 3 days
> *Pediatric:* <16 years: not recommended
> <18 years, <110 lb: not recommended

Duragesic® *Transdermal patch:* 12, 25, 50, 75, 100 mcg/hour (5/pck)

Transmucosal Opioid

Comment: For chronic severe pain. For management of breakthrough pain in patients with cancer who are already receiving and who are tolerant to opoid therapy. Opoid-tolerant patients are those taking oral morphine ≥60 mg/day, transdermal fentanyl ≥25 mcg/hr, oxycodone ≥30 mg/day, oral hydromorphone ≥8 mg/day, or equivalent, for ≥1 week

▶*fentanyl citrate* **(C)(II)** initially one 200 mcg unit placed between cheek and lower gum; move from side to side; suck (not chew); use 6 units before titrating; titrate dose as needed; max 4 units/day
> *Pediatric:* <16 years: not recommended

Actiq® *Unit:* 200, 400, 600, 800, 1200, 1600 mcg (24 units/pck)
Fentora® *Unit:* 100, 200, 400, 600, 800 mcg (24 units/pck)

Parenteral Opioid

▶*dezocine* **(C)** 5-20 mg IM q 3-6 hours prn; max 120 mg/day
> *Pediatric:* not recommended

Dalgan® *Vial:* 5, 10, 15 mg/ml (2 ml); 10 mg/ml (10 ml)

Parenteral Opioid (Agonist/Antagonist)

▶*pentazocine/naloxone* **(C)(IV)** 1-2 tabs q 3-4 hours prn; max 12 tabs/day
> *Pediatric:* <12 years: not recommended

Talwin®-NX *Tab: pent* 50 mg/*nal* 0.5*mg

Nasal Narcotic Analgesic

Pain

▶*butorphanol* **(C)(IV)** initially 1 spray (1 mg) in one nostril and may repeat after 60-90 minutes (elderly 90-120 minutes) in opposite nostril if needed or 1 spray in each nostril and may repeat in 3-4 hours
   Pediatric: <18 years: not recommended
   Butorphanol®Nasal Spray, Stadol®Nasal Spray *Nasal spray:* 10 mg/ml, 1 mg/actuation (2.5 ml)

Pancreatic Enzyme Deficiency

Comment: Seen in chronic pancreatitis, post-pancreatectomy, cystic fibrosis, steatorrhea, post-GI tract bypass surgery, and ductal obstruction from neoplasia. May sprinkle cap; however, do not crush or chew cap or tab.
▶*pancreatic enzymes* **(C)**
Comment: Contraindicated with pork protein hypersensitivity.
   Creon® 2-4 caps just prior to each meal or snack
      Pediatric: <6 years: 1-2 caps sprinkle on food during meals or snacks
      >6 years: same as adult
   Tab: **Creon®5:** *lipase* 5,000 units/*protease* 18,750 units/*amylase* 16,600 units ent-coat microtabs per cap
   Creon®10: *lipase* 10,000 units/*protease* 37,500 units/amylase 33,200 units ent-coat microtabs per cap
   Creon®20: *lipase* 20,000 units/*protease* 75,000 units/*amylase* 66,400 units ent-coat microtabs per cap
   Cotazym® 2 tabs just prior to each meal or snack
      Tab: lipase 1,000 units/*protease* 12,500 units/*amylase* 12,500 units ent-coat microtabs per tab
   Cotazym®-S 1-3 caps just prior to each meal or snack
      Tab: lipase 5,000 units/*protease* 20,000 units/*amylase* 20,000 units ent-coat microtabs per tab
   Donnazyme® 1-3 caps just prior to each meal or snack
      Cap: lipase 5,000 units/*protease* 20,000 units/*amylase* 20,000 units ent-coat microtabs per cap
   Ku-Zyme® 1-2 caps just prior to each meal or snack
      Cap: lipase 12,000 units/*protease* 15,000 units/*amylase* 15,000 units ent-coat microtabs per cap
   Kutrase® 1-2 caps just prior to each meal or snack
      Cap: lipase 12,000 units/*protease* 30,000 units/*amylase* 30,000 units ent-coat microtabs per cap
   Viokase® 1-2 tabs just prior to each meal or snack

Tab: **Viokase®8:** *lipase* 8,000 units/*protease* 30,000 units/*amylase* 30,000 units per tab

Viokase®16: *lipase* 16,000 units/*protease* 60,000 units/*amylase* 60,000 units per tab

Viokase®Powder 1/4 tsp (0.7 g) with meals

Pwdr: lipase 16,800 units/*protease* 70,000 units/*amylase* 70,000 units per 1/4 tsp (0.7 g)

Pancrease® 4,000-20,000 units or more *lipase* prior to each meal or snack

Pediatric: <6 months: not recommended

6 months-1 year: 2,000 units *lipase* prior to each meal or snack

1-6 years: 4,000-8,000 units or more *lipase* prior to each meal or snack

6-12 years: 4,000-12,000 units or more *lipase* prior to each meal or snack

Tab: **Pancrease®MT4:** *lipase* 4,000 units/*protease* 12,000 units/*amylase* 12,000 units ent-coat microtabs per cap

Pancrease®MT10: *lipase* 10,000 units/*protease* 30,000 units/*amylase* 30,000 units ent-coat microtabs per cap

Pancrease®MT16: *lipase* 16,000 units/*protease* 48,000 units/*amylase* 48,000 units ent-coat microtabs per cap

Pancrease®MT20: *lipase* 20,000 units/*protease* 44,000 units/*amylase* 56,000 units ent-coat microtabs per cap

Ultrase®MT 12 1-3 tabs just prior to each meal or snack

Tab: lipase 12,000 units/*protease* 39,000 units/*amylase* 39,000 units per ent-coat mini tab

Ultrase®MT 18 1-3 tabs just prior to each meal or snack

Tab: lipase 18,000 units/*protease* 58,500 units/*amylase* 58,500 units ent-coat mini tab

Ultrase®MT 20 1-3 tabs just prior to each meal or snack

Tab: lipase 20,000 units/*protease* 65,000 units/*amylase* 65,000 units ent-coat mini tab

Zymase® 1-3 caps just prior to each meal or snack

Cap: lipase 12,000 units/*protease* 24,000 units/*amylase* 24,000 units ent-coat microtabs per cap

Panic Disorder

Selective Serotonin Reuptake Inhibitors (SSRIs)

Panic Disorder

▶*fluoxetine* **(C)(G)**
    Prozac® initially 20 mg daily; may increase after 1 week; doses >20 mg/day should be divided into AM and noon doses; max 80 mg/day
        Pediatric: <8 years: not recommended
                8-17 years: initially 10 or 20 mg/day; start lower weight children at 10 mg/day; if starting at 10 mg daily, may increase after 1 week to 20 mg daily
        Tab: 10*mg; *Cap:* 10, 20, 40 mg; *Oral soln:* 20 mg/5 ml (4 oz; mint)
    Prozac®Weekly following daily fluoxetine therapy at 20 mg/day for 13 weeks, may initiate **Prozac®Weekly** 7 days after the last 20 mg fluoxetine dose
        Pediatric: not recommended
        Cap: 90 mg ent-coat del-rel pellets

▶*paroxetine maleate* **(D)(G)**
    Pediatric: not recommended
    Paxil® initially 20 mg daily in AM; may increase by 10 mg/day at weekly intervals as needed; max 60 mg/day
        Tab: 10*, 20*, 30, 40 mg
    Paxil®CR initially 25 mg daily in AM; may increase by 12.5 mg at weekly intervals as needed; max 62.5 mg/day
        Tab: 12.5, 25, 37.5 mg cont-rel ent-coat
    Paxil®Suspension initially 20 mg daily in AM; may increase by 10 mg/day at weekly intervals as needed; max 60 mg/day
        Oral susp: 10 mg/5 ml (250 ml; orange)

▶*sertraline* **(C)** initially 50 mg daily; increase at 1 week intervals if needed; max 200 mg daily
        Pediatric: <6 years: not recommended
                6-12 years: initially 25 mg daily; max 200 mg/day
                13-17 years: initially 50 mg daily; max 200 mg/day
    Zoloft® *Tab:* 15*, 50*, 100*mg; *Oral conc:* 20 mg per ml (60 ml, [dilute just before administering in 4 oz water, ginger ale, lemon-lime soda, lemonade, or orange juice]; alcohol 12%)

Serotonin-Norepinephrine Reuptake Inhibitor (Mixed Neurotransmitter Reuptake Inhibitor)

▶*venlafaxine* **(C)**
    Effexor® initially 75 mg/day in 2-3 doses; may increase at 4 day intervals in 75 mg increments to 150 mg/day; max 375 mg/day
        Pediatric: <18 years: not recommended
        Tab: 25, 37.5, 50, 75, 100 mg

Panic Disorder

Effexor®XR initially 75 mg q AM; may start at 37.5 mg daily x 4-7 days, then increase by increments of up to 75 mg/day at intervals of at least 4 days; usual max 375 mg/day
    Pediatric: not recommended
    Cap: 37.5, 75, 150 mg ext-rel

Tricyclic Antidepressants
▶*imipramine* **(C)(G)**
    Pediatric: not recommended
    Tofranil® initially 75 mg daily (max 200 mg); adolescents initially 30-40 mg daily (max 100 mg/day); if maintenance dose exceeds 75 mg daily, may switch to **Tofranil®PM** for divided or bedtime dose
        Tab: 10, 25, 50 mg
    Tofranil®PM initially 75 mg daily 1 hour before HS; max 200 mg
        Cap: 75, 100, 125, 150
    Tofranil®Injection 50 mg IM; lower dose for adolescents; switch to oral form as soon as possible
        Amp: 25 mg/2 ml (2 ml)

Benzodiazepines
▶*alprazolam* **(D)(IV)(G)**
    Niravam®, Xanax® initially 0.25-0.5 mg tid; may titrate every 3-4 days; max 4 mg/day
        Tab: 0.25*, 0.5*, 1*, 2*mg
    Xanax®XR initially 0.5-1 mg once daily, preferably in the AM; increase at interals of at least 3-4 days by up to 1 mg/day. Taper no faster than 0.5 mg every 3 days; max 10 mg/day. When switching from immediate-release *alprazolam*, give total daily dose of immediate-release once daily.
        Tab: 0.5, 1, 2, 3 mg

▶*chlordiazepoxide* **(D)(IV)**
    Librium® 50-100 mg q 6 hours prn; max 300 mg/day
        Cap: 5, 10, 25 mg
    Librium®Injectable 25-100 mg IM or IV tid-qid prn; max 300 mg/day
        Inj (pwdr for reconstitution): 100 mg

▶*clonazepam* **(D)(IV)** initially 0.25 mg bid; increase to 1 mg/day after 3 days; max 4 mg/day
    Pediatric: <18 years: not recommended
    Klonopin® *Tab:* 0.5*, 1, 2 mg
    Klonopin®Wafers dissolve in mouth with or without water
        Wafer: 0.125, 0.25, 0.5, 1, 2 mg orally-disintegrating

Parkinson's Disease

Dopamine Precursor
▶ *levodopa* **(C)** initially 0.5-1 g in divided doses; increase if needed q 3-7 days by 0.75 g/day; max 8 mg/day
    Dopar® *Tab:* 100, 250, 500 mg
    Larodopa® *Tab:* 100, 250, 500 mg

Dopamine Receptor Agonists
▶ *amantadine* **(C)** initially 100 mg bid; may increase after 1-2 weeks by 100 mg/day; max 400 mg/day in divided doses; for extrapyramidal effects 100 mg bid; max 300 mg/day in divided doses
    Symmetrel® *Cap:* 100 mg; *Syr:* 50 mg/5 ml (16 oz; raspberry)
▶ *bromocriptine* **(B)(G)** initially 1.25 mg bid to 2.5 mg tid with meals; increase as needed every 2-4 weeks by 2.5 mg/day; max 100 mg/day
    Parlodel® *Tab:* 2.5*mg; *Cap:* 5 mg
▶ *pramipexole* **(C)** initially 0.125 mg tid; increase at intervals q 5-7 days; max 1.5 mg tid
    Mirapex® *Tab:* 0.125, 0.25*, 0.5*, 1*, 1.5*mg
▶ *ropinirole* **(C)** initially 0.25 mg tid for first week; then 0.5 mg tid for second week; then 0.75 mg tid for third week; then 1 mg tid for fourth week; may increase by 1.5 mg/day at 1 week intervals to 9 mg/day; then increase up to 3 mg/day at 1 week intervals; max 24 mg/day
    Requip® *Tab:* 0.25, 0.5, 1, 2, 4, 5 mg

Dopa-Decarboxylase Inhibitors
Comment: Contraindicated in narrow-angle glaucoma. Use with caution with sympathomimetics and anti-hypertensive agents.
▶ *carbidopa/levodopa* **(C)** usually 400-1600 mg *levodopa*/day
    Pediatric: <18 years: not recommended
    Animet® initially 1 tab tid; increase dosage by 1 tab daily or qod
        Tab: carb 25 mg/*levo* 100 mg
    Sinemet®**10/100** initially 1 tab tid-qid; increase if needed daily or qod up to qid
        Tab: carb 10 mg/*levo* 100 mg*
    Sinemet®**25/100** initially 1 tab bid-tid; increase if needed daily or qod up to qid
        Tab: carb 25 mg/*lev* 100 mg*
    Sinemet®**25/250** 1 tab tid-qid
        Tab: carb 25 mg/*lev* 250 mg*
    Sinemet®**CR 25/100** initially one 25/100 tab bid; allow 3 days between dosage adjustments

Parkinson's Disease

    Tab: carb 25 mg/*levo* 100 mg cont-rel
Sinemet®CR 50/200 initially one 50/200 tab bid; allow 3 days between dosage adjustments
    Tab: carb 50 mg/*levo* 200 mg cont-rel*

Dopa-Decarboxylase Inhibitor/Dopamine Precursor/COMT Inhibitor

▶*carbidopa/levodopa/entacapone* **(C)** titrate individually with separate components; then, switch to corresponding strength levodopa and carbidopa; max 8 tabs/day
    Tab: **Stalevo®50**: *carb* 12.5 mg/*levo* 50 mg/*enta* 200 mg
        Stalevo®100: *carb* 12.5 mg/*levo* 100 mg/*enta* 200 mg
        Stalevo®150: *carb* 12.5 mg/*levo* 150 mg/*enta* 200 mg

MAO Inhibitors

▶*selegiline* **(C)** 5 mg at breakfast and at lunch; max 10 mg/day
    Atapryl® *Tab:* 5 mg
    Carbex®, **Eldepryl®** *Cap:* 5 mg
▶*selegiline* orally disintegrating **(C) 1.25** mg daily; max 2.5 mg/day
    Zelapar® *Tab:* 1.25 mg orally disintegrating (phenylalanine)

COMT Inhibitors

▶*entacapone* **(C)** 1 tab with each dose of *levodopa* or *carbidopa*; max 8 tabs/day
    Comtan® *Tab:* 200 mg

Comment: **Comtan®** is an adjunct to levodopa/carbidopa in patients with end-of-dose wearing off.

▶*tolcapone* **(C)** 100-200 mg tid; max 600 mg/day
    Tasmar® *Tab:* 100, 200 mg

Comment: Monitor LFTs every 2 weeks. Withdraw **Tasmar®** if no substantial improvement in the first 3 weeks of treatment.

Centrally-Acting Anticholinergics

▶*benztropine mesylate* **(C)** initially 0.5-1 mg q HS, increase if needed; for extrapyramidal disorders 1-4 mg daily-bid; max 6 mg/day
    Cogentin® *Tab:* 0.5*, 1*, 2*mg
▶*biperiden hydrochloride* **(C)** initially 1 tab tid-qid, then increase as needed; max 8 tabs/day
    Akineton® *Tab:* 2 mg
▶*procyclidine* **(C)** initially 2.5 mg tid; may increase as needed to 5 mg tid-qid every 3-5 days; max 15 mg/day
    Kemadrin® *Tab:* 5 mg
▶*trihexyphenidyl* **(C)(G)** initially 1 mg; increase as needed by 2 mg every 3-5 days; max 15 mg/day
    Artane® *Tab:* 2*, 5*mg

Paronychia (Periungal Abscess)

▶ *cephalexin* **(B)(G)** 500 mg bid x 10 days
    Pediatric: 25-50 mg/day in 2 doses x 10 days
  Keflex® *Cap:* 250, 500, 750 mg; *Oral susp:* 125, 250 mg/5 ml (100, 200 ml)
  Keftab® *Tab:* 500 mg
  Keftab®**K-pak** *Tab:* 20-500 mg tabs/pck

▶ *cloxacillin* **(B)** 250-500 mg q 6 hours x 10 days
    Pediatric: >1 month, <20 kg: 50-100 mg/kg/day in 4 doses q 6 hour x 10 days; max 4 g/day
    >1 month, >20 kg: same as adult
  Tegopen® *Tab:* 250, 500 mg; *Liq:* 125 mg/5 ml (100, 200 ml)

▶ *dicloxacillin* **(B)(G)** 500 mg q 6 hours x 10 days
    Pediatric: see page 586 for dose by weight
    12.5-25 mg/kg/day in 4 doses x 10 days
  Dynapen® *Cap:* 125, 250, 500 mg; *Oral susp:* 62.5 mg/5 ml (80, 100, 200 ml)

▶ *erythromycin base* **(B)(G)** 500 mg q 6 hours x 10 days
    Pediatric: see page 588 for dose by weight
    <45 kg: 30-50 mg in 2-4 doses x 10 days
    >45 kg: same as adult
  E-mycin® *Tab:* 250, 333 mg ent-coat
  Eryc® *Cap:* 250 mg ent-coat pellets
  Ery-Tab® *Tab:* 250, 333, 500 mg ent-coat
  PCE® *Tab:* 333, 500 mg

Pediculosis:
Pediculosis Humanus Capitis (Head Lice)
Phthirus (Pubic Lice)

▶ *lindane* **(C)(G)** apply, leave on for 4 minutes, then thoroughly wash off
    Pediatric: <2 years: not recommended
    >2 years: same as adult
  Kwell®**Shampoo** *Shampoo:* 1% (60 ml)

▶ *malathion* **(B)(G)** thoroughly wet hair and scalp; allow to dry naturally; shampoo and rinse after 8-12 hours; use a fine tooth comb to remove lice and nits; if lice persist after 7 to 9 days, may repeat treatment

Pediatric: same as adult
   Ovide® (OTC) *Lotn:* 59% (2 oz)
▶ *permethrin* **(B)(G)** apply to washed and towel-dried hair; allow to
Remain on for 10 minutes, then rinse off; repeat after 7 days if needed
   Pediatric: <2 months: not recommended
   >2 months: same as adult
   Nix® (OTC) *Crm rinse:* 1% (2 oz w. comb)
▶ *pyrethrins with piperonyl butoxide* **(C)(G)** apply and leave on for 10 minutes, then wash off
   A-200® *Shampoo: pyr 0.33%/pip but 3%*
   Rid®Mousse *Shampoo: pyr 0.33%/pip but 4%*
   Rid®Shampoo *Shampoo: pyr 0.33%/pip but 3%*

Comment: To remove nits, soak hair in equal parts white vinegar and water for 15-20 minutes.

Pelvic Inflammatory Disease (PID)

Comment: Treat all sexual partners. Empiric therapy requires concomitant treatment for chlamydia.

Adult Regimen A:
▶ *ofloxacin* **(C)(G)** 400 mg PO bid x 14 days
   Floxin® *Tab:* 200, 300, 400 mg
            or
▶ *levofloxacin* **(C)** 500 mg PO daily x 14 days (with or without *metronidazole* 500 mg PO bid x 14 days)
   Levaquin® *Tab:* 250, 500 mg
▶ *metronidazole* **(not for use in 1st; B in 2nd, 3rd)(G)** 500 mg bid x 14 days
   Flagyl®375 *Cap:* 375 mg
   Flagyl®ER *Tab:* 750 mg ext-rel
   Flagyl®, Protostat® *Tab:* 250*, 500* mg

Comment: Alcohol is contraindicated during treatment with oral *metronidazole* and for 72 hours after therapy due to a possible *disulfiram*-like reaction (nausea, vomiting, flushing, headache).

Adult Regimen B:
▶ *ceftriaxone* **(B)(G)** 250 mg IM x 1 dose
   Rocephin® *Vials* 250, 500 mg: 1, 2 g
            or
▶ *cefoxitin* **(B)(G)** 2 g IM x 1 dose
   Mefoxin® *Vial:* 1,2 g

PID

plus

probenecid **(B)(G)** 1 g po x 1 dose
    Benemid® 1 g 30 minutes before *cefoxitin*
▶*doxycycline* **(D)(G)** 100 mg bid x 14 days
    Adoxa® *Tab:* 50, 100 mg ent-coat
    Doryx® *Cap:* 100 mg
    Monodox® *Cap:* 50, 100 mg
    Vibramycin® *Cap:* 50, 100 mg; *Syr:* 50 mg/5 ml; (raspberry, sulfites); *Oral susp:* 25 mg/5 ml (raspberry-apple); *IV conc: doxy* 100 mg/*asc acid* 480 mg after dilution; *doxy* 200 mg/*asc acid* 960 mg after dilution
    Vibra-Tab® *Tab:* 100 mg film-coat

with or without

metronidazole **(not for use in 1st; B in 2nd, 3rd)** 500 mg PO bid x 14 days
    Flagyl®**375** *Cap:* 375 mg
    Flagyl®**ER** *Tab:* 750 mg ext-rel
    Flagyl®, **Protostat**® *Tab:* 250*, 500* mg

Comment: Doxycycline is contraindicated in pregnancy (discolors fetal tooth enamel). Alcohol is contraindicated during treatment with oral *metronidazole* and for 72 hours after therapy due to a possible *disulfiram*-like reaction (nausea, vomiting, flushing, headache).

Pediatric Regimen A:
▶*meropenem* **(A)** administer via IV infusion or IV bolus
    <3 months: not recommended
    >3 months with normal renal function:
        <50 mg/kg: 20 mg/kg q 8 hours
        >50 kg: 1 g q 8 hours
    Max 6 g/day
    Merrem® *Vial:* 500 mg; 1 g pwdr for reconstitution (sodium 3.92 mEq/g)

Pediatric Regimen B:
▶*clindamycin* (B)**(G)**
    Pediatric: see page 585 for dose by weight
        8-16 mg/kg/day in 3-4 doses or 20 mg/kg/day in 3-4 doses for severe infections
    Cleocin® *Cap:* 75 (tartrazine), 150 (tartrazine), 300 mg
    Cleocin®**Pediatric Granules** *Oral susp:* 75 mg/5 ml (100 ml; cherry)

Pediatric Regimen C (>8 years, only):

▶ *doxycycline* **(D)(G)**
    Pediatric: see page 587 for dose by weight
        >8 years, <100 lb: 1 mg/kg/day in 2 doses x 14 days
        or 2 mg/kg/day in 2 doses x 14 days for severe
        infection
        >8 years, >100 lb: 2 mg/kg/day in 2 doses x 10 days,
        then 1 mg/kg/day x 4 more days or 2 mg/kg/day x 14
        days for severe infection
        >8 years, >100 lb: same as adult
    Adoxa® *Tab:* 50, 100 mg ent-coat
    Doryx® *Cap:* 100 mg
    Monodox® *Cap:* 50, 100 mg
    Vibramycin® *Cap:* 50, 100 mg; *Syr:* 50 mg/5 ml (raspberry-apple) sulfites); *Oral susp:* 25 mg/5 ml (raspberry); *IV conc: doxy* 100 mg/*asc acid* 480 mg after dilution; *doxy* 200 mg/*asc acid* 960 mg after dilution
    Vibra-Tab® *Tab:* 100 mg film-coat

Comment: Doxycycline is contraindicated in pregnancy (discolors fetal tooth enamel).

Peptic Ulcer Disease (PUD)

Helicobacter pylori **Eradication Regimens** *see page 197*
H$_2$ Antagonists
▶ *cimetidine* **(B)(G)** 800 mg bid or 400 mg qid; max 2.4 g/day
    Pediatric: <16 years: not recommended
    Tagamet® *Tab:* 300, 400*, 800* mg
    Tagamet®HB (OTC) 1 tab ac as prophylaxis or 1 tab bid as treatment
        Tab: 200 mg
    Tagamet®HB Oral Suspension (OTC) 1 tsp ac as prophylaxis or 1 tsp bid as treatment
        Oral susp: 200 mg/20 ml (12 oz)
    Tagamet®Liquid *Liq:* 300 mg/5 ml (mint-peach, alcohol 2.8%)
▶ *famotidine* **(B)(G)** 20 mg bid; max 6 weeks
    Pediatric: 0.5 mg/kg/day q HS or in 2 doses; max 40 mg/day
    Pepcid® *Tab:* 20, 40 mg; *Oral susp:* 40 mg/5 ml (50 ml)
    Pepcid®AC (OTC) 1 tab ac; max 2 doses/day
        Tab/Rapid dissolving tab: 10 mg
    Pepcid®Complete (OTC) 1 tab ac; max 2 doses/day

Tab: fam 10 mg/$CaCO_2$ 800 mg/Mg hydroxide 165 mg

Pepcid®RPD *Tab:* 20, 40 mg rapid dissolving

▶ *nizatidine* **(B)(G)** 150 mg bid; max 12 weeks
   Pediatric: not recommended

Axid® *Cap:* 150, 300 mg

Axid®AR (OTC) 1 tab ac; max 150 mg/day
   Tab: 75 mg

▶ *ranitidine* **(B)(G)**
   Pediatric: <1 month: not recommended
      1 month-16 years: 2-4 mg/kg/day in 2 divided doses; max 300 mg/day
         Duodenal/Gastric Ulcer: 2-4 mg/kg/day divided bid; max 300 mg/day
         Erosive Esophagitis: 5-10 mg/kg/day divided bid; max 300 mg/day

Zantac® 150 mg bid or 300 mg q HS
   Tab: 150, 300 mg

Zantac®75 (OTC) 1 tab ac
   Tab: 75 mg

Zantac®Efferdose dissolve 25 mg tab in 5 ml water and dissolve 150 mg tab in 6-8 oz water
   Efferdose: 25, 150 mg effervescent (phenylalanine)

Zantac®Syrup *Syr:* 15 mg/ml (peppermint, alcohol 7.5%)

▶ *ranitidine bismuth citrate* **(C)** 400 mg bid
   Pediatric: not recommended

Tritec® *Tab:* 400 mg

Proton Pump Inhibitors

▶ *esomeprazole* **(B)** 20-40 mg daily; max 8 weeks
   Pediatric: not recommended

Nexium® *Cap:* 20, 40 mg del-rel

▶ *lansoprazole* **(B)** 15-30 mg daily
   Pediatric: <12 years: not recommended

Prevacid® *Cap:* 15, 30 mg ent-coat del-rel granules; may open and sprinkle; do not chew

Prevacid®for Oral Suspension
   Oral susp: 15, 30 mg ent-coat del-rel granules/pkt; mix in 2 tblsp water and drink immediately; 30 pkt/box (strawberry)

Prevacid®SoluTab *Tab:* 15, 30 mg orally disintegrating

▶ *omeprazole* **(C)(G)** 20 mg daily; max 4 weeks

Pediatric: not recommended
Prilosec® (OTC) *Cap:* 10, 20, 40 mg ent-coat del-rel granules; may open and sprinkle; do not chew
▶*pantoprazole* **(B)** 40 mg daily for up to 8 weeks; may repeat for 8 more weeks
Pediatric: not recommended
Protonix® *Tab:* 40 mg ent-coat del-rel
▶*rabeprazole* **(B)** 20 mg daily
Pediatric: not recommended
AcipHex® (OTC) *Tab:* 20 mg ent-coat del-rel

Antacids *see **GERD** page 177*

Other
▶*glycopyrrolate* **(B)** initially 1-2 mg bid-tid; maintenance 1 mg bid; max 8 mg/day
Pediatric: <12 years: not recommended
Robinul® *Tab:* 1 mg (dye-free)
Robinul®Forte *Tab:* 2 mg (dye-free)
Comment: Glycopyrrolate is an anticholinergic adjunct to PUD treatment.
▶*mepenzolate* **(B)(G)** 25-50 mg qid with meals and at HS
Cantil® *Tab:* 25 mg
▶*sucralfate* **(B)(G)** 1 g qid for active ulcer; 1 g bid for maintenance
Carafate® *Tab:* 1*g; *Oral susp:* 1 g/10 ml (14 oz)

Prophylaxis
▶*misoprostol* **(X)** 200 mg qid with food for prevention of NSAID-induced gastric ulcers
Cytotec® *Tab:* 100, 200 mg

Peripheral Vascular Disease
(PVD, Arterial Insufficiency, Intermittent Claudication)

Anti-platelet Therapy
▶*aspirin* **(D)(OTC)** 80 mg daily
Ecotrin® *Tab/Cap:* 81, 325, 500 mg ent-coat
▶*cilostazol* **(C)** 100 mg bid 1/2 hour before or 2 hours after breakfast or dinner; may reduce to 50 mg bid if used with CYP 3A4 (e.g., azole anti-fungals, macrolides, diltiazem, fluvoxamine, fluoxetine, nefazodine, sertraline) or CYP 2C19 (e.g., *omeprazole*) inhibitors
Pletal® *Tab:* 50, 100 mg
Comment: May be used with *aspirin*. Cautious use with other antiplatelet agents and anticoagulants.

PVD

▶*clopidogrel* **(B)** 75 mg daily
  Plavix® *Tab:* 75 mg
▶*dipyridamole* **(B)(G)** 25-100 mg tid-qid
  Persantine® *Tab:* 25, 50, 75 mg

Comment: Does not potentiate *warfarin* and may be taken concomitantly. Do not administer *dipyridamole* concomitantly with *aspirin*.

▶*pentoxifylline* **(C)** 400 mg tid with food
  PentoPak® *Tab:* 400 mg ext-rel
  Trental® *Tab:* 400 mg sust-rel
▶*ticlopidine* **(B)** 250 mg bid with food
  Teva®, **Ticlid**® *Tab:* 250 mg

Comment: Monitor for neutropenia, resolves after discontinuation.

▶*warfarin* **(X)** adjust dose to maintain INR in recommended range
*see **Anticoagulation Therapy** page 506*
  Coumadin® *Tab:* 1*, 2*, 2.5*, 5*, 7.5*, 10*mg
  Coumadin®**for Injection** *Vial:* 2 mg/ml (5 mg) pwdr for reconstitution

Comment: Treatment for over-*anticoagulation* with *warfarin* is vitamin K.

Pertussis (Whooping Cough)

Prophylaxis *see **Childhood Immunizations: Childhood** page 466*
Post-exposure Prophylaxis and Treatment

Comment: Antibiotics do not alter the course of illness, but they do prevent transmission. Infected persons should be isolated until after the fifth day of antibiotic treatment.

▶*erythromycin base* **(B)(G)** 1 g/day in divided doses x 14 days
  Pediatric: see page 588 for dose by weight
    40 mg/kg/day in divided doses x 14 days
  E-mycin® *Tab:* 250, 333 mg ent-coat
  Eryc® *Cap:* 250 mg ent-coat pellets
  Ery-Tab® *Tab:* 250, 333, 500 mg ent-coat
  PCE® *Tab:* 333, 500 mg
▶*erythromycin ethylsuccinate* **(B)(G)** 1 g/day in 4 divided doses x 14 days
  Pediatric: see page 589 for dose by weight
    40-50 mg/kg/day in 4 divided doses x 7 days; may double dose with severe infection; max 100 mg/kg/day
  Ery-Ped® *Oral susp*: 200 mg/5 ml (100, 200 ml; fruit); 400 mg/5 ml (60, 100, 200 ml; banana); *Oral drops*: 200, 400 mg/5 ml (50 ml;

fruit); *Chew tab:* 200 mg wafer (fruit)
> **E.E.S.®** *Oral susp:* 200, 400 mg/5 ml (100 ml; fruit)
> **E.E.S.®Granules** *Oral susp:* 200 mg/5 ml (100, 200 ml; cherry)
> **E.E.S.®400 Tablets** *Tab:* 400 mg

▶ *trimethoprim/sulfamethoxazole* **(C)(G)**
> *Pediatric: see page 597 for dose by weight*
>> <2 months: not recommended
>> >2 months: 40 mg/kg/day of *sulfamethoxazole*
>> in 2 doses bid x 10 days
>
> **Bactrim®, Septra®** 2 tabs bid x 10 days
>> *Tab:* trim 80 mg/sulfa 400 mg*
>
> **Bactrim®DS, Septra®DS** 1 tab bid x 10 days
>> *Tab:* trim 160 mg/sulfa 800 mg*
>
> **Bactrim®Pediatric Suspension, Septra®Pediatric Suspension**
> 20 ml bid x 10 days
>> *Oral susp:* trim 40 mg/sulfa 200 mg per 5 ml (100 ml; cherry) alcohol 0.3%)

Comment: Trimethoprim/sulfamethoxazole is not recommended in pregnancy or lactation.

Treatment
Same as Post-exposure Prophylaxis

Pharyngitis: Gonococcal

Comment: Treat all sexual contacts. Empiric therapy requires concomitant treatment for *chlamydia*.

Primary Therapy

▶ *azithromycin* **(B)(G)** 1 g x 1 dose
> **Zithromax®** *Tab:* 250, 500 mg; *Oral susp:* 100 mg/5 ml, (15 ml); 200 mg/5 ml (15, 22.5, 30 ml) (cherry-vanilla-banana); *Pkt:* 1 g for reconstitution (cherry-banana)

▶ *ceftriaxone* **(B)(G)** 125 mg IM x 1 dose
> *Pediatric:* <45 kg: 125 mg IM x 1 dose
>> >45 kg: same as adult
>
> **Rocephin®** *Vial:* 250, 500 mg; 1, 2 g

▶ *doxycycline* **(D)(G)** 100 mg bid x 7 days
> *Pediatric: see page 587 for dose by weight*
>> <8 years: not recommended
>> >8 years, <45 kg: 25 mg/kg/day in 1-2 doses x 7 days; max 200 mg/day

Pharyngitis: Gonococcal

>8 years, >45 kg: same as adult
>8 years, >100 lb: same as adult

Adoxa® *Tab:* 50, 100 mg ent-coat
Doryx® *Cap:* 100 mg
Monodox® *Cap:* 50, 100 mg
Vibramycin® *Cap:* 50, 100 mg; *Syr:* 50 mg/5 ml (raspberry-apple, sulfites); *Oral susp:* 25 mg/5 ml (raspberry); *IV conc: doxy* 100 mg/*asc acid* 480 mg after dilution; *doxy* 200 mg/*asc acid* 960 mg after dilution
Vibra-Tab® *Tab:* 100 mg film-coat

Comment: Doxycycline is contraindicated in pregnancy (discolors fetal tooth enamel).

Alternative Therapy

▶spectinomycin **(B)** 2 g IM x 1 dose
    Pediatric: <45 kg: 40 mg/kg/dose x 1 dose
        >45 kg: same as adult
Trobicin® *Vial:* 2.4 g

Pharyngitis: Streptococcal

▶*amoxicillin* **(B)(G)** 500-875 mg bid or 250-500 mg tid x 10 days
    Pediatric: see page 569 for dose by weight
        <40 kg (88 lb): 20-40 mg/kg/day in 3 doses x 10 days or 25-45 mg/kg/day in 2 doses x 10 days
        >40 kg: same as adult

Amoxil® *Cap:* 250, 500 mg; *Tab:* 875*mg; *Chew tab:* 125, 200, 250, 400 mg (cherry-banana-peppermint, phenylalanine); *Oral susp:* 125, 250 mg/5 ml (80, 100, 150 ml; strawberry); 200, 400 mg/5 ml (50, 75, 100 ml; bubble gum); *Oral drops:* 50 mg/ml (30 ml; bubble gum)
Trimox® *Cap:* 250, 500 mg; *Oral susp:* 125, 250 mg/5 ml (80, 100, 150 ml; raspberry-strawberry)

▶*amoxicillin/clavulanate* **(B)(G)** 500 mg tid or 875 mg bid x 10 days
    Pediatric: see pages 571-572 for dose by weight
        40-45 mg/kg/day divided tid x 10 days or
        90 mg/kg/day divided bid x 10 days

Augmentin® *Tab*: 250, 500, 875 mg; *Chew tab:* 125 mg (lemon-lime), 200 mg (cherry-banana, phenylalanine), 250 mg (lemon-lime), 400 mg (cherry-banana, phenylalanine); *Oral susp*: 125 mg/5 ml (banana), 250 mg/5 ml (orange) (75, 100, 150 ml); 200 mg/5 ml,

Pharyngitis: Streptococcal

400 mg/5 ml (50, 75, 100 ml; orange-raspberry, phenylalanine)
Augmentin®ES-600 *Oral susp:* 600 mg/5 ml (50, 75, 100, 150 ml; orange-raspberry, phenylalanine)
Augmentin®XR 2 tabs q 12 hours x 10 days
  Pediatric: <16 years: use other forms
  Tab: 1000 mg ext-rel
► *azithromycin* **(B)(G)** 500 mg x 1 dose on day 1, then 250 mg daily on days 2-5 or 500 mg daily x 3 days or **Zmax®** 2 g in a single dose
  Pediatric: see page 573 for dose by weight
    12 mg/kg/day x 5 days; max 500 mg/day
  Zithromax® *Tab:* 250, 500 mg; *Oral susp:* 100 mg/5 ml (15 ml); 200 mg/5 ml (15, 22.5, 30 ml) (cherry-vanilla-banana)
  Zithromax®Tri-pak *Tab:* 3-500 mg tabs/pck
  Zithromax®Z-pak *Tab:* 6-250 mg tabs/pck
  Zmax® *Oral susp:* 2 g ext rel (cherry-banana)
► *cefaclor* **(B)(G)** 250 mg tid or 375 mg bid x 5 days
  Pediatric: see page 575 for dose by weight
    20-40 mg/kg/day in 3 doses x 10 days
  Ceclor® *Pulvule:* 250, 500 mg; *Oral susp:* 125, 250 mg/5 ml (75, 150 ml); 187, 375 mg/5 ml (50, 100 ml) (strawberry)
  Ceclor®CD 375 mg q 12 hours x 5 days
    Pediatric: <16 years: not recommended
    Tab: 375, 500 mg ext-rel
  Ceclor®CDpak 500 mg q 12 hours x 7 days
    Pediatric: <16 years: not recommended
    Tab: 500 mg (14 tabs/CDpak)
  Raniclor® 500 mg q 12 hours x 7 days
    Pediatric: 20-40 mg/kg/day in 3 doses x 10 days
    Chew tab: 125, 187, 250, 375 mg
► *cefadroxil* **(B)** 1 g in 1-2 doses x 10 days
  Pediatric: see page 576 for dose by weight
    30 mg/kg/day in 2 doses x 10 days
  Duricef® *Cap:* 500 mg; *Tab:* 1 g; *Oral susp:* 250 mg/5 ml (100 ml); 500 mg/5 ml (75, 100 ml) (orange-pineapple)
► *cefdinir* **(B)** 300 mg bid x
  Pediatric: see page 574 for dose by weight
    <6 months: not recommended
    6 months-12 years: 14 mg/kg/day in 1-2 doses x 10 days
  Omnicef® *Cap:* 300 mg; *Oral susp:* 125 mg/5 ml (60, 100 ml;

Pharyngitis: Streptococcal

strawberry)

▶ *cefditoren pivoxil* **(B)** 200 mg bid x 10 days
    Pediatric: not recommended
  Spectracef® *Tab:* 200 mg
Comment: Contraindicated with milk protein allergy or carnitine deficiency.

▶ *cefixime* **(B)** 400 mg daily x 5 days
    Pediatric: see page 577 for dose by weight
        <6 months: not recommended
        6 months-12 years, <50 kg: 8 mg/kg/day in 1-2 doses x 10 days
        >12 years, >50 kg: same as adult
  Suprax®Oral Suspension *Oral susp:* 100 mg/5 ml (50, 75, 100 ml; strawberry)

▶ *cefpodoxime proxetil* **(B)** 100 mg bid x 5-7 days
    Pediatric: see page 578 for dose by weight
        <2 months: not recommended
        2 months-12 years: 10 mg/kg/day in 2 doses x 5-7 days
  Vantin® *Tab:* 100, 200 mg; *Oral susp:* 50, 100 mg/5 ml (50, 75, 100 ml; lemon-creme)

▶ *cefprozil* **(B)** 500 mg daily x 10 days
    Pediatric: see page 579 for dose by weight
        2-12 years: 7.5 mg/kg bid x 10 days
  Cefzil® *Tab:* 250, 500 mg; *Oral susp:* 125, 250 mg/5 ml (50, 75, 100 ml; bubble gum, phenylalanine)

▶ *ceftibuten* **(B)** 400 mg daily x 5 days
    Pediatric: see page 580 for dose by weight
        9 mg/kg daily x 5 days
  Cedax® *Cap:* 400 mg; *Oral susp:* 90 mg/5 ml (30, 60, 90, 120 ml); 180 mg/5 ml (30, 60, 120 ml; cherry)

▶ *cefuroxime axetil* **(B)(G)** 250 mg bid x 10 days
    Pediatric: see page 581 for dose by weight
        <3 months: not recommended
        >3 months: 20 mg/kg/day bid x 10 days
  Ceftin® *Tab:* 125, 250, 500 mg; *Oral susp:* 125, 250 mg/5 ml (50, 100 ml; tutti-frutti)

▶ *cephalexin* **(B)(G)** 500 mg bid x 10 days
    Pediatric: see page 582 for dose by weight
        25-50 mg/kg/day in 2 doses x 10 days
  Keflex® *Cap:* 250, 500, 750 mg; *Oral susp:* 125, 250 mg/5 ml (100, 200 ml)

Pharyngitis: Streptococcal

Keftab® *Tab:* 500 mg
Keftab®K-pak *Tab:* 20-500 mg tabs/pck

▶ *clarithromycin* **(C)(G)** 250 mg bid or 500 mg ext-rel daily x 10 days
    Pediatric: see page 584 for dose by weight
        <6 months: not recommended
        >6 months: 7.5 mg/kg bid x 10 days
Biaxin® *Tab:* 250, 500 mg
Biaxin®Oral Suspension *Oral susp:* 125, 250 mg/5 ml (50, 100 ml; fruit-punch)
Biaxin®XL *Tab:* 500 mg ext-rel

▶ *dirithromycin* **(C)** 500 mg daily x 10 days
    Pediatric: <12 years: not recommended
Dynabac® *Tab:* 250 mg

▶ *erythromycin base* **(B)(G)** 500 mg qid x 10 days
    Pediatric: see page 588 for dose by weight
        <45 kg: 30-50 mg in 2-4 doses x 10 days
        >45 kg: same as adult
E-mycin® *Tab:* 250, 333 mg ent-coat
Eryc® *Cap:* 250 mg ent-coat pellets
Ery-Tab® *Tab:* 250, 333, 500 mg ent-coat
PCE® *Tab:* 333, 500 mg

▶ *erythromycin estolate* **(B)(G)** 250-500 mg qid x 10 days
    Pediatric: see page 588 for dose by weight
        20-50 mg/kg q 6 hours x 10 days
Ilosone® *Pulvule:* 250 mg; *Tab:* 500 mg; *Liq:* 125, 250 mg/5 ml (100 ml)

▶ *erythromycin ethylsuccinate* **(B)(G)** 400 mg qid or 800 mg bid x 10 days
    Pediatric: see page 589 for dose by weight
        30-50 mg/kg/day in 4 divided doses x 7 days; may double dose with severe infection; max 100 mg/kg/day
Ery-Ped® *Oral susp:* 200 mg/5 ml (100, 200 ml; fruit); 400 mg/5 ml (60, 100, 200 ml; banana); *Oral drops:* 200, 400 mg/5 ml (50 ml; fruit); *Chew tab:* 200 mg wafer (fruit)
E.E.S.® *Oral susp:* 200, 400 mg/5 ml (100 ml; fruit)
E.E.S.®Granules *Oral susp:* 200 mg/5 ml (100, 200 ml; cherry)
E.E.S.®400 Tablets *Tab:* 400 mg

▶ *loracarbef* **(B)** 200 mg bid x 5 days
    Pediatric: see page 593 for dose by weight
        15 mg/kg/day in 2 doses x 5 days

Pharyngitis: Streptococcal

Lorabid® *Pulvule:* 200, 400 mg; *Oral susp:* 100 mg/5 ml (50, 100 ml); 200 mg/5 ml (50, 75, 100 ml) (strawberry bubble gum))
▶*penicillin G (benzathine)* **(B)(G)** 1.2 million units IM x 1 dose
    Pediatric: <60 lb: 300,000-600,000 units IM x 1 dose
        >60 lb: 900,000 units x 1 dose
  Bicillin®L-A *Cartridge-needle unit:* 600,000 units (1 ml); 1.2 million units (2 ml)
▶*penicillin G (benzathine and procaine)* **(B)(G)** 2.4 million units IM x 1 dose
    Pediatric: <30 lb: 600,000 units IM x 1 dose
        30-60 lb: 900,000-1.2 million units IM x 1 dose
  Bicillin®C-R *Cartridge-needle unit:* 600,000 units (1 ml); 1.2 million units; (2 ml); 2.4 million units (4 ml)
▶*penicillin v* **(B)(G)** 500 mg bid or 250 mg qid x 10 days
    Pediatric: see page 594 for dose by weight
        25-50 mg/kg day in 4 doses x 10 days
        >12 years: same as adult
  Pen-Vee®K *Tab:* 250, 500 mg; *Oral soln:* 125 mg/5 ml (100, 200 ml); 250 mg/5 ml (100, 150, 200 ml)
  Veetids® *Tab:* 250, 500 mg; *Oral soln:* 125, 250 mg/5 ml (100, 200 ml)
Comment: Post-treatment culture recommended if history of rheumatic fever.

Pheochromocytoma

Alpha-blocker
▶*phenoxybenzamine* **(C)** initially 10 mg bid; increase every other day as needed; usually 20-40 mg bid-tid
  Dibenzyline® *Cap:* 10 mg

Pinworm (*Enterobius vermicularis*)

Comment: Treatment of all family members is recommended.
Anthelmintics
▶*albendazole* **(C)** 400 mg x 1 dose; may repeat in 2-3 weeks if needed; take after a meal
  <60 kg: 15/mg/kg/day in 2 divided doses; max 800 mg/day
  >60 kg: same as adult
  Albenza® *Tab:* 200 mg
▶*mebendazole* **(C)(G)** 100 mg x 1 dose; may repeat in 2-3 weeks

if needed; take after a meal
> *Pediatric:* same as adult

Vermox® *Chew tab:* 100 mg

▶ *pyrantel pamoate* **(C)** 11 mg/kg x 1 dose; max 1 g/dose; may repeat in 2-3 weeks if needed; take after a meal
> *Pediatric:* 25-37 lb: 1/2 tsp x 1 dose
> 38-62 lb: 1 tsp x 1 dose
> 63-87 lb: 1½ tsp x 1 dose
> 88-112 lb: 2 tsp x 1 dose
> 113-137 lb: 2½ tsp x 1 dose
> 138-162 lb: 3 tsp x 1 dose
> 163-187 lb: 3½ tsp x 1 dose
> >187 lb: 4 tsp x 1 dose

Antiminth® **(OTC)** *Cap:* 180 mg; *Liq:* 50 mg/ml (30 ml); 144 mg/ml (30 ml); *Oral susp:* 50 mg/ml (60 ml)

Pin-X® **(OTC)**; *Cap:* 180 mg; *Liq:* 50 mg/ml (30 ml); 144 mg/ml (30 ml); *Oral susp:* 50 mg/ml (30 ml)

▶ *thiabendazole* **(C)** 50 mg/kg x 1 dose after a meal; max 3 g; may repeat in 2-3 weeks if needed; take after a meal
> *Pediatric:* same as adult

Mintezol® *Chew tab:* 500*mg (orange); *Oral susp:* 500 mg/5 ml (120 ml; orange)

Comment: Thiabendazole should not be used as first-line therapy for pinworms. May impair mental alertness.

Pityriasis Alba

Comment: Pityriasis alba is a chronic skin disorder seen in children with a genetic predisposition to atopic disease. Treatment is directed toward controlling roughness and pruritis. There is no known treatment for the associated skin pigment changes. Pityriasis alba resolves spontaneously and permanently in the 2nd or 3rd decade of life.

Topical Glucocorticosteroids *see page 483*

Topical Steroid/Antihistamine Combinations

▶ *hydrocortisone/chlorcyclizine* **(C)** apply sparingly 2-5 times/day
> *Pediatric:* same as adult

Mantadil® Cream *Crm:* 15 g

Coal Tar Preparations

▶ *coal tar* **(C)**
> *Pediatric:* same as adult

DHS® Shampoo (OTC) use twice weekly

Shampoo: 0.5% (4, 8, 16 oz); *Gel shampoo:* 0.5% (4, 8, 16 oz)
Fototar® (OTC) apply daily-qid
Crm: 2% (3 oz)
Zetar®Emulsion add 15-25 ml to lukewarm bath water, immerse for 15-20 minutes; use 3-7 times weekly
Emulsion: 30%; 300 mg/ml (6 oz)
Zetar®Shampoo massage into wet scalp, rinse, repeat; wait 5 minutes before rinsing second time
Shampoo: 1% (6 oz); *Oil:* 8 oz
Emollients and Other Moisturizing Agents
see **Dermatitis: Atopic** *page 136*

Pityriasis Rosea

Topical Glucocorticosteroids *see page 483*
Oral 1st Generation Antihistamines *see page 525*

Plague (*Yersinia pestis*)

Comment: Yersinia pestis is transmitted via the bite of a flea from an infected rodent or the bite, lick, or scratch of an infected cat. Untreated bubonic plague may progress to secondary pneumonic plague which may be transmitted via contaminated respiratory droplet spread.

▶*streptomycin* **(C)(G)** 15mg/kg IM bid x 10 days
Pediatric: same as adult
Amp: 1 g/2.5 ml or 400 mg/ml (2.5 ml)

Comment: For patients with renal impairment, reduce dose of *streptomycin* to 20 mg/kg/day if mild and 8 mg/kg/day q 3 days if advanced). For patients who are pregnant or who have hearing impairment, shorten the course of treatment to 3 days after fever has resolved.

▶*chloramphenicol* **(C)** 25 mg/kg IV followed by 60 mg/kg in 4 divided doses x 10 days
Pediatric: same as adult
Chloromycetin® *Vial:* 1 g

Comment: Chloramphenicol should only be used if safer agents are unavailable or the infective organism is resistant. *Chloramphenicol* is associated with hematologic toxicity including bone marrow depression and aplastic anemia.

▶*tetracycline* **(D)(G)** 500 mg qid or 25-50 mg/kg/day divided q 6 hours x 10 days

Pediatric: <8 years: not recommended
>8 years, <100 lb: 25-50 mg/kg/day divided q 6 hours, x 10 days
>8 years, >100 lb: same as adult

Achromycin®V *Cap:* 250, 500 mg
Sumycin® *Tab:* 250, 500 mg; *Cap:* 250, 500 mg; *Oral susp:* 125 mg/5 ml (100, 200 ml; fruit, sulfites)

Comment: Tetracycline is contraindicated in pregnancy (discolors fetal tooth enamel).

Pneumonia: Chlamydial

▶ *levofloxacin* **(C)**
Uncomplicated: 500 mg daily x 7 days
Complicated: 750 mg daily x 7 days
Pediatric: <18 years: not recommended
Levaquin® *Tab:* 250, 500, 750 mg

▶ *sparfloxacin* **(C)** 400 mg daily in a single dose on day 1, then 200 mg in a single dose on days 2-10
Zagam® *Tab:* 200 mg

▶ *trovafloxacin* **(C)** 200 mg x 14-21 days
Pediatric: <18 years: not recommended
Trovan® *Tab:* 100, 200 mg

Comment: Trovafloxacin is indicated only for life- or limb-threatening infection.

Pneumonia: Community Acquired (CAP)

Treatment
Age 3 months-5 years
▶ *amoxicillin* **(B)(G)**
Pediatric: see page 569 for dose by weight
<40 kg (88 lb): 20-40 mg/kg/day in 3 doses x 10 days or 25-45 mg/kg/day in 2 doses x 10 days
>40 kg: same as adult

Amoxil® *Cap:* 250, 500 mg; *Tab:* 875*mg; *Chew tab:* 125, 200, 250, 400 mg (cherry-banana-peppermint, phenylalanine); *Oral susp:* 125, 250 mg/5 ml (80, 100, 150 ml; strawberry); 200, 400 mg/5 ml (50, 75, 100 ml; bubble gum); *Oral drops:* 50 mg/ml (30 ml; bubble gum)

Pneumonia: CAP

    Trimox® *Cap:* 250, 500 mg; *Oral susp:* 125, 250 mg/5 ml (80, 100, 150 ml; raspberry-strawberry)
▶ *amoxicillin/clavulanate* **(B)(G)** 500 mg tid or 875 mg bid x 10 days
    Pediatric: see pages 571-572 for dose by weight
        40-45 mg/kg/day divided tid x 10 days or
        90 mg/kg/day divided bid x 10 days
    Augmentin® *Tab:* 250, 500, 875 mg; *Chew tab:* 125 mg (lemon-lime), 200 mg (cherry-banana, phenylalanine), 250 mg (lemon-lime), 400 mg (cherry-banana, phenylalanine); *Oral susp:* 125 mg/5 ml (banana), 250 mg/5 ml (orange) (75, 100, 150 ml); 200 mg/5 ml, 400 mg/5 ml (50, 75, 100 ml; orange-raspberry, phenylalanine)
    Augmentin®ES-600 *Oral susp:* 600 mg/5 ml (50, 75, 100, 150 ml; orange-raspberry, phenylalanine)
    Augmentin®XR 2 tabs q 12 hours x 10 days
        Pediatric: <16 years: use other forms
        Tab: 1000 mg ext-rel
▶ *azithromycin* **(B)(G)**
        Pediatric: see page 573 for dose by weight
            <6 months: not recommended
            >6 months: 10 mg/kg x 1 dose on day 1, then
            5 mg/kg/day on days 2-5; max 500 mg/day
    Zithromax® *Tab:* 250, 500 mg; *Oral susp:* 100 mg/5 ml (15 ml); 200 mg/5 ml (15, 22.5, 30 ml) (cherry-vanilla-banana)
    Zithromax®Tri-pak *Tab:* 3-500 mg tabs/pck
    Zithromax®Z-pak *Tab:* 6-250 mg tabs/pck
▶ *cefaclor* **(C)(G)**
    Pediatric: see page 575 for dose by weight
        20-40 mg/kg/day in 3 doses x 10 days
    Ceclor® *Pulvule:* 250, 500 mg; *Oral susp:* 125, 250 mg/5 ml (75, 150 ml); 187, 375 mg/5 ml (50, 100 ml) (strawberry)
    Ceclor®CD 375 mg q 12 hours x 7 days
        Pediatric: <16 years: not recommended
        Tab: 375, 500 mg ext-rel
    Ceclor®CDpak 500 mg q 12 hours x 7 days
        Pediatric: <16 years: not recommended
        Tab: 500 mg (14 tabs/CDpak)
    Raniclor® 500 mg q 12 hours x 7 days
        Pediatric: 20-40 mg/kg/day in 3 doses x 10 days
        Chew tab: 125, 187, 250, 375 mg
▶ *ceftriaxone* **(B)(G0**
        Pediatric: 50-75 mg/kg IM in 2 doses; max 2 g/day

Pneumonia: CAP

Rocephin® *Vial:* 250, 500 mg; 1, 2 g

▶*cephradine* **(B)** 500 mg q 6 hours or 1 g q 12 hours; max 4 g/day
> *Pediatric: see page 583 for dose by weight*
>> <9 months: not recommended
>> >9 months: 25-50 mg/kg/day divided q 6-12 hours; max 4 g/day

Velosef® *Cap:* 250, 500 mg; *Oral susp:* 125, 250 mg/5 ml (100, 200 ml)

▶*clarithromycin* **(C)** 500 mg q 12 hours or 500 mg ext-rel daily x 10 days
> *Pediatric: see page 584 for dose by weight*
>> <6 months: not recommended
>> >6 months: 7.5 mg/kg bid x 7-14 days

Biaxin® *Tab:* 250, 500 mg
Biaxin®Oral Suspension *Oral susp:* 125, 250 mg/5 ml (50, 100 ml; fruit-punch)
Biaxin®XL *Tab:* 500 mg ext-rel

▶*erythromycin base* **(B)(G)**
> *Pediatric: see page 588 for dose by weight*
>> <45 kg: 30-50 mg in 2-4 doses x 7-10 days
>> >45 kg: same as adult

E-mycin® *Tab:* 250, 333 mg ent-coat
Eryc® *Cap:* 250 mg ent-coat pellets
Ery-Tab® *Tab:* 250, 333, 500 mg ent-coat
PCE® *Tab:* 333, 500 mg

▶*erythromycin estolate* **(B)(G)**
> *Pediatric: see page 588 for dose by weight*
>> 30-50 mg/kg/day in divided doses x 10 days

Ilosone® *Pulvule:* 250 mg; *Tab:* 500 mg; *Liq:* 125, 250 mg/5 ml (100 ml)

Age 5-18 years

▶*amoxicillin* **(B)(G)** 875 mg bid or 500 mg tid x 10 days
> *Pediatric: see page 569 for dose by weight*
>> <40 kg (88 lb): 20-40 mg/kg/day in 3 doses x 10 days or 25-45 mg/kg/day in 2 doses x 10 days
>> >40 kg: same as adult

Amoxil® *Cap:* 250, 500 mg; *Tab:* 875*mg; *Chew tab:* 125, 200, 250, 400 mg (cherry-banana-peppermint, phenylalanine); *Oral susp:* 125, 250 mg/5 ml (80, 100, 150 ml; strawberry); 200, 400 mg/5 ml (50, 75, 100 ml; bubble gum); *Oral drops:* 50 mg/ml (30 ml; bubble gum)

Pneumonia: CAP

> **Trimox®** *Cap:* 250, 500 mg; *Oral susp:* 125, 250 mg/5 ml (80, 100, 150 ml; raspberry-strawberry)

▶ *amoxicillin/clavulanate* **(B)(G)** 500 mg tid or 875 mg bid x 10 days
> *Pediatric: see pages 571-572 for dose by weight*
>> 40-45 mg/kg/day divided tid x 10 days or
>> 90 mg/kg/day divided bid x 10 days
>
> **Augmentin®** *Tab:* 250, 500, 875 mg; *Chew tab:* 125 mg (lemon-lime), 200 mg (cherry-banana, phenylalanine), 250 mg (lemon-lime), 400 mg (cherry-banana, phenylalanine); *Oral susp:* 125 mg/5 ml (banana), 250 mg/5 ml (orange) (75, 100, 150 ml); 200 mg/5 ml, 400 mg/5 ml (50, 75, 100 ml; orange-raspberry, phenylalanine)
> **Augmentin®ES-600** *Oral susp:* 600 mg/5 ml (50, 75, 100, 150 ml; orange-raspberry, phenylalanine)
> **Augmentin®XR** 2 tabs q 12 hours x 10 days
>> *Pediatric:* <16 years: use other forms
>> *Tab:* 1000 mg ext-rel

▶ *azithromycin* **(B)(G)** weight-based or 500 mg x 1 dose on day 1, then 250 mg daily on days 2-5 or 500 mg daily x 3 days or **Zmax®** 2 g in a single dose
> *Pediatric: see page 573 for dose by weight*
>> 10 mg/kg x 1 dose on day 1, then 5 mg/kg/day on days 2-5; max 500 mg/day
>
> **Zithromax®** *Tab:* 250, 500 mg; *Oral susp:* 100 mg/5 ml (15 ml); 200 mg/5 ml (15, 22.5, 30 ml) (cherry-vanilla-banana)
> **Zithromax®Tri-pak** *Tab:* 3-500 mg tabs/pck
> **Zithromax®Z-pak** *Tab:* 6-250 mg tabs/pck
> **Zmax®** *Oral susp:* 2 g ext rel (cherry-banana)

▶ *cefaclor* **(B)(G)**
> *Pediatric: see page 575 for dose by weight*
>> 20-40 mg/kg/day in 3 doses x 10 days
>
> **Ceclor®** 250 mg tid x 7 days
>> *Pulvule:* 250, 500 mg; *Oral susp:* 125, 250 mg/5 ml (75, 150 ml); 187, 375 mg/5 ml (50, 100 ml) (strawberry)
>
> **Ceclor®CD** 375 mg q 12 hours x 7 days
>> *Pediatric:* <16 years: not recommended
>> *Tab:* 375, 500 mg ext-rel
>
> **Ceclor®CDpak** 500 mg q 12 hours x 7 days
>> *Pediatric:* <16 years: not recommended
>> *Tab:* 500 mg (14 tabs/CDpak)
>
> **Raniclor®** 500 mg q 12 hours x 7 days

Pneumonia: CAP

>   *Pediatric:* 20-40 mg/kg/day in 3 doses x 10 days
>   *Chew tab:* 125, 187, 250, 375 mg

▶*cefdinir* **(B)** 300 mg bid or 600 mg daily x 10 days
>   *Pediatric: see page 574 for dose by weight*
>   <6 months: not recommended
>   6 months-12 years: 14 mg/kg/day in 1-2 doses
>   x 10 days

Omnicef® *Cap:* 300 mg; *Oral susp:* 125 mg/5 ml (60, 100 ml; strawberry)

▶*cefpodoxime proxetil* **(B)** 200 mg bid x 14 days
>   *Pediatric: see page 578 for dose by weight*
>   2 months-12 years: 10 mg/kg/day in 2 doses x 14
>   days

Vantin® *Tab:* 100, 200 mg; *Oral susp:* 50, 100 mg/5 ml (50, 75, 100 ml; lemon-creme)

▶*ceftriaxone* **(B)**
>   *Pediatric:* 50-75 mg/kg IM in 2 doses; max 2 g/day

Rocephin® *Vial:* 250, 500 mg; 1, 2 g

▶*clarithromycin* **(C)** 7.5 mg/kg bid x 7-14 days
>   *Pediatric: see page 584 for dose by weight*
>   <6 months: not recommended
>   >6 months: 7.5 mg/kg bid x 7-14 days

Biaxin® *Tab:* 250, 500 mg
Biaxin®**Oral Suspension** *Oral susp:* 125, 250 mg/5 ml (50, 100 ml; fruit-punch)
Biaxin®**XL** *Tab:* 500 mg ext-rel

▶*dirithromycin* **(C)** 500 mg daily x 14 days
>   *Pediatric:* <12 years: not recommended

Dynabac® *Tab:* 250 mg

▶*erythromycin base* **(B)(G)** 500 mg q 6 hours x 10 days
>   *Pediatric: see page 588 for dose by weight*
>   <45 kg: 30-50 mg in 2-4 doses x 10 days
>   >45 kg: same as adult

E-mycin® *Tab:* 250, 333 mg ent-coat
Eryc® *Cap:* 250 mg ent-coat pellets
Ery-Tab® *Tab:* 250, 333, 500 mg ent-coat
PCE® *Tab:* 333, 500 mg

▶*erythromycin estolate* **(B)** 250 mg q 6 hours or 500 mg bid x 10 days
>   *Pediatric: see page 588 for dose by weight*
>   30-50 mg/kg/day in divided doses x 10 days

Ilosone® *Pulvule:* 250 mg; *Tab:* 500 mg; *Liq:* 125, 250 mg/5 ml

Pneumonia: CAP

(100 ml)

Age 18-60 years without co-morbidity

▶ *amoxicillin* **(B)(G)** 500-875 mg bid or 250-500 mg tid x 10 days

Amoxil® *Cap:* 250, 500 mg; *Tab:* 875*mg; *Chew tab:* 125, 200, 250, 400 mg (cherry-banana-peppermint, phenylalanine); *Oral susp:* 125, 250 mg/5 ml (80, 100, 150 ml; strawberry); 200, 400 mg/5 ml (50, 75, 100 ml; bubble gum); *Oral drops:* 50 mg/ml (30 ml; bubble gum)

Trimox® *Cap:* 250, 500 mg; *Oral susp:* 125, 250 mg/5 ml (80, 100, 150 ml; raspberry-strawberry)

▶ *amoxicillin/clavulanate* **(B)(G)** 500 mg tid or 875 mg bid x 10 days

Augmentin® *Tab:* 250, 500, 875 mg; *Chew tab:* 125 mg (lemon-lime), 200 mg (cherry-banana, phenylalanine), 250 mg (lemon-lime), 400 mg (cherry-banana, phenylalanine); *Oral susp:* 125 mg/5 ml (banana), 250 mg/5 ml (orange) (75, 100, 150 ml); 200 mg/5 ml, 400 mg/5 ml (50, 75, 100 ml; orange-raspberry, phenylalanine)

Augmentin®**ES-600** *Oral susp:* 600 mg/5 ml (50, 75, 100, 150 ml; orange-raspberry, phenylalanine)

Augmentin®**XR** 2 tabs q 12 hours x 10 days

Tab: 1000 mg ext-rel

▶ *azithromycin* **(B)(G)** 500 mg x 1 dose on day 1, then 250 mg daily on days 2-5 or 500 mg daily x 3 days or **Zmax**® 2 g in a single dose

Zithromax® *Tab:* 250, 500 mg; *Oral susp:* 100 mg/5 ml (15 ml); 200 mg/5 ml (15, 22.5, 30 ml) (cherry-vanilla-banana)

Zithromax®**Tri-pak** *Tab:* 3-500 mg tabs/pck

Zithromax®**Z-pak** *Tab:* 6-250 mg tabs/pck

Zmax® *Oral susp:* 2 g ext rel (cherry-banana)

▶ *cefaclor* **(B)(G)**

Ceclor® 250 mg tid x 7 days

Pulvule: 250, 500 mg; *Oral susp:* 125, 250 mg/5 ml (75, 150 ml); 187, 375 mg/5 ml (50, 100 ml) (strawberry)

Ceclor®**CD** 375 mg q 12 hours x 7 days

Pediatric: <16 years: not recommended

Tab: 375, 500 mg ext-rel

Ceclor®**CDpak** 500 mg q 12 hours x 7 days

Pediatric: <16 years: not recommended

Tab: 500 mg (14 tabs/CDpak)

Raniclor® 500 mg q 12 hours x 7 days

Pediatric: 20-40 mg/kg/day in 3 doses x 10 days

Chew tab: 125, 187, 250, 375 mg

▶ *cefdinir* **(B)** 300 mg bid or 600 mg daily x 10 days

Pneumonia: CAP

Omnicef® *Cap:* 300 mg; *Oral susp:* 125 mg/5 ml (60, 100 ml; strawberry)

▶ *cefpodoxime proxetil* **(B)** 200 mg bid x 14 days
    Vantin® *Tab:* 100, 200 mg; *Oral susp:* 50, 100 mg/5 ml (50, 75, 100 ml; lemon-creme)

▶ *ceftriaxone* **(B)(G)** 1-2 g IM daily; max 4 g
    Rocephin® *Vial:* 250, 500 mg; 1, 2 g

▶ *clarithromycin* **(C)(G)** 500 mg bid or 500 mg ext-rel daily x 7-14 days
    Biaxin® *Tab:* 250, 500 mg
    Biaxin®**Oral Suspension** *Oral susp:* 125, 250 mg/5 ml (50, 100 ml; fruit-punch)
    Biaxin®**XL** *Tab:* 500 mg ext-rel

▶ *dirithromycin* **(C)** 500 mg daily x 14 days
    Dynabac® *Tab:* 250 mg

▶ *doxycycline* **(D)(G)** 100 mg bid x 7-14 days
    Adoxa® *Tab:* 50, 100 mg ent-coat
    Doryx® *Cap:* 100 mg
    Monodox® *Cap:* 50, 100 mg
    Vibramycin® *Cap:* 50, 100 mg; *Syr:* 50 mg/5 ml (raspberry, sulfites); *Oral susp:* 25 mg/5 ml (raspberry-apple); *IV conc: doxy* 100 mg/*asc acid* 480 mg after dilution; *doxy* 200 mg/*asc acid* 960 mg after dilution
    Vibra-Tab® *Tab:* 100 mg film-coat

Comment: Doxycycline is contraindicated in pregnancy (discolors fetal tooth enamel).

▶ *ertapenem* **(B)** 1 g daily; CrCl <30 ml/min, 500 mg daily; treat x 3-10 days; may switch to an oral antibiotic after 3 days if warranted
    IV infusion: administer over 30 minutes
    IM injection: reconstitute with lidocaine only
    Ivanz® *Vial:* 1 g pwdr for reconstitution

▶ *erythromycin base* **(B)(G)** 500 mg q 6 hours x 14-21 days
    Pediatric: see page 588 for dose by weight
        <45 kg: 30-50 mg in 2-4 doses x 14-21 days
        >45 kg: same as adult
    E-mycin® *Tab:* 250, 333 mg ent-coat
    Eryc® *Cap:* 250 mg ent-coat pellets
    Ery-Tab® *Tab:* 250, 333, 500 mg ent-coat
    PCE® *Tab:* 333, 500 mg

▶ *erythromycin estolate* **(B)** 500 mg q 6 hours x 14-21 days
    Pediatric: see page 588 for dose by weight
        30-50 mg/kg/day in divided doses x 14-21 days

Pneumonia: CAP

> **Ilosone®** *Pulvule:* 250 mg; *Tab:* 500 mg; *Liq:* 125, 250 mg/5 ml (100 ml)

▶*levofloxacin* **(C)**
> Uncomplicated: 500 mg daily x 7-14 days
> Complicated: 750 mg daily x 7-14 days
>> *Pediatric:* <18 years: not recommended
>
> **Levaquin®** *Tab:* 250, 500, 750 mg

▶*linezolide* **(C)** 600 mg q 12 hours x 10-14 days
> **Zyvox®** *Tab:* 400, 600 mg; *Oral susp:* 100 mg/5 ml (150 ml); orange, phenylalanine)

▶*loracarbef* **(B)** 400 mg bid x 14 days
> **Lorabid®** *Pulvule:* 200, 400 mg; *Oral susp:* 100 mg/5 ml (50, 100 ml); 200 mg/5 ml (50, 75, 100 ml) (strawberry bubble gum)

▶*moxifloxacin* **(C)** 400 mg daily x 10 days
> **Avelox®** *Tab:* 400 mg

▶*ofloxacin* **(C)(G)** 400 mg bid x 10 days
> **Floxin®** *Tab:* 200, 300, 400 mg

▶*sparfloxacin* **(C)** 400 mg daily in a single dose on day 1, then 200 mg in a single dose on days 2-10
> **Zagam®** *Tab:* 200 mg

▶*telithromycin* **(C)** 2-400 mg tabs in a singe dose daily x 7-10 days
> **Ketek®** *Tab:* 400 mg

Comment: Telithromycin is contraindicated with PMHx hepatitis or jaundice associated with macrolide use.

▶*trovafloxacin* **(C)** 200 mg x 7-14 days
>> *Pediatric:* <18 years: not recommended
>
> **Trovan®** *Tab:* 100, 200 mg

Comment: Trovafloxacin is indicated only for life- or limb-threatening infection.

Age over 60 years *or presence of co-morbidity*

▶*amoxicillin/clavulanate* **(B)(G)** 500 mg tid or 875 mg bid x 10 days
> **Augmentin®** *Tab:* 250, 500, 875 mg; *Chew tab:* 125 mg (lemon-lime), 200 mg (cherry-banana, phenylalanine), 250 mg (lemon-lime), 400 mg (cherry-banana, phenylalanine); *Oral susp:* 125 mg/5 ml (banana), 250 mg/5 ml (orange) (75, 100, 150 ml); 200 mg/5 ml, 400 mg/5 ml (50, 75, 100 ml; orange-raspberry, phenylalanine)
> **Augmentin®ES-600** *Oral susp:* 600 mg/5 ml (50, 75, 100, 150 ml; orange-raspberry, phenylalanine)
> **Augmentin®XR** 2 tabs q 12 hours x 10 days
>> *Tab:* 1000 mg ext-rel

▶*azithromycin* **(B)(G)** 500 mg x 1 dose on day 1, then 250 mg daily on days 2-5 or 500 mg daily x 3 days or **Zmax®** 2 g in a single dose

Pneumonia: CAP

Zithromax® *Tab:* 250, 500 mg; *Oral susp:* 100 mg/5 ml (15 ml); 200 mg/5 ml (15, 22.5, 30 ml) (cherry-vanilla-banana)
Zithromax®Tri-pak *Tab:* 3-500 mg tabs/pck
Zithromax®Z-pak *Tab:* 6-250 mg tabs/pck
Zmax® *Oral susp:* 2 g ext rel (cherry-banana)

▶ *cefaclor* **(B)(G)** 250 mg tid x 7 days
Ceclor® *Pulvule:* 250, 500 mg; *Oral susp:* 125, 250 mg/5 ml (75, 150 ml); 187, 375 mg/5 ml (50, 100 ml) (strawberry)
Ceclor®CD 375 mg q 12 hours x 7 days
Tab: 375, 500 mg ext-rel
Ceclor®CDpak 500 mg q 12 hours x 7 days
Tab: 500 mg (14 tabs/CDpak)
Raniclor® 500 mg q 12 hours x 7 days
Chew tab: 125, 187, 250, 375 mg

▶ *cefdinir* **(B)** 300 mg bid or 600 mg daily x 10 days
Omnicef® *Cap:* 300 mg; *Oral susp:* 125 mg/5 ml (60, 100 ml; strawberry)

▶ *cefpodoxime proxetil* **(B)** 200 mg bid x 14 days
Vantin® *Tab:* 100, 200 mg; *Oral susp:* 50, 100 mg/5 ml (50, 75, 100 ml; lemon-creme)

▶ *ceftriaxone* **(B)(G)** 1-2 g IM daily; max 4 g
Rocephin® *Vial:* 250, 500 mg; 1, 2 g

▶ *clarithromycin* **(C)(G)** 500 mg bid x 7-14 days
Biaxin® *Tab:* 250, 500 mg
Biaxin®Oral Suspension *Oral susp:* 125, 250 mg/5 ml (50, 100 ml; fruit-punch)
Biaxin®XL *Tab:* 500 mg ext-rel

▶ *dirithromycin* **(C)** 500 mg daily x 14 days
Dynabac® *Tab:* 250 mg

▶ *levofloxacin* **(C)**
Uncomplicated: 500 mg daily x 7-14 days
Complicated: 750 mg daily x 7-14 days
Levaquin® *Tab:* 250, 500, 750 mg

▶ *loracarbef* **(B)** 400 mg bid x 14 days
Lorabid® *Pulvule:* 200, 400 mg; *Oral susp:* 100 mg/5 ml (50, 100 ml); 200 mg/5 ml (50, 75, 100 ml) (strawberry bubble gum)

▶ *sparfloxacin* **(C)** 400 mg daily in a single dose on day 1, then 200 mg in a single dose on days 2-10
Zagam® *Tab:* 200 mg

▶ *trimethoprim/sulfamethoxazole* **(C)(G)**

Pneumonia: CAP

Bactrim®, Septra® 2 tabs bid x 10 days
> *Tab: trim 80 mg/sulfa 400 mg**

Bactrim®DS, Septra®DS 1 tab bid x 10 days
> *Tab: trim 160 mg/sulfa 800 mg**

Bactrim®Pediatric Suspension, Septra®Pediatric Suspension 20 ml bid x 10 days
> *Oral susp: trim 40 mg/sulfa 200 mg per 5 ml (100 ml; cherry, alcohol 0.3%)*

Comment: *Trimethoprim/sulfamethoxazole* is not recommended in pregnancy or lactation.

▶*telithromycin* **(C)** 2-400 mg tabs in a singe dose daily x 7-10 days
> *Pediatric:* <18 years not recommended

Ketek® *Tab:* 400 mg

Comment: *Telithromycin* is contraindicated with PMHx hepatitis or jaundice associated with macrolide use.

▶*trovafloxacin* **(C)** 200 mg x 7-14 days
> *Pediatric:* <18 years: not recommended

Trovan® *Tab:* 100, 200 mg

Comment: *Trovafloxacin* is indicated only for life- or limb-threatening infection.

Pneumonia: Legionella

▶*ciprofloxacin* **(C)(G)** 500 mg bid x 14-21 days
Cipro® *Tab:* 100, 250, 500, 750 mg; *Oral susp:* 250, 500 mg/5 ml (100 ml; strawberry)

▶*clarithromycin* **(C)(G)** 500 mg bid or 500 mg ext-rel daily x 14-21 days
Biaxin® *Tab:* 250, 500 mg
Biaxin®Oral Suspension *Oral susp:* 125, 250 mg/5 ml (50, 100 ml; fruit-punch)
Biaxin®XL *Tab:* 500 mg ext-rel

▶*dirithromycin* **(C)** 500 mg daily x 14-21 days
Dynabac® *Tab:* 250 mg

▶*erythromycin base* **(B)(G)** 500 mg qid x 14-21 days
> *Pediatric: see page 588 for dose by weight*
>> <45 kg: 30-50 mg in 2-4 doses x 14-21 days
>> >45 kg: same as adult

E-mycin® *Tab:* 250, 333 mg ent-coat
Eryc® *Cap:* 250 mg ent-coat pellets
Ery-Tab® *Tab:* 250, 333, 500 mg ent-coat
PCE® *Tab:* 333, 500 mg

▶*erythromycin estolate* **(B)(G)** 1-2 g daily in divided doses x 14-21 days
> *Pediatric: see page 588 for dose by weight*
>> 30-50 mg/kg/day in divided doses x 14-21 days

Ilosone® *Pulvule:* 250 mg; *Tab:* 500 mg; *Liq:* 125, 250 mg/5 ml (100 ml)

▶*trimethoprim/sulfamethoxazole* **(C)(G)**
> *Pediatric: see page 597 for dose by weight*
>> <2 months: not recommended
>> >2 months: 40 mg/kg/day of *sulfamethoxazole* in 2 doses bid x 10 days

Bactrim®, Septra® 2 tabs bid x 10 days
Tab: trim 80 mg/*sulfa* 400 mg*
Bactrim®DS, Septra®DS 1 tab bid x 10 days
Tab: trim 160 mg/*sulfa* 800 mg*
Bactrim®Pediatric Suspension, Septra®Pediatric Suspension 20 ml bid x 10 days
Oral susp: trim 40 mg/*sulfa* 200 mg per 5 ml (100 ml; cherry, alcohol 0.3%)

Comment: Trimethoprim/sulfamethoxazole is not recommended in pregnancy or lactation.

Pneumonia: Mycoplasma

Anti-infectives

▶*azithromycin* **(B)(G)** 500 mg x 1 dose on day 1, then 250 mg daily on days 2-5 or 500 mg daily x 3 days or **Zmax®** 2 g in a single dose
Zithromax® *Tab:* 250, 500 mg; *Oral susp:* 100 mg/5 ml (15 ml); 200 mg/5 ml (15, 22.5, 30 ml) (cherry-vanilla-banana)
Zithromax®Tri-Pak *Tab:* 3-500 mg tabs/pck
Zithromax®Z-pak *Tab:* 6-250 mg tabs/pck
Zmax® *Oral susp:* 2 g ext rel (cherry-banana)

▶*clarithromycin* **(C)(G)** 500 mg bid or 500 mg ext-rel daily x 14-21 days
Biaxin® *Tab:* 250, 500 mg
Biaxin®Oral Suspension *Oral susp:* 125, 250 mg/5 ml (50, 100 ml; fruit-punch)
Biaxin® XL *Tab:* 500 mg ext-rel

▶*erythromycin base* **(B)(G)** 500 mg q 6 hours x 14-21 days
> *Pediatric: see page 588 for dose by weight*
>> <45 kg: 30-50 mg in 2-4 doses x 14-21 days
>> >45 kg: same as adult

Pneumonia: Mycoplasma

    E-mycin® *Tab:* 250, 333 mg ent-coat
    Eryc® *Cap:* 250 mg ent-coat pellets
    Ery-Tab® *Tab:* 250, 333, 500 mg ent-coat
    PCE® *Tab:* 333, 500 mg
▶*tetracycline* **(D)(G)** 500 mg qid
    Pediatric: see page 595 for dose by weight
        <8 years: not recommended
        >8 years, <100 lb: 25-50 mg/kg/day in 2-4 doses
        >8 years, >100 lb: same as adult
    Achromycin®V *Cap:* 250, 500 mg
    Sumycin® *Tab:* 250, 500 mg; *Cap:* 250, 500 mg; *Oral susp:* 125 mg/5 ml (100, 200 ml; fruit, sulfites)

Comment: Tetracycline is contraindicated in pregnancy (discolors fetal tooth enamel).

Pneumonia: Pneumococcal

Prophylaxis
▶*pneumococcal* vaccine **(C)** 0.5 ml IM or SC in deltoid x 1 dose
    Pneumovax®
        Pediatric: <2 years: not recommended
                >2 years: same as adult
        Vial: 25 mcg/0.5 ml (0.5 ml single-dose 10/pck; 2.5 ml)
    Pnu-Imune 23®
    Pediatric: <2 years: not recommended
               >2 years: same as adult
    Vial: 25 mcg/0.5 ml (0.5 ml single-dose 5/pck; 2.5 ml)

    Prevnar® not for adult
        Pediatric: total 4 doses: 2, 4, 6, and 12-15 months-of-age; may start at 6 weeks of age; administer first 3 doses 4-8 weeks apart and the 4th dose at least 2 months after the 3rd dose
        Vial: 25 mcg/0.5 ml (0.5 ml single-dose 5/pck; 2.5 ml)

Comment: Pneumococcal vaccine contains 23 polysaccharide isolates representing approximately 85-90% of common U.S. isolates. Administer the pneumococcal vaccine in the deltoid for toddlers and children.

Treatment
*see **CAP** page 337*

Poliomyelitis

Prophylaxis
▶*trivalent poliovirus vaccine, inactivated (type 1, 2, and 3)* **(C)**
> Pediatric: <6 weeks: not recommended
> >6 weeks: one dose at 2, 4, 6-18 months and 4-6 years of age

Ipol® 50.5 ml SC or IM in deltoid area

Polycystic Ovarian Syndrome (Stein-Leventhal Disease)

see **Contraceptives** page 470

Postherpetic Neuralgia

▶*gabapentin* **(C)(G)** 100 mg daily x 1 day, then 100 mg bid x 1 day, then 100 mg tid continuously; max 900 mg tid
> Pediatric: <3 years: not recommended
> 3-12 years: initially 10-15 mg/kg/day in 3 divided doses; max 12 hours between doses; titrate over 3 days
> 3-4 years: titrate to 40 mg/kg/day
> 5-12 years: titrate to 25-35 mg/kg/day; max 50 mg/kg/day

Neurontin® *Cap:* 100, 300, 400 mg; *Tab:* 600*, 800* mg; *Oral soln:* 250 mg/5 ml (480 ml; strawberry-anise)

Comment: Avoid abrupt cessation of *gabapentin*.

▶*pregabalin* **(C)(V)** (GABA analog) initially 150 mg daily divided bid or tid and may titrate within one week; max 600 mg divided bid or tid; discontinue over one week
> Pediatric: <18 years: not recommended

Lyrica® *Cap:* 25, 50, 75, 100, 150, 200, 225, 300 mg

Topical Analgesics
▶*capsaicin* cream **(NR)** apply tid-qid after lesions have healed
> Pediatric: <2 years: not recommended
> >2 years: same as adult

Axsain® *Crm:* 0.075% (1, 2 oz)
Capin® *Lotn:* 0.025, 0.075% (59 ml)

Postherpetic Neuralgia

    Capasicin®-P (OTC) *Crm:* 0.025% (1.5 oz); *Lotn:* 0.025% (2 oz)
    Capasicin®-HP (OTC) *Crm:* 0.075% (1.5 oz); *Lotn:* 0.075% (2 oz); *Crm:* 0.025% (45, 90 g)
    Dolorac® *Crm:* 0.025% (28 g)
    DoubleCap® (OTC) *Crm:* 0.05% (2 oz)
    R-Gel® *Gel:* 0.025% (15, 30 g)
    Zostrix® (OTC) *Crm:* 0.025% (0.7, 1.5, 3 oz)
    Zostrix®HP *Emol crm:* 0.075% (1, 2 oz)

▶*lidocaine* 5% patch **(B)** apply up to 3 patches at one time for up to 12 hours/24 hour period (12 hours on/12 hours off); patches may be cut into smaller sizes before removal of the release liner; do not reuse
    Pediatric: not recommended
    Lidoderm® *Patch:* 5% 10x14 cm (5/pck)

Oral Analgesics
▶*acetaminophen* **(B)(G)** see ***Fever*** *page 168*
▶*aspirin* **(D)(G)** see ***Fever*** *page 169*
Comment: Aspirin-containing medications are contraindicated with history of allergic-type reaction to *aspirin*, children and adolescents with *Varicella* or other viral illness, and 3rd trimester pregnancy.
▶*tramadol* **(C)(G)** 50-100 mg q 4-6 hours prn
    Pediatric: <16 years: not recommended
    Ultram® *Tab:* 50*mg
    Pediatric: <16 years: not recommended
    Ultram® ER *Tab:* 100, 200, 300 mg ext-rel
    Pediatric: <18 years: not recommended
▶*tramadol/acetaminophen* **(C)(G)** 2 tabs q 4-6 hours; max 8 tabs/day; max 5 days
    CrCl <30 ml/min: max 2 tabs q 12 hours; max 5 days
    Pediatric: not recommended
    Ultracet® *Tab:* tram 37.5/*acet* 325 mg

Oral Narcotic Analgesics see ***Pain*** *page 308*

Post-traumatic Stress Disorder (PTSD)

Selective Serotonin Reuptake Inhibitors (SSRIs)
▶*paroxetine maleate* **(D)(G)**
    Pediatric: not recommended
    Paxil® initially 20 mg daily in AM; may increase by 10 mg/day at weekly intervals as needed; max 60 mg/day
    Tab: 10*, 20*, 30, 40 mg

Paxil®CR initially 25 mg daily in AM; may increase by 12.5 mg at weekly intervals as needed; max 62.5 mg/day
> *Tab:* 12.5, 25, 37.5 mg cont-rel ent-coat

Paxil®Suspension initially 20 mg daily in AM; may increase by 10 mg/day at weekly intervals as needed; max 60 mg/day
> *Oral susp:* 10 mg/5 ml (250 ml; orange)

▶*sertraline* **(C)** initially 50 mg daily; increase at 1 week intervals if needed; max 200 mg daily
> *Pediatric:* <6 years: not recommended
> 6-12 years: initially 25 mg daily; max 200 mg/day
> 13-17 years: initially 50 mg daily; max 200 mg/day

Zoloft® *Tab:* 15*, 50*, 100*mg; *Oral conc:* 20 mg per ml (60 ml, [dilute just before administering in 4 oz water, ginger ale, lemon-lime soda, lemonade, or orange juice]; alcohol 12%)

Pregnancy

Prenatal Vitamins *see page 517*
Nausea/Vomiting
▶*promethazine* **(C)(G)** 12.5-50 mg po/IM/rectally q 4-6 hours po or rectally prn
> **Phenergan®** *Tab:* 12.5*, 25*, 50 mg; *Plain syr:* 6.25 mg/5 ml; *Fortis syr:* 25 mg/5 ml; *Rectal supp:* 12.5, 25, 50 mg; *Amp:* 25, 50 mg/ml (1 ml)

Premenstrual Dysphorphic Disorder (PMDD)
Premenstrual Syndrome (PMS)

NSAIDs *see Pain page 305*
Oral Non-narcotic Analgesics *see Pain page 308*
Oral Narcotic Analgesics *see Pain page 308*
Diuretics
▶*spironolactone* **(D)(G)** initially 50-100 mg daily or in divided doses; titrate at 2 week intervals
> *Pediatric:* not recommended
> **Aldactone®** *Tab:* 25, 50*, 100*mg

Antidepressants
▶*fluoxetine* **(C)(G)**

PMDD/PMS

Prozac® initially 20 mg daily; may increase after 1 week; doses >20 mg/day should be divided into AM and noon doses; max 80 mg/day
> *Pediatric:* <8 years: not recommended
> 8-17 years: initially 10 or 20 mg/day; start lower weight children at 10 mg/day; if starting at 10 mg daily, may increase after 1 week to 20 mg daily
> *Tab:* 10*mg; *Cap:* 10, 20, 40 mg; *Oral soln:* 20 mg/5 ml (4 oz; mint)

Prozac®Weekly following daily fluoxetine therapy at 20 mg/day for 13 weeks, may initiate **Prozac®Weekly** 7 days after the last 20 mg fluoxetine dose
> *Pediatric:* not recommended
> *Cap:* 90 mg ent-coat del-rel pellets

Sarafem® administer daily or 14 days before expected menses and through first full day of menses; initially 20 mg/day; max 80 mg/day
> *Cap:* 10, 20 mg

▶*paroxetine maleate* **(D)(G)**
> *Pediatric:* not recommended

Paxil® initially 20 mg daily in AM; may increase by 10 mg/day at weekly intervals as needed; max 60 mg/day
> *Tab:* 10*, 20*, 30, 40 mg

Paxil®CR initially 25 mg daily in AM; may increase by 12.5 mg at weekly intervals as needed; max 62.5 mg/day; may start 14 days before and continue through day one of menses
> *Tab:* 12.5, 25, 37.5 mg cont-rel ent-coat

Paxil®Suspension initially 20 mg daily in AM; may increase by 10 mg/day at weekly intervals as needed; max 60 mg/day
> *Oral susp:* 10 mg/5 ml (250 ml; orange)

▶*sertraline* **(C)**
> For 2 weeks prior to onset of menses, initially 50 mg daily x 3 days and then increase to 100 mg daily for remainder of the cycle or
> For full cycle, initially 50 mg daily, and may increase by 50 mg/day each cycle to max 150 mg/day
> *Pediatric:* not recommended

Zoloft® *Tab:* 25*, 50*, 100*mg; *Oral conc:* 20 mg per ml (60 ml; alcohol 12%) dilute just before administering in 4 oz water, ginger ale, lemon-lime soda, lemonade, or orange juice

▶*nortriptyline* **(D)(G)** initially 25 mg tid-qid; max 150 mg/day
> *Pediatric:* not recommended

Pamelor® *Cap:* 10, 25, 50, 75 mg; *Oral soln:* 10 mg/5 ml

Contraceptives *see page 470*
Calcium Supplements
▶*calcium* **(C)** 1200 mg/day
*see **Osteoporosis** page 293*

Prostatitis: Acute

▶*ciprofloxacin* **(C)(G)** 500 mg bid x 4 - 6 weeks
    Cipro® *Tab:* 100, 250, 500, 750 mg; *Oral susp:* 250, 500 mg/ 5 ml (100 ml; strawberry)
▶*norfloxacin* **(C)** 400 mg bid x 28 days
    Noroxin® *Tab:* 400 mg
▶*ofloxacin* **(C)(G)** 300 mg x bid x 6 weeks
    Floxin® *Tab:* 200, 300, 400 mg
▶*trimethoprim/sulfamethoxazole* **(C)(G)**
    Bactrim®, **Septra**® 2 tabs bid x 10 days
        Tab: trim 80 mg/*sulfa* 400 mg*
    Bactrim®**DS**, **Septra**®**DS** 1 tab bid x 10 days
        Tab: trim 160 mg/*sulfa* 800 mg*
    Bactrim®**Pediatric Suspension, Septra**®**Pediatric Suspension**
    20 ml bid x 10 days
        Oral susp: trim 40 mg/*sulfa* 200 mg per 5 ml (100 ml; cherry, alcohol 0.3%)
Comment: Trimethoprim/sulfamethoxazole is not recommended in pregnancy or lactation.

Prostatitis: Chronic

▶*carbenicillin* **(B)** 2 tabs qid x 4-12 weeks
    Geocillin® *Tab:* 382 mg
▶*ciprofloxacin* **(C)(G)** 500 mg bid x 3 or more months
    Cipro® *Tab:* 100, 250, 500, 750 mg; *Oral susp:* 250, 500 mg/ 5 ml (100 ml; strawberry)
    Cipro®**XR** *Tab:* 500, 1000 mg ext-rel
▶*ofloxacin* **(C)** 300 mg bid x 4-12 weeks
    Floxin® *Tab:* 200, 300, 400 mg
▶*norfloxacin* **(C)** 400 mg bid x 4-12 weeks
    Noroxin® *Tab:* 400 mg
▶*trimethoprim/sulfamethoxazole* **(C)(G)**

Prostatitis

    Bactrim®, Septra® 2 tabs bid x 10 days
        Tab: trim 80 mg/*sulfa* 400 mg*
    Bactrim®DS, Septra®DS 1 tab bid x 10 days
        Tab: trim 160 mg/*sulfa* 800 mg*
    Bactrim®Pediatric Suspension, Septra®Pediatric Suspension 20 ml bid x 10 days
        Oral susp: trim 40 mg/*sulfa* 200 mg per 5 ml (100 ml; cherry, alcohol 0.3%)

Comment: Trimethoprim/sulfamethoxazole is not recommended in pregnancy or lactation.

Suppression Therapy

▶ *trimethoprim/sulfamethoxazole* **(C)(G)**
    Bactrim®, Septra® 2 tabs bid x 10 days
        Tab: trim 80 mg/*sulfa* 400 mg*
    Bactrim®DS, Septra®DS 1 tab bid x 10 days
        Tab: trim 160 mg/*sulfa* 800 mg*
    Bactrim®Pediatric Suspension, Septra®Pediatric Suspension 20 ml bid x 10 days
        Oral susp: trim 40 mg/*sulfa* 200 mg per 5 ml (100 ml; cherry, alcohol 0.3%)

Comment: Trimethoprim/sulfamethoxazole is not recommended in pregnancy or lactation.

Pruritis

Moisturizing Agents
    Aquaphor®Healing Ointment (OTC) *Oint:* (1.75, 3.5, 14 oz) (alcohol)
    Eucerin®Daily Sun Defense (OTC) *Lotn:* 6 oz (fragrance-free)
Comment: **Eucerin®Daily Sun Defense** is a moisturizer with SPF 15.
    Eucerin®Facial Lotion (OTC) *Lotn:* 4 oz
    Eucerin®Light Lotion (OTC) *Lotn:* 8 oz
    Eucerin®Lotion (OTC) *Lotn:* 8, 16 oz
    Eucerin®Original Creme (OTC) *Crm:* 2, 4, 16 oz (alcohol)
    Eucerin®Plus Creme *Crm:* 4 oz
    Eucerin®Plus Lotion (OTC) *Lotn:* 6, 12 oz
    Eucerin®Protective Lotion (OTC) *Lotn:* 4 oz (alcohol)
Comment: **Eucerin®Protective Lotion** is a moisturizer with SPF 25.
    Lac-Hydrin®Cream (OTC) *Crm:* 280, 385 g
    Lac-Hydrin®Lotion (OTC) *Lotn:* 225, 400 g

Pruritis

Lubriderm®Dry Skin Scented (OTC) *Lotn:* 6, 10, 16, 32 oz
Lubriderm®Dry Skin Unscented (OTC) *Lotn:* 3.3, 6, 10, 16 oz (fragrance-free)
Lubriderm®Sensitive Skin Lotion (OTC) *Lotn:* 3.3, 6, 10, 16 oz (lanolin-free)
Lubriderm®Dry Skin (OTC) *Lotn (scented):* 2.5, 6, 10, 16 oz; *Lotn (fragrance-free):* 1, 2.5, 6, 10, 16 oz
Lubriderm®Bath & Shower Oil (OTC) 1-2 capsful in bath or rub onto wet skin as needed, then rinse
    Oil: 8 oz
Moisturel® apply as needed
    Crm: 4, 16 oz; *Lotn:* 8, 12 oz; *Clnsr:* 8.75 oz

Oatmeal Colloids
    Aveeno® (OTC) add to bath as needed
        Regular: 1.5 oz (8/pck); *Moisturizing:* 0.75 oz (8/pck)
    Aveeno®Oil (OTC) add to bath as needed
        Oil: 8 oz
    Aveeno®Moisturizing (OTC) apply as needed
        Lotn: 2.5, 8, 12 oz; *Crm:* 4 oz
    Aveeno®Cleansing Bar (OTC) *Bar:* 3 oz
    Aveeno®Gentle Skin Cleanser (OTC) *Liq clnsr:* 6 oz

Topical Oil
▶*fluocinolone acetomide* 0.01% topical oil **(C)**
        Pediatric: <6 years: not recommended
                >6 years: apply sparingly bid for up to 4 weeks
    Derma-Smoothe®/FS Topical Oil apply sparingly tid
        Topical oil: 0.01% (4 oz; peanut oil)

Topical Analgesics
▶*capsaicin* (NR)**(G)** cream apply tid-qid prn
        Pediatric: <2 years: not recommended
                >2 years: apply sparingly tid-qid prn
    Axsain® *Crm:* 0.075% (1, 2 oz)
    Capin® *Lotn:* 0.025, 0.075% (59 ml)
    Capzasin®-P (OTC) *Crm:* 0.025% (1.5 oz); *Lotn:* 0.025% (2 oz)
    Capzasin®-HP (OTC) *Crm:* 0.075% (1.5 oz); *Lotn:* 0.075% (2 oz)
    Dolorac® *Crm:* 0.025% (28 g)
    DoubleCap® (OTC) *Crm:* 0.05% (2 oz)
    R-Gel® *Gel:* 0.025% (15, 30 g)
    Zostrix® (OTC) *Crm:* 0.025% (0.7, 1.5, 3 oz)
    Zostrix®HP (OTC) *Emol crm:* 0.075% (1, 2 oz)

Pruritis

Comment: Provides some relief by 1-2 weeks; optimal benefit may take 4-6 weeks.

▶*doxepin* **(B)** cream apply to affected area qid at intervals of at least 3-4 hours; max 8 days

    Pediatric: not recommended

Prudoxin® *Crm:* 5% (45 g)
Zonalon® *Crm:* 5% (30, 45 g)

▶*tacrolimus* **(C)** apply to affected area bid; continue for 1 week after clearing

    Pediatric: <2 years: not recommended
    2-15 years: use 0.03% strength; apply to affected area bid; continue for 1 week after clearing

Protopic® *Oint:* 0.03, 0.1% (30, 60 g)

Topical Anesthetic

▶*lidocaine* 3% cream **(B)** apply bid-tid prn

    Pediatric: reduce dosage commensurate with age, body weight, and physical condition

LidaMantle® *Crm:* 3% (1 oz)

Oral 1st Generation Antihistamines *see page 525*
Topical Glucocorticosteroids *see page 483*
Topical Steroid/Antihistamine Combinations

▶*hydrocortisone/chlorcyclizine* **(C)** apply sparingly 2-5 times/day

Mantadil®Cream *Crm:* 15 g

Parenteral Glucocorticosteroids *see page 389*
Oral Glucocorticosteroids *see page 387*

Pseudogout

NSAIDs *see **Pain** page 305*
Oral Non-narcotic Analgesics *see **Pain** page 308*
Oral Narcotic Analgesics *see **Pain** page 308*
Topical Analgesics *see **Pain** page 308*
Parenteral Glucocorticosteroids *see page 389*
Oral Glucocorticosteroids *see page 387*
Topical Anesthetic *see page 383*
Topical Anesthetic/Steroid Combinations *see page 480*

Pseudomembranous Colitis

Comment: Staphylococcal enterocolitis and antibiotic-associated pseudo-

membranous colitis caused by *C. difficile*.
- ▶*vancomycin* **(B, caps; C, susp)** 500 mg-2 g in 3-4 doses x 7-10 days; cmax 2 g/day
    Pediatric: 40 mg/kg/day in 3-4 doses x 7-10 days; max 2 g/day
- ▶*metronidazole* **(not for use in 1st; B in 2nd, 3rd)(G)** 500 mg bid x 14 days
    Flagyl®375 *Cap:* 375 mg
    Flagyl®ER *Tab:* 750 mg ext-rel
    Flagyl®, Protostat® *Tab:* 250*, 500* mg

Comment: Alcohol is contraindicated during treatment with oral *metronidazole* and for 72 hours after therapy due to a possible *disulfiram*-like reaction (nausea, vomiting, flushing, headache).

Psittacosis

- ▶*tetracycline* **(D)(G)** 250 mg qid or 500 mg tid x 7-14 days
    Pediatric: see page 595 for dose by weight
        <8 years: not recommended
        >8 years, <100 lb: 25-50 mg/kg/day in 4 doses x 7-14 days
        >8 years, >100 lb: same as adult
    Achromycin®V *Cap:* 250, 500 mg
    Sumycin® *Tab:* 250, 500 mg; *Cap:* 250, 500 mg; *Oral susp:* 125 mg/5 ml (100, 200 ml; fruit, sulfites)

Comment: Tetracycline is contraindicated in pregnancy (discolors fetal tooth enamel).

Psoriasis

Emollients see ***Dermatitis: Atopic*** *page 136*
Topical Glucocorticosteroids *see page 483*
Vitamin D-3 Derivatives
- ▶*calcipotriene* **(C)**
    Dovonex® apply bid to lesions and gently rub in completely
        Pediatric: not recommended
        Crm/Oint: 0.005% (30, 60 g)
    Dovonex®Scalp Solution apply bid to lesions and rub in completely

Psoriasis

> *Pediatric:* not recommended
> *Soln:* 0.005% (60 ml)

Vitamin D-3 Derivative/Corticosteroid

▶*calcipotriene/betamethasone* **(C)**
> *Pediatric:* <18 years: not recommended
>
> **Taclonex®** apply to affected area and gently rub in completely daily for 4 weeks; limit treatment area to 30% of body surface area; do not occlude; do not use on face, axillae, groin, or atrophic skin; max 100 g/week
>
> *Pediatric:* not recommended
> *Oint:* calci 0.005%/beta 0.064% (15, 30, 60 g)

Immunosuppressant

▶*alefacept* **(B)** 7.5 mg IV bolus IV or 15 mg IM once weekly x 12 weeks; may retreat x 12
> *Pediatric:* not recommended
>
> **Amevive®**
> *IV dose pack:* 7.5 mg single-use (w. 10 ml sterile water diluent [use 0.6 ml]; 1, 4/pck)
> *IM dose pack:* 15 mg single-use (w. 10 ml sterile water diluent [use 0.6 ml]; 1, 4/pck)

Comment: CD4+ and T-lymphycyte count should be checked prior to initiating treatment with *alefacept* and then monitored. Treatment should be withheld if CD4+ T-lymphocyte counts are below 250 cells/mcl.

▶*cyclosporine* **(C)** 1.25 mg/kg bid; may increase after 4 weeks by 0.5 mg/kg/day; then adjust at 2 week intervals; max 4 mg/kg/day; administer with meals
> *Pediatric:* <18 years: not recommended
>
> **Neoral®** *Cap:* 25, 100 mg (alcohol)
>
> **Neoral®Oral Solution** *Oral soln:* 100 mg/ml (50 ml) may dilute in room temperature apple juice or orange juice (alcohol)

Antimitotics

▶*anthralin* **(C)**
> *Pediatric:* not recommended
>
> **Drithocreme®** initially 0.1% strength daily; adjust based on response
> *Crm:* 0.1, 0.25, 0.5, 1% (50 g)
>
> **Dritho-Scalp®** initially 0.25% strength daily x 1 week; adjust as tolerated
> *Crm:* 0.25, 0.5% (50 g)
>
> **Micanol®** apply daily
> *Crm:* 1% (50 g)

Retinoids

▶*acitretin* **(X)** 25-50 mg daily with main meal
    Pediatric: not recommended
  Soriatane® *Cap:* 10, 25 mg

▶*tazarotene* **(X)(G)** apply daily at HS
    Pediatric: not recommended
  Avage®Cream*Crm:* 0.1% (30 g)
  Tazorac®Cream *Crm:* 0.05, 0.1% (15, 30, 60 g)
  Tazorac®Gel *Gel:* 0.05, 0.1% (30, 100 g)

Coal Tar Preparations

▶*coal tar* **(C)(G)**
    Pediatric: same as adult
  DHS®Shampoo (OTC) use twice weekly
    Shampoo: 0.5% (4, 8, 16 oz); *Gel shampoo:* 0.5%
  Fototar® (OTC) apply daily-qid
    Crm: 2% (3 oz)
  Zetar®Emulsion add 15-25 ml to lukewarm bath water, immerse for 15-20 minutes; use 3-7 times weekly
    Emulsion: 30%; 300 mg/ml (6 oz)
  Zetar®Shampoo massage into wet scalp, rinse, repeat; wait 5 minutes before rinsing second time
    Shampoo: 1% (6 oz)

Pyelonephritis: Acute

Outpatient Treatment

▶*amoxicillin/clavulanate* **(B)(G)** 500 mg tid or 875 mg bid x 10-14 days
    Pediatric: see pages 571-572 for dose by weight
        40-45 mg/kg/day divided tid x 10-14 days or
        90 mg/kg/day divided bid x 10-14 days
  Augmentin® *Tab:* 250, 500, 875 mg; *Chew tab:* 125 mg (lemon-lime), 200 mg (cherry-banana, phenylalanine), 250 mg (lemon-lime), 400 mg (cherry-banana, phenylalanine); *Oral susp:* 125 mg/5 ml (banana), 250 mg/5 ml (orange) (75, 100, 150 ml); 200 mg/5 ml, 400 mg/5 ml (50, 75, 100 ml; orange-raspberry, phenylalanine)
  Augmentin®ES-600 *Oral susp:* 600 mg/5 ml (50, 75, 100, 150 ml) (orange-raspberry, phenylalanine)
  Augmentin®XR 2 tabs q 12 hours x 10 days

Pyelonephritis: Acute

> *Pediatric:* <16 years: use other forms
> *Tab:* 1000 mg ext-rel

▶ *cephalexin* **(B)(G)** 1-4 g/day in 4 doses x 10-14 days
> *Pediatric: see page 582 for dose by weight*
> 25-50 mg/kg/day in 4 doses x 10-14 days

Keflex® *Cap:* 250, 500, 750 mg; *Oral susp:* 125, 250 mg/5 ml (100, 200 ml)
Keftab® *Tab:* 500 mg
Keftab®**K-pak** *Tab:* 20-500 mg tabs/K-pak

▶ *ciprofloxacin* **(C)(G)** 500 mg bid or 1000 mg XR daily x 3-14 days
> *Pediatric:* <18 years: not recommended

Cipro® *Tab:* 100, 250, 500, 750 mg; *Oral susp:* 250, 500 mg/5 ml (100 ml; strawberry)

▶ *levofloxacin* **(C)**
Uncomplicated: 500 mg daily x 10 days
Complicated: 750 mg daily x 10 days
> *Pediatric:* <18 years: not recommended

Levaquin® *Tab:* 250, 500, 750 mg

▶ *loracarbef* **(B)** 400 mg bid x 14 days
> *Pediatric: see page 593 for dose by weight*
> 15 mg/kg/day in 2 doses x 14 days

Lorabid® *Pulvule:* 200, 400 mg; *Oral susp:* 100 mg/5 ml (50, 100 ml); 200 mg/5 ml (50, 75, 100 ml); (strawberry bubble gum)

▶ *trimethoprim/sulfamethoxazole* **(C)(G)** bid x 10 days
> *Pediatric: see page 597 for dose by weight*
> <2 months: not recommended
> >2 months: 40 mg/kg/day of *sulfamethoxazole*
> in 2 doses bid x 10 days

Bactrim®, **Septra**® 2 tabs bid x 10 days
> *Tab: trim* 80 mg/*sulfa* 400 mg*

Bactrim®**DS, Septra**®**DS** 1 tab bid x 10 days
> *Tab: trim* 160 mg/*sulfa* 800 mg*

Bactrim®**Pediatric Suspension, Septra**®**Pediatric Suspension**
20 ml bid x 10 days
> *Oral susp: trim* 40 mg/*sulfa* 200 mg per 5 ml (100 ml; cherry, alcohol 0.3%)

Comment: Trimethoprim/sulfamethoxazole is not recommended in pregnancy or lactation.

Rabies

Pre-exposure Prophylaxis
Comment: Postpone pre-exposure prophylaxis during acute febrile illness or infection. Have *epinephrine* 1:1000 readily available.

▶*rabies immune globulin, human* (HRIG) **(C)** 3 injections of 1 ml IM each on day 0, 7, and either day 21 or 28; booster doses 1 ml IM every 2 years
> *Pediatric:* same as adult (except for infants administer in the vastus lateralis muscle)

Imovax® *Vial:* 2.5 u/ml (1 ml, single dose)

Post-exposure Prophylaxis
Comment: Have *epinephrine* 1:1000 readily available.

▶*rabies immune globulin, human* (HRIG) **(C)** 20 IU/kg infiltrated into wound area as much as feasible, then remaining dose administered IM at site remote from vaccine administration
> *Pediatric:* same as adult

Bayrab®, Imogam®Rabies *Vial:* 150 IU/ml (2, 10 ml)

▶*rabies vaccine, human diploid cell* **(C)**
Not previously immunized: administer first dose 1 ml in the deltoid as soon as possible after exposure, then repeat on days 3, 7, 14, 28 or 30, and 90; administer 1st dose with rabies immune globulin. Previously immunized: only 2 doses are administered, immediately after exposure and again 3 days later ; no rabies immune globulin is needed).
> *Pediatric:* same as adult (except for infants administer in vastus lateralis muscle)

Imovax®, RabAvert® *Vial:* 2.5 IU/ml (2.5 IU of freeze-dried vaccine w. diluent)

▶**Tetanus prophylaxis**
*see **Tetanus** page 397 for patients not previously immunized*

Respiratory Syncytial Virus (RSV)

Prophylaxis
▶*palivizumab* 15 mg/kg IM administered monthly throughout the RSV season

Synagis® *Vial:* 100 mg/ml
*see **Bronchiolitis** page 83*

Restless Legs Syndrome

▶*gabapentin* **(C)** 100 mg daily x 1 day, then 100 mg bid x 1 day, then 100 mg tid continuously; max 900 mg tid
   Neurontin® *Tab:* 600*, 800*mg; *Cap:* 100, 300, 400 mg; *Oral soln:* 250 mg/5 ml (480 ml; strawberry-anise)
Comment: Avoid abrupt cessation of *gabapentin*.
Dopamine agonist
▶*ropinirole* **(C)** take once daily 1-3 hours prior to bedtime; initially 0.25 mg on days 1 and 2; then, 0.5 mg on days 3-7; increase by 0.5 mg/day at 1 week intervals to 3 mg; max 4 mg/day
   Requip® *Tab:* 0.25, 0.5, 1, 2, 3, 4, 5 mg

Retinitis: *Cytomegalovirus*

▶*cidofovir* **(C)** administer via IV infusion over 1 hour; pre-treat with oral *probenecid* (2 g, 3 hours prior to starting the *cidofovir* infusion and 1 g, 2 and 8 hours after the infusion is ended) and 1 liter of IV NaCl should be infused immediately before each dose of *cidofovir* (a 2nd liter of NaCl should also be infused either during or after each dose of *cidofovir* if a fluid load is tolerable).
   Induction: 5 mg/kg once weekly for 2 consecutive weeks
   Maintenance: 5 mg/kg once every 2 weeks; reduce to 3 mg/kg if serum Cr increases 0.3-0.4 mg/dL above baseline; discontinue if serum Cr increases to >0.5 mg/dL above baseline or if >3+ proteinuria develops
      Pediatric: not recommended
   Vistide® *Vial:* 75 mg/ml (5 ml; preservative-free)
Comment: Cidofovir is a nucleoside analogue indicated for treatment of AIDS-related *cytomegalovirus* (CMV) retinitis.
▶*valganciclovir* **(C)** take with food
   Induction: 900 mg bid x 21 days
   Maintenance: 900 mg daily; CrCl <60 ml/min reduce dose (see mfr literature; hemodialysis or CrCl <10 ml/min not recommended (use *ganicyclovir*)
      Pediatric: not recommended
   Valcyte® *Tab:* 450 mg (preservative-free)
Comment: Valganciclovir is a nucleoside analogue and prodrug of *ganiciclovir* indicated for treatment of AIDS-related *cytomegalovirus* (CMV) retinitis.

Rheumatoid Arthritis (RA)

NSAIDs see *Pain* page 305
Oral Non-narcotic Analgesics see *Pain* page 308
Oral Narcotic Analgesics see *Pain* page 308
Topical Analgesics see *Pain* page 308
Parenteral Glucocorticosteroids see page 389
Oral Glucocorticosteroids see page 387
Topical Anesthetics see page 383
Topical Anesthetics/Steroid Combinations see page 480
COX-2 Inhibitors
Comment: Contraindicated with history of asthma, urticaria, and allergic-type reactions to aspirin, other NSAIDs, and sulfonamides.
▶*celecoxib* (**C; not for use in 3rd**) 100-400 mg daily-bid; max 800 mg/day
> *Pediatric:* <18 years: not recommended
> **Celebrex®** *Cap:* 100, 200 mg

DMARDs (Disease Modifying Anti-rheumatic Drugs)
Comment: DMARDs include penicillamine, gold salts (*auranofin, aurothioglucose*), immunosuppressants, and *hydroxychloroquine*. The drugs reduce ESR, reduce RF, and favorably affect the outcome of RA. Immunosuppressants may require 6 weeks to affect benefits and 6 months for full improvement.
▶*adalimumab* (**B**) (tumor necrosing factor [TNF]-alpha blocker) 40 mg SC every other week; may increase to SC weekly
> *Pediatric:* <18 years: not recommended
> **Humira®** *Prefilled syringe:* 40 mg/0.8 ml single-dose (preservative-free)
▶*anakinra* (**B**) (interleukin-1 receptor antagonist) 100 mg SC daily
> *Pediatric:* not recommended
> **Kineret®** *Prefilled syringe:* 100 mg/single-dose syringe (7, 28/pk) (preservative-free)

Comment: **Kineret®** is preservative-free. Do not save unused portion.
▶*auranofin* (**C**) (gold salt) 3 mg bid or 6 mg daily; if inadequate response after 6 months, increase to 3 mg tid
> *Pediatric:* not recommended
> **Ridaura®** *Vial:* 100 mg/20 ml
▶*azathioprine* (immunosuppressant) (**D**) 1 mg/kg/day in 1 or more doses; may increase by 0.5 mg/kg/day q 4 weeks; max 2.5 mg/kg/day; minimum trial to ascertain effectiveness is 12 weeks

Pediatric: not recommended
Imuran® Tab 50*mg

▶*cyclosporine* **(C)** (immunosuppressant) 1.25 mg/kg bid; may increase after 4 weeks by 0.5 mg/kg/day; then adjust at 2 week intervals; max 4 mg/kg/day; administer with meals
Pediatric: not recommended
Neoral® *Cap:* 25, 100 mg (alcohol)
Neoral®Oral Solution *Oral soln:* 100 mg/ml (50 ml) may dilute in room temperature apple juice or orange juice (alcohol)

▶*etanercept* **(B)** (tumor necrosing factor [TNF]-blocker) 25 mg SC twice weekly, 72-96 hours apart or 50 mg SC weekly
Pediatric: <4 years: not recommended
4-17 years: 0.4 mg/kg SC twice weekly, 72-96 hours apart (max 25 mg/dose) or 0.8 mg/kg SC weekly (max 50 mg/dose)
Enbrel® *Vial:* 25 mg (single-use, 4/pck)

Comment: Etanercept reduces pain, morning stiffness, and swelling. May be taken in combination with *methotrexate*. Live vaccines should not be administered concurrently. *Do not* administer with active infection.

▶*hydroxychloroquine* **(C)** 400-600 mg/day
Pediatric: not recommended
Plaquenil® *Tab:* 200 mg

Comment: May require several weeks to achieve beneficial effects. If no improvement in 6 months, discontinue.

▶*infliximab* **(X)** (tumor necrosis factor-alpha blocker) administer by IV infusion over at least 2 hours; 3 mg/kg at weeks 0, 2, 6; then every 8 weeks; may increase to 10 mg/kg or administer every 4 weeks
Pediatric: not recommended
Remicade® *Vial:* 100 mg pwdr for IV infusion single-use (preservative-free)

Comment: Use *infliximab* concomitantly with *methotrexate* when there has been insufficient response to *methotrexate* alone.

▶*leflunomide* **(X)** initially 100 mg daily x 3 days; maintenance dose 20 mg daily; max 20 mg daily
Pediatric: <18 years: not recommended
Arava® *Tab:* 10, 20, 100 mg

▶*methotrexate* **(X)** 7.5 mg x 1 dose per week or 2.5 mg x 3 at 12 hour intervals once a week; max 20 mg/week; therapeutic response begins in 3-6 weeks
Pediatric: not recommended

Rheumatrex® *Tab:* 2.5*mg (5, 7.5, 10, 12.5, 15 mg/week, 4/card unit-of-use dose pack)
Trexall® *Tab:* 5*, 7.5*, 10*, 15*mg (5, 7.5, 10, 12.5, 15 mg/week, 4/card unit-of-use dose pack)

▶ *penicillamine* **(D)** 125-250 mg daily initially; may increase by 125-250 mg/day q 1-3 months; max 1.5 g/day
> *Pediatric:* not recommended

Cuprimine® *Cap:* 125, 250 mg
Depen® *Tab:* 250 mg

▶ *sodium hyaluronate* 20 mg as intra-articular injection weekly x 5 weeks
> *Pediatric:* not recommended

Hyalgan® *Prefilled syringe:* 20 mg/2 ml

Comment: Remove joint effusion and inject with *lidocaine* if possible before injecting **Hyalgan®**.

▶ *sulfasalazine* **(C; D in 2nd, 3rd)(G)** initially 0.5 g daily-bid; gradually increase every 4 days; usual maintenance 2-3 g/day in equally divided doses at regular intervals; max 4 g/day
> *Pediatric:* <6 years: not recommended
> 6-16 years: initially 1/4 to 1/3 of maintenance dose; increase weekly; maintenance 30-50 mg/kg/day in 2 equally divided doses at regular intervals; max 2 g/day

Azulfidine® *Tab:* 500 mg
Azulfidine®EN *Tab:* 500 mg ent-coat

Topical Analgesics

▶ *capsaicin* cream **(NR)(G)** apply tid-qid
> *Pediatric:* <2 years: not recommended
> >2 years: same as adult

Axsain® *Crm:* 0.075% (1, 2 oz)
Capin® *Lotn:* 0.025, 0.075% (59 ml)
Capzasin®-P (OTC) *Crm:* 0.025% (1.5 oz); *Lotn:* 0.025% (2 oz)
Capzasin®-HP (OTC) *Crm:* 0.075% (1.5 oz); *Lotn:* 0.075% (2 oz)
Dolorac® *Crm:* 0.025% (28 g)
DoubleCap® (OTC) *Crm:* 0.05% (2 oz)
R-Gel® *Gel:* 0.025% (15, 30 g)
Zostrix® (OTC) *Crm:* 0.025% (0.7, 1.5, 3 oz)
Zostrix®HP (OTC) *Emol crm:* 0.075% (1, 2 oz)

Comment: Provides some relief by 1-2 weeks; optimal benefit may take 4-6 weeks.

▶*trolamine salicylate*
    Mobisyl® apply tid-qid
        Crm: 10%

Rhinitis: Allergic

Leukotriene Receptor Antagonists
Comment: For prophylaxis and chronic treatment, only. Not for primary (rescue) treatment of acute asthma attack.
▶*montelukast* **(B)** 10 mg daily
        Pediatric: <2 years: not recommended
                    2-5 years: 1 chew tab or granule pkt daily
                    6-14 years: 5 mg daily
    Singulair® *Tab:* 10 mg
    Singulair®Chewable *Chew tab:* 4, 5 mg (cherry, phenylalanine)
    Singulair®Oral Granules take within 15 minutes of opening pkt; may mix with applesauce, carrots, rice, or ice cream
        Granules: 4 mg/pkt
▶*zafirlukast* **(B)** 20 mg bid, 1 hour ac or 2 hours pc
        Pediatric: <7 years: not recommended
                    7-11 years: 10 mg bid 1 hour ac or 2 hours pc
    Accolate® *Tab:* 10, 20 mg
▶*zileuton* **(C)** 1 tab qid
        Pediatric: <12 years: not recommended
    Zyflo® *Tab:* 600 mg
Nasal Glucocorticosteroids
▶*beclomethasone* **(C)**
    Beconase® 1 spray in each nostril bid-qid
        Pediatric: <6 years: not recommended
                    6-12 years: 1 spray in each nostril tid
        Nasal spray: 42 mcg/actuation (6.7 g, 80 sprays; 16.8 g, 200 sprays)
    Beconase®AQ 1-2 sprays in each nostril bid
        Pediatric: <6: not recommended
                    >6 years: same as adult
        Nasal spray: 42 mcg/actuation (25 g, 200 sprays)
    Beconase®Inhalation Aerosol 1-2 sprays in each nostril bid-qid
        Pediatric: <6: not recommended
                    6-12 years: 1 spray in each nostril tid

Rhinitis: Allergic

> *Nasal spray:* 42 mcg/actuation (6.7 g, 80 sprays; 16.8 g, 200 sprays)

Vancenase®AQ 1-2 sprays in each nostril bid
> *Pediatric:* <6 years: not recommended
> >6 years: same as adult
> *Nasal spray:* 84 mcg/actuation (25 g, 200 sprays)

Vancenase®AQ DS 1-2 sprays in each nostril daily
> *Pediatric:* <6 years: not recommended
> >6 years: same as adult
> *Nasal spray:* 84, 168 mcg/actuation (19 g, 120 sprays)

Vancenase®Pockethaler 1 spray in each nostril bid-qid
> *Pediatric:* <6: not recommended
> >6 years: 1 spray in each nostril tid
> *Pockethaler:* 42 mcg/actuation (7 g, 200 sprays)

▶ *budesonide* **(C)**
> **Rhinocort®** initially 2 sprays in each nostril bid in the AM and PM, or 4 sprays in each nostril in the AM; max 4 sprays each nostril/day; use lowest effective dose
> > *Pediatric:* <6 years: not recommended
> > >6 years: same as adult
> > *Nasal spray:* 32 mcg/actuation (7 g, 200 sprays)
>
> **Rhinocort®Aqua Nasal Spray** initially 1 spray in each nostril daily; max 4 sprays in each nostril daily
> > *Pediatric:* <6 years: not recommended
> > 6-12 years: initially 1 spray in each nostril daily; max 2 sprays in each nostril daily
> > *Nasal spray:* 32 mcg/actuation (10 ml, 60 sprays)

▶ *dexamethasone* **(C)** 2 sprays in each nostril bid-tid; max 12 sprays/day; maintain at lowest effective dose
> *Pediatric:* <6 years: not recommended
> 6-12 years: 1-2 sprays in each nostril bid; max 8 sprays/day; maintain at lowest effective dose

Dexacort®Turbinaire
> *Nasal spray:* 84 mcg/actuation (12.6 g, 170 sprays)

▶ *fluticasone propionate* **(C)(G)** initially 2 sprays in each nostril daily or 1 spray bid; maintenance 1 spray daily
> *Pediatric:* <4 years: not recommended
> >4 years: initially 1 spray in each nostril daily; may increase to 2 sprays in each nostril daily; maintenance 1 spray in each nostril daily; max 2 sprays in each nostril/day

Rhinitis: Allergic

Flonase® *Nasal spray:* 50 mcg/actuation (16 g, 120 sprays)

▶*flunisolide* **(C)** 2 sprays in each nostril bid; may increase to 2 sprays in each nostril tid; max 8 sprays/nostril/day

    Pediatric: <6 years: not recommended
    6-14 years: initially 1 spray in each nostril tid or 2 sprays in each nostril bid; max 4 sprays/nostril/day

Nasalide® *Nasal spray:* 25 mcg/actuation (25 ml; 200 sprays)
Nasarel® *Nasal spray:* 25 mcg/actuation (25 ml; 200 sprays)

▶*mometasone furoate* **(C)** 2 sprays in each nostril daily

    Pediatric: <2 years: not recommended
    2-11 years: 1 spray in each nostril daily; max 2 sprays in each nostril daily

Nasonex® *Nasal spray:* 50 mcg/actuation (17 g, 120 sprays)

▶*triamcinolone acetonide* **(C)** initially 2 sprays in each nostril daily; max 4 sprays in each nostril daily, or 2 sprays in each nostril bid, or 1 spray in each nostril qid; maintain at lowest effective dose

    Pediatric: <6 years: not recommended
    >6 years: 1 spray in each nostril daily; max 2 sprays in each nostril daily

Nasacort® *Nasal spray:* 55 mcg/actuation (10 g, 100 sprays)
Nasacort®AQ *Nasal spray:* 55 mcg/actuation (16.5 g, 120 sprays)
Tri-Nasal® *Nasal spray:* 50 mcg/actuation (15ml, 120 sprays)

Nasal Mast Cell Stabilizers

▶*cromolyn sodium* **(B)(OTC)** 1 spray in each nostril tid-qid; max 6 sprays in each nostril/day

    Pediatric: <2 years: not recommended
    >2 years: same as adult

Children's NasalCrom®, NasalCrom® *Nasal spray:* 5.2 mg/spray (13 ml, 100 sprays; 26 ml, 200 sprays)

Comment: Begin 1-2 weeks before exposure to known allergen. May take 2-4 weeks to achieve maximum effect.

Nasal Antihistamine

▶*azelastine* **(C)** 2 sprays in each nostril bid

    Pediatric: <5 years: not recommended
    5-12 years: 1 spray in each nostril bid

Astelin®Ready Spray *Nasal spray:* 137 mcg/actuation (30 ml, 200 sprays)

Nasal Anticholinergics

▶*ipratropium bromide* **(B)**

Atrovent®Nasal Spray 0.03% 2 sprays in each nostril bid-tid

    Pediatric: <6 years: not recommended

Rhinitis: Allergic

>6 years: same as adult
Nasal spray: 21 mcg/actuation (30 ml, 345 sprays)
Atrovent®Nasal Spray 0.06% 2 sprays in each nostril tid-qid; max 5-7 days
Pediatric: <5 years: not recommended
5-11 years: 2 sprays in each nostril tid
>11 years: same as adult
Nasal spray: 42 mcg/actuation (15 ml, 165 sprays)

Comment: Avoid use with narrow-angle glaucoma, prostate hyperplasia, and bladder neck obstruction

Nasal Saline Drops/Sprays
Comment: Homemade saline nose drops: 1/4 tsp salt added to 8 oz boiled, then cooled water.

▶*saline* spray
Pediatric: same as adult
Afrin®Moisturizing Saline Mist, Afrin®Saline Mist w/Eucalyptol and Menthol (OTC) 2-6 sprays in each nostril prn
Squeeze bottle: 45 ml

Nasal Sympathomimetics
▶*oxymetazoline* **(C)(OTC)(G)**
12-hour formulation: 2-3 drops or sprays in each nostril q 10-12 hours prn; max 2 doses/day.
Pediatric: <6 years: not recommended
>6 years: same as adult
4-hour formulation: 2-3 drops or sprays q 4 hours prn
Pediatric: not recommended
Afrin®12-Hour Extra Moisturizing Nasal Spray
Afrin®12-Hour Nasal Spray Pump Mist
Afrin®12-Hour Original Nasal Spray
Afrin®12-Hour Original Nose Drops
Afrin®12-Hour Severe Congestion Nasal Spray
Afrin®12-Hour Sinus Nasal Spray
Nasal spray: 0.05% (45 ml); *Nasal drops:* 0.05% (45 ml)
Afrin®4-Hour Nasal Spray
Neo-Synephrine®12 Hour Nasal Spray
Neo-Synephrine®12 Hour Extra Moisturizing Nasal Spray
Nasal spray: 0.05% (15 ml)

▶*phenylephrine* **(C)(G)**
Afrin®Allergy Nasal Spray (OTC) 2-3 sprays in each nostril q 4 hours prn

Rhinitis: Allergic

> *Pediatric:* <12 years: not recommended
> *Nasal spray:* 0.5% (15 ml)

Afrin®Nasal Decongestant Children's Pump Mist (OTC)
> *Pediatric:* <6 years: not recommended
> >6 years: 2-3 sprays in each nostril q 4 hours prn
> *Nasal spray:* 0.25% (15 ml)

Neo-Synephrine®Extra Strength (OTC) 2-3 sprays or drops in each nostril q 4 hours prn
> *Pediatric:* <12 years: not recommended
> *Nasal spray:* 0.1% (15 ml); *Nasal drops:* 0.1% (15 ml)

Neo-Synephrine®Mild Formula (OTC) 2-3 sprays or drops in each nostril q 4 hours prn
> *Pediatric:* <6 years: not recommended
> >6 years: same as adult
> *Nasal spray:* 0.25% (15 ml)

Neo-Synephrine®Regular Strength (OTC) 2-3 sprays or drops in each nostril q 4 hours prn
> *Pediatric:* <12 years: not recommended
> *Nasal spray:* 0.5% (15 ml); *Nasal drops:* 0.5% (15 ml)

▶*tetrahydrozoline* **(C)**
Tyzine® 2-4 drops or 3-4 sprays in each nostril q 3-8 hours prn
> *Pediatric:* <6 years: not recommended
> >6 years: same as adult
> *Nasal spray:* 0.1% (15 ml); *Nasal drops:* 0.1% (30 ml)

Tyzine®Pediatric Nasal Drops 2-3 sprays or drops in each nostril q 3-6 hours prn
> *Nasal drops:* 0.05% (15 ml)

Oral 1st Generation Antihistamines *see page 525*
Oral 2nd Generation Antihistamines *see page 527*
Oral Antihistamine/Decongestant Combinations *see page 531*
Oral Decongestant/Expectorant Combinations *see page 537*
Parenteral Glucocorticosteroids *see page 389*
Oral Glucocorticosteroids *see page 387*

Rhinitis Medicamentosa

Nasal Glucocorticosteroids see *Allergic Rhinitis* page 366
Oral 1st Generation Antihistamines *see page 525*
Oral Decongestants *see page 528*
Oral Antihistamine/Decongestant Combinations *see page 531*

Rhinitis: Medicamentosa

Oral Decongestant/Expectorant Combinations *see page 537*
Comment: The nasal/oral regimen selected should be instituted with concurrent weaning from the nasal decongestant.

Afrin®4-Hour Nasal Spray
Neo-Synephrine®12 Hour Nasal Spray
Neo-Synephrine®12 Hour Extra Moisturizing Nasal Spray
> *Nasal spray:* 0.05% (15 ml)

▶ *phenylephrine* **(C)(G)**

Afrin®Allergy Nasal Spray (OTC) 2-3 sprays in each nostril q 4 hours prn
> *Pediatric:* <12 years: not recommended
> *Nasal spray:* 0.5% (15 ml)

Afrin®Nasal Decongestant Children's Pump Mist (OTC)
> *Pediatric:* <6 years: not recommended
> >6 years: 2-3 sprays in each nostril q 4 hours prn
> *Nasal spray:* 0.25% (15 ml)

Neo-Synephrine®Extra Strength (OTC) 2-3 sprays or drops in each nostril q 4 hours prn
> *Pediatric:* <12 years: not recommended
> *Nasal spray:* 0.1% (15 ml); *Nasal drops:* 0.1% (15 ml)

Neo-Synephrine®Mild Formula (OTC) 2-3 sprays or drops in each nostril q 4 hours prn
> *Pediatric:* <6 years: not recommended
> >6 years: same as adult
> *Nasal spray:* 0.25% (15 ml)

Neo-Synephrine®Regular Strength (OTC) 2-3 sprays or drops in each nostril q 4 hours prn
> *Pediatric:* <12 years: not recommended
> *Nasal spray:* 0.5% (15 ml); *Nasal drops:* 0.5% (15 ml)

▶ *tetrahydrozoline* **(C)**

Tyzine® 2-4 drops or 3-4 sprays in each nostril q 3-8 hours prn
> *Pediatric:* <6 years: not recommended
> >6 years: same as adult
> *Nasal spray:* 0.1% (15 ml); *Nasal drops:* 0.1% (30 ml)

Tyzine®Pediatric Nasal Drops 2-3 sprays or drops in each nostril q 3-6 hours prn
> *Nasal drops:* 0.05% (15 ml)

Rhinitis: Vasomotor

▶*azelastine* **(C)** 2 sprays in each nostril bid
>*Pediatric:* <5 years: not recommended
>5-12 years: 1 spray in each nostril bid

Astelin®Ready Spray
>*Nasal spray:* 137 mcg/actuation (30 ml, 200 sprays)

▶*cyproheptadine* **(B)** initially 4 mg tid, usual range 12-16 mg/day; max 0.5 mg/kg per day
>*Pediatric:* < 2 years: not recommemded
>2-6 years: 2 mg 2-3 times/day: max 12 mg daily
>7-14 years: 4 mg 2-3 times/day: max 16 mg daily

Periactin® *Tab:* 4*mg

Roseola (*Exanthem Subitum*)

Antipyretics *see Fever page 168*

Rocky Mountain Spotted Fever (*Rickettsia rickettseii*)

▶*doxycycline* **(D)(G)** 200 mg on first day; then 100 mg bid x 7-10 days
>*Pediatric:* <8 years: not recommended
>>8 years, <100 lb: 2-2.5 mg/kg q 12 hours x 7-10
>>8 years, >100 lb: same as adult

Adoxa® *Tab:* 50, 100 mg ent-coat
Doryx® *Cap:* 100 mg
Monodox® *Cap:* 50, 100 mg
Vibramycin® *Cap:* 50, 100 mg; *Syr:* 50 mg/5 ml; (raspberry, sulfites); *Oral susp:* 25 mg/5 ml (raspberry-apple); *IV conc: doxy* 100 mg/*asc acid* 480 mg after dilution; *doxy* 200 mg/*asc acid* 960 mg after dilution
Vibra-Tab® *Tab:* 100 mg film-coat

Comment: Doxycycline is contraindicated in pregnancy (discolors fetal tooth enamel).

▶*tetracycline* **(D)** 500 mg q 6 hours x 7-10 days
>*Pediatric: see page 595 for dose by weight*
><8 years: not recommended
>>8 years, <100 lb: 10 mg/kg/day q 6 hours x 7-10 days

>8 years, >100 lb: same as adult
Achromycin®V *Cap:* 250, 500 mg
Sumycin® *Tab:* 250, 500 mg; *Cap:* 250, 500 mg; *Oral susp:* 125 mg/5 ml (100, 200 ml; fruit, sulfites)

Comment: Tetracycline is contraindicated in pregnancy (discolors fetal tooth enamel).

Rotavirus Gastroenteritis

Comment: RotaTeq® targets the most common strains of rotavirus (G1, G2, G3, G4) which are responsible for more than 90% of rotavirus disease in the U.S.
▶*rotavirus vaccine, live* not recommended for adults
    Pediatric: <6 weeks or >32 weeks: not recommended
    >6 weeks and <32 weeks: administer 1st dose at 6-12 weeks of age; administer 2nd and 3rd doses at 4-10 week intervals for a total of 3 doses; if an incomplete dose is administered, do not administer a replacement dose, but continue with the remaining doses in the recommended series

RotaTeq® *Oral susp:* 2 ml single-use tube (fetal bovine serum [trace], preservative-free, thimerosal-free)

Roundworm (*Ascariasis*)

Anthelmintics
▶*albendazole* **(C)** 400 mg bid x 7 days; take after a meal
    Pediatric: <2 years: 200 mg daily x 3 days; may repeat in 3 weeks
    2-12 years: 400 mg daily x 3 days; may repeat in 3 weeks
Albenza® *Tab:* 200 mg
▶*mebendazole* **(C)(G)** 100 mg bid x 3 days; may repeat in 2-3 weeks if Needed; take after a meal
    Pediatric: same as adult (chew or crush and mix with food)
Vermox® *Chew tab:* 100 mg
▶*pyrantel pamoate* **(C)** 11 mg/kg daily x 3 days; max 1 g/dose; take after a meal
    Pediatric: 25-37 lb: 1/2 tsp x 1 dose

Roundworm

>38-62 lb: 1 tsp x 1 dose
>63-87 lb: 1½ tsp x 1 dose
>88-112 lb: 2 tsp x 1 dose
>113-137 lb: 2½ tsp x 1 dose
>138-162 lb: 3 tsp x 1 dose
>163-187 lb: 3½ tsp x 1 dose
>\>187 lb: 4 tsp x 1 dose

Antiminth® **(OTC)** *Cap:* 180 mg; *Liq:* 50 mg/ml (30 ml); 144 mg/ml (30 ml); *Oral susp:* 50 mg/ml (60 ml)
Pin-X® **(OTC)** *Cap:* 180 mg; *Liq:* 50 mg/ml (30 ml); 144 mg/ml (30 ml); *Oral susp:* 50 mg/ml (30 ml)

▶*thiabendazole* **(C)** 25 mg/kg bid x 7 days; max 1.5 g/dose; take after a meal

>*Pediatric:* same as adult
>><30 lb: consult mfr literature
>>\>30 lb 2 doses/day with meals
>>30-50 lbs: 250 mg bid with meals
>>\>50 lb: 10 mg/lb/dose bid with meals; max 3g/day

Mintezol® *Chew tab:* 500*mg (orange); *Oral susp:* 500 mg/5 ml (120 ml; orange)

Comment: Thiabendazole is not for prophylaxis. May impair mental alertness.

Rubella (German Measles)

Prophylaxis
▶*rubella virus, live, attenuated/neomycin* vaccine **(C)**
>**Meruvax II®** 25 mcg SC
>>*Pediatric:* <12 months: not recommended (if vaccinated <12 months, revaccinate at 12 months)
>>\>12 months: 25 mcg SC

▶ *Measles, mumps, rubella, live, attenuated, neomycin vaccine* **(C)**
>**MMR II®** 25 mcg SC (preservative-free)

Comment: Contraindications: hypersensitivity to *neomycin* or eggs, primary or acquired immune deficiency, immunosuppressant therapy, bone marrow or lymphatic malignancy, and pregnancy (within 3 months following vaccination).
*see **Immunizations: Childhood** page 466*

Treatment
▶*immune globulin* (Ig) 0.25 ml/kg IM (0.5 mg/kg in immunocompromised children)
***Antipyretics** see **Fever** page 168*

Rubeola (Red Measles)

Prophylaxis
▶ *Measles, mumps, rubella, live, attenuated, neomycin vaccine* **(C)**
   MMR II 25 mcg SC (preservative-free)
Comment: Contraindications: hypersensitivity to neomycin or eggs, primary or acquired immune deficiency, immunosuppressant therapy, bone marrow or lymphatic malignancy, and pregnancy (within 3 months following vaccination).
*see **Immunizations: Childhood** page 466*
Treatment
▶ *immune globulin* (Ig) 0.25 ml/kg IM (0.5 mg/kg in immuno-compromised children)
*Antipyretics see **Fever** page 168*

Salmonellosis

▶ *ampicillin* **(B)** 500 mg qid x 10-14 days
        Pediatric: see page 570 for dose by weight
            50-100 mg/kg/day in 4 doses x 10-14 days
   Omnipen®, Principen® *Cap:* 250, 500 mg; *Oral susp:* 125, 250 mg/5 ml (100, 150, 200 ml; fruit)
▶ *ciprofloxacin* **(C)(G)** 500 mg bid x 3-5 days
        Pediatric: <18 years: not recommended
   Cipro® *Tab:* 100, 250, 500, 750 mg; *Oral susp:* 250, 500 mg/5 ml (100 ml; strawberry)
▶ *trimethoprim/sulfamethoxazole* **(C)(G)**
        Pediatric: see page 597 for dose by weight
            <2 months: not recommended
            >2 months: 40 mg/kg/day of *sulfamethoxazole*
        in 2 doses bid x 10 days
   Bactrim®, Septra® 2 tabs bid x 10 days
     Tab: trim 80 mg/*sulfa* 400 mg*
   Bactrim®DS, Septra®DS 1 tab bid x 10 days
     Tab: trim 160 mg/*sulfa* 800 mg*
   Bactrim®Pediatric Suspension, Septra®Pediatric Suspension
   20 ml bid x 10 days
     Oral susp: trim 40 mg/*sulfa* 200 mg per 5 ml (100 ml; cherry, alcohol 0.3%)
Comment: Trimethoprim/sulfamethoxazole is not recommended in pregnancy or lactation.

Scabies (*Sarcoptes scabei*)

▶*crotamiton* (C) massage into skin from chin down; repeat in 24 hours
    Pediatric: not recommended
  Eurax® *Lotn:* 10% (60 g); *Crm:* 10% (60 g)

▶*lindane* (B)(G) 1 oz of lotion or 30 g of cream apply to all skin surfaces from neck down to the soles of the feet; leave on x 8 hours, then wash off thoroughly; may repeat if needed in 14 days
    Pediatric: <2 months: not recommended
             >2 months: same as adult
  Kwell® *Lotn:* 1% (60, 473 ml); *Crm:* 1% (60 g); *Shampoo:* 1% (60, 473 ml)

▶*permethrin* (B)(G) massage into skin from head to soles of feet; leave on x 8-14 hours, then rinse off
    Pediatric: <2 months: not recommended
             >2 months: same as adult
  Acticin®, **Elimite**® *Crm:* 5% (60 g)

Scarlet Fever (Scarlatina)

Comment: Microorganism responsible for scarlet fever is Group A Beta-hemolytic Streptococcus (GABHS). Strep cultures and screens will be positive.

▶*azithromycin* (B) 500 mg x 1 dose on day 1, then 250 mg daily on days 2-5 or 500 mg daily x 3 days or **Zmax**® 2 g in a single dose
    Pediatric: see page 573 for dose by weight
             12 mg/kg/day x 5 days; max 500 mg/day
  Zithromax® *Tab:* 250, 500 mg; *Oral susp:* 100 mg/5 ml (15 ml); 200 mg/5 ml (15, 22.5, 30 ml) (cherry-vanilla-banana); *Pkt:* 1 g for reconstitution (cherry-banana)
  Zithromax®**Tri-pak** *Tab:* 3-500 mg tabs/pck
  Zithromax®**Z-pak** *Tab:* 6-250 mg tabs/pck
  Zmax® *Oral susp:* 2 g ext-rel (cherry-banana)

▶*cefadroxil* (B)
    Pediatric: see page 576 for dose by weight
             15-30 mg/kg/day in 2 doses x 10 days
  Duricef® *Cap:* 500 mg; *Tab:* 1 g; *Oral susp:* 250 mg/5 ml (100 ml); 500 mg/5 ml (75, 100 ml) (orange-pineapple)

▶*cephalexin* (B)(G)
    Pediatric: see page 582 for dose by weight
             25-50 mg/kg/day in 2 doses x 10 days

Scarlet Fever

    Keflex® *Cap:* 250, 500, 750 mg; *Oral susp:* 125, 250 mg/5 ml (100, 200 ml)
    Keftab® *Tab:* 500 mg
    Keftab®K-pak *Tab:* 20-500 mg tabs/K-pak

▶ *clarithromycin* **(C)(G)** 250 mg bid or 500 mg ext-rel daily x 10 days
        Pediatric: see page 584 for dose by weight
            <6 months: not recommended
            >6 months: 7.5 mg/kg bid x 10 days
    Biaxin® *Tab:* 250, 500 mg
    Biaxin®Oral Suspension *Oral susp:* 125, 250 mg/5 ml (50, 100 ml; fruit-punch)
    Biaxin®XL *Tab:* 500 mg ext-rel

▶ *clindamycin* **(B)** 150-300 mg q 6 hours x 10 days
        Pediatric: 8-16 mg/kg/day in 3-4 doses x 10 days
    Cleocin® *Cap:* 75 (tartrazine), 150 (tartrazine), 300 mg
    Cleocin®Pediatric Granules *Oral susp:* 75 mg/5 ml (100 ml; cherry)

▶ *erythromycin estolate* **(B)(G)** 250 mg q 6 hours x 10 days
        Pediatric: see page 588 for dose by weight
            20-50 mg/kg q 6 hours x 10 days
    Ilosone® *Pulvule:* 250 mg; *Tab:* 500 mg; *Liq:* 125, 250 mg/5 ml (100 ml)

▶ *erythromycin ethylsuccinate* **(B)(G)** 400 mg qid or 800 mg bid x 10 days
        Pediatric: see page 589 for dose by weight
            30-50 mg/kg/day in 4 divided doses x 10 days; may double dose with severe infection; max 100 mg/kg/day
    Ery-Ped® *Oral susp:* 200 mg/5 ml (100, 200 ml; fruit); 400 mg/5 ml (60, 100, 200 ml; banana); *Oral drops:* 200, 400 mg/5 ml (50 ml; fruit); *Chew tab:* 200 mg wafer (fruit)
    E.E.S.® *Oral susp:* 200, 400 mg/5 ml (100 ml; fruit)
    E.E.S.®Granules *Oral susp:* 200 mg/5 ml (100, 200 ml; cherry)
    E.E.S.®400 Tablets *Tab:* 400 mg

▶ *penicillin G (benzathine and procaine)* **(B)(G)** 2.4 million units IM x 1 dose
        Pediatric: <30 lb: 600,000 units IM x 1 dose
            30-60 lb: 900,000-1.2 million units IM x 1 dose
    Bicillin®C-R Cartridge-needle unit: 600,000 units (1 ml); 1.2 million units; (2 ml); 2.4 million units (4 ml)

Scarlet Fever

▶*penicillin v* **(B)** 250 mg tid x 10 days
    Pediatric: see page 594 for dose by weight
        25-50 mg/kg day in 4 doses x 10 days
        >12 years: same as adult
  Pen-Vee®K *Tab:* 250, 500 mg; *Oral soln:* 125 mg/5 ml (100, 200 ml); 250 mg/5 ml (100, 150, 200 ml)
  Veetids® *Tab:* 250, 500 mg; *Oral soln:* 125, 250 mg/5 ml (100, 200 ml)

Seizure Disorder

Status Epilepticus *see* **Status Epilepticus** *page 390*
Oral Anti-convulsants *see page 390*

Shigellosis

▶*azithromycin* **(B)** 500 mg x 1 dose on day 1, then 250 mg daily on days 2-5 or 500 mg daily x 3 days or **Zmax®** 2 g in a single dose
    Pediatric: see page 573 for dose by weight
        <6 months: not recommended
        >6 months: 10 mg/kg x 1 dose on day 1, then
        5 mg/kg/day on days 2-5; max 500 mg/day
  Zithromax® *Tab:* 250, 500 mg; *Oral susp:* 100 mg/5 ml (15 ml); 200 mg/5 ml (15, 22.5, 30 ml) (cherry-vanilla-banana)
  Zithromax®Tri-pak *Tab:* 3-500 mg tabs/pck
  Zithromax®Z-pak *Tab:* 6-250 mg tabs/pck
  Zmax® *Oral susp:* 2 g ext-rel (cherry-banana)
▶*ciprofloxacin* **(C)(G)** 500 mg bid x 3 days
    Pediatric: <18 years: not recommended
  Cipro® *Tab:* 100, 250, 500, 750 mg; *Oral susp:* 250, 500 mg/5 ml (100 ml; strawberry)
▶*ofloxacin* **(C)(G)** 400 mg bid x 3 days
    Pediatric: <18 years: not recommended
  Floxin® *Tab:* 200, 300, 400 mg
▶*tetracycline* **(D)** 250-500 mg qid x 5 days
    Pediatric: see page 595 for dose by weight
        <8 years: not recommended
        >8 years, <100 lb: 25-50 mg/kg/day in 4 doses x 5 days
        >8 years, >100 lb: same as adult

Achromycin®V *Cap:* 250, 500 mg
Sumycin® *Tab:* 250, 500 mg; *Cap:* 250, 500 mg; *Oral susp:* 125 mg/5 ml (100, 200 ml; fruit, sulfites)

Comment: Tetracycline is contraindicated in pregnancy (discolors fetal tooth enamel).

▶ *trimethoprim/sulfamethoxazole* **(C)(G)**
   Bactrim®, Septra® 2 tabs bid x 10 days
      Tab: trim 80 mg/*sulfa* 400 mg*
   Bactrim®DS, Septra®DS 1 tab bid x 10 days
      Tab: trim 160 mg/*sulfa* 800 mg*
   Bactrim®Pediatric Suspension, Septra®Pediatric Suspension
   20 ml bid x 10 days
      Oral susp: trim 40 mg/*sulfa* 200 mg per 5 ml (100 ml; cherry, alcohol 0.3%)

Comment: Trimethoprim/sulfamethoxazole is not recommended in pregnancy or lactation.

Sinusitis/Rhinosinusitis: Acute Bacterial

Anti-infectives

▶ *amoxicillin* **(B)(G)** 500-875 mg bid or 250-500 mg tid x 10 days
   Pediatric: see page 569 for dose by weight
      <40 kg (88 lb): 20-40 mg/kg/day in 3 doses x 10 days or 25-45 mg/kg/day in 2 doses x 10 days
   Amoxil® *Cap:* 250, 500 mg; *Tab:* 875*mg; *Chew tab:* 125, 200, 250, 400 mg (cherry-banana-peppermint, phenylalanine); *Oral susp:* 125, 250 mg/5 ml (80, 100, 150 ml; strawberry); 200, 400 mg/5 ml (50, 75, 100 ml; bubble gum); *Oral drops:* 50 mg/ml (30 ml; bubble gum)
   Trimox® *Cap:* 250, 500 mg; *Oral susp:* 125 mg/5 ml, 250 mg/5 ml (80, 100, 150 ml; raspberry-strawberry)

▶ *amoxicillin/clavulanate* **(B)(G)** 500 mg tid or 875 mg bid x 10 days
   Pediatric: see pages 571-572 for dose by weight
      40-45 mg/kg/day divided tid x 10 days or
      90 mg/kg/day divided bid x 10 days
   Augmentin® *Tab:* 250, 500, 875 mg; *Chew tab:* 125 mg (lemon-lime), 200 mg (cherry-banana, phenylalanine), 250 mg (lemon-lime), 400 mg (cherry-banana, phenylalanine); *Oral susp:* 125 mg/5 ml (banana), 250 mg/5 ml (orange) (75, 100, 150 ml); 200 mg/5 ml, 400 mg/5 ml (50, 75, 100 ml; orange-raspberry, phenylalanine)

Sinusitis/Rhinosinusitis

> **Augmentin®ES-600** *Oral susp:* 600 mg/5 ml (50, 75, 100, 150 ml) (orange-raspberry, phenylalanine)
> **Augmentin®XR** 2 tabs q 12 hours x 10 days
> > *Pediatric:* <16 years: use other forms
> > *Tab:* 1000 mg ext-rel

▶ *cefaclor* **(B)(G)**
> **Ceclor®** 250 mg tid or 375 mg bid x 10 days
> > *Pediatric: see page 575 for dose by weight*
> > > 20-40 mg/kg/day in 3 doses x 10 days
> >
> > *Pulvule*: 250, 500 mg; *Oral susp:* 125, 250 mg/5 ml (75, 150 ml); 187, 375 mg/5 ml (50, 100 ml) (strawberry)
>
> **Ceclor®CD** 500 mg q 12 hours x 10days
> > *Pediatric:* <16 years: not recommended
> > *Tab:* 375, 500 mg ext-rel
>
> **Ceclor®CDpak** 500 mg q 12 hours x 10 days
> > *Pediatric:* <16 years: not recommended
> > *Tab:* 500 mg (14 tabs/CDpak)
>
> **Raniclor®** 500 mg q 12 hours x 10 days
> > *Pediatric:* 20-40 mg/kg/day in 3 doses x 10 days
> > *Chew tab:* 125, 187, 250, 375 mg

▶ *cefdinir* **(B)** 300 mg bid or 600 mg daily x 10 days
> > *Pediatric: see page 574 for dose by weight*
> > > <6 months: not recommended
> > > 6 months-12 years: 14 mg/kg/day in 1-2 doses x 10 days
>
> **Omnicef®** *Cap:* 300 mg; *Oral susp:* 125 mg/5 ml (60, 100 ml) (strawberry)

▶ *cefixime* **(B)** 400 mg daily x 10 days
> > *Pediatric: see page 577 for dose by weight*
> > > <6 months: not recommended
> > > 6 months-12 years, <50 kg: 8 mg/kg/day in 1-2 doses x 10 days
> > > >12 years, >50 kg: same as adult
>
> **Suprax®Oral Suspension** *Oral susp:* 100 mg/5 ml (50, 75, 100 ml; strawberry)

▶ *cefpodoxime* 200 mg bid x 10 days
> > *Pediatric: see page 578 for dose by weight*
> > > <2 months: not recommended
> > > 2 months-12 years: 10 mg/kg/day (max 400 mg/dose) or 5 mg/kg/day bid (max 200 mg/dose) x 10 days

Sinusitis/Rhinosinusitis

Vantin® *Tab:* 100, 200 mg; *Oral susp:* 50, 100 mg/5 ml (50, 75, 100 mg; lemon-creme)

▶ *cefprozil* **(B)** 250-500 mg bid x 10 days
　　Pediatric: see page 579 for dose by weight
　　　　2-12 years: 7.5 mg/kg bid x 10 days
Cefzil® *Tab:* 250, 500 mg; *Oral susp:* 125, 250 mg/5 ml (50, 75, 100 ml; bubble gum, phenylalanine)

▶ *ceftibuten* **(B)** 400 mg daily x 10 days
　　Pediatric: see page 580 for dose by weight
　　　　9 mg/kg daily x 10 days; max 400 mg/day
Cedax® *Cap:* 400 mg; *Oral susp:* 90 mg/5 ml (30, 60, 90, 120 ml); 180 mg/5 ml (30, 60, 120 ml) (cherry)

▶ *cefuroxime axetil* **(B)(G)** 250 mg bid x 10 days
　　Pediatric: see page 581 for dose by weight
　　　　<3 months: not recommended
　　　　3 months-12 years: 20-30 mg/kg/day in 2 doses
　　　　x 10 days
Ceftin® *Tab:* 125, 250, 500 mg; *Oral susp:* 125, 250 mg/5 ml (50, 100 ml; tutti-frutti)

▶ *ciprofloxacin* **(C)** 500 mg bid x 10 days
　　Pediatric: <18 years: not recommended
Cipro® *Tab:* 100, 250, 500, 750 mg; *Oral susp:* 250, 500 mg/ 5 ml (100 ml; strawberry)

▶ *clarithromycin* **(C)(G)** 500 mg bid or 1000 mg ext-rel daily x 10 days
　　Pediatric: see page 584 for dose by weight
　　　　<6 months: not recommended
　　　　>6 months: 7.5 mg/kg bid x 10 days
Biaxin® *Tab:* 250, 500 mg
Biaxin®Oral Suspension *Oral susp:* 125, 250 mg/5 ml (50, 100 ml; fruit-punch)
Biaxin®XL *Tab:* 500 mg ext-rel

▶ *levofloxacin* **(C)**
　Uncomplicated: 500 mg daily x 10-14 days
　Complicated: 750 mg daily x 10-14 days
　　Pediatric: <18 years: not recommended
Levaquin® *Tab:* 250, 500, 750 mg

▶ *loracarbef* **(B)** 400 mg bid x 10 days
　　Pediatric: see page 593 for dose by weight
　　　　15 mg/kg/day in 2 doses x 10 days
Lorabid® *Pulvule*: 200, 400 mg; *Oral susp:* 100 mg/5 ml (50, 100 ml); 200 mg/5 ml (50, 75, 100 ml); (strawberry bubble gum)

Sinusitis/Rhinosinusitis

▶*moxifloxacin* **(C)** 400 mg daily x 10 days
    Pediatric: <18 years: not recommended
  Avelox® *Tab:* 400 mg
▶*trimethoprim/sulfamethoxazole* **(C)(G)**
    Pediatric: see page 597 for dose by weight
        <2 months: not recommended
        >2 months: 40 mg/kg/day of *sulfamethoxazole*
        in 2 doses bid x 10 days
  Bactrim®, Septra® 2 tabs bid x 10 days
    Tab: trim 80 mg/*sulfa* 400 mg*
  Bactrim®DS, Septra®DS 1 tab bid x 10 days
    Tab: trim 160 mg/*sulfa* 800 mg*
  Bactrim®Pediatric Suspension, Septra®Pediatric Suspension
  20 ml bid x 10 days
    Oral susp: trim 40 mg/*sulfa* 200 mg per 5 ml (100 ml; cherry, alcohol 0.3%)

Comment: Trimethoprim/sulfamethoxazole is not recommended in pregnancy or lactation.

▶*trovafloxacin* **(C)** 200 mg daily x 10 days
    Pediatric: <18 years: not recommended
  Trovan® *Tab:* 100, 200 mg

Comment: Trovafloxacin is indicated only for life- or limb-threatening infection.

Decongestants *see page 528*
Expectorants *see page 529*
Decongestant/Expectorant Combinations *see page 537*
Nasal Glucocorticosteroids *see **Rhinitis: Allergic** page 366*

Sjogren's Syndrome (Dry Mouth)

Muscarinic Agonist
▶*cevimeline* **(C)** 30 mg tid
  Evoxac® *Cap:* 30 mg

Comment: Cevimeline is contraindicated in acute iritis, narrow angle glaucoma, and uncontrolled asthma.

Synthetic Saliva
▶*synthetic saliva* **(NR)(OTC)** spray oral mucosa prn
  Salivart® *Oral spray:* 75 g (2.48 oz)

Skin: Calloused

Keratolytics
▶*salicylic acid* **(C)(OTC)** apply lotion, cream or gel to affected area daily-bid; apply patch to affected area and leave on x 48 hours with max 5 applications/14 days
    Pediatric: <12 years: not recommended
▶*urea* **(C)**
    Pediatric: <12 years: not recommended
  Carmol®40 apply to affected area with applicator stick provided daily-tid; smooth over until cream is absorbed; protect surrounding tissue; may cover with adhesive bandage or gauze secured with adhesive tape
    Crm/Gel: 40% (30 g)
  Keratol®40 apply to affected area with applicator stick provided daily-tid; smooth over until cream is absorbed; protect surrounding tissue; may cover with adhesive bandage or gauze secured with adhesive tape
    Crm: 40% (1, 3, 7 oz); *Gel:* 40% (15 ml); *Lotn:* 40% (8 oz)
Comment: The moisturizing effect of **Carmol®40** and **Keratol®40** is enhanced by applying while the skin is still moist (after washing or bathing).

Skin Infection: Bacterial
(Carbuncle, Folliculitis, Furuncle)

Comment: Abscesses usually require surgical incision and drainage.
Anti-bacterial Skin Cleansers
  Dial® soap **(OTC)** bid
  Lever 2000®Antibacterial soap **(OTC)** bid
▶*chlorhexidine gluconate*
  Hibiclens® after wetting skin, apply minimal amount and wash gently, then rinse thoroughly.
    Liq clnsr: 4, 8 oz
Comment: **Hibiclens®** should not be used in areas with wounds which involve more than the superficial layers of skin.
▶*hexachlorophene* **(C)**
  pHisoHex® dispense 5 ml into wet hand, work up into lather, then apply to area to be cleansed; rinse thoroughly
    Liq clnsr: 5, 16 oz

Skin Infection: Bacterial

Topical Anti-infectives
▶*mupirocin* **(B)(G)** apply to lesions bid
    Pediatric: same as adult
  Bactroban® *Oint:* 2% (22 g); *Crm:* 2% (15, 30 g)
  Centany® *Oint:* 2% (15, 30 g)
▶*polymixin B/neomycin* **(C)** oint apply daily-tid
  Neosporin® **(OTC)** *Oint:* 15 g

Oral Anti-infectives
▶*amoxicillin* **(B)(G)** 500-875 mg bid or 250-500 mg tid x 10 days
    Pediatric: see page 569 for dose by weight
        <40 kg (88 lb): 20-40 mg/kg/day in 3 doses x 10 days or 25-45 mg/kg/day in 2 doses x 10 days
  Amoxil® *Cap:* 250, 500 mg; *Tab:* 875*mg; *Chew tab:* 125, 200, 250, 400 mg (cherry-banana-peppermint, phenylalanine); *Oral susp:* 125, 250 mg/5 ml (80, 100, 150 ml; strawberry); 200, 400 mg/5 ml (50, 75, 100 ml; bubble gum); *Oral drops:* 50 mg/ml (30 ml; bubble gum)
  Trimox® *Cap:* 250, 500 mg; *Oral susp:* 125 mg/5 ml, 250 mg/5 ml (80, 100, 150 ml; raspberry-strawberry)
▶*azithromycin* **(B)** 500 mg x 1 dose on day 1, then 250 mg daily on days 2-5 or 500 mg daily x 3 days or **Zmax®** 2 g in a single dose
    Pediatric: see page 573 for dose by weight
        12 mg/kg/day x 5 days; max 500 mg/day
  Zithromax® *Tab:* 250, 500 mg; *Oral susp:* 100 mg/5 ml (15 ml); 200 mg/5 ml (15, 22.5, 30 ml) (cherry-vanilla-banana); *Pkt:* 1 g for reconstitution (cherry-banana)
  Zithromax®Tri-pak *Tab:* 3-500 mg tabs/pck
  Zithromax®Z-pak *Tab:* 6-250 mg tabs/pck
  Zmax® *Oral susp:* 2 g ext rel (cherry-banana)
▶*cefaclor* **(B)(G)**
  Ceclor® 250 mg tid or 375 mg bid x 10 days
    Pediatric: see page 575 for dose by weight
        20-40 mg/kg/day in 3 doses x 10 days
  Pulvule: 250, 500 mg; *Oral susp:* 125, 250 mg/5 ml (75, 150 ml); 187, 375 mg/5 ml (50, 100 ml) (strawberry)
  Ceclor®CD 500 mg q 12 hours x 10 days
    Pediatric: <16 years: not recommended
    Tab: 375, 500 mg ext-rel
  Ceclor®CDpak 500 mg q 12 hours x 10 days
    Pediatric: <16 years: not recommended
    Tab: 500 mg (14 tabs/CDpak)

Skin Infection: Bacterial

Raniclor® 500 mg q 12 hours x 10 days
    Pediatric: 20-40 mg/kg/day in 3 doses x 10 days
    Chew tab: 125, 187, 250, 375 mg

▶*cefadroxil* **(B)** 1-2 g in 1-2 doses x 10 days
    Pediatric: see page 576 for dose by weight
        15-30 mg/kg/day in 2 doses x 10 days
  Duricef® *Cap:* 500 mg; *Tab:* 1 g; *Oral susp:* 250 mg/5 ml (100 ml); 500 mg/5 ml (75, 100 ml) (orange-pineapple)

▶*cefdinir* **(B)** 300 mg bid x 10 days
    Pediatric: see page 574 for dose by weight
        <6 months: not recommended
        6 months-12 years: 14 mg/kg/day in 1-2 doses x 10 days
  Omnicef® *Cap:* 300 mg; *Oral susp:* 125 mg/5 ml (60, 100 ml) (strawberry)

▶*cefditoren pivoxil* **(B)** 200 mg bid x 10 days
    Pediatric: not recommended
  Spectracef® *Tab:* 200 mg
Comment: Contraindicated with milk protein allergy or carnitine deficiency.

▶*cefpodoxime* **(B)** *proxetil* 400 mg bid x 7-14 days
    Pediatric: see page 578 for dose by weight
        <2 months: not recommended
        2 months-12 years: 10 mg/kg/day (max 400 mg/dose) or 5 mg/kg/day bid (max 200 mg/dose) x 7-14 days
  Vantin® *Tab:* 100, 200 mg; *Oral susp:* 50, 100 mg/5 ml (50, 75, 100 mg; lemon-creme)

▶*cefprozil* **(B)** 250-500 mg bid or 500 mg daily x 10 days
    Pediatric: see page 579 for dose by weight
        2-12 years: 7.5 mg/kg bid x 10 days
  Cefzil® *Tab:* 250, 500 mg; *Oral susp:* 125, 250 mg/5 ml (50, 75, 100 ml; bubble gum, phenylalanine)

▶*ceftriaxone* **(B)(G)** 1-2 g IM daily; max 4 g/day
  Rocephin®
    Pediatric: 50-75 mg/kg IM in 1-2 doses; max 2 g/day
    Vial: 250, 500 mg; 1, 2 g

▶*cefuroxime axetil* **(B)(G)** 250-500 mg bid x 10 days
    Pediatric: see page 581 for dose by weight
        <3 months: not recommended
        3 months-12 years: 20-30 mg/kg/day in 2 doses x 10 days

Skin Infection: Bacterial

Ceftin® *Tab:* 125, 250, 500 mg; *Oral susp:* 125, 250 mg/5 ml (50, 100 ml; tutti-frutti)

▶*cephalexin* **(B)(G)** 500 mg bid x 10 days
> *Pediatric: see page 582 for dose by weight*
> 25-50 mg/kg/day in 4 doses x 10 days

Keflex® *Cap:* 250, 500, 750 mg; *Oral susp:* 125, 250 mg/5 ml (100, 200 ml)
Keftab® *Tab:* 500 mg
Keftab®K-pak *Tab:* 20-500 mg tabs/K-pak

▶*clarithromycin* **(C)(G)** 250-500 mg bid or 500-1000 mg extended-Release daily x 7-14 days
> *Pediatric: see page 584 for dose by weight*
> <6 months: not recommended
> >6 months: 7.5 mg/kg bid x 7-14 days

Biaxin® *Tab:* 250, 500 mg
Biaxin®Oral Suspension *Oral susp:* 125, 250 mg/5 ml (50, 100 ml; fruit-punch)
Biaxin®XL *Tab:* 500 mg ext-rel

▶*dicloxacillin* **(B)** 500 mg qid x 10 days
> *Pediatric: see page 586 for dose by weight*
> 12.5-25 mg/kg/day in 4 doses x 10 days

Dynapen® *Cap:* 125, 250, 500 mg; *Oral susp:* 62.5 mg/5 ml (80, 100, 200 ml)

▶*dirithromycin* **(C)** 500 mg daily x 5-7 days
> *Pediatric:* <12 years: not recommended

Dynabac® *Tab:* 250 mg

▶*doxycycline* **(D)(G)** 200 mg on first day; then 100 mg in 1-2 doses x 9 days
> *Pediatric:* <8 years: not recommended
> >8 years, <100 lb: 2 mg/lb on first day in 2 doses, followed by 1 mg/lb/day in 1-2 doses x 9 days
> >8 years, >100 lb: same as adult

Adoxa® *Tab:* 50, 100 mg ent-coat
Doryx® *Cap:* 100 mg
Monodox® *Cap:* 50, 100 mg
Vibramycin® *Cap:* 50, 100 mg; *Syr:* 50 mg/5 ml; (raspberry, sulfites); *Oral susp:* 25 mg/5 ml (raspberry-apple); *IV conc: doxy* 100 mg/*asc acid* 480 mg after dilution; *doxy* 200 mg/*asc acid* 960 mg after dilution
Vibra-Tab® *Tab:* 100 mg film-coat

Skin Infection: Bacterial

Comment: Doxycycline is contraindicated in pregnancy (discolors fetal tooth enamel).

▶*erythromycin base* **(B)(G)** 250-500 mg tid x 10 days
    Pediatric: see page 588 for dose by weight
        30-50 mg/kg/day in 2-4 doses x 10 days
  E-Mycin® *Tab:* 250 mg; 333 mg ent-coat
  Eryc® *Cap:* 250 mg ent-coat
  Ery-Tab® *Tab:* 250, 333, 500 mg ent-coat
  PCE® *Tab:* 333, 500 mg

▶*erythromycin ethylsuccinate* **(B)(G)** 400 mg qid x 10 days
    Pediatric: see page 589 for dose by weight
        30-50 mg/kg/day in 4 divided doses x 10 days; may double dose with severe infection; max 100 mg/kg/day
  Ery-Ped® *Oral susp:* 200 mg/5 ml (100, 200 ml; fruit); 400 mg/5 ml (60, 100, 200 ml; banana); *Oral drops:* 200, 400 mg/5 ml (50 ml; fruit); *Chew tab:* 200 mg wafer (fruit)
  E.E.S.® *Oral susp:* 200, 400 mg/5 ml (100 ml; fruit)
  E.E.S.®Granules *Oral susp:* 200 mg/5 ml (100, 200 ml; cherry,
  E.E.S.®400 Tablets *Tab:* 400 mg

▶*erythromycin estolate* **(B)(G)** 250-500 mg q 6 hours x 10 days
    Pediatric: see page 588 for dose by weight
        20-50 mg/kg q 6 hours x 10 days
  Ilosone® *Pulvule:* 250 mg; *Tab:* 500 mg; *Liq:* 125, 250 mg/5 ml (100 ml)

▶*levofloxacin* **(C)**
  Uncomplicated: 500 mg daily x 7-10 days
  Complicated: 750 mg daily x 7-10 days
    Pediatric: <18 years: not recommended
  Levaquin® *Tab:* 250, 500, 750 mg

▶*linezolide* **(C)** 400-600 mg q 12 hours x 10-14 days
    Pediatric: not recommended
  Zyvox® *Tab:* 400, 600 mg; *Oral susp:* 100 mg/5 ml (150 ml) (orange, phenylalanine)

▶*loracarbef* **(B)** 200 mg bid x 7 days
    Pediatric: see page 593 for dose by weight
        15 mg/kg/day in 2 doses x 7 days
  Lorabid® *Pulvule:* 200, 400 mg; *Oral susp:* 100 mg/5 ml (50, 100 ml); 200 mg/5 ml (50, 75, 100 ml) (strawberry bubble gum)

▶*minocycline* **(D)(G)** 200 mg on first day; then 100 mg q 12 hours x 9 more days

Skin Infection: Bacterial

> *Pediatric:* <8 years: not recommended
> >8 years, <100 lb: 2 mg/lb on first day in 2 doses, followed by 1 mg/lb/ q 12 hours x 9 more days
> >8 years, >100 lb: same as adult
>
> **Minocin**® *Cap:* 100 mg ent-coat

Comment: Minocycline is contraindicated in pregnancy (discolors fetal tooth enamel).

▶ *moxifloxacin* **(C)** 400 mg daily x 10 days
> *Pediatric:* <18 years: not recommended
>
> **Avelox**® *Tab:* 400 mg

▶ *ofloxacin* **(C)(G)** 400 mg bid x 10 days
> *Pediatric:* <18 years: not recommended
>
> **Floxin**® *Tab:* 200, 300, 400 mg

▶ *tetracycline* **(D)** 500 mg qid x 10 days
> *Pediatric: see page 595 for dose by weight*
> <8 years: not recommended
> >8 years, <100 lb: 25-50 mg/kg/day in 4 doses x 10 days
> >8 years, >100 lb: same as adult
>
> **Achromycin**®V *Cap:* 250, 500 mg
> **Sumycin**® *Tab:* 250, 500 mg; *Cap:* 250, 500 mg; *Oral susp:* 125 mg/5 ml (100, 200 ml; fruit, sulfites)

Comment: Tetracycline is contraindicated in pregnancy (discolors fetal tooth enamel).

▶ *trovafloxacin* **(C)** 100 mg daily x 7-10 days
> *Pediatric:* <18 years: not recommended
>
> **Trovan**® *Tab:* 100, 200 mg

Comment: Trovafloxacin is indicated only for life- or limb-threatening infection.

Sleep Apnea

Anti-narcoleptic Agent
▶ *modafinil* **(C)(IV)** 100-200 mg q AM; max 400 mg/day
> *Pediatric:* <16 years: not recommended
>
> **Provigil**® *Tab:* 100, 200*mg

Comment: Modafinil promotes wakefulness in patients with excessive sleepiness due to obstructive sleep apnea/hypopnea syndrome.

Sleepiness: Excessive

Anti-narcoleptic Agent
▶*modafinil* **(C)(IV)** 100-200 mg q AM; max 400 mg/day
>*Pediatric:* <16 years: not recommended
>**Provigil®** *Tab:* 100, 200*mg

Comment: **Provigil®** promotes wakefulness in patients with narcolepsy, shift work sleep disorder, and excessive sleepiness due to obstructive sleep apnea/hypopnea syndrome.

Smallpox *(Variola major)*

Prophylaxis
▶*vaccina virus* vaccine (dried, calf lymph type) **(C)**
>*Pediatric:* < 12 months: not recommended
>12 months-18 years, non-emergency: not recommended

>**DRYvax®**
>>*Kit:* vial dried smallpox vaccine (1), 0.25 ml diluent in syringe (1), vented needle (1), 100 individually wrapped Bifurcated needles (5 needles/strip, 20 strips) (polymyxin B sulfate, dihydrostreptomycin sulfate, chlortetracycline HCL, neomycin sulfate, glycerin, phenol)

Comment: **Dryvax®** is a dried live vaccine with approximately 100 million infectious vaccina viruses (pock-forming units [pfu] per ml. Contact with immunosuppressed individuals should be avoided until the scab has separated from the skin (2 to 3 weeks) and/or a protective occlusive dressing covers the inoculation site. Scarification only. Do not inject IV, IM, or SC. Revaccination is recommended every 10 years.

Sprain

Comment: RICE: Rest; Ice; Compression; Elevation.
NSAIDs *see **Pain** page 305*
Oral Non-narcotic Analgesics *see **Pain** page 308*
Oral Narcotic Analgesics *see **Pain** page 308*
Topical Analgesics *see **Pain** page 308*
Parenteral Glucocorticosteroids *see page 389*

Sprain

Oral Glucocorticosteroids *see page 387*
Topical Anesthetic *see page 383*
Topical Anesthetic/Steroid Combinations *see page 480*

Status Asthmaticus

▶*epinephrine* **(C)** 0.3-0.5 mg (0.3-0.5 ml of a 1:1000 soln) SC q 20-30 minutes as needed up to 3 doses
        Pediatric: <2 years: 0.05-0.1 ml
                2-6 years: 0.1 ml
                6-12 years: 0.2 ml
                All: q 20-30 minutes as needed up to 3 doses

Emergency Treatment Kit
▶*epinephrine* **(C)** 0.3 ml IM in thigh; may repeat if needed
        Pediatric: 0.01 mg/kg IM in thigh; may repeat if needed
    EpiPen® *EpiPen 0.3 mg:* auto-injector with *epi* 1:1000, 0.3 ml (1, 2/box)
    EpiPen®Jr. *EpiPen Jr. 0.15 mg:* auto-injector with *epi* 1:2000, 0.3 ml (1, 2/box)

Inhaled Anticholinergics
▶*ipratropium bromide* **(C)**
    Atrovent® 2 inhalations qid; additional inhalations as required; max 12 inhalations/day
        Pediatric: not recommended
        Inhaler: 18 mcg/actuation (14 g, 200 inh)
    Atrovent®Inhalation Solution 500 mcg tid-qid prn by nebulizer
        Pediatric: not recommended
        Inhal soln: 0.02% (500 mcg in 2.5 ml; 25/box)

Parenteral Glucocorticosteroids *see page 389*
Oral Glucocorticosteroids *see page 387*

Status Epilepticus

▶*diazepam* injectable **(D)(IV)** initially 5-10 mg IV in large vein; may repeat q 10-15 minutes; max 30 mg; may repeat in 2-4 hours if needed; do not dilute; may give IM if IV not accessible
        Pediatric: 1 month-5 years: 0.2-0.5 mg IV q 2-5 minutes; max 5 mg
                >5 years: 1 mg IV q 2-5 minutes; max 10 mg; may repeat in 2-4 hours if needed

Valium®Injectable *Vial:* 5 mg/ml (10 ml); *Amp:* 5 mg/ml (2 ml); *Prefilled syringe:* 5 mg/ml (5 ml)
▶*lorazepam* injectable **(D)(IV)** 4 mg IV over 2 minutes (dilute first); may repeat in 10-15 minutes; may give IM if needed (undiluted)
   Pediatric: <18 years: not recommended
   Ativan®Injectable *Vial:* 2 mg/ml (1, 10 ml); *Tubex:* 2 mg/ml (0.5 ml); *Cartridge:* 2, 4 mg/ml (1 ml)
▶*phenytoin* injectable **(D)(G)** 10-15 mg/kg IV, not to exceed 50 mg/minute; follow with 100 mg orally or IV q 6-8 hours; do not dilute in IV fluid
   Pediatric: 15-20 mg/kg IV, not to exceed 1-2 mg/kg/minute
   Dilantin® *Vial:* 50 mg/ml (2, 5 ml); *Amp:* 50 mg/ml (2 ml)

Comment: Monitor *phenytoin* serum levels. Therapeutic serum level: 10-20 g/ml. Side effects include gingival hyperplasia.

Oral Anti-convulsants for Routine Management of Seizure Disorder
see *Seizure Disorder* page 483

Stye (Hordeolum)

▶*erythromycin* ophthalmic ointment **(B)** 1 cm up to 6 times/day
   Pediatric: same as adult
   Ilotycin®Ophthalmic Ointment *Ophth oint:* 5 mg/g (1/8 oz)
▶*erythromycin* ophthalmic solution **(B)** initially 1-2 drops q 1-2 hours; may then increase dose interval
   Pediatric: same as adult
   Isopto Cetamide®Ophthalmic Solution *Ophth soln:* 15% (15 ml)
▶*gentamicin* ophthalmic ointment **(C)** 1 cm bid-tid
   Pediatric: same as adult
   Garamycin®Ophthalmic Ointment *Ophth oint:* 3 mg/g (3.5 g)
   Genoptic®Ophthalmic Ointment *Ophth oint:* 3 mg/g (3.5 g)
   Gentacidin®Ophthalmic Ointment *Ophth oint:* 3 mg/g (3.5 g)
▶*polymixin/bacitracn* ophthalmic ointment **(C)** apply 1/2 inch q 3-4 hours
   Pediatric: same as adult
   Polysporin® *Ophth oint: poly* 10,000 U/*bac* 500 units per g (3.75 g)
▶*polymyxin B/bacitracin/neomycin* ophthalmic ointment **(C)(G)** apply 1/2 inch q 3-4 hours
   Pediatric: same as adult
   Neosporin®Ophthalmic Ointment *Ophth oint: poly* B 10,000 U/*bac* 400 U/*neo* 3.5 mg/g (3.75 g)

Stye

▶*polymyxin B/neomycin/gramicidin* ophthalmic solution **(C)** 1-2 drops 2-3 times q 1 hour, then 1-2 drops bid-qid x 7-10 days
    Pediatric: same as adult
  Neosporin®Ophthalmic Solution *Ophth soln: poly* 10,000 U/*neo* 1.75 mg/*gram* 0.025 mg/ml (10 ml)

▶*sodium sulfacetamide* ophthalmic solution and ointment **(C)**
  Bleph-10®Ophthalmic Solution 2 drops q 4 hour x 7-14 days
    Pediatric: <2 years: not recommended
                >2 years: 1-2 drops q 2-3 hours during the day
    Ophth soln: 10% (2.5, 5, 15 ml; benzalkonium chloride)
  Bleph-10®Ophthalmic Ointment apply 1/2 inch qid and HS
    Pediatric: <2 years: not recommended
                >2 years: apply 1/4-1/3 inch qid and HS
    Ophth oint: 10% (3.5 g; phenylmercuric acetate)
  Sulamyd®Ophthalmic Solution 1 drop of 30% soln or 1-2 drops of 10% soln q 2 hours
    Pediatric: same as adult
    Ophth soln: 10% (5, 15 ml); 30% (15 ml; parabens)
  Sulamyd®Ophthalmic Ointment apply 1/2 inch qid and HS
    Pediatric: same as adult
    Ophth oint: 10% (3.5 g; parabens)

Sunburn

▶*prednisone* **(C)(G)** 10 mg qid x 4-6 days if severe and extensive
▶*silver sulfadiazine* **(C)(G)** apply topically to burn daily-bid
    Pediatric: not recommended
  Silvadene® *Crm:* 1% (20, 50, 85, 400, 1000 g jar; 20 g tube)

Syphilis (*Treponema pallidum*)

Comment: Treat all sexual contacts. Consider testing for other STDs.
Primary, secondary, and early latent <1 year
Primary Therapy
▶*penicillin G (benzathine)* **(B)(G)** 2.4 million units IM x 1 dose
    Pediatric: 50,000 units/kg IM x 1 dose; max 2.4 million units
  Bicillin®L-A *Cartridge-needle unit:* 600,000 million units (1 ml); 1.2 million units (2 ml); 2.4 million units (4 ml)
If Penicillin allergic

Syphilis

▶*doxycycline* **(D)(G)** 100 mg bid x 14 days
>   *Pediatric:* <8 years: not recommended
>   >8 years, <100 lb: 2 mg/lb on first day in 2 doses, followed by 1 mg/lb/day in 1-2 doses x 14 days
>   >8 years, >100 lb: same as adult

Adoxa® *Tab:* 50, 100 mg ent-coat
Doryx® *Cap:* 100 mg
Monodox® *Cap:* 50, 100 mg
Vibramycin® *Cap:* 50, 100 mg; *Syr:* 50 mg/5 ml (raspberry, sulfites); *Oral susp:* 25 mg/5 ml (raspberry-apple); *IV conc: doxy* 100 mg/*asc acid* 480 mg after dilution; *doxy* 200 mg/*asc acid* 960 mg after dilution
Vibra-Tab® *Tab:* 100 mg film-coat

Comment: Doxycycline is contraindicated in pregnancy (discolors fetal tooth enamel).

▶*minocycline* **(D)(G)** 200 mg on first day; then 100 mg q 12 hours x 9 more days
>   *Pediatric:* <8 years: not recommended
>   >8 years, <100 lb: 2 mg/lb on first day in 2 doses, followed by 1 mg/lb/ q 12 hours x 9 more days
>   >8 years, >100 lb: same as adult

Minocin® *Cap:* 100 mg ent-coat

Comment: Minocycline is contraindicated in pregnancy (discolors fetal tooth enamel).

▶*tetracycline* **(D)(G)** 500 mg qid x 14 days
>   *Pediatric: see page 595 for dose by weight*
>   <8 years: not recommended
>   >8 years, <100 lb: 25-50 mg/kg/day in 2-4 doses x 14 days
>   >8 years, >100 lb: same as adult

Achromycin®V *Cap:* 250, 500 mg
Sumycin® *Tab:* 250, 500 mg; *Cap:* 250, 500 mg; *Oral susp:* 125 mg/5 ml (100, 200 ml; fruit, sulfites)

Comment: Tetracycline is contraindicated in pregnancy (discolors fetal tooth enamel).

Alternative Therapy

▶*ceftriaxone* **(B)** 1 g IM daily x 8-10 days
>   *Pediatric:* use in children only if allergic to penicillin

Rocephin®
Vial: 250, 500 mg; 1, 2 g

Syphilis

▶ *erythromycin base* **(B)** 500 mg qid x 14 days
    Pediatric: see page 588 for dose by weight
        30-50 mg/kg/day in 2-4 doses x 14 days; use in
        children only if allergic to penicillin

  E-Mycin® *Tab:* 250 mg; 333 mg ent-coat
  Eryc® *Cap:* 250 mg ent-coat
  Ery-Tab® *Tab:* 250, 333, 500 mg ent-coat
  PCE® *Tab:* 333, 500 mg

▶ *erythromycin estolate* **(B)(G)** 500 mg q 6 hours x 10 days
    Pediatric: see page 588 for dose by weight
        20-50 mg/kg q 6 hours x 10 days

  Ilosone® *Pulvule:* 250 mg; *Tab:* 500 mg; *Liq:* 125, 250 mg/5 ml (100 ml)

Latent >1 year, of unknown duration, and tertiary
Primary Therapy

▶ *penicillin G (benzathine)* **(B)(G)** 2.4 million units IM weekly x 3 doses
    Pediatric: 50,000 unit/kg IM weekly x 3 doses; max 2.4
        million units

  Bicillin®L-A *Cartridge-needle unit:* 600,000 million units (1 ml); 1.2 million units (2 ml); 2.4 million units (4 ml)

If Penicillin allergic

▶ *doxycycline* **(D)(G)** 100 mg bid x 4 weeks
    Pediatric: <8 years: not recommended
        >8 years, <100 lb: 2 mg/lb on first day in 2 doses,
        followed by 1 mg/lb/day in 1-2 doses x 4 weeks
        >8 years, >100 lb: same as adult

  Adoxa® *Tab:* 50, 100 mg ent-coat
  Doryx® *Cap:* 100 mg
  Monodox® *Cap:* 50, 100 mg
  Vibramycin® *Cap:* 50, 100 mg; *Syr:* 50 mg/5 ml (raspberry, sulfites); *Oral susp:* 25 mg/5 ml (raspberry-apple); *IV conc: doxy* 100 mg/*asc acid* 480 mg after dilution; *doxy* 200 mg/*asc acid* 960 mg after dilution
  Vibra-Tab® *Tab:* 100 mg film-coat

Comment: Doxycycline is contraindicated in pregnancy (discolors fetal tooth enamel).

▶ *minocycline* **(D)(G)** 100 mg q 12 hours x 10 days
    Pediatric: <8 years: not recommended
        >8 years, <100 lb: 2 mg/lb on first day in 2 doses,
        followed by 1 mg/lb/ q 12 hours x 9 more days
        >8 years, >100 lb: same as adult

Minocin® *Cap:* 100 mg ent-coat
Comment: Minocycline is contraindicated in pregnancy (discolors fetal tooth enamel).
▶*tetracycline* **(D)** 500 mg qid x 4 weeks
    Pediatric: see page 595 for dose by weight
        <8 years: not recommended
        >8 years, <100 lb: 25-50 mg/kg/day in 2-4 doses x 4 weeks
        >8 years, >100 lb: same as adult
  Achromycin®V *Cap:* 250, 500 mg
  Sumycin® *Tab:* 250, 500 mg; *Cap:* 250, 500 mg; *Oral susp:* 125 mg/5 ml (100, 200 ml; fruit, sulfites)
Comment: Tetracycline is contraindicated in pregnancy (discolors fetal tooth enamel).

Temporal Arteritis

Parenteral Glucocorticosteroids *see page 389*
Oral Glucocorticosteroids *see page 387*

Temporomandibular Joint (TMJ) Disorder

NSAIDs *see **Pain** page 305*
Oral Non-narcotic Analgesics *see **Pain** page 308*
Oral Narcotic Analgesics *see **Pain** page 308*
Topical Analgesics *see **Pain** page 308*
Parenteral Glucocorticosteroids *see page 389*
Oral Glucocorticosteroids *see page 387*
Topical Anesthetics *see page 383*
Topical Anesthetics/Steroid Combinations *see page 480*

Testosterone Deficiency

Comment: Testosterone is contraindicated in male breast cancer and prostate cancer. *Testosterone* replacement therapy is indicated in males with primary or hypogonadotropic hypogonadism.
Oral Androgens
▶*fluoxymesterone* **(X)(III)** for hypogonadism, 5-20 mg daily; for delayed puberty, use low dose and limit duration to 4-6 months

Pediatric: use by specialist only
Halotestin® *Tab:* 2*, 5*, 10*mg (tartrazine)

▶*methyltestosterone* **(X)(III)** usually 10-50 mg daily; for delayed puberty, use low dose and limit duration to 4-6 months
Android® *Cap:* 10 mg

▶*testosterone* **(X)(III)** 30 mg q 12 hours to gum region, just above the incisor tooth on either side of the mouth; hold system in place for 30 sec; rotate sites with each application
Striant® *Tab, buccal:* 30 mg (6 blister pks; 10 buccal systems/blister pck)

Topical Androgens
Comment: Pregnant and nursing women must avoid skin contact with application sites on men.

▶*testosterone* **(X)(III)**
Pediatric: <18 years: not recommended
AndroGel® initially apply 5 g daily in the AM to clean, dry, intact skin of the upper arms, and/or abdomen; no not apply to scrotum; may increase by 2.5 g q 2 weeks as needed; wash hands after application; allow gel to dry before skin is allowed to touch clothing
Gel: 2.5, 5 g (30 pkts)
Testim® initially apply 5 g daily in the AM to clean, dry, intact skin of the shoulders and/or upper arms; do not apply to the genitals or abdomen; may increase to 10 g after 2 weeks; do not wash site for at least 2 hours after application
Gel: 1%, clear, hydroalcoholic (5 mg/5 g, 5 g single-use tube)

Transdermal Androgen Transdermal Systems
▶*testosterone* **(X)(III)**
Androderm® initially apply 5 mg nightly at approximately 10 PM to clean, dry area of arm, back, or upper buttocks; leave on x 24 hours; may increase to 7.5 mg or decrease to 2.5 mg based on confirmed AM serum testosterone concentrations
Pediatric: <15 years: not recommended
Transdermal patch: 2.5, 5 mg/day
Testostoderm® apply one patch every 22-24 hours to clean, dry scrotal skin that has been shaved; if scrotal area is inadequate, use 4 mg/day strength
Pediatric: <18 years: not recommended
Transdermal patch: 4, 6 mg/day
Testostoderm®**TTS** apply one patch every 22-24 hours to clean, dry scrotal skin that has been shaved; if scrotal area is inadequate, use 4 mg/day strength

Pediatric: <18 years: not recommended
Transdermal patch: 5 mg/day (alcohol)

Tetanus

Prophylaxis
see ***Appendix M: Immunizations: Childhood** page 466*
Post-exposure Prophylaxis in Previously Non-immunized Persons
▶*tetanus immune globulin, human* **(C)** 3000-6000 units IM
    Baytet®, Hyper-tet® *Vial:* 250 units single dose; *Prefilled syringe:* 250 units
▶*tetanus toxoid* vaccine **(C)** 0.5 cc IM x 3 dose series
    Vial: 5 Lf units/0.5 ml (0.5, 5 ml); *Prefilled syringe:* 5 Lf units/0.5 ml (0.5 ml)

Threadworm (*Strongyloidiasis*)

Anthelmintics
▶*albendazole* **(C)** 400 mg bid x 7 days; take after a meal
    Pediatric: <2 years: 200 mg daily x 3 days; may repeat in 3 weeks
              2-12 years: 400 mg daily x 3 days; may repeat in 3 weeks
  Albenza® *Tab:* 200 mg
▶*mebendazole* **(C)(G)** 100 mg bid x 3 days; may repeat in 2-3 weeks if needed; take after a meal
    Pediatric: same as adult (chew or crush and mix with food)
  Vermox® *Chew tab:* 100 mg
▶*pyrantel pamoate* **(C)** 11 mg/kg x 1 dose; max 1 g/dose; take after a meal
    Pediatric: 25-37 lb: 1/2 tsp x 1 dose
               38-62 lb: 1 tsp x 1 dose
               63-87 lb: 1½ tsp x 1 dose
               88-112 lb: 2 tsp x 1 dose
               113-137 lb: 2½ tsp x 1 dose
               138-162 lb: 3 tsp x 1 dose
               163-187 lb: 3½ tsp x 1 dose
               >187 lb: 4 tsp x 1 dose
  Antiminth® **(OTC)** *Cap:* 180 mg; *Liq:* 50 mg/ml (30 ml); 144 mg/ml (30 ml); *Oral susp:* 50 mg/ml (60 ml)

Threadworm

    Pin-X®(OTC) *Cap:* 180 mg; *Liq:* 50 mg/ml (30 ml); 144 mg/ml (30 ml); *Oral susp:* 50 mg/ml (30 ml)

▶*thiabendazole* **(C)** 25 mg/kg bid x 7 days; max 1.5 g/dose; take after a meal
    Pediatric: same as adult
        <30 lb: consult mfr literature
        >30 lb 2 doses/day with meals
        30-50 lbs: 250 mg bid with meals
        >50 lb: 10 mg/lb/dose bid with meals; max 3g/day
    Mintezol® *Chew tab:* 500*mg (orange); *Oral susp:* 500 mg/5 ml (120 ml; orange)

Comment: Thiabendazole is not for prophylaxis. May impair mental alertness.

Tinea Capitis

Comment: Tinea capitis must be treated with an oral anti-fungal.

▶*griseofulvin, microsize* **(C)(G)** 1 g daily x 4-6 weeks or longer
    Pediatric: see page 592 for dose by weight
        <30 lb: 5 mg/lb/day
        30-50 lb: 125-250 mg/day
        >50 lb: 250-500 mg/day
        5 mg/lb/day x 4-6 weeks or longer
    Grifulvin®V *Tab:* 250, 500 mg; *Oral susp:* 125 mg/5 ml (120 ml; alcohol 0.02%)

▶*griseofulvin, ultramicrosize* **(C)(G)** 375 mg/day in 1 or more doses x 4-6 weeks or longer
    Pediatric: <2 years: not recommended
        >2 years: 3.3 mg/lb/day in 1 or more doses x 4-6 weeks or longer
    Fulvicin®P/G *Tab:* 125, 165, 250, 330 mg
    Grisactin® *Tab:* 250, 330 mg
    Grisactin®Ultra *Cap:* 250 mg
    Gris-PEG® *Tab:* 125, 250 mg

Comment: Griseofulvin should be taken with fatty foods (e.g., milk, ice cream). Liver enzymes should be monitored.

▶*ketoconazole* **(C)(G)** initially 200 mg daily; max 400 mg/day x 4 weeks
    Pediatric: <2 years: not recommended
        >2 years: 3.3-6.6 mg/kg daily x 4 weeks
    Nizoral® *Tab:* 200 mg

For severe kerion

▶ *prednisone* **(C)** 1 mg/kg/day for 7-14 days
see **Oral Glucocorticosteroids** page 387

Tinea Corporis (Ringworm)

Topical Anti-fungals
▶ *butenafine* **(B)(G)** apply bid x 1 week or daily x 4 weeks
    Pediatric: <12 years: not recommended
  Lotrimin®Ultra (C)(OTC) *Crm:* 1% (12, 24 g)
  Mentax® *Crm:* 1% (15, 30 g)
Comment: Butenafine is a benzylamine, not an "azole." Fungicidal activity continues for at least 5 weeks after last application.
▶ *ciclopirox* **(B)**
  Loprox®Cream apply bid; max 4 weeks
    Pediatric: <10 years: not recommended
        >10 years: same as adult
    Crm: 0.77% (15, 30, 90 g)
  Loprox®Lotion apply bid; max 4 weeks
    Pediatric: <10 years: not recommended
        >10 years: same as adult
    Lotn: 0.77% (30, 60 ml)
  Loprox®Gel apply bid; max 4 weeks
    Pediatric: <16 years: not recommended
    Gel: 0.77% (30, 45 g)
▶ *clotrimazole* **(B)(G)** apply to affected area bid x 7 days
    Pediatric: same as adult
  Fungoid® *Crm:* 1% (45 g); *Soln:* 1% (1 oz w. dropper)
  Lotrimin® *Crm:* 1% (15, 30, 45 g)
  Lotrimin®AF (OTC) *Crm:* 1% (12 g); *Lotn:* 1% (10 ml); *Soln:* 1% (10 ml)
▶ *econazole* **(C)** apply daily x 14 days
    Pediatric: same as adult
  Spectazole® *Crm:* 1% (15, 30, 85 g)
▶ *ketoconazole* **(C)** apply daily x 14 days
    Pediatric: not recommended
  Nizoral®Cream *Crm:* 2% (15, 30, 60 g)
▶ *miconazole 2%* **(C)** apply bid x 2 weeks
    Pediatric: same as adult
  Lotrimin®AF Spray Liquid (OTC) *Spray liq:* 2% (113 g; alcohol 17%)

Tinea Corporis

Lotrimin®AF Spray Powder (OTC) *Spray pwdr:* 2% (90 g; (alcohol 10%)
Monistat-Derm® *Crm:* 2% (1, 3 oz); *Spray liq:* 2% (3.5 oz); *Spray pwdr:* 2% (3 oz)

▶*naftifine* **(B)**
    Pediatric: not recommended
Naftin®Cream apply daily x 14 days
    Crm: 1% (15, 30, 60 g)
Naftin®Gel apply bid x 14 days
    Gel: 1% (20, 40, 60 g)

▶*oxiconazole nitrate* **(B)** apply daily-bid x 2 weeks
    Pediatric: same as adult
Oxistat® *Crm:* 1% (15, 30, 60 g); *Lotn:* 1% (30 ml)

▶*sulconazole* **(C)** apply daily-bid x 3 weeks
    Pediatric: not recommended
Exelderm® *Crm:* 1% (15, 30, 60 g); *Lotn:* 1% (30 mg)

▶*terbinafine* **(B)(G)**
    Pediatric: <12 years: not recommended
Lamisil®Cream (OTC) apply to affected and surrounding area daily-bid x 1-4 weeks until significantly improved
    Crm: 1% (15, 30 g)
Lamisil®AT Cream (OTC) apply to affected and surrounding area daily-bid x 1-4 weeks until significantly improved
    Crm: 1% (15, 30 g)
Lamisil®Solution (OTC) apply to affected and surrounding area daily x 1 week
    Soln: 1% (30 ml spray bottle)

Topical Anti-fungal/Steroid Combinations

▶*clotrimazole/betamethasone* **(C)** apply bid x 2 weeks; max 4 weeks
    Pediatric: <12 years: not recommended
Lotrisone® *Crm:* clotrim 10 mg/*beta* 0.5 mg (15, 45 g); *Lotn:* clotrim 10 mg/*beta* 0.5 mg (30 ml)

Systemic Anti-fungals

▶*griseofulvin, microsize* **(C)(G)** 500 mg/day x 2-4 weeks; max 1 g/day
    Pediatric: see page 592 for dose by weight
        <30 lb: 5 mg/lb/day
        30-50 lb: 125-250 mg/day
        >50 lb: 250-500 mg/day
Grifulvin®V *Tab:* 250, 500 mg; *Oral susp:* 125 mg/5 ml (120 ml; alcohol 0.02%)

▶ *griseofulvin, ultramicrosize* **(C)(G)** 375 mg/day in 1 or more doses x 2-4 weeks
       Pediatric: <2 years: not recommended
                >2 years: 3.3 mg/lb/day in 1 or more doses
   Fulvicin®P/G *Tab:* 125, 165, 250, 330 mg
   Grisactin® *Tab:* 250, 330 mg
   Grisactin®Ultra *Cap:* 250 mg
   Gris-PEG® *Tab:* 125, 250

Comment: Griseofulvin should be taken with fatty foods (e.g., milk, ice cream). Liver enzymes should be monitored.

▶ *ketoconazole* **(C)** initially 200 mg daily; max 400 mg/day x 4 weeks
       Pediatric: <2 years: not recommended
                >2 years: 3.3-6.6 mg/kg/day x 4 weeks
   Nizoral® *Tab:* 200 mg

Tinea Cruris (Jock Itch)

Topical Anti-fungals

▶ *butenafine* **(B)(G)** apply bid x 1 week or daily x 4 weeks
       Pediatric: <12 years: not recommended
   Lotrimin®Ultra (C)(OTC) *Crm:* 1% (12, 24 g)
   Mentax® *Crm:* 1% (15, 30 g)

Comment: Butenafine is a benzylamine, not an "azole." Fungicidal activity continues for at least 5 weeks after last application.

▶ *ciclopirox* **(B)**
   Loprox®Cream apply bid; max 4 weeks
       Pediatric: <10 years: not recommended
                >10 years: same as adult
       Crm: 0.77% (15, 30, 90 g)
   Loprox®Lotion apply bid; max 4 weeks
       Pediatric: <10 years: not recommended
                >10 years: same as adult
       Lotn: 0.77% (30, 60 ml)
   Loprox®Gel apply bid; max 4 weeks
       Pediatric: <16 years: not recommended
       Gel: 0.77% (30, 45 g)

▶ *clotrimazole* **(B)(G)** apply to affected area bid x 7 days
       Pediatric: same as adult
   Fungoid® *Crm:* 1% (45 g); *Soln:* 1% (1 oz w. dropper)
   Lotrimin® *Crm:* 1% (15, 30, 45 g)

Tinea Cruris

Lotrimin®AF (OTC) *Crm:* 1% (12 g); *Lotn:* 1% (10 ml); *Soln:* 1% (10 ml)

▶ *econazole* **(C)** apply daily x 2 weeks
  Pediatric: same as adult
  Spectazole® *Crm:* 1% (15, 30, 85 g)

▶ *ketoconazole* **(C)(G)** apply daily x 2 weeks
  Pediatric: not recommended
  Nizoral®Cream *Crm:* 2% (15, 30, 60 g)

▶ *miconazole 2%* **(C)(G)** apply daily x 2 weeks
  Pediatric: same as adult
  Lotrimin®AF Spray Liquid (OTC) *Spray liq:* 2% (113 g; alcohol 17%)
  Lotrimin®AF Spray Powder (OTC) *Spray pwdr:* 2% (90 g; alcohol 10%)
  Monistat-Derm® *Crm:* 2% (1, 3 oz); *Spray liq:* 2% (3.5 oz); *Spray pwdr:* 2% (3 oz)

▶ *naftifine* **(B)**
  Pediatric: not recommended
  Naftin®Cream apply daily x 2 weeks
    Crm: 1% (15, 30, 60 g)
  Naftin®Gel apply bid x 2 weeks
    Gel: 1% (20, 40, 60 g)

▶ *oxiconazole nitrate* **(B)** apply daily-bid x 2 weeks
  Pediatric: same as adult
  Oxistat® *Crm:* 1% (15, 30, 60 g); *Lotn:* 1% (30 ml)

▶ *sulconazole* **(C)** apply daily-bid x 3 weeks
  Pediatric: not recommended
  Exelderm® *Crm:* 1% (15, 30, 60 g); *Lotn:* 1% (30 mg)

▶ *terbinafine* **(B)(G)**
  Pediatric: <12 years: not recommended
  Lamisil®Cream (OTC) apply bid x 1-4 weeks
    Crm: 1% (15, 30 g)
  Lamisil®AT Cream (OTC) apply to affected and surrounding area daily-bid x 1-4 weeks until significantly improved
    Crm: 1% (15, 30 g)
  Lamisil®Solution (OTC) apply to affected and surrounding area daily x 1 week
    Soln: 1% (30 ml spray bottle)

▶ *tolnaftate* **(C)(OTC)(G)** apply sparingly bid x 2-4 weeks
  Pediatric: <2 years: not recommended

Tinactin® *Crm:* 1% (15, 30 g); *Pwdr:* 1% (45, 90 g); *Soln:* 1% (10 ml); *Aerosol liq:* 1% (4 oz); *Aerosol pwdr:* 1% (3.5, 5 oz)

▶*undecylenate acid* **(NR)** apply bid x 4 weeks

    Pediatric: same as adult

Desenex® **(OTC)** *Pwdr:* 25% (1.5, 3 oz); *Spray pwdr:* 25% (2.7 oz) *Oint:* 25% (0.5, 1 oz)

Topical Anti-fungal/Anti-inflammatory Agents

▶*clotrimazole/betamethasone* **(C)(G)** apply bid x 4 weeks; max 4 weeks

    Pediatric: <12 years: not recommended

    Crm: clotrim 10 mg/*beta* 0.5 mg (15, 45 g); *Lotn:* clotrim 10 mg/*beta* 0.5 mg (30 ml)

Systemic Anti-fungals

▶*griseofulvin, microsize* **(C)(G)** 1 g daily x 2 weeks

    Pediatric: see page 592 for dose by weight

        <30 lb: 5 mg/lb/day

        30-50 lb: 125-250 mg/day

        >50 lb: 250-500 mg/day

        5 mg/lb/day x 4-6 weeks or longer

Grifulvin®V *Tab:* 250, 500 mg; *Oral susp:* 125 mg/5 ml (120 ml; alcohol 0.02%)

▶*griseofulvin, ultramicrosize* **(C)** 375 mg/day in 1 or more doses x 2 weeks

    Pediatric: <2 years: not recommended

        >2 years: 3.3 mg/lb/day in 1 or more doses

Fulvicin®P/G *Tab:* 125, 165, 250, 330 mg

Grisactin® *Tab:* 250, 330 mg

Grisactin®Ultra *Cap:* 250 mg

Gris-PEG® *Tab:* 125, 250 mg

Comment: Griseofulvin should be taken with fatty foods (e.g., milk, ice cream). Liver enzymes should be monitored.

▶*ketoconazole* **(C)** initially 200 mg daily; max 400 mg daily x 4 weeks

    Pediatric: <2 years: not recommended

        >2 years: 3.3-6.6 mg/kg/day

Nizoral® *Tab:* 200 mg

Tinea Pedis (Athlete's Foot)

Topical Anti-fungals

▶*butenafine* **(B)(G)** apply bid x 1 week or daily x 4 weeks

Tinea Pedis

> *Pediatric:* <12 years: not recommended
> **Lotrimin®Ultra (C)(OTC)** *Crm:* 1% (12, 24 g)
> **Mentax®** *Crm:* 1% (15, 30 g)

Comment: Butenafine is a benzylamine, not an "azole." Fungicidal activity continues for at least 5 weeks after last application.

▶ *burrow's* **(NR)** wet dressings
▶ *ciclopirox* **(B)**
> **Loprox®Cream** apply bid; max 4 weeks
> > *Pediatric:* <10 years: not recommended
> > >10 years: same as adult
> > *Crm:* 0.77% (15, 30, 90 g)
>
> **Loprox®Lotion** apply bid; max 4 weeks
> > *Pediatric:* <10 years: not recommended
> > >10 years: same as adult
> > *Lotn:* 0.77% (30, 60 ml)
>
> **Loprox®Gel** apply bid; max 4 weeks
> > *Pediatric:* <16 years: not recommended
> > *Gel:* 0.77% (30, 45 g)

▶ *clotrimazole* **(C)(G)** apply bid to affected area x 4 weeks
> *Pediatric:* same as adult
> **Desenex®** *Crm:* 1% (0.5 oz)
> **Fungoid®** *Crm:* 1% (45 g)
> *Soln:* 1% (1 oz w. dropper)
> **Lotrimin®** *Crm:* 1% (15, 30, 45, 90 g); *Lotn:* 1% (30 ml); *Soln:* 1% (10, 30 ml)
> **Lotrimin®AF (OTC)** *Crm:* 1% (15, 30, 45, 90 g); *Lotn:* 1% (20 ml); *Soln:* 1% (20 ml)

▶ *econazole* **(C)** apply daily x 4 weeks
> *Pediatric:* same as adult
> **Spectazole®** *Crm:* 1% (15, 30, 85 g)

▶ *ketoconazole* **(C)** apply daily x 6 weeks
> *Pediatric:* not recommended
> **Nizoral®Cream** *Crm:* 2% (15, 30, 60 g)

▶ *miconazole 2%* **(C)(G)** apply daily x 2 weeks
> *Pediatric:* same as adult
> **Lotrimin®AF Spray Liquid (OTC)** *Spray liq:* 2% (113 g; alcohol 17%)
> **Lotrimin®AF Spray Powder (OTC)** *Spray pwdr:* 2% (90 g; alcohol 10%)
> **Monistat-Derm®** *Crm:* 2% (1, 3 oz); *Spray liq:* 2% (3.5 oz); *Spray pwdr:* 2% (3 oz)

Tinea Pedis

▶*naftifine* (**B**)
  Pediatric: not recommended
  Naftin®Cream apply daily x 4 weeks
    Crm: 1% (15, 30, 60 g)
  Naftin®Gel apply bid x 4 weeks
    Gel: 1% (20, 40, 60 g)
▶*oxiconazole nitrate* (**B**) apply daily-bid x 4 weeks
  Pediatric: same as adult
  Oxistat® *Crm:* 1% (15, 30, 60 g); *Lotn:* 1% (30 ml)
▶*sertaconazole* (**C**) apply daily-bid x 4 weeks
  Pediatric: <12 years: not recommended
  Ertaczo® *Crm:* 2% (15, 30 g)
▶*sulconazole* (**C**) apply daily-bid x 4 weeks
  Pediatric: not recommended
  Exelderm® *Crm:* 1% (15, 30, 60 g); *Lotn:* 1% (30 mg)
▶*terbinafine* (**B**)(**G**)
  Pediatric: <12 years: not recommended
  Lamisil®Cream (OTC) apply bid x 1-4 weeks
    Crm: 1% (15, 30 g)
  Lamisil®AT Cream (OTC) apply to affected and surrounding area daily-bid x 1-4 weeks until significantly improved
    Crm: 1% (15, 30 g)
  Lamisil®Solution (OTC) apply to affected and surrounding area bid x 1 week
    Soln: 1% (30 ml spray bottle)
▶*tolnaftate* (**C**)(**OTC**)(**G**) apply sparingly bid x 2-4 weeks
  Pediatric: <2 years: not recommended
       >2 years: same as adult
  Tinactin® *Crm:* 1% (15, 30 g); *Pwdr:* 1% (45, 90 g); *Soln:* 1% (10 ml); *Aerosol liq:* 1% (4 oz); *Aerosol pwdr:* 1% (3.5, 5 oz)

Topical Anti-fungal/Anti-inflammatory Combinations
▶*clotrimazole/betamethasone* (**C**) apply bid x 4 weeks; max 4 weeks
  Pediatric: <12 years: not recommended
  Lotrisone® *Crm:* clotrim 10 mg/beta 0.5 mg (15, 45 g); *Lotn:* clotrim 10 mg/beta 0.5 mg (30 ml)

Systemic Anti-fungals
▶*griseofulvin, microsize* (**C**)(**G**) 1 g daily x 4-8 weeks
  Pediatric: see page 592 for dose by weight
       <30 lb: 5 mg/lb/day
       30-50 lb: 125-250 mg/day

Tinea Pedis

>50 lb: 250-500 mg/day
5 mg/lb/day x 4-6 weeks or longer

Grifulvin®V *Tab:* 250, 500 mg; *Oral susp:* 125 mg/5 ml (120 ml); alcohol 0.02%)

▶*griseofulvin, ultramicrosize* **(C)** 750 mg/day in 1 or more doses x 4-6 weeks

Pediatric: <2 years: not recommended
>2 years: 3.3 mg/lb/day in 1 or more doses

Fulvicin®P/G *Tab:* 125, 165, 250, 330 mg
Grisactin® *Tab:* 250, 330 mg
Grisactin®Ultra *Cap:* 250 mg
Gris-PEG® *Tab:* 125, 250

Comment: Griseofulvin should be taken with fatty foods (e.g., milk, ice cream). Liver enzymes should be monitored.

▶*ketoconazole* **(C)** initially 200 mg daily; max 400 mg/day x 4 weeks

Pediatric: <2 years: not recommended
>2 years: 3.3-6.6 mg/kg daily x 4 weeks

Nizoral® *Tab:* 200 mg

Tinea Versicolor

Comment: Resolution may take 3-6 months.

Topical Anti-fungals

▶*butenafine* **(G)** apply daily x 2 weeks

Pediatric: <12 years: not recommended

Lotrimin®Ultra (C)(OTC) *Crm:* 1% (12, 24 g)
Mentax® **(B)** *Crm:* 1% (15, 30 g)

Comment: Butenafine is a benzylamine, not an "azole." Fungicidal activity continues for at least 5 weeks after last application.

▶*ciclopirox* **(B)**

Loprox®Cream apply bid; max 4 weeks

Pediatric: <10 years: not recommended
>10 years: same as adult

Crm: 0.77% (15, 30, 90 g)

Loprox®Lotion apply bid; max 4 weeks

Pediatric: <10 years: not recommended
>10 years: same as adult

Lotn: 0.77% (30, 60 ml)

Loprox®Gel apply bid; max 4 weeks

Pediatric: <16 years: not recommended

Tinea Versicolor

>16 years: same as adult
    Gel: 0.77% (30, 45 g)
▶ *clotrimazole* **(B)(G)** apply bid x 7 days
    Pediatric: same as adult
  Fungoid® *Crm:* 1% (45 g); *Soln:* 1% (1 oz w. dropper)
  Lotrimin® *Crm:* 1% (15, 30, 45 g)
  Lotrimin®**AF (OTC)** *Crm:* 1% (12 g); *Lotn:* 1% (10 ml); *Soln:* 1% (10 ml)
▶ *econazole* **(C)** apply daily x 2 weeks
    Pediatric: same as adult
  Spectazole® *Crm:* 1% (15, 30, 85 g)
▶ *miconazole* 2% **(C)(G)** apply daily x 2 weeks
    Pediatric: same as adult
  Lotrimin®**AF Spray Liquid (OTC)** *Spray liq:* 2% (113 g; alcohol 17%)
  Lotrimin®**AF Spray Powder (OTC)** *Spray pwdr:* 2% (90 g; alcohol 10%)
  Monistat-Derm® *Crm:* 2% (1, 3 oz); *Spray liq:* 2% (3.5 oz); *Spray pwdr:* 2% (3 oz)
▶ *ketoconazole* **(C)(G)**
    Pediatric: not recommended
  Nizoral®**Cream** apply daily x 2 weeks
    Crm: 2% (15, 30, 60 g)
  Nizoral®**Shampoo** lather into area and leave on 5 minutes x 1 application
    Shampoo: 2% (4 oz)
▶ *oxiconazole nitrate* **(B)** apply daily x 2 weeks
    Pediatric: same as adult
  Oxistat® *Crm:* 1% (15, 30, 60 g); *Lotn:* 1% (30 ml)
▶ *selenium sulfide* lotion **(C)(G)** apply daily-tid and allow to dry for 10 minutes, then rinse; repeat daily x 7 days
    Pediatric: not recommended
  Selsun®**Rx** *Lotn:* 2.5% (4 oz)
▶ *selenium sulfide* shampoo **(C)(G)** apply after shower, allow to dry, leave on overnight, then scrub off vigorously in AM; repeat in 1 week and again q 3 months until resolution occurs
    Pediatric: same as adult
  Selsun®**Shampoo** *Shampoo:* 1% (120, 210, 240, 330 ml); 2.5% (120 ml)
▶ *sulconazole* **(C)** apply daily-bid x 3 weeks

Tinea Versicolor

    Pediatric: not recommended
  Exelderm® *Crm:* 1% (15, 30, 60 g); *Lotn:* 1% (30 mg)
▶*terbinafine* **(B)** apply bid to affected and surrounding area x 1 week
    Pediatric: <12 years: not recommended
  Lamisil®Solution (OTC) *Soln:* 1% (30 ml spray bottle)

Oral Anti-fungals
▶*ketoconazole* **(C)** initially 200 mg daily; max 400 mg/day x 4 weeks
    Pediatric: <2 years: not recommended
        >2 years: 3.3-6.6 mg/kg daily x 4 weeks
  Nizoral® *Tab:* 200 mg

Tobacco Dependence
Nicotine Withdrawal Syndrome

Non-nicotine Products
Alpha$_4$-beta$_2$ nicotinic acetylcholine receptor partial agonist
▶*varenicline* **(C)**
    Pediatric: <18 years: not recommended
  Chantix® set target quit date; begin therapy 1 week prior to target quit date; take after eating with a full glass of water; initially 0.5 mg once daily for 3 days; then, 0.5 mg bid x 4 days; then 1 mg bid; treat x 12 weeks; may continue treatment for 12 more weeks
    Tab: 0.5, 1 mg
    Starting Month Pak: 0.5 mg x 11 tabs + 1 mg x 42 tabs
    Continuing Month Pak: 1 mg x 56 tabs

Aminoketones
▶*bupropion* **(B)(G)**
    Pediatric: <18 years: not recommended
  Wellbutrin® initially 100 mg bid for at least 3 days; may Increase to 375 or 400 mg/day after several weeks; then after at least 3 more days, 450 mg in 4 doses; max 450 mg/day, 150 mg/single dose
    Tab: 75, 100 mg
  Wellbutrin®SR initially 150 mg in AM for at least 3 days; increase to 150 mg bid if well tolerated; usual dose 300 mg/day; max 400 mg/day
    Tab: 100, 150 mg sust-rel
  Wellbutrin®XL initially 150 mg in AM for at least 3 days; increase to 150 mg bid if well tolerated; usual dose 300 mg/day; max 400 mg/day

Tobacco Dependence

    Tab: 150, 300 mg sust-rel

  Zyban® 150 mg daily x 3 days, then 150 mg bid x 7-12 weeks; max 300 mg/day

    Pediatric: <18 years: not recommended

    Tab: 150 mg sust-rel

Comment: Contraindications to *bupropion* include seizure disorder, eating disorder, concurrent MAOI and alcohol use. Smoking should be discontinued after the 7th day of therapy with *bupropion*. Avoid bedtime dose.

Transdermal Nicotine Systems (D)

  Habitrol® (OTC) initially one 21 mg/24 hour patch/day x 4-6 weeks, then one 14 mg/24 hour patch/day x 2-4 weeks, then one 7 mg/24 hour patch/day x 2-4 weeks, then discontinue

    Pediatric: not recommended

    Transdermal patch: 7, 14, 21 mg/24 hour

  Nicoderm®CQ (OTC) initially one 21 mg/24 hour patch/day x 6 weeks, then one 14 mg/24 hour patch/day x 2 weeks, then one 7 mg/24 hour patch/day x 2 weeks

    Pediatric: not recommended

    Transdermal patch: 7, 14, 21 mg/24 hour

Comment: **Nicoderm®CQ** is available as a clear patch.

  Nicotrol®Step-down Patch (OTC) 1 patch/day x 6 weeks

    Pediatric: not recommended

    Transdermal patch: 5, 10, 15 mg/16 hour (7/pck)

  Nicotrol®Transdermal (OTC) 1 patch/day x 6 weeks

    Pediatric: not recommended

    Transdermal patch: 15 mg/16 hour (7/pck)

  Prostep® initially one 22 mg/24 hour patch/day x 4-8 weeks, then discontinue, or one 11 mg/24 hour patch/day x 2-4 additional weeks

    Pediatric: not recommended

    Transdermal patch: 11, 22 mg/24 hour (7/pck)

Nicotine Gum

▶*nicotine polacrilex* **(D)** chew one piece of gum slowly and intermittently over 30 minutes q 1-2 hours x 6 weeks then q 2-4 hours x 3 weeks then q 4-8 hours x 3 weeks; max 24 pieces/day; 2 mg if smoked <25 cigarettes/day; 4 mg if smoked >24 cigarettes/day.

    Pediatric: not recommended

  Nicorette® (OTC) *Gum squares:* 2, 4 mg (108 piece starter kit and 48 piece refill) (orange, mint, or original, sugar-free)

Tobacco Dependence

Nicotine Lozenge
▶*nicotine polacrilex* **(D)** dissolve over 20-30 minutes; minimize swallowing; do not eat or drink for 15 min before and during use
    Use 2 mg lozenge if first cigarette smoked >30 minutes after waking
    Use 4 mg lozenge if first cigarette smoked within 30 min of waking
    1 lozenge q 1-2 hours (at lest 9/day) x 6 weeks; then q 2-4 hours x 3 weeks; then q 4-8 hours x 3 weeks; then stop; max 5 lozenges/6 hours and 20 lozenges/day
    Pediatric: <18 years: not recommended
  Commit®Lozenge (OTC) *Loz:* 2, 4 mg (72/pck; phenylalanine)

Nicotine Inhalation Products
▶*nicotine* 0.5 mg aqueous nasal spray **(D)**
    Pediatric: not recommended
  Nicotrol®NS 1-2 doses/hour nasally; max 5 doses/hour or 40 doses/day; usual max 3 months
    Nasal spray: 0.5 mg/spray; 10 mg/ml (10 ml, 200 doses)

▶*nicotine* 10 mg inhalation system **(D)**
    Pediatric: not recommended
  Nicotrol®Inhaler individualize therapy; at least 6 cartridges/day x 3-6 weeks; max 16 cartridges/day x first 12 weeks, then reduce gradually over 12 more weeks
    Inhaler: 10 mg/cartridge, 4 mg delivered (42 cartridge/pck; menthol)

Comment: **Nicotrol®Inhaler** is a smoking replacement; to be used with decreasing frequency. Smoking should be discontinued before starting therapy. Side effects include cough, nausea, mouth, or throat irritation. This system delivers nicotine, but no tars or carcinogens. Each cartridge lasts about 20 minutes with frequent continuous puffing and provides nicotine equivalent to 2 cigarettes.

Tonsillitis: Acute

▶*amoxicillin* **(B)(G)** 500-875 mg bid or 250-500 mg tid x 10 days
    Pediatric: see page 569 for dose by weight
        <40 kg (88 lb): 20-40 mg/kg/day in 3 doses x 10 days or 25-45 mg/kg/day in 2 doses x 10 days
  Amoxil® *Cap:* 250, 500 mg; *Tab:* 875*mg; *Chew tab:* 125, 200, 250, 400 mg (cherry-banana-peppermint, phenylalanine); *Oral susp:* 125, 250 mg/5 ml (80, 100, 150 ml; strawberry); 200, 400 mg/5 ml (50, 75, 100 ml; bubble gum); *Oral drops:* 50 mg/ml (30 ml; bubble gum)
  Trimox® *Cap:* 250, 500 mg; *Oral susp:* 125 mg/5 ml, 250 mg/5 ml

Tonsillitis:Acute

(80, 100, 150 ml; raspberry-strawberry)

▶ *azithromycin*
(B) 500 mg x 1 dose on day 1, then 250 mg daily on days 2-5 or 500 mg daily x 3 days or **Zmax®** 2 g in a single dose
> *Pediatric: see page 573 for dose by weight*
> 12 mg/kg/day x 5 days; max 500 mg/day

Zithromax® *Tab:* 250, 500 mg; *Oral susp:* 100 mg/5 ml (15 ml); 200 mg/5 ml (15, 22.5, 30 ml) (cherry-vanilla-banana); *Pkt:* 1 g for reconstitution (cherry-banana)
Zithromax®Tri-pak *Tab:* 3-500 mg tabs/pck
Zithromax®Z-pak *Tab:* 6-250 mg tabs/pck
Zmax® *Oral susp:* 2 g ext rel (cherry-banana)

▶ *cefaclor* **(B)(G)**
Ceclor® 250 mg tid or 375 mg bid x 10 days
> *Pediatric: see page 575 for dose by weight*
> 20-40 mg/kg/day in 3 doses x 10 days
> *Pulvule:* 250, 500 mg; *Oral susp:* 125, 250 mg/5 ml (75, 150 ml); 187, 375 mg/5 ml (50, 100 ml) (strawberry)

Ceclor®CD 500 mg q 12 hours x 10 days
> *Pediatric:* <16 years: not recommended
> *Tab:* 375, 500 mg ext-rel

Ceclor®CDpak 500 mg q 12 hours x 10 days
> *Pediatric:* <16 years: not recommended
> *Tab:* 500 mg (14 tabs/CDpak)

Raniclor® 500 mg q 12 hours x 10 days
> *Pediatric:* 20-40 mg/kg/day in 3 doses x 10 days
> *Chew tab:* 125, 187, 250, 375 mg

▶ *cefadroxil* **(B)** 1 g in 1-2 doses x 10 days
> *Pediatric: see page 576 for dose by weight*
> 30 mg/kg/day in 2 doses x 10 days

Duricef® *Cap:* 500 mg; *Tab:* 1 g; *Oral susp:* 250 mg/5 ml (100 ml); 500 mg/5 ml (75, 100 ml) (orange-pineapple)

▶ *cefdinir* **(B)** 300 mg bid x 5-10 days or 600 mg daily x 10 days
> *Pediatric: see page 574 for dose by weight*
> <6 months: not recommended
> 6 months-12 years: 14 mg/kg/day in 1-2 doses x 10 days

Omnicef® *Cap:* 300 mg; *Oral susp:* 125 mg/5 ml (60, 100 ml) (strawberry)

▶ *cefditoren pivoxil* **(B)** 200 mg bid x 10 days
> *Pediatric:* <12 years: not recommended

Tonsillitis: Acute

Spectracef® *Tab:* 200 mg
Comment: Contraindicated with milk protein allergy or carnitine deficiency.
▶ *ceftibuten* **(B)** 200 mg daily x 10 days
> *Pediatric: see page 579 for dose by weight*
>> 9 mg/kg daily x 10 days; max 400 mg/day

Cedax® *Cap:* 400 mg; *Oral susp:* 90 mg/5 ml (30, 60, 90, 120 ml); 180 mg/5 ml (30, 60, 120 ml) (cherry)

▶ *cefixime* **(B)** 400 mg daily x 10 days
> *Pediatric: see page 577 for dose by weight*
>> <6 months: not recommended
>> 6 months-12 years, <50 kg: 8 mg/kg/day in 1-2 doses x 10 days
>> >12 years, >50 kg: same as adult

Suprax®Oral Suspension *Oral susp:* 100 mg/5 ml (50, 75, 100 ml; strawberry)

▶ *cefpodoxime proxetil* **(B)** 200 mg bid x 5-7 days
> *Pediatric: see page 578 for dose by weight*
>> <2 months: not recommended
>> 2 months-12 years: 10 mg/kg/day (max 400 mg/dose) or 5 mg/kg/day bid (max 200 mg/dose) x 5-7 days

Vantin® *Tab:* 100, 200 mg; *Oral susp:* 50, 100 mg/5 ml (50, 75, 100 mg; lemon-creme)

▶ *cefprozil* **(B)** 500 mg daily x 10 days
> *Pediatric: see page 579 for dose by weight*
>> 2-12 years: 7.5 mg/kg bid x 10 days

Cefzil® *Tab:* 250, 500 mg; *Oral susp:* 125, 250 mg/5 ml (50, 75, 100 ml; bubble gum, phenylalanine)

▶ *cephalexin* **(B)(G)** 250 mg tid x 10 days
> *Pediatric: see page 582 for dose by weight*
>> 25-50 mg/kg/day in 4 doses x 10 days

Keflex® *Cap:* 250, 500, 750 mg; *Oral susp:* 125, 250 mg/5 ml (100, 200 ml)
Keftab® *Tab:* 500 mg
Keftab®K-pak *Tab:* 20-500 mg tabs/K-pak

▶ *clarithromycin* **(C)(G)** 250 mg bid or 500 mg ext-rel daily x 10 days
> *Pediatric: see page 584 for dose by weight*
>> <6 months: not recommended
>> >6 months: 7.5 mg/kg bid x 10 days

Biaxin® *Tab:* 250, 500 mg
Biaxin®Oral Suspension *Oral susp:* 125, 250 mg/5 ml (50, 100 ml); fruit-punch)
Biaxin®XL *Tab:* 500 mg ext-rel
▶ *dirithromycin* **(C)** 500 mg daily x 10 days
    Pediatric: <12 years: not recommended
    Dynabac® *Tab:* 250 mg
▶ *erythromycin base* **(B)(G)** 300-400 mg tid x 10 days
    Pediatric: see page 588 for dose by weight
        30-50 mg/kg/day in 2-4 doses x 10 days
    E-Mycin® *Tab:* 250 mg; 333 mg ent-coat
    Eryc® *Cap:* 250 mg ent-coat
    Ery-Tab® *Tab:* 250, 333, 500 mg ent-coat
    PCE® *Tab:* 333, 500 mg
▶ *loracarbef* **(B)** 200 mg bid x 10 days
    Pediatric: see page 593 for dose by weight
        15 mg/kg/day in 2 doses x 10 days
    Lorabid® *Pulvule:* 200, 400 mg; *Oral susp:* 100 mg/5 ml (50, 100 ml); 200 mg/5 ml (50, 75, 100 ml); (strawberry bubble gum)
▶ *penicillin v* **(B)(G)** 250 mg tid x 10 days
    Pediatric: see page 594 for dose by weight
        25-50 mg/kg day in 4 doses x 10 days
        >12 years: same as adult
    Pen-Vee®K *Tab:* 250, 500 mg; *Oral soln:* 125 mg/5 ml (100, 200 ml); 250 mg/5 ml (100, 150, 200 ml)
    Veetids® *Tab:* 250, 500 mg; *Oral soln:* 125, 250 mg/5 ml (100, 200 ml)

Trichinosis

Anthelmintics
▶ *albendazole* **(C)** 400 mg as bid x 15 days; take after a meal
    Pediatric: <2 years: 200 mg daily x 3 days; may repeat in 3 weeks
        2-12 years: 400 mg daily x 3 days; may repeat in 3 weeks
    Albenza® *Tab:* 200 mg
▶ *mebendazole* **(C)(G)** 200-400 mg tid x 3 days, then 400-500 mg tid x 10 days; take wit
    Pediatric: same as adult (chew or crush and mix with food)

Trichinosis

Vermox® *Chew tab:* 100 mg
▶*pyrantel pamoate* **(C)** 11 mg/kg x 1 dose; max 1 g/dose; take after a meal

    Pediatric: 25-37 lb: 1/2 tsp x 1 dose
              38-62 lb: 1 tsp x 1 dose
              63-87 lb: 1½ tsp x 1 dose
              88-112 lb: 2 tsp x 1 dose
              113-137 lb: 2½ tsp x 1 dose
              138-162 lb: 3 tsp x 1 dose
              163-187 lb: 3½ tsp x 1 dose
              >187 lb: 4 tsp x 1 dose

    Antiminth® **(OTC)** *Cap:* 180 mg; *Liq:* 50 mg/ml (30 ml); 144 mg/ml (30 ml); *Oral susp:* 50 mg/ml (60 ml)
    Pin-X® **(OTC)** *Cap:* 180 mg; *Liq:* 50 mg/ml (30 ml); 144 mg/ml (30 ml); *Oral susp:* 50 mg/ml (30 ml)

▶*thiabendazole* **(C)** 25 mg/kg bid x 7 days; max 1.5 g/dose; take after a meal

    Pediatric: same as adult
              <30 lb: consult mfr literature
              >30 lb 2 doses/day with meals
              30-50 lbs: 250 mg bid with meals
              >50 lb: 10 mg/lb/dose bid with meals; max 3g/day

    Mintezol® *Chew tab:* 500*mg (orange); *Oral susp:* 500 mg/5 ml (120 ml; orange)

Comment: Thiabendazole is not for prophylaxis.

Trichomoniasis (*Trichomonas vaginalis*)

Comment: Treat all sexual contacts.

Primary Therapy
▶*metronidazole* **(not for use in 1st; B in 2nd, 3rd)(G)** 1 g bid x 1 day or 2 g x 1 dose

    Pediatric: not recommended
    Flagyl®375 *Cap:* 375 mg
    Flagyl®ER *Tab:* 750 mg ext-rel
    Flagyl®, Protostat® *Tab:* 250*, 500*mg

Comment: Alcohol is contraindicated during treatment with oral *metronidazole* and for 72 hours after therapy due to a possible *disulfiram*-like reaction (nausea, vomiting, flushing, headache).

▶*tinidazole* **(not for use in 1st; B in 2nd, 3rd)** 2 g in a single dose; take with food
> *Pediatric:* <3 years: not recommended
> >3 years: 50 mg/kg in a single dose; take with food; max 2 g

Tindamax® *Tab:* 250*, 500*mg

Alternative Therapy

▶*metronidazole* **(not for use in 1st; B in 2nd, 3rd)(G)** 250 mg tid or 500 mg bid x 7 days

Flagyl®**375** *Cap:* 375 mg
Flagyl®**ER** *Tab:* 750 mg ext-rel
Flagyl®, **Protostat**® *Tab:* 250*, 500*mg

Comment: Oral *metronidazole* is contraindicated in the 1st trimester of pregnancy. Alcohol is contraindicated during treatment with oral *metronidazole* and for 72 hours after therapy due to a possible *disulfiram*-like reaction (nausea, vomiting, flushing, headache). For treatment failures, retreat with *metronidazole* 500 mg x 7 days. For repeated failure, treat with *metronidazole* 2 g in a single dose x 3-5 days.

Trigeminal Neuralgia (Tic Douloureux)

▶*baclofen* **(C)(G)** initially 5-10 mg tid with food; usual dose 10-80 mg/day

Atrofen® *Tab:* 10, 20 mg

▶*carbamazepine* **(C)**

Carbatrol® initially 200 mg bid; may increase weekly as needed by 200 mg/day; usual maintenance 800 mg-1.2 g/day
> *Pediatric:* <12 years: max <35 mg/kg/day; use extended-release form above 400 mg/day
> 12-15 years: max 1 g/day in 2 doses
> >15 years: usual maintenance 1.2 g/day in 2 doses

Cap: 200, 300 mg ext-rel

Tegretol® initially 100 mg bid or 1/2 tsp susp qid; may increase dose by 100 mg q 12 hours or by 1/2 tsp susp q 6 hours; usual maintenance 400-800 mg/day; max 1200 mg/day
> *Pediatric:* <6 years: initially 10-20 mg/kg/day in 2 divided doses; increase weekly as needed in 3-4 divided doses; max 35 mg/kg/day in 3-4 divided doses
> >6 years: initially 100 mg bid; increase weekly as needed by 100 mg/day in 3-4 divided doses; max 1 g/day in 3-4 divided doses

Trigeminal Neuralgia

>   *Tab:* 200*mg; *Chew tab:* 100*mg; *Oral susp:* 100 mg/5 ml
>   (450 ml; citrus-vanilla)
>
>   **Tegretol®XR** initially 200 mg bid; may increase weekly by
>   200 mg/day in 2 doses
>
>   >   *Pediatric:* <6 years: use other forms
>   >   >6 years: initially 100 mg bid; may increase weekly
>   >   by 100 mg/day in 2 doses; max 1 g/day
>
>   *Tab:* 100, 200, 400 mg ext-rel

▶*clonazepam* **(D)(IV)(G)** initially 0.25 mg bid; increase to 1 mg/day
after 3 days

>   *Pediatric:* <10 years, <30 kg: initially 0.1-0.3 mg/kg/day; may
>   increase up to 0.05 mg/kg/day bid-tid; usual
>   maintenance 0.1-0.2 mg/kg/day tid
>
>   **Klonopin®** *Tab:* 0.5*, 1, 2 mg
>
>   **Klonopin®Wafers** dissolve in mouth with or without water
>
>   *Wafer:* 0.125, 0.25, 0.5, 1, 2 mg orally-disintegrating

▶*divalproex sodium* **(D)** initially 250 mg bid; gradually increase to
max of 1000 mg/day if needed

>   *Pediatric:* <10 years: not recommended
>   >10 years: same as adult
>
>   **Depakene®** *Cap:* 250 mg; *Syr:* 250 mg/5 ml
>   **Depakote®** *Tab:* 125, 250 mg
>   **Depakote®ER** *Tab:* 250, 500 mg ext-rel
>   **Depakote®Sprinkle** *Cap:* 125 mg

▶*phenytoin* **(D)** 400 mg/day in divided doses

>   **Dilantin®** *Cap:* 30, 100 mg; *Oral susp:* 125 mg/5 ml (8 oz);
>   *Infatab:* 50 mg

Comment: Monitor *phenytoin* serum levels. Therapeutic serum level: 10-20
g/ml. Side effects include gingival hyperplasia.

▶*valproic acid* **(D)** initially 15 mg/kg/day; may increase weekly by
5-10 mg/kg/day; max 60 mg/kg/day or 250 mg/day

>   **Depakene®** *Cap:* 250 mg; *Syr:* 250 mg/5 ml

Tuberculosis (TB)

Screening

▶*purified protein derivative (PPD)* **(C)** 0.1 ml intradermally; examine
inoculation site for induration at 48 to 72 hours.

>   *Pediatric:* same as adult

Aplisol®, **Tubersol®** *Soln:* 5 US units/0.1 ml (1, 5 ml)

Anti-tubercular Agents

Comment: Avoid *streptomycin* in pregnancy. *Pyridoxine* (vitamin B-6) 25 mg daily x 6 months should be administered concomitantly with *INH* for prevention of side effects. *Rifampin* and *rifapentine* produce red-orange discoloration of body tissues and body fluids and may stain contact lenses.

▶*ethambutol (EMB)* **(B)(G)**
   Myambutol® *Tab:* 100, 400*mg
▶*isoniazid (INH)* **(C)** *Tab:* 300*mg
▶*pyrazinamide (PZA)* **(C)** *Tab:* 500*mg
▶*rifampin (RIF)* **(C)(G)**
   Rifadin®, **Rimactane®** *Cap:* 150, 300 mg
▶*rifapentine* **(C)**
   Priftin® *Tab:* 150 mg
▶*streptomycin (SM)* **(C)(G)** *Amp:* 1 g/2.5 ml or 400 mg/ml (2.5 ml)

Combination Products

▶*rifampin/isoniazid* **(C)**
   Rifamate® *Cap: rif* 300 mg/*iso* 150 mg
▶*rifampin/isoniazid/pyrazinamide* **(C)**
   Rifater® *Tab: rif* 120 mg/*iso* 50 mg/*pyr* 300 mg

Prophylaxis after exposure to tuberculosis, with negative PPD

▶*isoniazid* **(C)** 300 mg daily in a single dose x at least 6 months
   Pediatric: 10-20 mg/kg/day x 9 months

Prophylaxis after exposure, with new PPD conversion

▶*isoniazid* **(C)** 300 mg daily in a single dose x 12 months
   Pediatric: 10-20 mg/kg/day x 9 months
   Tab: 100, 300*mg; *Syr:* 50 mg/5 ml; *Inj:* 100 mg/ml
▶*rifampin* **(C)** 600 mg daily + isoniazid 300 mg daily **(C)** x 4 months
   Pediatric: rifampin 10-20 mg/kg + *isoniazid* 10-20 mg/kg daily
   x 4 months

Adult Treatment Options

Option 1

▶*rifampin* 600 mg + *isoniazid* 300 mg + *pyrazinamide* 2 g + *ethambutol* 15-25 mg/kg or *streptomycin* 1 g daily x 8 weeks; then *isoniazid* 300 mg + *rifampin* 600 mg daily x 16 weeks, or *isoniazid* 900 mg + *rifampin* 600 mg 2-3 times/week x 16 weeks

Option 2

▶*rifampin* 600 mg + *isoniazid* 300 mg + *pyrazinamide* 2 g + *ethambutol* 15-25 mg/kg or *streptomycin* 1 g daily x 2 weeks; then *rifampin* 600 mg + *isoniazid* 900 mg + *pyrazinamide* 4 g + *ethambutol* 50 mg/kg or *streptomycin* 1.5 g 2 times/week x 6 weeks;

TB

then *isoniazid* 300 mg + *rifampin* 600 mg daily x 16 weeks, or 2 times/week x 16 weeks

Option 3
▶ *rifampin* 600 mg + *isoniazid* 900 mg + *pyrazinamide* 3 g + *ethambutol* 25-30 mg/kg or *streptomycin* 1.5 g 3 times/week x 6 months

Option 4 (for smear and culture negative pulmonary TB in adult)
▶ Options 1, 2, or 3 x 8 weeks; then *isoniazid* 300 mg + *rifampin* 600 mg for daily x 16 weeks; then *rifampin* 600 mg + *isoniazid* 300 mg + *pyrazinamide* 2 g + *ethambutol* 15-25 mg/kg or *streptomycin* 1 g daily x 8 weeks, or 2-3 times/week x 8 weeks

Option 5 (when pyrazinamide is contraindicated)
▶ *rifampin* 600 mg + *isoniazid* 300 mg + *ethambutol* 15-25 mg/kg + *streptomycin* 1 g daily x 4-8 weeks; then *isoniazid* 300 mg + *rifampin* 600 mg daily x 24 weeks, or 2 times/week x 24 weeks

Pediatric Treatment Options
Option 1
▶ *rifampin* 10-20 mg/kg + *isoniazid* 10-20 mg/kg + *pyrazinamide* 15-20 mg/kg + *ethambutol* 15-25 mg/kg or *streptomycin* 20-40 mg/kg daily x 8 weeks; then *isoniazid* 10-20 mg/kg + *rifampin* 10-20 mg/kg daily x 16 weeks, or *isoniazid* 20-40 mg/kg + *rifampin* 10-20 mg/kg 2-3 times/ week x 16 weeks

Option 2
▶ *rifampin* 10-20 mg/kg + *isoniazid* 10-20 mg/kg + *pyrazinamide* 15-30 mg/kg + *ethambutol* 15-25 mg/kg or *streptomycin* 20-40 mg/kg daily x 2 weeks; then *rifampin* 10-20 mg/kg + *isoniazid* 20-40 mg/kg + *pyrazinamide* 50-70 mg/kg + *ethambutol* 50 mg/kg or *streptomycin* 25-30 mg/kg 2 times/week x 6 weeks; then *isoniazid* 10-20 mg/kg + *rifampin* 10-20 mg/kg daily x 16 weeks, or *rifampin* 10-20 mg/kg + *isoniazid* 20-40 mg/kg 2 times/week x 16 weeks

Option 3
▶ *rifampin* 10-20 mg/kg + *isoniazid* 20-40 mg/kg + *pyrazinamide* 50-70 mg/kg + *ethambutol* 25-30 mg/kg or *streptomycin* 25-30 mg/kg 3 times/week x 6 months

Option 4 (when pyrazinamide is contraindicated)
▶ *rifampin* 10-20 mg/kg + *isoniazid* 10-20 mg/kg + *ethambutol* 15-25 mg/kg + *streptomycin* 20-40 mg/kg daily x 4-8 weeks; then *isoniazid* 10-20 mg/kg + *rifampin* 10-20 mg/kg daily x 24 weeks, or *rifampin* 10-20 mg/kg + *isoniazid* 20-40 mg/kg 2 times/week x 24 weeks

Type 1 Diabetes Mellitus

Comment: Target glycosolated hemoglobin (HbA_{1c}) is <7%. Addition of daily ACE-I and/or ARB therapy is strongly recommended for renal protection.

Insulins

Rapid-Acting Insulins

▶*insulin aspart* **(C)** onset <15 minutes; peak 1-3 hours; duration 3-5 hours; administer 5-10 minutes prior to a meal; SC only
> *Pediatric:* <3 years: not recommended
> >3 years: same as adult

NovoLog® *Vial:* 100 U/ml (10 ml); *PenFill cartridge:* 100 U/ml (3 ml, 5/pk)

▶*insulin glulisine* **(B)** *(rDNA origin)* onset <15 minutes; peak 1 hour; duration 2-4 hours; administer up to 15 minutes before, or within 20 minutes after starting a meal; SC only; may administer via insulin pump; *do not* dilute or mix with other insulins in pump
> *Pediatric:* not recommended

Apidra® *Vial:* 100 U/ml (10 ml); *Cartridge:* 100 U/ml (3 ml, 5/pck; m-cresol)

▶*insulin human* **(B)** *(rDNA origin)* onset $\leq$10-20 minutes; peak 2 hours; duration 6 hours; administer $\leq$10 minutes before meals; initially 0.05 mg/kg by oral inhalation per premeal dose (round down to nearest mg); 1 mg blister approx = 3 IU SC regular insulin; 3 blisters approx = 8 IU SC regular insulin; use fewest number of blisters per dose
> *Pediatric: <18 years:* not recommended

Exubera® *Blisters:* 1, 3 mg/blister dry pwdr for oral inhal (90, w/ 2 release units); Combination pack 90 x 1 mg + 90 x 3 mg w/ 2 release units)

Comment: Use **Exubera®** with extreme caution with underlying lung diasease (e.g., asthma, COPD); not recommended with baseline FEV_1 <70% predicted.

▶*insulin lispro (human)* **(B)** onset <15 minutes; peak 1 hour; duration 3.5-4.5 hours; administer up to 15 minutes before, or immediately after, a meal; SC only
> *Pediatric:* <3 years: not recommended
> >3 years: same as adult

Humalog® *Vial:* 100 U/ml (10 ml); *Cartridge:* 100 U/ml (1.5 ml); *Prefilled disposable pen:* 100 U/ml (3 ml, 5/pck)

▶*insulin regular* **(B)**

Humulin®R (OTC) (human) onset 30 minutes; peak 2-4 hours; duration 6-8 hours; SC, IV, or IM

Type I Diabetes Mellitus

> *Vial:* 100 U/ml (10 ml)

Humulin®R U-500 (human) onset 30-60 minutes; peak 3-4 hours; duration up to 24 hours; SC only; for in-hospital use only
> *Vial:* 500 U/ml (20 ml)

Iletin®II Regular (OTC) (pork) onset 30 minutes; peak 2-4 hours; duration 6-8 hours; SC, IV or IM
> *Vial:* 100 U/ml (10 ml)

Novolin®R (OTC) (human) onset 30 minutes; peak 2.5-5 hours; duration 8 hours; SC, IV, or IM
> *Vial:* 100 U/ml (10 ml); *PenFill cartridge:* 100 U/ml (1.5 ml, 5/pck); *Prefilled syringe:* 100 U/ml (1.5 ml, 5/pck)

▶*pramlintide* **(C)** (amylin analogue/amilynomimetic) administer immediately before major meals (≥250 kcal or ≥30 g carbohydrates); Initially 15 mcg; titrate in 15 mcg increments for 3 days if no significant nausea occurs; if nausea occurs at 45 or 60 mcg, reduce to 30 mcg; if not tolerated, consider discontinuing therapy Maintenance: 60 mcg (30 mcg *only* if 60 mcg not tolerated
Symlin® *Vial:* 0.6 mg/ml (5 ml; cresol, mannitol)

Comment: **Symlin®** is indicated as adjunct to mealtime insulin with or without a sulfonylurea and/or metformin when blood glucose control is sub-optimal despite optimal insulin therapy. *Do not* mix with insulin. When initiating **Symlin®**, reduce preprandial short/rapid-acting insulin dose by 50% and monitor pre- and post-prandial and bedtime blood glucose. *Do not* use in patients with poor compliance, HbA1c is >9%, recurrent hypoglycemia requiring assistance in the previous 6 months, or if taking a prokinetic drug. With Type 2 DM, initial therapy is 60 mcg/dose and max is 120 mcg/dose.

Rapid-Acting and Intermediate-Acting Insulin
Insulin Aspart Protamine Suspension/Insulin Aspart Combinations
▶*insulin aspart protamine suspension 70%/insulin aspart 30%* **(B)**
NovoLog®Mix 70/30 (OTC) (human) onset 15 min; peak 1-4 hours; duration up to 24 hours; SC only
> *Vial:* 100 U/ml (10 ml)

NovoLog®Mix 70/30 FlexPen (OTC) *FlexPen prefilled disposable pen:* 100 U/ml (3 ml, 5/pck); *PenFill cartridge:* 100 U/ml (3 ml, 5/pck)

Long-Acting Insulins
▶*insulin detemir* **(C)** (human) onset 1 hour; no peak; duration 24 hours; SC only
> *Pediatric:* <6 years: not recommended

Levemir® initially 0.1-0.2 units/kg once daily in the evening or 10 units 1-2 times daily

Type I Diabetes Mellitus

Vial: 100 U/ml (10 ml); *FlexPen:* 100 U/ml (3 ml, 5/pck; m-cresol)

▶ *insulin isophane suspension (NPH)* **(B)**

Humulin® **(OTC)** (human) onset 1-2 hours; peak 6-12 hours; duration 18-24 hours; SC only

Vial: 100 U/ml (10 ml); *Prefilled disposable pen:* 100 U/ml (3 ml, 5/pck)

Novolin®N (OTC) (human) onset 1.5 hours; peak 4-12 hours; duration 24 hours; SC only

Vial: 100 U/ml (10 ml); *PenFill cartridge:* 1.5 ml (5/pck); *Prefilled disposable syringe:* 1.5 ml (5/pck)

Iletin®II NPH (OTC) (pork) onset 1-2 hours; peak 6-12 hours; duration 18-26 hours; SC only

Vial: 100 U/ml (10 ml)

▶ *insulin glargine* **(C)** (human) administer daily at HS as basal insulin; initial average starting dose 10 units for insulin-naive patients; when switching from once-daily NPH or ultralente insulin, initial dose of insulin glargine should be on a unit-for-unit basis; when switching from twice-daily NPH insulin, start at 20% lower than the previous total daily NPH dose; SC only

Pediatric: <6 years: not recommended
>6 years: same as adult

Lantus® *Vial:* 100 U/ml (10 ml); *Cartridge:* 100 U/ml (3 ml, for use in the OptiPen One Insulin Delivery Device) (5/box)

▶ *insulin zinc suspension (lente)* **(B)**

Humulin®L (OTC) (human) onset 1-3 hours; peak 6-12 hours; duration 18-24 hours; SC only

Vial: 100 U/ml (10 ml)

Iletin®II Lente (OTC) (pork) onset 1-3 hours; peak 6-12 hours; duration 18-26 hours; SC only

Vial: 100 U/ml (10 ml)

Novolin®L (OTC) (human) onset 2.5 hours; peak 7-15 hours; duration 22 hours; SC only

Vial: 100 U/ml (10 ml)

Ultra long-acting Insulin

▶ *insulin extended zinc suspension (ultralente)* **(B)**

Humulin®U (OTC) (human) onset 4-6 hours; peak 8-20 hours; duration 24-48 hours; SC only

Vial: 100 U/ml (10 ml)

Insulin Lispro Protamine/Insulin Lispro Combinations

Type I Diabetes Mellitus

▶ *insulin lispro protamine 75%/insulin lispro 25%* **(B)**
  Pediatric: <18 years: not recommended
  Humalog®Mix 75/25 (human) onset 15 minutes; peak 30 minutes 1 hour; duration 24 hours; SC only
  Vial: 100 U/ml (10 ml); *Prefilled disposable pen:* 100 U/ml (3 ml 5/pck)

▶ *insulin lispro protamine 50%/insulin lispro 50%* **(B)**
  Pediatric: <18 years: not recommended
  Humalog Mix®50/50 (human) onset 15 minutes; peak 2.3 hours; range 1-5 hours; SC only
  Vial: 100 U/ml (10 ml); *Cartridge:* 100 U/ml (3 ml); *Prefilled disposable pen:* 100 U/ml (3 ml 5/pck)

Insulin Isophane Suspension (NPH)/Insulin Regular Combinations

▶ *NPH 70%/regular 30%* **(B)**
  Pediatric: same as adult
  Humulin®70/30 (OTC) (human) onset 30 minutes; peak 2-12 hours; duration up to 24 hours; SC only
  Vial: 100 U/ml (10 ml)
  Novolin®70/30 (OTC) (human) onset 30 minutes; peak 2-12 hours; duration up to 24 hours; SC only
  Vial: 100 U/ml (10 ml)

▶ *NPH 50%/regular 50%* **(B)**
  Pediatric: same as adult
  Humulin®50/50 (OTC) (human) onset 30 minutes; peak 3-5 hours; duration up to 24 hours; SC only
  Vial: 100 U/ml (10 ml)

Ultra long-acting Insulin

▶ *insulin extended zinc suspension (ultralente)* **(B)**
  Humulin®U (OTC) (human) onset 4-6 hours; peak 8-20 hours; duration 24-48 hours; SC only
  Vial: 100 U/ml (10 ml)

Insulin Lispro Protamine/Insulin Lispro Combinations

▶ *insulin lispro protamine 75%/insulin lispro 25%* **(B)**
  Pediatric: <18 years: not recommended
  Humalog®Mix 75/25 (human) onset 15 minutes; peak 30 minutes-1hour; duration 24 hours; SC only
  Vial: 100 U/ml (10 ml); *Prefilled disposable pen:* 100 U/ml (3 ml, 5/pck)

▶ *insulin lispro protamine 50%/insulin lispro 50%* **(B)**
  Pediatric: <18 years: not recommended
  Humalog®Mix 50/50 (human) onset 15 minutes; peak 2.3 hours;

range 1-5 hours; SC only
Vial: 100 U/ml (10 ml); *Cartridge:* 100 U/ml (3 ml); *Prefilled disposable pen:* 100 U/ml (3 ml 5/pck)

Insulin Isophane Suspension (NPH)/Insulin Regular Combinations
▶ *NPH 70%/regular 30%* **(B)**
Pediatric: same as adult
Humulin®70/30 (OTC) (human) onset 30 minutes; peak 2-12 hours; duration up to 24 hours; SC only
Vial: 100 U/ml (10 ml)
Novolin®70/30 (OTC) (human) onset 30 minutes; peak 2-12 hours; duration up to 24 hours; SC only
Vial: 100 U/ml (10 ml)
▶ *NPH 50%/regular 50%* **(B)**
Pediatric: same as adult
Humulin®50/50 (OTC) (human) onset 30 minutes; peak 3-5 hours; duration up to 24 hours; SC only
Vial: 100 U/ml (10 ml)

Type 2 Diabetes Mellitus

Comment: Normal fasting glucose is <100 mg/dL. Impaired glucose tolerance is a risk factor for type 2 diabetes and a marker for cardiovascular disease risk; it occurs early in the natural history of these two diseases. Impaired fasting glucose is >100 mg/dL and <125 mg/dL. Impaired glucose tolerance is OGTT, 2 hour post-load 75 g glucose >140 mg/dL and <200 mg/dL. Target preprandial glucose is 80 mg/dL to 120 mg/dL. Target bedtime glucose is 100mg/dL to 140 mg/dL. Target glycosolated hemoglobin (HbA1c) is <7.0%. Addition of daily ACE-I and/or ARB therapy is strongly recommended for renal protection. Consider diabetes screening at age 25 years for persons in high-risk groups (non-Caucasian, positive family history for DM, obesity). Hypertension and hyperlipidemia are common co-morbid conditions. Macrovascular complications include cerebral vascular disease, coronary artery disease, and peripheral vascular disease. Microvascular complications include retinopathy, nephropathy, neuropathy, and cardiomyopathy. Oral hypoglycemics are *contraindicated* in pregnancy.

Insulins
see *Type 1 Diabetes Mellitus* page 419
Sulfonylureas
Comment: Sulfonylureas are secretagogues (i.e., stimulate pancreatic insulin secretion); therefore, the patient taking a sulfonylurea should be alerted to the risk for hypoglycemia. Action is dependent on functioning beta cells in the pancreatic islets.

Type 2 Diabetes Mellitus

1st Generation Sulfonylureas

▶*chlorpropamide* **(C)(G)** initially 250 mg/day with breakfast; max 750 mg
    Pediatric: not recommended
  Diabinese® *Tab:* 100*, 250*mg

▶*tolazamide* **(C)(G)** initially 100-250 mg/day with breakfast; increase by 100-250 mg/day at weekly intervals; maintenance 100 mg-1 g/day; max 1 g/day
    Pediatric: not recommended
  Tolinase® *Tab:* 100, 250, 500 mg

▶*tolbutamide* **(C)** initially 1-2 g in divided doses; max 2 g/day
    Pediatric: not recommended
  Orinase® *Tab:* 500 mg

2nd Generation Sulfonylureas

▶*glimepiride* **(C)** initially 1-2 mg daily with breakfast; after reaching dose of 2 mg, increase by 2 mg at 1-2 week intervals as needed; usual maintenance 1-4 mg daily; max 8 mg/day
    Pediatric: not recommended
  Amaryl® *Tab:* 1*, 2*, 4*mg

▶*glipizide* **(C)(G)**
    Pediatric: not recommended
  Glucotrol® initially 5 mg before breakfast; increase by 2.5-5 mg every few days if needed; max 15 mg/day; max 40 mg/day in divided doses
    Tab: 2.5, 5, 10 mg
  Glucotrol®**XL** initially 5 mg with breakfast; usual range 5-10 mg/day; max 20 mg/day
    Tab: 2.5, 5, 10 mg ext-rel

▶*glyburide* **(C)(G)** initially 2.5-5 mg/day with breakfast; increase by 2.5 mg at weekly intervals; maintenance 1.25-20 mg/day in 1-2 doses; max 20 mg/day
    Pediatric: not recommended
  DiaBeta®, **Micronase**® *Tab:* 1.25*, 2.5*, 5*mg

▶*glyburide, micronized* **(B)**
    Pediatric: not recommended
  Glynase®**PresTab** initially 1.5-3 mg/day with breakfast; increase by 1.5 mg at weekly intervals if needed; usual maintenance 0.75-12 mg/day in single or divided doses; max 12 mg/day
    Tab: 1.5*, 3*, 6*mg

Alpha-Glucosidase Inhibitors
Comment: Alpha-glucosidase inhibitors block the enzyme that breaks down carbohydrates in the small intestine, delaying digestion and absorption of complex carbohydrates, and lowering peak post-prandial glycemic concentrations. Use as monotherapy or in combination with a sulfonylurea. Contraindicated in inflammatory bowel disease, colon ulceration, and intestinal obstruction. Side effects include flatulence, diarrhea, and abdominal pain.

▶ *acarbose* **(B)** initially 25 mg tid ac, increase at 4-8 week intervals; or initially 25 mg daily, increase gradually to 25 mg tid; usual range 50-100 mg tid; max 100 mg tid
   Pediatric: not recommended
   Precose® *Tab:* 25, 50, 100 mg

▶ *miglitol* **(B)** initially 25 mg tid at the start of each main meal, titrated to 50 mg tid at the start of each main meal; max 100 mg tid
   Glyset® *Tab:* 25, 50, 100 mg

Biguanide
Comment: The biguanides decrease gluconeogenesis by the liver in the presence of insulin. Action is dependent on the presence of circulating insulin. Lower hepatic glucose production leads to lower overnight, fasting, and pre-prandial plasma glucose levels. Common side effects include GI distress, nausea, vomiting, bloating, and flatulence which usually eventually resolve. Contraindicated with renal impairment. As monotherapy or (in adult only) with a sulfonylurea or insulin.

▶ *metformin* **(B)(G)** take with meals
   Fortamet® initially 1000 mg daily; may increase by 500 mg/day at 1 week intervals; max 2.5 g/day
      Pediatric: <17 years: not recommended
      Tab: 500, 1000 mg ext-rel
   Glucophage® initially 500 mg bid; may increase by 500 mg/day at 1 week intervals; max 1 g bid or 2.5 g in 3 doses; or initially 850 mg daily in AM; may increase by 850 mg/day in divided doses at 2 week intervals; max 850 mg tid
      Pediatric: <10 years: not recommended
                  10-16 years: use only as monotherapy; dose same as adult
      Tab: 500, 850, 1000*mg
   Glumetza® initially 1000 mg once daily; may increase by 500 mg/day at week intervals; max 2 g/day
      Pediatric: <18 years: not recommended
      Tab: 500 mg ext-rel
   Glucophage®XR initially 500 mg bid; may increase by 500

mg/day at 1 week intervals; max 1 g bid
>   *Pediatric:* <10 years: not recommended
>   10-16 years: use immediate release form
>   *Tab:* 500, 750 mg ext-rel
> **Riomet®XR** initially 500 mg bid; may increase by 500 mg/day at 1 week intervals; max 2 g/day in divided doses
>   *Pediatric:* <10 years: not recommended
>   >10 years: monotherapy only
>   *Oral soln:* 500 mg/ml (4 oz; cherry)

Meglitinides

Comment: Sulfonylureas are secretagogues (i.e., stimulate pancreatic insulin secretion) in response to a meal. Action is dependent on functioning beta cells in the pancreatic islets. Use as monotherapy or in combination with *metformin*.

▶ *nateglinide* **(C)** 60-120 mg tid ac 1 to 30 minutes prior to start of the meal
>   *Pediatric:* not recommended
>   **Starlix®** *Tab:* 60, 120 mg

▶ *repaglinide* **(C)** initially 0.5 mg with 2-4 meals/day; take 30 minutes ac; titrate by doubling dose at intervals of at least 1 week; range 0.5-4 mg with 2-4 meals/day; max 16 mg/day
>   *Pediatric:* not recommended
>   **Prandin®** *Tab:* 0.5, 1, 2 mg

Thiazolidinediones

Comment: The "TZDs" decrease hepatic gluconeogenesis and reduce insulin resistance (i.e., increase glucose uptake and utilization by the muscles). Liver function tests are indicated before initiating these drugs. Do not start if ALT more than 3 times greater than normal. Recheck ALT monthly for the first six months of therapy, then every two months for the remainder of the first year and periodically thereafter. Liver function tests should be obtained at the first symptoms suggestive of hepatic dysfunction (nausea, vomiting, fatigue, dark urine, anorexia, abdominal pain).

▶ *pioglitazone* **(C)** initially 15 or 30 mg daily; max 45 mg/day as a monotherapy; usual max 30 mg/day in combination with *metformin*, insulin, or a sulfonylurea
>   *Pediatric:* <18 years: not recommended
>   **Actos®** *Tab:* 15, 30, 45 mg

▶ *rosiglitazone* **(C)** initially 4 mg/day in 1 or 2 divided doses; may increase after 8-12 weeks; max 8 mg/day as a monotherapy or combination therapy with *metformin* or a sulfonylurea
>   *Pediatric:* <18 years: not recommended
>   **Avandia®** *Tab:* 2, 4, 8 mg

2nd Generation Sulfonylurea/Biguanide Combinations
Comment: **Metaglip**® and **Glucovance**® are combination secretagogues (sulfonylureas) and insulin sensitizers (biguanides). Sulfonylurea: Action is dependent on functioning beta cells in the pancreatic islets; patient should be alerted to the risk for hypoglycemia. Biguanide: Common side effects include GI distress, nausea, vomiting, bloating, and flatulence which usually eventually resolve. Take with food. Contraindicated with renal impairment.

▶*glipizide/metformin* **(C)** take with meals
 Pediatric: not recommended
 Primary therapy: 2.5/250 daily or if FBS is 280-320 mg/dl, may start at 2.5/250 bid; may increase by 1 tab/day every 2 weeks; max: 10/2000 per day in 2 divided doses
 Second Line Therapy: 2.5/500 or 5/500 bid; may increase by up to 5/500 every 2 weeks; max: 20/2000 per day
 Same precautions as *glipizide* and *metformin*
 Metaglip®
  Tab: **Metaglip**®**2.5/250**: *glip* 2.5 mg/*met* 250 mg
  Metaglip®**2.5/500**: *glip* 2.5 mg/*met* 500 mg
  Metaglip®**5/500**: *glip* 5 mg/*met* 500 mg

▶*glyburide/metformin* **(B)** take with meals
 Pediatric: not recommended
 Primary therapy (initial therapy if HgbA$_{1c}$ <9.0%): initially 1.25/250 daily; max *glyburide* 20 mg and *metformin* 2000 mg per day.
 Primary therapy (initial therapy if HbA$_{1c}$ >9.0% or FBS >200): initially 1.25/250 bid; max *glyburide* 20 mg and *metformin* 2000 mg per day
 Second line therapy (initial therapy if HbA$_{1c}$ >7.0%): initially 2.5/500 or 5/500 bid; max *glyburide* 20 mg and *metformin* 2000 mg per day
 Previously treated with a sulfonylurea and *metformin*: dose to approximate total daily doses of *glyburide* and *metformin* already being taken
 Max: *glyburide* 20 mg and *metformin* 2000 mg per day
 Same precautions as *glyburide* and *metformin*
 Glucovance®
  Tab: **Glucovance**®**1.25/250**: *glyb* 1.25 mg/*met* 250 mg
  Glucovance®**2.5/500**: *glyb* 2.5 mg/*met* 500 mg
  Glucovance®**5/500**: *glyb* 5 mg/*met* 500 mg

Thiazlidinedione/Biguanide Combination
▶*pioglitazone/metformin* **(C)** take in divided doses with meals
 Pediatric: not recommended

Type 2 Diabetes Mellitus

Previously on *metformin* alone: initially 15mg/500mg or 5mg/850mg once or twice daily

Previously on *pioglitazone* alone: initially 15mg/500mg bid or

Previously on *pioglitazone* and *metformin*: switch on a mg/mg basis; may increase after 8-12 weeks

Max: *pioglitazone* 45 mg and *metformin* 2550 mg per day

Same precautions as *pioglitazone* and *metformin*

Actoplus Met®

Tab: **ActoplusMet® 15/500**: *pio* 15 mg/*met* 500 mg

ActoplusMet® 15/850: *pio* 15 mg/*met* 850 mg

▶*rosiglitazone/metformin* **(C)** take in divided doses with meals

Pediatric: not recommended

Previously on *metformin* alone: add rosiglitazone 4 mg/day; may increase after 8-12 weeks

Previously on *rosiglitazone* alone: add *metformin* 1000 mg/day; may increase after 1-2 weeks

Previously on *rosiglitazone* and *metformin*: switch on a mg/mg basis; may increase *rosiglitazone* by 4 mg and/or *metformin* by 500 mg per day

Max: *rosiglitazone* 8 mg and *metformin* 2000 mg per day

Same precautions as *rosiglitazone* and *metformin*

Avandamet®

Tab: **Avandamet®1/500**: *rosi* 1 mg/*met* 250 mg

Avandamet®2/500: *rosi* 2 mg/*met* 500 mg

Avandamet®4/500: *rosi* 4 mg/*met* 500 mg

Avandamet®2/1000: *rosi* 2 mg/*met* 1000 mg

Avandamet®4/1000: *rosi* 4 mg/*met* 1000 mg

Thiazlidinedione/Sulfonylurea Combination

▶*pioglitazone/glimepiride* **(C)** take 1 dose daily with first meal of the day

Previously on *sulfonylurea* alone: initially 30mg/2mg

Previously on *pioglitazone* and *glimepiride*: switch on a mg/mg basis

Max: *pioglitazone* 30 mg and *glimepiride* 4 mg per day

Same precautions as *pioglitazone* and *glimepiride*

Pediatric: <18 years: not recommended

Duetact®

Tab: **Duetact®30mg/2mg**: *pio* 30 mg/*glim* 2 mg

Duetact®30mg/4mg: *pio* 30 mg/*glim* 4 mg

▶*rosiglitazone/glimepiride* **(C)** take 1 dose daily with first meal of the day

Previously on *sulfonylurea* alone: initially 4mg/1mg or 4mg/2mg
Previously on *rosiglitazone* and *glimepiride*: switch on a mg/mg basis
Max: *rosiglitazone* 8 mg and *glimepiride* 4 mg per day
Same precautions as *rosiglitazone* and *glimepiride*
    Pediatric: <18 years: not recommended
Avandaryl®
    Tab: **Avandaryl®4mg/1mg**: *rosi* 4 mg/*glim* 1 mg
          Avandaryl®4mg/2mg: *rosi* 4 mg/*glim* 2 mg
          Avandaryl®4mg/4mg: *rosi* 4 mg/*glim* 4 mg

Incretin mimetic
▶*exenatide* **(C)** administer by SC injection into the thigh, abdomen, or upper arm within 60 minutes before AM and PM meals; initially 5 mcg/dose; may increase to 10 mcg/dose after one month
    Pediatric: not recommended
    Byetta® *Prefilled pen:* 250 mcg/ml (5, 10 mcg/dose; 60 doses, needles not included; m-cresol, mannitol)

Comment: **Byetta®** is an adjunct to metformin and/or sulfonylurea when glycemic control is not adequate. **Byetta®** is *not* a substitute for insulin, *not* for treatment of DKA, and *not* for post-prandial administration.

Dipeptidyl Peptidase-4 (DPP-4) Inhibitor
▶*sitagliptin* **(B)** 100 mg daily (as monotherapy or as combination therapy with metforman or a TZD)
    Januvia® *Tab:* 25, 50, 100 mg

Typhoid Fever (*Salmonella typhi*)

Pre-exposure Prophylaxis
▶*typhoid* vaccine, oral, live, attenuated strain
    Vivotif Berna® 1 cap qod, 1 hour before a meal, with a lukewarm (not >body temperature) or cold drink for a total of 4 doses; do not crush or chew; complete therapy at least 1 week prior to expected exposure; re-immunization recommended every 5 years if repeated exposure
    Pediatric: <6 years: not recommended
               >6 years: same as adult
    Cap: enteric coated
▶*typhoid Vi polysaccharide* vaccine **(C)**
    Typhim Vi® 0.5 ml IM in deltoid; re-immunization recommended every 2 years if repeated exposure

Typhoid Fever

Pediatric: <2 years: not recommended
>2 years: same as adult
Vial: 20, 50 dose; *Prefilled syringe:* 0.5 ml

Comment: Febrile illness may require delaying administration of the vaccine. Have *epinephrine* 1:1000 readily available.

Treatment
1st Line

▶*amoxicillin* **(B)(G)** 500 mg qid
Pediatric: see page 569 for dose by weight
<40 kg (88 lb): 20-40 mg/kg/day in 3 doses
days or 25-45 mg/kg/day in 2 doses

Amoxil® *Cap:* 250, 500 mg; *Tab:* 875*mg; *Chew tab:* 125, 200, 250, 400 mg (cherry-banana-peppermint, phenylalanine); *Oral susp:* 125, 250 mg/5 ml (80, 100, 150 ml; strawberry); 200, 400 mg/5 ml (50, 75, 100 ml; bubble gum); *Oral drops:* 50 mg/ml (30 ml; bubble gum)

Trimox® *Cap:* 250, 500 mg; *Oral susp:* 125 mg/5 ml, 250 mg/5 ml (80, 100, 150 ml; raspberry-strawberry)

▶*amoxicillin/clavulanate* **(B)(G)** 500 mg qid
Pediatric: see pages 571-572 for dose by weight
40-45 mg/kg/day divided tid or
90 mg/kg/day divided bid

Augmentin® *Tab:* 250, 500, 875 mg; *Chew tab:* 125 mg (lemon-lime), 200 mg (cherry-banana, phenylalanine), 250 mg (lemon-lime), 400 mg (cherry-banana, phenylalanine); *Oral susp:* 125 mg/5 ml (banana), 250 mg/5 ml (orange) (75, 100, 150 ml); 200 mg/5 ml, 400 mg/5 ml (50, 75, 100 ml; orange-raspberry, phenylalanine)

Augmentin®ES-600 *Oral susp:* 600 mg/5 ml (50, 75, 100, 150 ml) (orange-raspberry, phenylalanine)

Augmentin®XR 2 tabs q 12 hours x 10 days
Pediatric: <16 years: use other forms
Tab: 1000 mg ext-rel

▶*ampicillin* **(B)** 500 mg qid
Pediatric: see page 570 for dose by weight
50-100 mg/kg/day in 4 doses

Omnipen®, Principen® *Cap:* 250, 500 mg; *Oral susp:* 125, 250 mg/5 ml (100, 150, 200 ml; fruit)

▶*trimethoprim/sulfamethoxazole* **(C)(G)**
Pediatric: see page 597 for dose by weight
<2 months: not recommended
>2 months: 40 mg/kg/day of *sulfamethoxazole*

Typhoid Fever

in 2 doses bid x 10 days
Bactrim®, Septra® 2 tabs bid x 10 days
  Tab: trim 80 mg/*sulfa* 400 mg*
Bactrim®DS, Septra®DS 1 tab bid x 10 days
  Tab: trim 160 mg/*sulfa* 800 mg*
Bactrim®Pediatric Suspension, Septra®Pediatric Suspension
20 ml bid x 10 days
  Oral susp: trim 40 mg/*sulfa* 200 mg per 5 ml (100 ml; cherry, alcohol 0.3%)

Comment: Trimethoprim/sulfamethoxazole is not recommended in pregnancy or lactation.

Alternate Regimen
▶*azithromycin* **(B)** 1 g daily
  Pediatric: see page 573 for dose by weight
    12 mg/kg/day x 5 days; max 500 mg/day
  Zithromax® *Tab:* 250, 500 mg; *Oral susp:* 100 mg/5 ml (15 ml); 200 mg/5 ml (15, 22.5, 30 ml) (cherry-vanilla-banana);
  Pkt: 1 g for reconstitution (cherry-banana)
  Zithromax®Tri-pak *Tab:* 3-500 mg tabs/pck
  Zithromax®Z-pak *Tab:* 6-250 mg tabs/pck
  Zmax® *Oral susp:* 2 g ext rel (cherry-banana)
▶*cefixime* **(B)** 400 mg daily
  Pediatric: see page 577 for dose by weight
    <6 months: not recommended
    6 months-12 years, <50 kg: 8 mg/kg/day in 1-2 doses
    >12 years, >50 kg: same as adult
  Suprax®Oral Suspension *Oral susp:* 100 mg/5 ml (50, 75, 100 ml; strawberry)
▶*ciprofloxacin* **(C)(G)** 500 mg bid
  Pediatric: <18 years: not recommended
  Cipro® *Tab:* 100, 250, 500, 750 mg; *Oral susp:* 250, 500 mg/5 ml (100 ml; strawberry)
▶*norfloxacin* **(C)** 400 mg bid
  Pediatric: <18 years: not recommended
  Noroxin® *Tab:* 400 mg
▶*ofloxacin* **(C)(G)** 400 mg bid x 10 days
  Pediatric: <18 years: not recommended
  Floxin® *Tab:* 200, 300, 400 mg

Ulcer

Ulcer: Diabetic, Neuropathic Lower Extremity

Debriding/Capillary Stimulant Agent
  Granulex® (*trypsin* 0.1 mg/*balsam peru* 72.5 mg/castor oil 650 mg per 0.82 ml) apply at least twice daily; may cover with a wet bandage
  Aerosol liq: (2, 4 oz)

Growth Factor
▶*becaplermin* **(C)** apply daily with a cotton swab or tongue depressor; then cover with saline moistened gauze dressing; rinse after 12 hours; then recover with a clean saline dressing
  Regranex® *Gel:* 0.01% (2, 7.5, 15 g; parabens)

Comment: Store in refrigerator; do not freeze. Not for use in wounds that close by primary intention.

Ulcer: Pressure/Decubitus

Debriding/Capillary Stimulant Agent
  Granulex® (*trypsin* 0.1 mg/*balsam peru* 72.5 mg/castor oil 650 mg per 0.82 ml) apply at least twice daily; may cover with a wet bandage
  Aerosol liq: (2, 4 oz)

Growth Factor
▶*becaplermin* **(C)** apply daily with a cotton swab or tongue depressor; then cover with saline moistened gauze dressing; rinse after 12 hours; then recover with a clean saline dressing
  Regranex® *Gel:* 0.01% (2, 7.5, 15 g; parabens)

Comment: Store in refrigerator; do not freeze. Not for use in wounds that close by primary intention.

Ulcerative Colitis

Comment: Standard treatment regimen is anti-infective, anti-spasmodic, and bowel rest; progressing to clear liquids; then to high fiber.

▶*hydrocortisone* **(C)**
  Cortenema® 1 enema q HS x 21 days or until symptoms controlled
  Enema: 100 mg/60 ml (1, 7/pck)
  Cortifoam® 1 applicatorful daily-bid x 2-3 weeks and every second day thereafter until symptoms are controlled

Aerosol: 80 mg/applicator (14 application/container)

Comment: Use *hydrocortisone* foam as adjunctive therapy in the distal portion of the rectum when hydrocortisone enemas cannot be retained.

▶*balsalazide* **(B)** 2.25 g 3 times per week x 8 weeks; max 12 weeks
  Pediatric: not recommended
 Colasal® *Cap:* 750 mg

Comment: Balsalazide 6.75 g provides 2.4 g of mesalazine to the colon.

▶*mesalamine* **(B)**
 Asacol® 800 mg tid x 6 weeks; maintenance 1.6 g/day in divided doses
  Tab: 400 mg delayed-release
 Pentasa® 1 g qid for up to 8 weeks
  Cap: 250 mg controlled-release
 Rowasa® 4 g rectally by enema q HS; retain for 8 hours x 3-6 weeks
  Enema: 4 g/60 ml (7/pck)
 Rowasa® 1 supp rectally bid x 3-6 weeks; retain for 1-3 hours or longer
  Rectal supp: 500 mg (12, 24/pck)

▶*osalazine* **(C)** 1 g/day in 2 divided doses
 Dipentum® *Cap:* 250 mg

▶*sulfasalazine* **(B; D in 2nd, 3rd)(G)**
  Pediatric: <2 years: not recommended
    2-16 years: initially 40-60 mg/kg/day in 3 to 6 divided doses; max 30 mg/kg/day in 4 ivided doses; max 2 g/day
 Azulfidine® initially 1-2 g/day; increase to 3-4 g/day in divided doses pc until clinical symptoms controlled; maintenance 2 g/day; max 4 g/day
  Tab: 500 mg
 Azulfidine®EN initially 500 mg in the PM x 7 days; then 500 mg bid x 7 days; then 500 mg in the AM and 1 g in the PM x 7 days; then 1 g bid; max 4 g/day
  Tab: 500 mg ent-coat

Parenteral Glucocorticosteroids *see page 389*
Oral Glucocorticosteroids *see page 387*
Anti-diarrheal Agents
▶*difenoxin/atropine* **(C)** 2 tabs, then 1 tab after each loose stool or 1 tab q 3-4 hours; max 8 tabs/day x 2 days
 Motofen® *Tab: dif* 1 mg/*atro* 0.025 mg

Ulcerative Colitis

▶*diphenoxylate/atropine* **(C)(G)** 2 tabs or 10 ml qid
  Lomotil® *Tab: diphen* 2.5 mg/*atro* 0.025 mg; *Liq: diphen* 2.5 mg/*atro* 0.025 mg/5 ml (2 oz w. dropper)
▶*loperamide* **(B)(G)**
  Imodium® (OTC) 4 mg initially, then 2 mg after each loose stool; max 16 mg/day
    Cap: 2 mg
  Imodium®A-D (OTC) 4 mg initially, then 2 mg after each loose stool; usual max 8 mg/day x 2 days
    Cplt: 2 mg; *Liq:* 1 mg/5 ml (2, 4 oz)
  Imodium®Advanced (OTC) 2 tabs chewed after first loose stool, then 1 after the next loose stool; max 4 tabs/day
    Chew tab: loperamide 2 mg/simethicone 125 mg

Urethritis: Gonococcal

Comment: Empiric therapy requires concomitant treatment for chlamydia. Treat all sexual contacts.

▶*azithromycin* **(B)** 1 g x 1 dose
  Zithromax® *Tab:* 250, 500 mg; *Oral susp:* 100 mg/5 ml (15 ml); 200 mg/5 ml (15, 22.5, 30 ml) (cherry-vanilla-banana); *Pkt:* 1 g for reconstitution (cherry-banana)
  Zithromax®Tri-pak *Tab:* 3-500 mg tabs/pck
  Zithromax®Z-pak *Tab:* 6-250 mg tabs/pck
  Zmax® *Oral susp:* 2 g ext rel (cherry-banana)
▶*cefixime* **(B)** 400 mg x 1 dose
    Pediatric: see page 577 for dose by weight
        <6 months: not recommended
        6 months-12 years, <50 kg: 8 mg/kg/day in 1-2 doses x 10 days
        >12 years, >50 kg: same as adult
  Suprax®Oral Suspension *Oral susp:* 100 mg/5 ml (50, 75, 100 ml; strawberry)
▶*ceftriaxone* **(B)(G)** 125 mg IM x 1 dose
  Rocephin® *Vial:* 250, 500 mg; 1, 2 g
▶*ciprofloxacin* **(C)(G)** 500 mg bid x 1 dose
    Pediatric: <18 years: not recommended
    Pediatric: <18 years: not recommended
  Cipro® *Tab:* 100, 250, 500, 750 mg; *Oral susp:* 250, 500 mg/5 ml (100 ml; strawberry)

▶*norfloxacin* **(C)** 800 mg x 1 dose
    Pediatric: <18 years: not recommended
  Noroxin® *Tab:* 400 mg
▶*ofloxacin* **(C)(G)** 400 mg bid x 10 days
    Pediatric: <18 years: not recommended
  Floxin® *Tab:* 200, 300, 400 mg

Urethritis: Nongonococcal

Primary Therapy
▶*azithromycin* **(B)** 1 g x 1 dose
  Zithromax® *Tab:* 250, 500 mg; *Oral susp:* 100 mg/5 ml (15 ml); 200 mg/5 ml (15, 22.5, 30 ml) (cherry-vanilla-banana); *Pkt:* 1 g for reconstitution (cherry-banana)
▶*doxycycline* **(D)(G)** 100 mg bid x 7 days
    Pediatric: <8 years: not recommended
             >8 years, <100 lb: 2 mg/lb on first day in 2 doses, followed by 1 mg/lb/day in 1-2 doses x 7 days
              >8 years, >100 lb: same as adult
  Adoxa® *Tab:* 50, 100 mg ent-coat
  Doryx® *Cap:* 100 mg
  Monodox® *Cap:* 50, 100 mg
  Vibramycin® *Cap:* 50, 100 mg; *Syr:* 50 mg/5 ml (raspberry, sulfites); *Oral susp:* 25 mg/5 ml (2 oz) (raspberry-apple); *IV conc: doxy* 100 mg/*asc acid* 480 mg after dilution; *doxy* 200 mg/*asc acid* 960 mg after dilution
  Vibra-Tab® *Tab:* 100 mg film-coat
Comment: Doxycycline is contraindicated in pregnancy (discolors fetal tooth enamel).
▶*erythromycin base* **(B)** 500 mg qid x 7 days or 250 mg qid x 14 days
    Pediatric: see page 588 for dose by weight
              30-50 mg/kg/day in 2-4 doses x 14 days
  E-Mycin® *Tab:* 250 mg; 333 mg ent-coat
  Eryc® *Cap:* 250 mg ent-coat
  Ery-Tab® *Tab:* 250, 333, 500 mg ent-coat
  PCE® *Tab:* 333, 500 mg
▶*erythromycin ethylsuccinate* **(B)(G)** 800 mg po qid x 7 days or 400 mg qid x 14 days
    Pediatric: see page 589 for dose by weight
              30-50 mg/kg/day in 4 divided doses x 7-14 days;

Urethritis: Nongonococcal

> may double dose with severe infection; max 100 mg/kg/day

Ery-Ped® *Oral susp:* 200 mg/5 ml (100, 200 ml; fruit); 400 mg/5 ml (60, 100, 200 ml; banana); *Oral drops:* 200, 400 mg/5 ml (50 ml; fruit); *Chew tab:* 200 mg wafer (fruit)
E.E.S.® *Oral susp:* 200, 400 mg/5 ml (100 ml; fruit)
E.E.S.®Granules *Oral susp:* 200 mg/5 ml (100, 200 ml; cherry,
E.E.S.®400 Tablets *Tab:* 400 mg

▶ *minocycline* **(D)(G)** 200 mg on first day; then 100 mg q 12 hours x 9 more days
> *Pediatric:* <8 years: not recommended
> >8 years, <100 lb: 2 mg/lb on first day in 2 doses, followed by 1 mg/lb/ q 12 hours x 9 more days
> >8 years, >100 lb: same as adult

Minocin® *Cap:* 100 mg ent-coat

Comment: Minocycline is contraindicated in pregnancy (discolors fetal tooth enamel).

▶ *ofloxacin* **(C)(G)** 400 mg bid x 10 days
> *Pediatric:* <18 years: not recommended

Floxin® *Tab:* 200, 300, 400 mg

Urethritis: Recurrent/Persistent

▶ *erythromycin base* **(B)** 500 mg qid x 7 days
> *Pediatric:* see page 588 for dose by weight
> 30-50 mg/kg/day in 2-4 doses x 7 days

E-Mycin® *Tab:* 250 mg; 333 mg ent-coat
Eryc® *Cap:* 250 mg ent-coat
Ery-Tab® *Tab:* 250, 333, 500 mg ent-coat
PCE® *Tab:* 333, 500 mg

▶ *erythromycin ethylsuccinate* **(B)(G)** 800 mg po tid x 7 days
> *Pediatric:* see page 589 for dose by weight
> 30-50 mg/kg/day in 4 divided doses x 7 days; may double dose with severe infection; max 100 mg/kg/day

Ery-Ped® *Oral susp:* 200 mg/5 ml (100, 200 ml; fruit); 400 mg/5 ml (60, 100, 200 ml; banana); *Oral drops:* 200, 400 mg/5 ml (50 ml; fruit); *Chew tab:* 200 mg wafer (fruit)
E.E.S.® *Oral susp:* 200, 400 mg/5 ml (100 ml; fruit)

E.E.S.®Granules *Oral susp:* 200 mg/5 ml (100, 200 ml; cherry)
E.E.S.®400 Tablets *Tab:* 400 mg

Urinary Retention: Unobstructive

▶*bethanechol* **(C)** 10-30 mg tid
   Urecholine® *Tab:* 5, 10, 25, 50 mg
Comment: Contraindicated in presence of urinary obstruction. *Atropine* 0.4 mg administered SC reverses *bethanechol* toxicity.

Urinary Tract Infection (UTI, Cystitis: Acute)

Anti-infectives: Therapy in Adult Female with Uncomplicated UTI
▶*amoxicillin/clavulanate* **(B)(G)** 500 mg tid or 875 mg bid x 3 days
   Augmentin® *Tab:* 250, 500, 875 mg; *Chew tab:* 125 mg (lemon-lime), 200 mg (cherry-banana, phenylalanine), 250 mg (lemon-lime), 400 mg (cherry-banana, phenylalanine); *Oral susp:* 125 mg/5 ml (banana), 250 mg/5 ml (orange) (75, 100, 150 ml); 200 mg/5 ml, 400 mg/5 ml (50, 75, 100 ml; orange-raspberry, phenylalanine)
   Augmentin®ES-600 *Oral susp:* 600 mg/5 ml (50, 75, 100, 150 ml) (orange-raspberry, phenylalanine)
   Augmentin®XR 2 tabs q 12 hours x 10 days
      Pediatric: <16 years: use other forms
      Tab: 1000 mg ext-rel
▶*cephradine* **(B)** 500 mg q 12 hours x 3 days; max 4 g/day
      Pediatric: see page 583 for dose by weight
            <9 months: not recommended
            >9 months: 25-50 mg/kg/day divided q 6-12
            hours x 3 days; max 4 g/day
   Velosef® *Cap:* 250, 500 mg; *Oral susp:* 125, 250 mg/5 ml (100, 200 ml)
▶*ciprofloxacin* **(C)(G)**
      Pediatric: <18 years: not recommended
   Cipro® 100 mg bid x 3 days
      Tab: 100, 250, 500, 750 mg; *Cystitis Pack:* 100 mg tabs (6/pck)
      Oral susp: 250, 500 mg/5 ml (100 ml; strawberry)
▶*fosfomycin* **(B)** 1 pkt in 3-4 oz cold water x 1 dose
   Monurol® *Single-dose pkts:* 1-3 g (mandarin orange, sucrose)
▶*levofloxacin* **(C)** 250 mg daily x 3 days
      Pediatric: <18 years: not recommended

UTI

    Levaquin® *Tab:* 250, 500 mg
▶*norfloxacin* **(C)** 400 mg daily x 3 days
    Noroxin® *Tab:* 400 mg
▶*ofloxacin* **(C)(G)** 200 mg q 12 hours x 3 days
    Floxin® *Tab:* 200, 300, 400 mg
    Floxin®UroPak *Tab:* 200 mg (6/pck)
▶*trimethoprim* **(C)(G)**
    Primsol® 100 mg q 12 hours or 200 mg daily x 10 days
        Pediatric: <6 months: not recommended
                    >6 months: 10 mg/kg/day in 2 doses divided
                    q 12 hours x 10 days
        Oral soln: 50 mg/5 ml (bubble gum, dye-free, alcohol-free)
    Proloprim® 100 mg q 12 hours or 200 mg daily x 10 days
        Pediatric: not recommended
        Tab: 100, 200 mg
    Trimpex® 100 mg q 12 hours or 200 mg daily x 10 days
        Pediatric: not recommended
        Tab: 100 mg
▶*trimethoprim/sulfamethoxazole* **(C)(G)**
        Pediatric: see page 597 for dose by weight
                <2 months: not recommended
                >2 months: 40 mg/kg/day of *sulfamethoxazole*
                in 2 doses bid x 10 days
    Bactrim®, Septra® 2 tabs bid x 10 days
        Tab: trim 80 mg/*sulfa* 400 mg*
    Bactrim®DS, Septra®DS 1 tab bid x 10 days
        Tab: trim 160 mg/*sulfa* 800 mg*
    Bactrim®Pediatric Suspension, Septra®Pediatric Suspension
    20 ml bid x 10 days
        Oral susp: trim 40 mg/*sulfa* 200 mg per 5 ml (100 ml; cherry, alcohol 0.3%)

Comment: Trimethoprim/sulfamethoxazole is not recommended in pregnancy or lactation.

Anti-infectives: Standard Regimen for UTI
▶*acetylsulfisoxazole* **(C)(G)**
    Gantrisin® initial dose 2-4 g; then 4-8 g/day in 4-6 doses x 7 days
        Tab: 500 mg
    Gantrisin®Pediatric: <2 months: not recommended
                        >2 months: initial dose 75 mg/kg/day; then
                        150 mg/kg/day in 4-6 doses x 7 days; max 6

g/day
Oral susp: 500 mg/5 ml (4, 16 oz); *Syr:* 500 mg/5 ml (16 oz)

▶ *amoxicillin* **(B)(G)** 500-875 mg bid or 250-500 mg tid x 7 days
Pediatric: see page 569 for dose by weight
<40 kg (88 lb): 20-40 mg/kg/day in 3 doses x 7 days or 25-45 mg/kg/day in 2 doses x 7 days

Amoxil® *Cap:* 250, 500 mg; *Tab:* 875*mg; *Chew tab:* 125, 200, 250, 400 mg (cherry-banana-peppermint, phenylalanine); *Oral susp:* 125, 250 mg/5 ml (80, 100, 150 ml; strawberry); 200, 400 mg/5 ml (50, 75, 100 ml; bubble gum); *Oral drops:* 50 mg/ml (30 ml; bubble gum)

Trimox® *Cap:* 250, 500 mg; *Oral susp:* 125 mg/5 ml, 250 mg/5 ml (80, 100, 150 ml; raspberry-strawberry)

▶ *amoxicillin/clavulanate* **(B)(G)** 500-800 mg bid or 250 mg tid x 7 days

Pediatric: see pages 571-572 for dose by weight
40-45 mg/kg/day divided tid x 7 days or
90 mg/kg/day divided bid x 7 days

Augmentin® *Tab:* 250, 500, 875 mg; *Chew tab:* 125 mg (lemon-lime), 200 mg (cherry-banana, phenylalanine), 250 mg (lemon-lime), 400 mg (cherry-banana, phenylalanine); *Oral susp:* 125 mg/5 ml (banana), 250 mg/5 ml (orange) (75, 100, 150 ml); 200 mg/5 ml, 400 mg/5 ml (50, 75, 100 ml; orange-raspberry, phenylalanine)

Augmentin®**ES-600** *Oral susp:* 600 mg/5 ml (50, 75, 100, 150 ml; orange-raspberry, phenylalanine)

Augmentin®**XR** 2 tabs q 12 hours x 10 days
Pediatric: <16 years: use other forms
Tab: 1000 mg ext-rel

▶ *ampicillin* **(B)** 500 mg qid x 7-14 days
Pediatric: see page 570 for dose by weight
50-100 mg/kg/day in 4 doses x 7-14 days

Omnipen®, **Principen**® *Cap:* 250, 500 mg; *Oral susp:* 125, 250 mg/5 ml (100, 150, 200 ml; fruit)

▶ *carbenicillin* **(B)** 1-2 tabs qid x 7-14 days
Pediatric: not recommended
Geocillin® *Tab:* 382 mg

▶ *cefaclor* **(B)(G)**
Ceclor® 250 mg tid or 375 mg bid x 7days
Pediatric: see page 575 for dose by weight
20-40 mg/kg/day in 3 doses x 7 days

UTI

        Pulvule: 250, 500 mg; *Oral susp:* 125, 250 mg/5 ml (75, 150 ml); 187, 375 mg/5 ml (50, 100 ml) (strawberry)

Ceclor®CD 500 mg q 12 hours x 7 days
    Pediatric: <16 years: not recommended
    Tab: 375, 500 mg ext-rel

Ceclor®CDpak 500 mg q 12 hours x 7 days
    Pediatric: <16 years: not recommended
    Tab: 500 mg (14 tabs/CDpak)

Raniclor® 500 mg q 12 hours x 7 days
    Pediatric: 20-40 mg/kg/day in 3 doses x 7 days
    Chew tab: 125, 187, 250, 375 mg

▶*cefadroxil* **(B)** 1-2 g in 1-2 doses x 10 days
    Pediatric: see page 576 for dose by weight
        30 mg/kg/day in 2 doses x 10 days

Duricef® *Cap:* 500 mg; *Tab:* 1 g; *Oral susp:* 250 mg/5 ml (100 ml); 500 mg/5 ml (75, 100 ml) (orange-pineapple)

▶*cefixime* **(B)** 400 mg daily x 10 days
    Pediatric: see page 577 for dose by weight
        <6 months: not recommended
        6 months-12 years, <50 kg: 8 mg/kg/day in 1-2 doses x 10 days
        >12 years, >50 kg: same as adult

Suprax®Oral Suspension *Oral susp:* 100 mg/5 ml (50, 75, 100 ml; strawberry)

▶*cefpodoxime proxetil* **(B)** 100 mg bid x 7 days
    Pediatric: see page 578 for dose by weight
        <2 months: not recommended
        2 months-12 years: 10 mg/kg/day (max 400 mg/dose) or 5 mg/kg/day bid (max 200 mg/dose) x 7 days

Vantin® *Tab:* 100, 200 mg; *Oral susp:* 50, 100 mg/5 ml (50, 75, 100 mg; lemon-creme)

▶*cefuroxime axetil* **(B)(G)** 125-250 mg bid x 7-10 days
    Pediatric: see page 581 for dose by weight
        <3 months: not recommended
        3 months-12 years: 20-30 mg/kg/day in 2 doses x 7-10 days

Ceftin® *Tab:* 125, 250, 500 mg; *Oral susp:* 125, 250 mg/5 ml (50, 100 ml; tutti-frutti)

▶*cephalexin* **(B)(G)** 500 mg bid x 7-10 days
    Pediatric: see page 582 for dose by weight

UTI

25-50 mg/kg/day in 4 doses x 7-10 days
Keflex® *Cap:* 250, 500, 750 mg; *Oral susp:* 125, 250 mg/5 ml (100, 200 ml)
Keftab® *Tab:* 500 mg
Keftab®K-pak *Tab:* 20-500 mg tabs/K-pak

▶*cephradine* **(B)** 500 mg q 12 hours or 1 g q 12 hours or 1 g q 6 hours x 7-10 days; max 4 g/day
  Pediatric: see page 583 for dose by weight
    <9 months: not recommended
    >9 months: 25-50 mg/kg/day divided q 6-12
    Hours x 7-10 days; max 4 g/day
Velosef® *Cap:* 250, 500 mg; *Oral susp:* 125, 250 mg/5 ml (100, 200 ml)

▶*ciprofloxacin* **(C)(G)** 500 mg bid or 1000 mg XR daily x 3-14 days
  Pediatric: <18 years: not recommended
Cipro® *Tab:* 100, 250, 500, 750 mg; *Oral susp:* 250, 500 mg/5 ml (100 ml; strawberry)

▶*doxycycline* **(D)(G)** 100 mg bid x 7-10 days
  Pediatric: <8 years: not recommended
    >8 years, <100 lb: 2 mg/lb on first day in 2 doses, followed by 1 mg/lb/day in 1-2 doses x 7-10 days
    >8 years, >100 lb: same as adult
Adoxa® *Tab:* 50, 100 mg ent-coat
Doryx® *Cap:* 100 mg
Monodox® *Cap:* 50, 100 mg
Vibramycin® *Cap:* 50, 100 mg; *Syr:* 50 mg/5 ml (raspberry, sulfites); *Oral susp:* 25 mg/5 ml (raspberry-apple); *IV conc: doxy* 100 mg/*asc acid* 480 mg after dilution; *doxy* 200 mg/*asc acid* 960 mg after dilution
Vibra-Tab® *Tab:* 100 mg film-coat

Comment: Doxycycline is contraindicated in pregnancy (discolors fetal tooth enamel).

▶*enoxacin* **(C)** 200 mg q 12 hours x 7 days
  Pediatric: <18 years: not recommended
Penetrex® *Tab:* 200, 400 mg

▶*levofloxacin* **(C)** 250 mg daily x 7-10 days
  Pediatric: <18 years: not recommended
Levaquin® *Tab:* 250, 500 mg

▶*lomefloxacin* **(C)** 400 mg daily x 10 days
  Pediatric: <18 years: not recommended

UTI

Maxaquin® *Tab:* 400 mg

▶*minocycline* **(D)(G)** 100 mg q 12 hours x 10 days
    Pediatric: <8 years: not recommended
    >8 years, <100 lb: 2 mg/lb on first day in 2 doses, followed by 1 mg/lb/ q 12 hours x 9 more days
    >8 years, >100 lb: same as adult
  Minocin® *Cap:* 100 mg ent-coat

Comment: Minocycline is contraindicated in pregnancy (discolors fetal tooth enamel).

▶*nalidixic acid* **(B)** 1 g qid x 7-14 days
    Pediatric: <3 months: not recommended
    >3 months: 25 mg/lb/day in 4 doses x 7-14 days
  NegGram® *Tab:* 250, 500 mg; 1 g; *Cap:* 250, 500 mg; *Oral susp:* 250 mg/5 ml

▶*nitrofurantoin* **(B)(G)**
  Furadantin® 50-100 mg qid x 7-10 days
    Pediatric: see page 593 for dose by weight
      <1 month: not recommended
      >1 month: 5-7 mg/kg/day in 4 doses x 7-10 days
    Oral susp: 25 mg/5 ml (60 ml)
  Macrobid® 100 mg q 12 hours x 7-10 days
    Pediatric: <12 years: not recommended
    Cap: 100 mg
  Macrodantin® 50-100 mg qid x at least 7 days; long-term use 50-100 mg q HS
    Cap: 25, 50, 100 mg

▶*norfloxacin* **(C)** 400 mg x 7-10 days
    Pediatric: <18 years: not recommended
  Noroxin® *Tab:* 400 mg

▶*ofloxacin* **(C)(G)** 200 mg q 12 hours x 7-10 days
    Pediatric: <18 years: not recommended
  Floxin® *Tab:* 200, 300, 400 mg

▶*trimethoprim* **(C)(G)**
  Primsol® 100 mg q 12 hours or 200 mg daily x 10 days
    Pediatric: <6 months: not recommended
      >6 months: 10 mg/kg/day in 2 doses divided q 12 hours x 10 days
    Oral soln: 50 mg/5 ml (bubble gum, dye-free, alcohol-free)
  Proloprim® 100 mg q 12 hours or 200 mg daily x 10 days
    Pediatric: not recommended

Tab: 100, 200 mg
Trimpex® 100 mg q 12 hours or 200 mg daily x 10 days
Pediatric: not recommended
Tab: 100 mg
▶*trimethoprim/sulfamethoxazole* **(C)(G)**
Pediatric: see page 597 for dose by weight
<2 months: not recommended
>2 months: 40 mg/kg/day of *sulfamethoxazole*
in 2 doses bid x 10 days
Bactrim®, Septra® 2 tabs bid x 10 days
Tab: trim 80 mg/*sulfa* 400 mg*
Bactrim®DS, Septra®DS 1 tab bid x 10 days
Tab: trim 160 mg/*sulfa* 800 mg*
Bactrim®Pediatric Suspension, Septra®Pediatric Suspension
20 ml bid x 10 days
Oral susp: trim 40 mg/*sulfa* 200 mg per 5 ml (100 ml; cherry, alcohol 0.3%)
Comment: Trimethoprim/sulfamethoxazole is not recommended in pregnancy or lactation.

Parenteral Therapy
▶*ertapenem* **(B)** 1 g daily; CrCl <30 ml/min, 500 mg daily; treat x 10-14 days; may switch to an oral antibiotic after 3 days if warranted
IV infusion: administer over 30 minutes
IM injection: reconstitute with lidocaine only
Pediatric: <18 years: not recommended
Ivanz® *Vial:* 1 g pwdr for reconstitution

Long-term Prophylactic/Suppression Therapy
▶*methenamine hippurate* **(C)** 1 tab bid
Pediatric: <6 years: not recommended
6-12 years: 1/2 tab bid
Hiprex®, Urex® *Tab:* 1 g

Urinary Tract Analgesics/Anti-spasmodics
▶*flavoxate* **(B)** 100-200 mg tid-qid
Pediatric: <12 years: not recommended
Urispas® *Tab:* 100 mg
▶*hyoscyamine* **(C)(G)** 1-2 tabs qid
Cystospaz® 1-2 tabs qid
Tab: 0.15 mg
IB-Stat® 1 oral spray q 12 hours
Oral spray: 0.125 mg/ml
Levbid® 1-2 tabs q 12 hours prn; max 4 tabs/day

Pediatric: <12 years: not recommended
Tab: 0.375*mg ext-rel

Levsin® 1-2 tabs q 4 hours prn; max 12 tabs/day
Pediatric: <6 years: not recommended
6-12 years: 1 tab q 4 hours prn
Tab: 0.125*mg

Levsin®Drops 1-2 ml q 4 hours prn; max 60 ml/day
Pediatric: 3.4 kg: 4 drops q 4 hours prn; max 24 drops/day
5 kg: 5 drops q 4 hours prn; max 30 drops/day
7 kg: 6 drops q 4 hours prn; max 36 drops/day
10 kg: 8 drops q 4 hours prn; max 40 drops/day
Oral drops: 0.125 mg/ml (15 ml; orange, alcohol 5%)

Levsin®Elixir 5-10 ml q 4 hours prn
Pediatric: <10 kg: use drops
10-19 kg: 1.25 ml q 4 hours prn
20-39 kg: 2.5 ml q 4 hours prn
40-49 kg: 3.75 ml q 4 hours prn
>50 kg: 5 ml q 4 hours prn
Elix: 0.125 mg/5 ml (16 oz; orange, alcohol 20%)

Levsinex®SL 1-2 tabs q 4 hours SL or po; max 12 tabs/day
Pediatric: 2-12 years: ½-1 tab q 4 hours; max 6 tabs/day
Tab: 0.125 mg sublingual

Levsinex®Timecaps 1-2 caps q 12 hours; may adjust to 1 cap q 8 hours
Pediatric: 2-12 years: 1 cap q 12 hours; max 2 caps/day
Cap: 0.375 mg time-rel

NuLev® dissolve 1-2 tabs on tongue, with or without water, q 4 hours prn; max 12 tabs/day
Pediatric: <2 years: not recommended
2-12 years: dissolve ½-1 tab on tongue, with or without water, q 4 hours prn; max 6 tabs/day
Tab: 0.125 mg orally-disintegrating (mint, phenylalanine)

Symax®SL 1-2 tabs SL q 4 hours prn
Pediatric: <2 years: not recommended
2-12 years: ½-1 tab SL q 4 hours prn
SL tab: 0.125 mg

Symax®SR 1 tab q 12 hours prn
Pediatric: <12 years: not recommended
SL tab: 0.375 mg

▶*methenamine/phenyl salicylate/methylene blue/benzoic acid/ atropine sulfate/hyoscyamine* **(C)(G)** 2 tabs qid

Pediatric: <6 years: not recommended

Urised® *Tab:* meth 40.8 mg/*phenyl salic* 18.1 mg/*meth blue* 5.4 mg/*benz acid* 4.5 mg/*atro sulf* 0.03 mg/*hyoscy* 0.03 mg

Comment: **Urised®** imparts a blue-green color to urine which may stain fabrics.

▶*phenazopyridine* **(B)(G)** 95-200 mg q 6 hours prn; max 2 days
  Pediatric: not recommended

Azo Standard®, **Prodium®**, **Uristat®** (OTC) *Tab:* 95 mg
Pyridium®, **Urogesic®** *Tab:* 100, 200 mg

Comment: Phenazopyridine imparts an orange-red color to urine which may stain fabrics.

Prophylactic/Suppression Therapy

▶*metheramine hippurate* **(C)** 1 g bid
  Pediatric: <6 years: 0.25 g/30 lb qid
            6-12 years: 25-50 mg/kg/day in 2 doses or 0.5-1 g bid

Hiprex® *Tab:* 1 g; *Oral susp:* 500 mg/5 ml (480 ml)

Urolithiasis (Renal Calculi, Kidney Stones)

NSAIDs *see **Pain** page 308*
Oral Non-narcotic Analgesics *see **Pain** page 308*
Oral Narcotic Analgesics *see **Pain** page 308*
Parenteral Narcotics
▶*buprenorphine* **(C)** 0.3 mg IM q 6 hours prn
  Buprenex® *Amp:* 0.3 mg/ml (1 ml)
▶*meperidine* **(B; D in 2nd, 3rd)(II)(G)** 50-100 mg IM q 3-4 hours prn
  Demerol® *Tubex®:* 25, 50, 75, 100 mg/ml (2 ml); *Vial:* 25 mg/ml (1 ml); 50 mg/ml (1, 30 ml); 75 mg/ml; (1 ml); 100 mg/ml (1, 20 ml)
  Amp: 25, 50, 75, 100 mg/ml (1 ml)
▶*morphine sulfate* **(C)(II)(G)** 10-15 mg q 3-4 hours prn
  Vial: 1 mg/ml (1, 60 ml); 5 mg/ml (1 ml); 8 mg/ml (1 ml);
  10 mg/ml (1, 2, 10 ml); 15 mg/ml (1, 20 ml); *Amp:* 8 mg/ml (1 ml); 10 mg/ml (1 ml); 15 mg/ml (1 ml)

Prevention of Calcium Stones
▶*hydrochlorothiazide* **(B)(G)** 50 mg bid
  Hydrodiuril® *Tab:* 25*, 50*mg
  Microzide® *Cap:* 12.5 mg
  Oretic® *Tab:* 25, 50 mg
▶*potassium citrate* **(C)** 15-20 mEq bid
  Polycitra-K® *Oral crystals:* 30 mEq (unit dose pkts); *Oral soln:*

Urolithiasis

10 mEq/5 ml
▶*sodium cellulose phosphate* **(C)** 2.5-5.0 g with each meal
   Calcibind® *Pwdr:* 300 g
Prevention of Cystine Stone
▶*penicillamine* **(D)** 1-4 g/day
     Pediatric: not recommended
   Cuprimine® *Cap:* 125, 250 mg
   Depen® *Titratable tab:* 250 mg
▶*potassium citrate* **(C)**
   Polycitra-K® 30 mEq qid
     Oral crystals: 30 mEq (unit dose pkts); *Oral soln:* 10 mEq/5 ml

Prevention of Uric Acid Stones
▶*allopurinol* **(C)(G)** 200-300 mg in 1-3 doses; max 800 mg/day
   Zyloprim® *Tab:* 100*, 300* mg
▶*potassium citrate* **(C)**
   Polycitra-K® 30 mEq qid
     Oral crystals: 30 mEq (unit dose pkts); *Oral soln:* 10 mEq/5 ml

Urticaria: Chronic Idiopathic (CIU)

Mild
Oral 2nd Generation Antihistamines *see page 527*
Moderate/Severe
Oral 1st Generation Antihistamines *see page 525*

Urticaria: Acute (Hives)

Mild/Moderate
Oral 1st Generation Antihistamines *see page 525*
Topical Glucocorticosteroids *see page 527*
Oral Glucocorticosteroids *see page 387*
Severe
Parenteral Antihistamines
▶*diphenhydramine* **(C)(G)** 25-50 mg IM immediately; then q 6 hours
     Pediatric: 1.25 mg/kg up to 25 mg IM x 1 dose; then q 6 hours
   Benadryl®Injectable *Vial:* 50 mg/ml (1 ml single-use); 50 mg/ml (10 ml multidose); *Amp:* 10 mg/ml (1 ml); *Prefilled syringe:* 50 mg/ml (1 ml)

Parenteral Glucocorticosteroids *see page 389*
▶*epinephrine* **(C)** 1:1000 0.01 ml/kg SC; max 0.3 ml
   Pediatric: 0.01 mg/kg SC

Vaginal Irritation: External

▶**Replens®Vaginal Moisturizer (NR)(OTC)** apply as needed; for external use only
   Bottle: 2 oz
▶**Vagisil®Intimate Moisturizer (NR)(OTC)** apply as needed; for external use only
   Bottle: 2 oz
Comment: **Vagisil®** has no effect on condom integrity.

Vertigo

▶*meclizine* **(B)(G)** 25-100 mg/day in divided doses
   Antivert® *Tab:* 12.5, 25, 50*mg; *Amp:* 50 mg/ml (1 ml); *Vial:* 50 mg/ml (1 ml single-use); 50 mg/ml (10 ml multidose)
   Bonine® (OTC) *Cap:* 15, 25, 30 mg

Vitamin/Mineral Deficiency
Vitamin /Mineral Prophylaxis

Adult *see page 509*
Infants and Children *see page 514*
Pregnancy *see page 517*
Fluoride Deficiency *see **Fluoridation, Water <0.6 ppm** page 174*

Vitiligo

Repigmentation Enhancement
▶*methoxsalen* **(C)** Apply to well-defined area of vitiligo; then expose area to source of UVA (ultraviolet A) or sunlight; initial exposure no more than 1/2 predicted minimal erythemal dose; repeat weekly
   Pediatric: <12 years: not recommended
   Oxsoralen® *Lotn:* 1% (30 ml)

Vitiligo

Comment: Methoxsalen may only be applied by a healthcare provider. Do not dispense to patient.

▶*trioxsalen* **(C)** 10 mg daily, taken 2-4 hours before ultraviolet light exposure; max 14 days and 28 tabs

    Pediatric: <12 years: not recommended

Trisoralen® *Tab:* 5 mg

Depigmenting Agents *see Hyperpigmentation page 212*

Wart: Common (*Verruca vulgaris*)

▶*salicylic acid* **(NR)(G)**
    DuoFilm® (OTC) apply daily-bid; max 12 weeks; *Liq:* 17% (1/2 oz w. applicator)
    DuoFilm®Patch for Kids (OTC) apply 1 patch q 48 hours; max 12 weeks
        Patch: 40% (18/pck)
    Occlusal®HP (OTC) apply daily-bid; max 12 weeks
        Liq: 17% (10 ml w. applicator)
    Wart-Off® (OTC) apply one drop at a time to sufficiently cover wart, let dry; repeat 1-2 times daily; max 12 weeks
        Liq: 17% (0.45 oz)

Wart: Plantar (*Verruca plantaris*)

▶*salicylic acid* **(NR)(G)**
    DuoPlant®Gel (OTC) apply daily-bid; max 12 weeks
        Gel: 17% (1/2 oz)
    Mediplast® cut to size of wart and apply; remove q 1-2 days, peel keratin, and reapply; repeat as long as needed
    Occlusal®-HP (OTC) apply daily-bid; max 12 weeks
        Liq: 17% (10 ml w. applicator)
    Wart-Off® (OTC) apply one drop at a time to sufficiently cover wart, let dry; repeat 1-2 times daily; max 12 weeks
        Liq: 17% (0.45 oz)

▶*trichloroacetic acid* **(NR)** apply after wart is pared and repeat weekly

Warts: Venereal
(Human Papilloma Virus [HPV], Condyloma Acuminata)

Comment: Due to the increased risk of cervical cancer with HPV, Pap smears should be done q 3 months during active disease and then q 3-6 months for the next 2 years.

Patient-applied Agents
- ▶*imiquimod* **(B)** rub into lesion before bedtime and remove with soap and water 8 hours later; treat 3 times per week; max 16 weeks
    Aldara® *Crm:* 5% (250 mg single-use pkts; 12/box)
- ▶*podofilox* **(C)** apply bid (q 12 hours) x 3 days; then discontinue for 4 days; may repeat if needed; max treatment 4 cycles
    Pediatric: not recommended
    Condylox® *Soln:* 0.5% (3.5 ml); *Gel:* 0.5% (3.5 g)

Provider-administered Agents
- ▶*interferon alfa-n3* **(C)** 0.05 ml injected into base of wart twice weekly for up to 8 weeks; max 0.5 ml/session (20 warts/session)
    Alferon N® *Vial:* 5 million units/ml (1 ml)
- ▶*interferon alfa-2b* **(C)** 0.1 ml injected into base of wart three times weekly for up to 3 weeks; max 0.5 ml/session (5 warts/session)
    Intron A® *Vial:* 1 million units/0.1 ml (0.5, 1 ml)
- ▶*podophyllin* **(C)** 10-25% in tincture of benzoin apply directly to warts, leave on 1-4 hours, then wash off; repeat q 7 days if needed
    Podocon-25® *Liq:* 25% (15 ml w. applicator tip)

Comment: Contraindicated in pregnancy.

- ▶*trichloroacetic acid (TCA) 80-90%* apply to warts; repeat weekly if needed

Comment: Preferred treatment during pregnancy. Immediate application of sodium bicarbonate paste following treatment decreases pain.

Whipworm (*Trichuriasis*)

Anthelmintics
- ▶*albendazole* **(C)** 400 mg as a single dose; may repeat in 3 weeks; take after a meal
    Pediatric: <2 years: 200 mg daily x 3 days; may repeat in 3 weeks
    2-12 years: 400 mg daily x 3 days; may repeat in 3 weeks

Whipworm

Albenza® *Tab:* 200 mg
▶ *mebendazole* **(C)(G)** 100 mg bid x 3 days; may repeat in 2-3 weeks if needed; take after a meal
    Pediatric: same as adult (chew or crush and mix with food)
Vermox® *Chew tab:* 100 mg
▶ *pyrantel pamoate* **(C)** 11 mg/kg x 1 dose; max 1 g/dose; take after a meal
    Pediatric: 25-37 lb: 1/2 tsp x 1 dose
                38-62 lb: 1 tsp x 1 dose
                63-87 lb: 1½ tsp x 1 dose
                88-112 lb: 2 tsp x 1 dose
                113-137 lb: 2½ tsp x 1 dose
                138-162 lb: 3 tsp x 1 dose
                163-187 lb: 3½ tsp x 1 dose
                >187 lb: 4 tsp x 1 dose
Antiminth® **(OTC)** *Cap:* 180 mg; *Liq:* 50 mg/ml (30 ml); 144 mg/ml (30 ml); *Oral susp:* 50 mg/ml (60 ml)
Pin-X® **(OTC)** *Cap:* 180 mg; *Liq:* 50 mg/ml (30 ml); 144 mg/ml (30 ml); *Oral susp:* 50 mg/ml (30 ml)
▶ *thiabendazole* **(C)** 25 mg/kg bid x 7 days; max 1.5 g/dose; take after a meal
    Pediatric: same as adult
                <30 lb: consult mfr literature
                >30 lb 2 doses/day with meals
                30-50 lbs: 250 mg bid with meals
                >50 lb: 10 mg/lb/dose bid with meals; max 3g/day
Mintezol® *Chew tab:* 500*mg (orange); *Oral susp:* 500 mg/5 ml (120 ml; orange)
Comment: Thiabendazole is not for prophylaxis. May impair mental alertness.

Wound: Infected, Non-surgical, Minor

Tetanus Prophylaxis
Previously Immunized (within previous 5 years)
▶ *tetanus toxoid* vaccine **(C)** 0.5 ml IM x 1 dose
    Vial: 5 Lf units/0.5 ml (0.5, 5 ml); *Prefilled syringe:* 5 Lf units/0.5 ml (0.5 ml)
Not Previously Immunized, see **Tetanus** page 397
Topical Anti-infectives

▶ *mupirocin* **(B)(G)** apply to lesions bid
> *Pediatric:* same as adult

Bactroban® *Oint:* 2% (22 g); *Crm:* 2% (15, 30 g)
Centany® *Oint:* 2% (15, 30 g)

Oral Anti-infectives

▶ *azithromycin* **(B)** 500 mg x 1 dose on day 1, then 250 mg daily on days 2-5 or 500 mg daily x 3 days or **Zmax**® 2 g in a single dose
> *Pediatric: see page 573 for dose by weight*
> 10 mg/kg x 1 dose on day 1, then 5 mg/kg/day on days 2-5; max 500 mg/day

Zithromax® *Tab:* 250, 500 m; *Oral susp:* 100 mg/5 ml (15 ml); 200 mg/5 ml (15, 22.5, 30 ml) (cherry-vanilla-banana)
Zithromax®**Tri-pak** *Tab:* 3-500 mg tabs/pck
Zithromax®**Z-pak** *Tab:* 6-250 mg tabs/pck
Zmax® *Oral susp:* 2 g ext rel (cherry-banana)

▶ *amoxicillin/clavulanate* **(B)(G)** 500-875 mg bid or 250-500 mg tid x 10 days
> *Pediatric: see pages 571-572 for dose by weight*
> 40-45 mg/kg/day divided tid x 10 days or
> 90 mg/kg/day divided bid x 10 days

Augmentin® *Tab:* 250, 500, 875 mg; *Chew tab:* 125 mg (lemon-lime), 200 mg (cherry-banana, phenylalanine), 250 mg (lemon-lime), 400 mg (cherry-banana, phenylalanine); *Oral susp:* 125 mg/5 ml (banana), 250 mg/5 ml; (orange) (75, 100, 150 ml); 200 mg/5 ml, 400 mg/5 ml (50, 75, 100 ml; orange-raspberry, phenylalanine)
Augmentin®**ES-600** *Oral susp:* 600 mg/5 ml (50, 75, 100, 150 ml; orange-raspberry, phenylalanine)
Augmentin®**XR** 2 tabs q 12 hours x 10 days
> *Pediatric:* <16 years: use other forms
> *Tab:* 1000 mg ext-rel

▶ *cefaclor* **(B)(G)**
Ceclor® 250 mg tid or 375 mg bid x 10 days
> *Pediatric: see page 575 for dose by weight*
> 20-40 mg/kg/day in 3 doses x 10 days
> *Pulvule:* 250, 500 mg; *Oral susp:* 125, 250 mg/5 ml (75, 150 ml); 187, 375 mg/5 ml (50, 100 ml) (strawberry)

Ceclor®**CD** 500 mg q 12 hours x 10days
> *Pediatric:* <16 years: not recommended
> *Tab:* 375, 500 mg ext-rel

Ceclor®**CDpak** 500 mg q 12 hours x 10 days

Pediatric: <16 years: not recommended
Tab: 500 mg (14 tabs/CDpak)
Raniclor® 500 mg q 12 hours x 10 days
Pediatric: 20-40 mg/kg/day in 3 doses x 10 days
Chew tab: 125, 187, 250, 375 mg

▶ *cefadroxil* 1 g/day in 1-2 doses x 10 days
Pediatric: see page 576 for dose by weight
15-30 mg/kg/day in 2 doses x 10 days
Duricef® *Cap:* 500 mg; *Tab:* 1 g; *Oral susp:* 250 mg/5 ml (100 ml); 500 mg/5 ml (75, 100 ml); (orange-pineapple)

▶ *cefdinir* **(B)** 300 mg bid or 600 mg daily x 10 days
Pediatric: see page 574 for dose by weight
<6 months: not recommended
6 months-12 years: 14 mg/kg/day in 1-2 doses x 10 days
Omnicef® *Cap:* 300 mg; *Oral susp:* 125 mg/5 ml (60, 100 ml; (strawberry)

▶ *cefpodoxime proxetil* **(B)** 400 mg bid x 7-14 days
Pediatric: see page 578 for dose by weight
<2 months: not recommended
2 months-12 years: 10 mg/kg/day (max 400 mg/dose) or 5 mg/kg/day bid (max 200 mg/dose) x 7-14 days
Vantin® *Tab:* 100, 200 mg; *Oral susp:* 50, 100 mg/5 ml (50, 75, 100 mg; lemon-creme)

▶ *cefprozil* **(B)** 250-500 mg q 12 hours or 500 mg daily x 10 days
Pediatric: see page 579 for dose by weight
2-12 years: 7.5 mg/kg bid x 10 days
Cefzil® *Tab:* 250, 500 mg; *Oral susp:* 125, 250 mg/5 ml (50, 75, 100 ml; bubble gum, phenylalanine)

▶ *cephalexin* **(B)(G)** 2 g 1 hour before procedure
Pediatric: see page 582 for dose by weight
50 mg/kg/day in 4 doses x 10 days
Keflex® *Cap:* 250, 500, 750 mg; *Oral susp:* 125, 250 mg/5 ml (100, 200 ml)
Keftab® *Tab:* 500 mg
Keftab®K-pak *Tab:* 20-500 mg tabs/K-pak

▶ *clarithromycin* **(C)(G)** 500 mg or 500 mg ext-rel 1 hour before procedure
Pediatric: see page 584 for dose by weight

Biaxin® *Tab:* 250, 500 mg
Biaxin®Oral Suspension *Oral susp:* 125, 250 mg/5 ml (50, 100 ml; fruit-punch)
Biaxin®XL *Tab:* 500 mg ext-rel

▶ *dirithromycin* **(C)** 500 mg daily x 7 days
　　Pediatric: <12 years: not recommended
　Dynabac® *Tab:* 250 mg

▶ *erythromycin base* **(B)(G)** 500 mg qid x 14 days
　　Pediatric: see page 588 for dose by weight
　　　　30-50 mg/kg/day in 2-4 doses x 10 days
　E-Mycin® *Tab:* 250 mg; 333 mg ent-coat
　Eryc® *Cap:* 250 mg ent-coat
　Ery-Tab® *Tab:* 250, 333, 500 mg ent-coat
　PCE® *Tab:* 333, 500 mg

▶ *levofloxacin* **(C)**
　Uncomplicated: 500 mg daily x 7 days
　Complicated: 750 mg daily x 7 days
　　Pediatric: <18 years: not recommended
　Levaquin® *Tab:* 250, 500, 750 mg

▶ *loracarbef* **(B)** 200-400 mg bid x 7 days
　　Pediatric: see page 593 for dose by weight
　　　　15 mg/kg/day in 2 doses x 7 days
　Lorabid® *Pulvule:* 200, 400 mg; *Oral susp:* 100 mg/5 ml (50, 100 ml); 200 mg/5 ml (50, 75, 100 ml); (strawberry bubble gum)

▶ *ofloxacin* **(C)** 400 mg bid x 10 days
　　Pediatric: <18 years: not recommended
　Floxin® *Tab:* 200, 300, 400 mg

Wrinkles: Facial
(Crow's Feet, Frown Lines, Smile Lines)

Topical Retinoids
Comment: Wash affected area with a soap-free cleanser; pat dry and wait 20 to 30 minutes; then apply sparingly to affected area. Use only once daily in the PM. Avoid eyes, ears, nostrils, and mouth.

▶ *adapalene* **(C)**
　　Pediatric: <12 years: not recommended
　Differin® *Crm:* 0.1% (15, 45 g); *Gel:* 0.1% (15, 45 g); *Pad:* 0.1% (30/pk; alcohol 30%)
　Differin®Solution *Soln:* 0.1% (30 ml; alcohol 30%)

Wrinkles: Facial

▶*tazarotene* **(X)** apply daily at HS
    Pediatric: not recommended
  Avage®Cream *Crm:* 0.1% (5, 30 g)
  Tazorac®Cream *Crm:* 0.05, 0.1% (15, 30, 60 g)
  Tazorac®Gel *Gel:* 0.05, 0.1% (30, 100 g)
▶*tretinoin* **(C)** apply daily at HS
    Pediatric: <12 years: not recommended
  Avita® *Crm/Gel:* 0.025% (20, 45 g)
  Renova® *Crm:* 0.02% (40 g); 0.05% (40, 60 g)
  Retin-A®Cream *Crm:* 0.025, 0.05, 0.1% (20, 45 g)
  Retin-A®Gel *Gel:* 0.01, 0.025% (15, 45 g; alcohol 90%)
  Retin-A®Liquid *Liq:* 0.05% (28 ml; alcohol 55%)
  Retin-A®Micro Microspheres: 0.04, 0.1% (20, 45 g)

Comment: Effective for mitigation of fine wrinkles, mottled hyperpigmentation, and tactile roughness of skin. No mitigating effect on deep wrinkles, skin yellowing, letigines, telangiectasia, skin laxity, keratinocytic atypia, melanocytic atypia, or dermal elastosis. Avoid sun exposure. Cautious use of concomitant astringents, alcohol-based products, sulfur-containing products, salicylic acid-containing products, soap, and other topical agents.

Xerosis

Moisturizing Agents
  Aquaphor®Healing Ointment (OTC) *Oint:* 1.75, 3.5, 14 oz (alcohol)
  Eucerin®Daily Sun Defense (OTC) *Lotn:* 6 oz (fragrance-free)

Comment: **Eucerin®Daily Sun Defense** is a moisturizer with SPF 15 sunscreen.

  Eucerin®Facial Lotion (OTC) *Lotn:* 4 oz
  Eucerin®Light Lotion (OTC) *Lotn:* 8 oz
  Eucerin®Lotion (OTC) *Lotn:* 8, 16 oz
  Eucerin®Original Creme (OTC) *Crm:* 2, 4, 16 oz (alcohol)
  Eucerin®Plus Creme *Crm:* 4 oz
  Eucerin®Plus Lotion (OTC) *Lotn:* 6, 12 oz
  Eucerin®Protective Lotion (OTC) *Lotn:* 4 oz (alcohol)

Comment: **Eucerin®Protective** is a moisturizer with SPF 25 sunscreen.

  Lac-Hydrin®Cream (OTC) *Crm:* 280, 385 g
  Lac-Hydrin®Lotion (OTC) *Lotn:* 225, 400 g
  Lubriderm®Dry Skin Scented (OTC) *Lotn:* 6, 10, 16, 32 oz
  Lubriderm®Dry Skin Unscented (OTC) *Lotn:* 3.3, 6, 10, 16 oz (fragrance-free)
  Lubriderm®Sensitive Skin Lotion (OTC) *Lotn:* 3.3, 6, 10, 16 oz

(lanolin-free)
Lubriderm®Dry Skin (OTC) *Lotn:* 2.5, 6, 10, 16 oz (scented); *Lotn:* 1, 2.5, 6, 10, 16 oz (fragrance-free)
Lubriderm®Bath & Shower Oil (OTC) 1-2 capsful in bath or rub onto wet skin as needed, then rinse
Oil: 8 oz
Moisturel® apply as needed
Crm: 4, 16 oz; *Lotn:* 8, 12 oz; *Clnsr:* 8.75 oz

Topical Oil
▶*fluocinolone acetomide* 0.01% topical oil **(C)**
Pediatric: <6 years: not recommended
>6 years: apply sparingly bid for up to 4 weeks
Derma-Smoothe®/FS Topical Oil apply sparingly tid
Topical oil: 0.01% (4 oz; peanut oil)

Zollinger-Ellison Syndrome

Proton Pump Inhibitors
Comment: If hepatic impairment, or if patient is Asian, consider reducing the PPI dosage.
▶*esomeprazole* **(B)** 20-40 mg daily; max 8 weeks
Pediatric: not recommended
Nexium® *Cap:* 20, 40 mg del-rel
▶*lansoprazole* **(B)** 15-30 mg daily
Pediatric: <12 years: not recommended
Prevacid® *Cap:* 15, 30 mg ent-coat del-rel granules; may open and sprinkle; do not chew
Prevacid®for Oral Suspension *Oral susp:* 15, 30 mg ent-coat del-rel granules/pkt; mix in 2 tblsp water and drink immediately; 30 pkt/box (strawberry)
Prevacid®SoluTab *Tab:* 15, 30 mg orally disintegrating
▶*omeprazole* **(C)** initially 60 daily; adjust up to 120 mg tid; if >80 mg/day give in divided doses
Pediatric: not recommended
Prilosec® (OTC) *Cap:* 10, 20, 40 mg ent-coat del-rel granules; may open and sprinkle
▶*pantoprazole* **(B)** initially 40 mg bid; max 240 mg/day
Pediatric: not recommended
Protonix® *Tab:* 40 mg ent-coat del-rel

Zollinger-Ellison Syndrome

▶ *rabeprazole* **(B)** initially 60 mg daily; then titrate; may give in divided doses; max 100 mg daily or 60 mg bid
    Pediatric: not recommended
  AcipHex® (OTC) *Tab:* 20 mg ent-coat del-rel

SECTION II

APPENDIXES

Appendix A: FDA Pregnancy Categories

Category	Description
A	Controlled studies in women have failed to demonstrate risk to the fetus in the first trimester of pregnancy and there is no evidence of risk in later trimesters.
B	Animal reproduction studies have not demonstrated risk to the fetus, but there are no controlled studies in pregnant women, or animal studies have demonstrated an adverse effect, but controlled studies in pregnant women have not documented risk to the fetus in the first trimester of pregnancy and there is no evidence of risk in later trimesters.
C	Risk to the fetus cannot be ruled out. Animal reproduction studies have demonstrated adverse effects on the fetus (i.e., teratogenic or embryocidal effects or other) but there are no controlled studies in pregnant women or controlled studies in women and animals are not available.
D	There is positive evidence of human fetal risk, but benefits from use by pregnant women may be acceptable despite the potential risk (e.g. if the drug is needed in a life-threatening situation or for a serious disease for which safer drugs cannot be used or are ineffective.
X	Studies in animals or humans have demonstrated fetal abnormalities or there is evidence of fetal risk based on human experience, or both, and the risk of using the drug in pregnant women clearly outweighs any possible benefit. The drug is contraindicated in women who are pregnant or who may become pregnant.

Appendix B: U.S. Schedule of Controlled Substances

Schedule	Description
I	High potential for abuse and of no currently accepted medical use. Not obtainable by prescription, but may be legally procured for research, study, <u>or</u> instructional use. (Examples: *heroin, LSD, marijuana, mescaline, peyote*)
II	High abuse potential and high liability for severe psychological <u>or</u> physical dependence potential. Prescription required and cannot be refilled. Prescription must be written in ink <u>or</u> typed and signed. A verbal prescription may be allowed in an emergency by the dispensing pharmacist, but must be followed by a written prescription within 72 hours. Includes opium derivatives, other opioids, and short-acting barbiturates.
III	Potential for abuse is less than that for drugs in schedules I and II. Moderate to low physical dependence and high psychological dependence potential. Prescription required. May be refilled up to 5 times in 6 months. Prescription may be verbal (telephone) <u>or</u> written. Includes certain stimulants and depressants not included in the above schedules, and preparations containing limited quantities of certain opioids.
IV	Lower potential for abuse than Schedule III drugs. Prescription required. May be refilled up to 5 times in 6 months. Prescription may be verbal (telephone) <u>or</u> written.

Schedule	Description
V	Abuse potential less than that for Schedule IV drugs. Preparations contain limited quantities of certain narcotic drugs. Generally intended for antitussive and antidiarrheal purposes and may be distributed without a prescription provided that: 1. such distribution is made only by a pharmacist; 2. not more than 240 ml <u>or</u> not more than 48 solid dosage units of any substance containing opium, nor more than 120 ml <u>or</u> not more than 24 solid dosage units of any other controlled substance may be distributed at retail to the same purchaser in any given 48-hour period without a valid prescription order; 3. the purchaser is at least 18 years old; 4. the pharmacist knows the purchaser <u>or</u> requests suitable identification; 5. the pharmacist keeps an official written record of: name and address of purchaser, name and quantity of controlled substance purchased, date of sale, initials of dispensing pharmacist. This record is to be made available for inspection and copying by the U.S. officers authorized by the Attorney General; 6. other federal, state, <u>or</u> local law does not require a prescription order. Under jurisdiction of the Federal Controlled Substances Act. Refillable up to 5 times within 6 months.

Appendix C: JNC-VII Hypertension Evaluation & Treatment Recommendations

Appendix C.1: Blood Pressure Classification

Classification	SBP mmHg		DBP mmHg
Normal	<120	and	<80
Prehypertension	120-139	or	80-89
Hypertension, Stage 1	140-159	or	90-99
Hypertension, Stage 2	≥160	or	≥100

Appendix C.2: Identifiable Causes of Hypertension

Sleep apnea
Chronic kidney disease
Primary aldosteronism
Renovascular disease
Excess sodium ingestion
Herbal supplements
Cushing's syndrome or steroid therapy
Pheochromocytoma
Coarctation of the aorta
Thyroid or parathyroid disease
Excess alcohol consumption
Drugs (illicit, oral contraceptives, NSAIDs, sympathomimetics)

Appendix C.3 CVD Risk Factors

Hypertension
Obesity (BMI ≥30 kg/m^2)
Dyslipidemia
Diabetes Mellitus
Cigarette smoking
Physical inactivity
Microalbuminuria, estimated GFR <60 mL/min
Age (men >55 yrs, women >65 yrs)
Family History of premature CVD (men <55 yrs, women <65 yrs)

Appendix C.4: Diagnostic Workup of Hypertension

Assess risk factors and co-morbidities
Reveal identifiable causes of hypertension
Assess for presence of target organ damage
History and physical examination
Urinalysis, blood glucose, hematocrit, lipid panel, potassium, creatinine, calcium, (*optional* urine albumin/Cr ratio), EKG

Appendix C.5: Compelling Indications for Individual Drug Classes

Heart Failure
- Thiazide Diuretic
- Beta Blocker
- Angiotensin Converting Enzyme Inhibitor
- Angiotensin Receptor Blocker
- Aldosterone Antagonist

Post Myocardial Infarction
- Beta Blocker
- Angiotensin Converting Enzyme Inhibitor
- Aldosterone Antagonist

High Risk for Cardiovascular Disease (CVD)
- Thiazide Diuretic
- Beta Blocker
- Angiotensin Converting Enzyme Inhibitor
- Calcium Channel Blocker

Diabetes Mellitus
- Thiazide Diuretic
- Beta Blocker
- Angiotensin Converting Enzyme Inhibitor
- Angiotensin Receptor Blocker
- Calcium Chanel Blocker

Chronic Kidney Disease
- Angiotensin Converting Enzyme Inhibitor
- Angiotensin Receptor Blocker

Recurrent Stroke Prevention
- Thiazide Diuretic
- ACE Inhibitor

Appendix C.6: Initial Drug Choices Without Compelling Indications

Stage 1 Hypertension	Stage 2 Hypertension
Thiazide diuretic for most; may consider an ACEI, ARB, BB, CCB, <u>or</u> a combination	2-drug combination for most (usually thiazide-type <u>and</u> ACEI, <u>or</u> ARB, <u>or</u> BB, <u>or</u> CCB)

Appendix D: Target Lipid Recommendations

Appendix D.A: Target TC, TG, HDL-C	
Total Cholesterol	<200 mg/dL
Triglycerides	<150 mg/dL
High Density Lipoproteins (HDL)	>40 mg/dL (male) >45 mg/dL (female)

Appendix D.B: Target LDL-C†			
Risk Assessment††	**LDL Target**	**Initiate TLC†††**	**Initiate Drug Therapy**
0 - 1	<160 mg/dL	≥160 mg/dL	≥190 mg/dL *optional* at 160-189 mg/dL
2 or more plus 10 year risk <10%	<130 mg/dL	≥130 mg/dL	≥160 mg/dL
2 or more plus 10 year risk <20%	<130 mg/dL <100 mg/dL optional	≥130 mg/dL	≥130 mg/dL
CHD or CHD risk equivalents 10 year risk >20%	<100 mg/dL <70 mg/dL optional	≥100 mg/dL	≥100 mg/dL

† Treatment decisions based on LDL cholesterol
†† Risk factors include age (men ≥45 years and women ≥55 years)
††† Therapeutic Lifestyle Changes (e.g., exercise, weight loss, low fat diet)

Adapted from the National Cholesterol Education Program Expert Panel on Detection, Evaluation, and Treatment of High Blood Cholesterol in Adults (Adult Treatment Panel III, 2004).

Appendix E: Effects of Selected Drugs on Insulin Activity

Hyper- and Hypo-glycemic Drug Effects	
Drugs that May Cause Hyperglycemia	**Drugs that May Cause Hypoglycemia**
Calcium channel blockers Thiazide diuretics Glucocorticosteroids Nicotinic acid Oral contraceptives Phenytoin Sympathomimetics Diazoxide	Alcohol Beta-blockers MAO inhibitors Salicylates NSAIDs Warfarin Phenylbutazone

Appendix F: Glycosolated Hemoglobin (HbA$_{1C}$) & Average Blood Glucose Equivalent

HbA$_{1C}$ and Average Blood Glucose Equivalent			
HbA$_{1C}$	**GLU**	**HbA$_{1C}$**	**GLU**
4%	60 mg/dL	14%	360 mg/dL
5%	90 mg/dL	15%	390 mg/dL
6%	120 mg/dL	16%	420 mg/dL
7%	150 mg/dL	17%	450 mg/dL
8%	180 mg/dL	18%	480 mg/dL
9%	210 mg/dL	19%	510 mg/dL
10%	240 mg/dL	20%	540 mg/dL
11%	270 mg/dL	21%	570 mg/dL
12%	300 mg/dL	22%	600 mg/dL
13%	330 mg/dL	23%	630 mg/dL

Appendix G: Childhood Immunizations

Comment:
- Prior to age 1 yr, administer IM vaccinations in the vastus lateralis muscle.
- After age 1 yr, administer IM vaccinations in the deltoid muscle and SC vaccinations in the posterolateral upper arm.
- The **HBV** (hepatitis B virus) 3-dose series is initiated at birth. Administer 2nd dose at 1-2 months. Administered the 3rd dose at age ≥ 24 weeks.
- Infants born to HVsAG-positive mothers should be tested for HBsAG and antibody to HBsAg after completion of the **HBV** series (at age 9-18 months).
- **DTaP** (diphtheria, tetanus toxoid, acellular pertussis); minimum age 6 wks.
- **IPV** (inactivated poliovirus vaccine); minimum age 4 wks.
- **Hib** (*hemophilus influenzae* type b conjugate vaccine); minimum age 6 mos.
- **MMR** (measles, mumps, rubella); minimum age 12 mos.
- **Td** (tetanus and Diphtheria toxoid); minimum age ≥ 7 yrs.
- **Var** (*varicella* vaccine); minimum age 12 mos.
- **Var** should be offered to children at age 11-12 years who have not had chickenpox. After age 12 yrs, give 2 doses at least 4 weeks apart.
- **PCV** (pneumococcal vaccine); minimum age 6 wks.
- **DTaP** and **IPV** can be initiated as early as 4 weeks in areas of high endemicity or outbreak.
- **DTaP** and **IPV** should be administered at or before school entry.
- An all-**IPV** schedule is recommended to eliminate the risk of vaccine-associated paralytic polio (VAPP) associated with OPV.
- **MMR** should be administered at 12 months in high-risk areas. If indicated, tuberculin testing can be done at the same visit.
- **MMR** should be administered at age 11-12 years unless 2 doses were given after the first birthday. The interval between doses should be at least 4 weeks.
- The 4th dose of **DTaP** vaccine can be administered as early as age 12 months, provided that the interval between doses 3 and 4 is at least 6 months.
- **Hib** is not recommended if age ≥ 5 years.
- **DTaP** should not be administered at or after the 7th birthday.
- Older infants and children previously vacccinated with **PCV** should receive 3 doses (if age 7-11 mos), 2 doses (if age 12-23 mos), or 1 dose (if age ≥ 24 mos).
- **PCV** does not replace 23-valent pneumococcal polysaccharide in children age ≥ 24 mos.
- **HBV** should be offered to all children who have not received the full series.
- **Td** should be repeated every 10 years throughout life (<u>or</u> if at-risk injury ≥ 5 years after previous dose).
- **HAV** vaccine is recommended for all children at 1 year (12-23 months) of age.
- The **HAV** 2-dose series should be administered at least 6 months apart
- **Men** should be administered to all children at the 11-12 year-old visit as well as to unvaccinated adolescents 15 years-of-age (usually at high school entry).

- **Men** should be administered to all college freshmen living in dormitories.
- Use MPSV4 for children aged 2-10 years and MCV4 for older children, although MPSV4 is an acceptable alternative for **men** prophylaxis.
- **Rotavirus vaccine** is a live attenuated oral vaccine for infants >6 weeks or <32 weeks *only*. Administer the 1st dose at 6-12 weeks of age; administer 2nd and 3rd doses at 4-10 week intervals for a total of 3 doses. If an incomplete dose is administered, *do not* administer a replacement dose, but continue with the remaining doses in the recommended series.
- Influenza vaccine should be administered annually.

Appendix G.1: Recommended Childhood Immunization Schedule											
Type	Birth	1 mo	2 mos	4 mos	6 mos	6-18 mos	12-15 mos	15-18 mos	4-6 yrs	11-12 yrs
HBV	▓	▓			▓					
DTaP			▓	▓	▓			▓	▓	
IPV			▓	▓		▓			▓	
Hib			▓	▓	▓		▓			
MMR							▓		▓	
Td										▓
Var							▓			
PVC			▓	▓	▓		▓			
HAV										
Men										▓

Shaded box=immunization due

Appendix G.2: Childhood Immunization Catch-up Schedule				
	← Minimum Interval Between Doses →			
Type	#1 to #2	#2 to #3	#3 to #4	#4 to #5
HBV	4 weeks	8 weeks (16 weeks after #1)		
DTaP	4 weeks	4 weeks	6 months	6 months
IPV	4 weeks	4 weeks	4 weeks	
MMR	4 weeks			
Var	4 weeks			
Rotavirus	4 weeks	4 weeks; do not administer >32 weeks of age		

PCV	4 weeks (if #1 at age <12 mo and current age <24 mo); 8 weeks (as last dose if #1 at age >12 mo <u>or</u> current age 24-59 mo); No more doses needed if healthy and #1 at age ≥24 mo	4 weeks if age <12 mo; 8 weeks (as last dose if age ≥12 mo); No more doses needed if healthy and previous dose at age ≥24 mo	8 weeks (as last dose; only necessary for age 12 mo-5 yr who received 3 doses before age 12 mo)	
Hib	4 weeks (if #1 at age <12 mo); 8 weeks (as last dose if #1 at age 12-14 mo); No more doses needed if healthy and #1 at age ≥15 mo	4 weeks if age 12 mo; 8 weeks (as last dose if age ≥12 mo); No more doses needed if previous dose at age ≥15 mo	8 weeks (as last dose; only necessary for age 12 mo-2 yr who received 3 doses before age 12 mo)	

Appendix G.3: Contraindications to Vaccines	
All vaccines	Previous anaphylactic reaction to the vaccine. Moderate <u>or</u> severe illness with <u>or</u> without fever.
DTP/DTaP	Encephalopathy within 7 days of administration of previous dose.
HBV	Anaphylactic reaction to baker's yeast.
Influenza	Allergy to eggs
IPV	Anaphylactic reaction to neomycin <u>or</u> streptomycin
Pneumococcal	Hypersensitivity to diphtheria toxoid
MMR	Pregnancy, immunodeficiency, anaphylactic reaction to eggs <u>or</u> neomycin
Meningococcal	
Rotavirus	<6 months <u>or</u> >32 months

Appendix G.4: Route of Administration and Dosage of Vaccines		
Vaccine	**Route**	**Dose**
HBV	IM	0.5 ml: age <20 mo 1.0 ml: age >20 mo
DTaP, Dtap, DTP	IM	0.5 ml
Hib	IM	0.5 ml
Influenza	IM	0.5 ml
MMR	SC	0.5 ml
Pneumococcal	IM/SC	0.5 ml
IPV	SC	0.5 ml
Td	IM	0.5 ml
Varicella	SC	0.5 ml
Meningococcal	SC/IM (*see pkg insert*)	0.5 ml
Rotavirus	PO	2 ml

Appendix G.5: Adverse Reactions to Vaccines		
Vaccine	**Signs & Symptoms**	**Treatment**
Inactivated antigens: DTP, Dtap, DTaP, Td, IPV Live attenuated viruses: MMR, Meningococcal, Rotavirus	Local tenderness Erythema Swelling Low-grade fever Drowsiness Fretfulness Decreased appetite Prolonged crying Unusual cry	*acetaminophen* <u>or</u> *ibuprofen* for age <u>and/or</u> weight; *aspirin* and *aspirin*-containing products are *contraindicated*

Appendix H: Contraceptives (Non-Barrier)

Comment:
- All oral and parenteral contraceptives are pregnancy category X.
- No oral or parenteral contraceptives protect against STDs.
- **Absolute contraindications**:
    - HTN >35 years-of-age
    - DM >35 years-of-age
    - LDL-C >160 or TG >250
    - Known or suspected pregnancy
    - Known or suspected carcinoma of the breast
    - Known or suspected carcinoma of the endometrium
    - Known or suspected estrogen-dependent neoplasia
    - Undiagnosed abnormal genital bleeding
    - Cerebral vascular or coronary artery disease
    - Cholestatic jaundice of pregnancy or jaundice with prior use
    - Hepatic adenoma or carcinoma or benign liver tumor
    - Active or past history of thrombophlebitis or thromboembolic disorder
- **Relative contraindications**:
    - Lactation
    - Asthma
    - Ulcerative colitis
    - Migraine or vascular headache
    - Cardiac or renal dysfunction
    - Gestational diabetes, pre-diabetes, diabetes mellitus
    - Diastolic BP 90 mmHg or greater or hypertension by any other criteria
    - Psychic depression
    - Varicose veins
    - Smoker >35 years-of-age
    - Sickle-cell or sickle-hemoglobin C disease
    - Cholestatic jaundice during pregnancy, active gallbladder disease
    - Hepatitis or mononucleosis during the preceding year
    - First-order family history of fatal or non-fatal rheumatic CVD or diabetes prior to age 50 years
    - Drug(s) with known interaction(s)
    - Elective surgery or immobilization within 4 weeks
    - Age >50 years
- Start the first pill on the first Sunday after menses begins. Thereafter, each new pill pack will be started on a Sunday.
- If 1 pill is missed, take it as soon as possible and the next pill at the regular time.

- If 2 pills are missed, take both pills as soon as possible and then two pills the following day. A barrier method should be used for the remainder of the pill pack.
- If 3 pills are missed before 10th cycle day, resume taking OCs on a regular schedule and take precautions.
- If 3 pills are missed after the 10th cycle day, discard the current pill pack and begin a new one 7 days after the last pill was taken.
- If very low-dose OCs are used or if combination OCs are begun after the 5th day of the menstrual cycle, an additional method of birth control should be used for the first 7 days of OC use.
- If nausea occurs as a side effect, select an OC with lower *estrogen* content.
- If breakthrough bleeding occurs during the first half of the cycle, select an OC with higher *progesterone* content.
- Symptoms of a serious nature include loss of vision, diplopia, unilateral numbness, weakness, or tingling, severe chest pain, severe pain in left arm or neck, severe leg pain, slurring of speech, and abdominal tenderness or mass.

Appendix H.1: Combined Oral Contraceptives

Combined Oral Contraceptive	Estrogen (mcg)	Progesterone (mg)
Alesse®-21, Alesse®-28 (X)(G) *ethinyl estradiol/levonorgestrel*	20	0.1
Apri® (X)(G) *ethinyl estradiol/desogestrel*	30	0.15
Aranelle® (X)(G) *ethinyl estradiol/norethindrone*	35	0.5
Aviane® (X)(G) *ethinyl estradiol/levonorgestrel*	20	0.1
Balziva (X)(G) *ethinyl estradiol/norethindrone*	35	0.4
Brevicon®-21, Brevicon®-28 (X) *ethinyl estradiol/norethindrone*	35	0.5
Cryselle® (X)(G) *ethinyl estradiol/norgestrel*	30	0.3
Cyclessa® (X)(G) *ethinyl estradiol/desogestrel*	25 25 25	0.1 0.125 0.15
Demulen®1/35-21, Demulen®1/35-28 (X)(G) *ethinyl estradiol/ethynodiol diacetate*	35	1
Demulen®1/50-21, Demulen®1/50-28 (X)(G) *ethinyl estradiol/ethynodiol diacetate*	50	1

Appendix H.1: Combined Oral Contraceptives

Combined Oral Contraceptive	Estrogen (mcg)	Progesterone (mg)
Desogen® (X)(G) *ethinyl estradiol/desogestrel diacetate*	30	0.15
Enpresse® (X)(G) *ethinyl estradiol/levonorgestrel*	30 40 30	0.050 0.075 0.125
Estrostep®Fe (X) *ethinyl estradiol/norethindrone* plus *ferrous fumarate* 75 mg	20 30 35	1 1 1
Junel®1/20 (X)(G) *ethinyl estradiol/norethindrone*	20	1
Junel®1.5/30 (X)(G) *ethinyl estradiol/norethindrone*	30	1.5
Junel®Fe 1/20 (X)(G) *ethinyl estradiol/norethindrone* plus *ferrous fumarate* 75 mg	20	1
Junel®Fe 1.5/30 (X)(G) *ethinyl estradiol/norethindrone* plus *ferrous fumarate* 75 mg	30	1.5
Jenest®-28 (X) *ethinyl estradiol/norethindrone*	35 35	0.5 1
Kariva® (X)(G) *ethinyl estradiol/desogestrel*	20 10	0.15
Kelnor®1/35 (X)(G) *ethinyl estradiol/ethynodiol diacetate*	35	1
Lessina®28 (X)(G) *ethinyl estradiol/levonorgestrel*	20	0.1
Levlen®21, Levlen®28 (X) *ethinyl estradiol/levonorgestrel*	30	0.15
Levlite®28 (X)(G) *ethinyl estradiol/levonorgestrel*	20	0.1
Levora®-21, Levora®-28 (X) *ethinyl estradiol/levonorgestrel*	30	0.15
Loestrin®1/20 (X)(G) *ethinyl estradiol/norethindrone*	20	1
Loestrin®1.5/30 (X)(G) *ethinyl estradiol/norethindrone*	30	1.5
Loestrin®Fe 1/20 (X)(G) *ethinyl estradiol/norethindrone* plus *ferrous fumarate* 75 mg	20	1
Loestrin®Fe 1.5/30 (X)(G) *ethinyl estradiol/norethindrone* plus *ferrous fumarate* 75 mg (4 tabs)	30	1.5

Appendix H.1: Combined Oral Contraceptives

Combined Oral Contraceptive	Estrogen (mcg)	Progesterone (mg)
Low-Ogestrel®-21, Low-Ogestrel®-28 (X)(G) *ethinyl estradiol/norgestrel*	30	0.3
Lo/Ovral®-21, Lo/Ovral®-28 (X)(G) *ethinyl estradiol/norgestrel*	30	0.3
Mircette® (X)(G) *ethinyl estradiol/desogestrel diacetate*	20 10	0.15
Microgestin®Fe 1/20 (X) *ethinyl estradiol/norethindrone* plus *ferrous fumarate* 75 mg	20	1
Microgestin®Fe 1.5/30 (X) *ethinyl estradiol/norethindrone* plus *ferrous fumarate* 75 mg	30	1.5
Modicon®0.5/35-28 (X)(G) *ethinyl estradiol/norethindrone*	35	0.5
Necon®0.5/35-21, Necon®0.5/35-28 (X) *ethinyl estradiol/norethindrone*	35	0.5
Necon®1/35-21, Necon®1/35-28 (X) *ethinyl estradiol/norethindrone*	35	0.5
Necon®10/11-21, Necon®10/11-28 (X) *ethinyl estradiol/norethindrone*	35 35	0.5 1
Necon®1/50-21, Necon®1/50-28 (X) *mestranol/norethindrone*	50	1
Nelova®0.5/35-21, Nelova®0.5/35-28 (X) *ethinyl estradiol/norethindrone*	35	0.5
Nelova®1/35-21, Nelova®1/35-28 (X) *ethinyl estradiol/norethindrone*	35	1
Nelova®10/11-21, Nelova®10/11-21-28) (X) *ethinyl estradiol/norethindrone*	35 35	0.5 1
Nelova®1/50-21, Nelova®1/50-28 (X) *mestranol/norethindrone*	50	1
Nordette®-21, Nordette®-28 (X)(G) *ethinyl estradiol/levonorgestrel*	30	0.15
Norethin®1/50 (X) *mestranol/norethindrone*	50	1
Norinyl®1+35-21, Norinyl®1+35-28 (X) *ethinyl estradiol/norethindrone*	35	1
Norinyl®1+50-21, Norinyl®1+50-28 (X) *mestranol/norethindrone*	50	1
Nortrel®0.5/35 (X)(G) *ethinyl estradiol/norethindrone*	35	0.5
Nortrel®1/35-21, Nortrel®1/35-28 (X)(G) *ethinyl estradiol/norethindrone*	35	1

Appendix H.1: Combined Oral Contraceptives		
Combined Oral Contraceptive	Estrogen (mcg)	Progesterone (mg)
Nortrel®7/7/7-28 (X)(G) *ethinyl estradiol/norethindrone*	35 35 35	0.5 0.75 1
Ortho-Cept®28 (X)(G) *ethinyl estradiol/desogestrel*	30	0.15
Ortho-Cyclen®28 (X)(G) *ethinyl estradiol/norgestimate*	35	0.25
Ortho-Novum®1/35-21, Ortho-Novum® 1/35-28 (X)(G) *ethinyl estradiol/norethindrone*	35	1
Ortho-Novum®1/50-21, Ortho-Novum®1/50-28 *mestranol/norethindrone*	50	1
Ortho-Novum®7/7/7-28 (X)(G) *ethinyl estradiol/norethindrone*	35 35 35	0.5 0.75 1
Ortho-Novum®10/11-28 *ethinyl estradiol/norethindrone*	35 35	0.5 1
Ortho Tri-Cyclen®21, Ortho Tri-Cyclen ®28 (X)(G) *ethinyl estradiol/norgestimate*	35 35 35	0.18 0.215 0.25
Ortho Tri-Cyclen®Lo (X) *ethinyl estradiol/norgestimate*	25 25 25	0.18 0.215 0.25
Ovcon®35 Chewable (X) *ethinyl estradiol/norethindrone*	35	0.4
Ovcon®35-21, Ovcon®35-28 (X) *ethinyl estradiol/norethindrone*	35	0.4
Ovcon®50-28, Ovcon®50-28 (X) *ethinyl estradiol/norethindrone*	50	1
Ovral®-21, Ovral®-28 (X) *ethinyl estradiol/norgestrel*	50	0.5
Portia® (X)(G) *ethinyl estradiol/levonorgestrel*	30	0.15
Sprintec®28 (X)(G) *ethinyl estradiol/norgestimate*	35	0.25
Tri-Levlen®21, Tri-Levlen®28 (X) *ethinyl estradiol/levonorgestrel*	30 40 30	0.05 0.075 0.125
Tri-Norinyl®21, Tri-Norinyl®28 (X)(G) *ethinyl estradiol/norethindrone*	35 35 35	0.5 1 0.5

Appendix H.1: Combined Oral Contraceptives

Combined Oral Contraceptive	Estrogen (mcg)	Progesterone (mg)
Triphasil®-21, Triphasil®-28 (X)(G) *ethinyl estradiol/levonorgestrel*	30 40 30	0.050 0.075 0.125
Tri-Sprintec® (X)(G) *ethinyl estradiol/norgestimate*	35 35 35	0.18 0.215 0.25
Trivora® (X) *ethinyl estradiol/levonorgestrel*	30 40 30	0.05 0.075 0.125
Velivet® (X)(G) *ethinyl estradiol/desogestrel*	25 25 25	0.1 0.125 0.15
Yasmin® (X) *ethinyl estradiol/drospirenone*	30	3
Yaz® (X) *ethinyl estradiol/drospirenone*	20	3
Zovia®1/35-21, Zovia®1/35-28 (X) *ethinyl estradiol/ethynodiol diacetate*	35	1
Zovia®1/50-21, Zovia®1/50-28 (X) *ethinyl estradiol/ethynodiol diacetate*	50	1

Appendix H.2: 91 day Combined (Extended Cycle) Oral Contraceptives

▶ *ethinyl estradiol/levonorgestrel* **(X)** 1 tab daily x 91 days; repeat
  Jolessa® (G)*Tab: levonorgest* 15 mcg/*eth est* 30 mcg (84)
  + inert tabs (7) (91 tabs/pck)
  Quasense® *Tab: levonorgest* 15 mcg/*eth est* 30 mcg (84)
  + inert tabs (7) (91 tabs/pck)
  Seasonale® *Tab: levonorgest* 15 mcg/*eth est* 30 mcg (84)
  + inert tabs (7) (91 tabs/pck)
  Seasonique® *Tab: levnorgest* 15 mcg/*eth est* 30 mcg (84)
  + *eth est* 10 mcg (7) (91 tabs/pck)

Appendix H.2: Progesterone-only Contraceptives ("Mini-Pill")

Brand	Progesterone	mcg
Comment: Take progestin-only pills at the same time each day (within 3 hours). If a pill is missed, another method of contraception should be used for the remainder of the pill pack.		
Camila®	*norethindrone* **(X)(G)**	35
Errin®	*norethindrone* **(X)(G)**	35
Micronor®	*norethindrone* **(X)(G)**	35
Nor-QD®	*norethindrone* **(X)(G)**	35
Ovrette®	*norgestrel* **(X)**	7.5

Appendix H.3: Injectable Contraceptives

Injectable Progesterone

▶*medroxyprogesterone* **(X)**
    Depo-Provera® 150 mg deep IM q 3 months
        Vial: 150 mg/ml (1 ml)
        Prefilled syringe: 150 mg/ml
    Depo-SubQ® 104 mg SC q 3 months
        Prefilled syringe: 104 mg/ml (0.65 ml; parabens)

Comment: Administer first dose within 5 days of onset of normal menses, within 5 days postpartum if not breastfeeding, or at 6 weeks postpartum if breast-feeding exclusively. Do not use for >2 years unless other methods are inadequate.

Injectable Progesterone/Estradiol

▶*medroxyprogesterone/estradiol* **(X)**
    Lunelle®Monthly Contraceptive Injection 0.5 ml deep IM into deltoid, gluteous maximus, or anterior thigh q 28-30 days
        Vial: medroxy 250 mcg/*est* 50 mcg per 0.5 ml (0.5 ml)

Comment: Administer first dose within 5 days of onset of normal menses or a complete first-trimester abortion. Administer no earlier than 4 weeks postpartum if not breastfeeding or 6 weeks if breastfeeding. Administer within 7 days of last active pill when switching from an oral to an injectible contraceptive. Maximum 33 days between doses. Pregnancy test is required if more than 13 weeks since last injection. Mechanism of action: suppresses LH surge which suppresses ovulation. Side effect: scant to absent menses.

Appendix H.4: Transdermal Contraceptive
Ethinyl Estradiol/Norelgestromin

▶ *ethinyl estradio/norelgestromin* **(X)** apply one patch once weekly x 3 weeks; then 1 patch-free week; then repeat

Ortho Evra® *Transdermal patch:* eth est 20 mcg/*norel* 150 mcg per day (1, 3/pck)

Comment: Apply the transdermal patch to the abdomen, buttock, upper-outer arm, or upper torso. Do not apply the transdermal patch to the breast. Rotate the site (however, may use the same anatomical area).

Appendix H.5: Contraceptive Vaginal Ring
Etonogestrel/Ethinyl Estradiol

▶ *etonogestrel/ethinyl estradiol* **(X)** insert 1 ring vaginally and leave in place for 3 weeks; then remove for 1 ring-free week; the repeat

NuvaRing® *Vag ring:* eton 120 mcg/*eth est* 15 mcg per day (1, 3/pck)

Comment: The vaginal ring should be inserted prior to, or on 5th day, of the menstrual cycle. Use of a back up method is recommended during the first week. When switching from oral contraceptives, the vaginal ring should be inserted anytime within 7 days after the last active tablet and no later than the day a new pill pack would have been started (no back up method is needed). If the ring is accidently expelled for less than 3 hours, it should be rinsed with cool to lukewarm water and reinserted promptly. If ring removal lasts for more than 3 hours, an additional contraceptive method should be used. If the ring is lost, a new ring should be inserted and the regimen continued without alteration.

Appendix H.6: Subdermal Contraceptive
Levonorgestrel

▶ *levonorgestrel* **(X)** 6-36 mg (total 216 mg) implants subdermally; remove and replace q 5 years
Norplant® *Implants:* 6-36 mg implants (total 216 mg) for subdermal insertion (1 kit w/ sterile supplies)

Comment: Implants must be inserted within 7 days of the onset of menses. A complete physical examination is required annually. Remove if pregnancy, thromboembolic disorder including thrombophlebitis, jaundice, visual disturbances. Not for use by patients with hypertension, diabetes, hyperlipidemia, impaired liver function, epilepsy, asthma, migraine, depression, cardiac or renal insufficiency, thromboembolic disorder including thrombophlebitis, prolonged immobilization, or who are smokers.

Appendix H.7: Emergency Contraception

Comment: Emergency contraception must be started within 72 hours after unprotected intercourse following a negative urine hCG pregnancy test. If vomiting occurs within 1 hour of taking a dose, repeat the dose.

▶ *ethinyl estradiol/levonorgestrel* **(X)**
Preven® 2 tabs as soon as possible after unprotected intercourse, then 2 more 12 hours after first dose
Tab: eth est 50 mcg/lev 250 mcg (4/pck)
Pregnancy test: 1 hCG home pregnancy test
Yuzpe Regimen® *Tab:* eth est 50 mcg/lev 250 mcg (4/pck)
▶ *levonorgestrel* **(X)**
Plan B® 1 tab as soon as possible after unprotected intercourse and 1 tab 12 hours after first dose
Tab: lev 0.75 mg (2/pck)
Pregnancy test: 1 hCG home pregnancy test

Brand	# Pills/Dose (2 doses 12 hrs apart)	*ethinyl estradiol* mcg/dose	Progestin mcg/dose
Alesse®	5 pink	100	500*
Aviane®	5 orange	100	500*
Cryselle®	4 white	120	1200*

Brand	# Pills/Dose (2 doses 12 hrs apart)	*ethinyl estradiol* mcg/dose	Progestin mcg/dose
Lessina®	5 pink	100	500*
Levlen®	4 light orange	120	600*
Levlite®	5 pink	120	600*
Levora®	4 white	120	600*
Lo-Ovral®	4 white	120	1200*
Nordette®	4 light orange	120	600*
Ovral®	2 white	100	500**
Portia®	4 pink	120	600*
Preven®	2 blue	100	500*
Tri-Levlen®	4 yellow	120	500*
Triphasal®	4 yellow	120	500*
Trivora®	4 pink	120	500*

* *levonorgestrel*
** *norgestrel*

Appendix I: Anesthetic Agents for Local infiltration & Dermal/Mucosal Membrane Application

Anesthetic Agents and Indications	
Brand/*generic*	**Indication(s)**
Anamantle®HC *lidocaine 3%/hydrocortisone 0.5%*	Hemorrhoids, pruritis ani, anal fissure; apply bid
Decadron®Phosphate with Xylocaine® *dexamethasone 4 mg/lidocaine 10 mg/ml (5 ml)*	Local infiltration by injection
Dyclone®0.5%, 1% *dyclonine 0.5%, 0.1%*	Local infiltration by injection
Duranest® *etidocaine 1%*	Mouth, pharynx, larynx, trachea, esophagus, anogenital area, urethra
Duranest®with Epinephrine *etidocaine 1% with 1:200,000 epinephrine*	Local infiltration by injection
Ela-Max®4% Cream *lidocaine 4%*	Minor wounds, burns, injections, minor procedures, insect bites
Ela-Max®5% Cream *lidocaine 5%*	Anorectal irritation and pain
Emla®Cream, Emla®Anesthetic Disc *lidocaine 2.5%/prilocaine 2.5%*	Intact skin, external genital mucous membranes
LidaMantle® *lidocaine 3% adhesive patch* **Lidoderm®** *lidocaine 5% adhesive patch*	Adhesive patch for abrasion, minor burn, pruritis, postherpetic neuralgia; max 12 out of 24 hours
Ophthaine® *proparacaine 0.5% ophthalmic solution*	Examination/removal of foreign body (eye)
Synera®Topical Patch *lidocaine 70 mg/tetracaine 70 mg*	Local dermal analgesic for venous access or skin lesion removal
Xylocaine®Jelly (5, 10, 20, 30 ml) *lidocaine 2% aqueous*	For painful Urethritis
Xylocaine®Ointment (3.5, 35 g) *lidocaine 5% water miscible*	For the oropharyngeal mucosa
Xylocaine®Viscous (50 ml) *lidocaine 2% viscous solution*	Oral swish or gargle
Zostrix® *capsaicin 0.025% emolient cream*	For neuralgic pain, including postherpetic neuralgia and diabetic neuropathy; avoid broken or irritated skin, eyes, and mucous membranes

Appendix J: Oral Non-Steroidal Antiinflammatory Drugs

Oral NSAIDs by Classification				
(Gastrointestinal Adverse Effects: + mild, ++ frequent, +++ more frequent/severe)				
Generic Name	**Trade Name**	**mg/Day**	**Doses per Day**	**GI AE**
Heterocarboxylic acid				
aspirin (D)	Bayer®, Easprin®, Ecotrin®	1000-6000	2-4	+++
diflunisal (C)	Dolobid®	500-1500	2	+++
magnesium choline salicylate (C)	Trilisate®	1500-4000	2-4	+
meclofenamate sodium (B/D)	Meclofen®	200-400	4	++
salsalate (D)	Disalcid®, Mono-gesic®, Salflex®	1500-5000	2-4	+
Phenylacetic acid				
diclofenac (B)	Cataflam®, Voltaren®, Voltaren® XR			
Phenylacetic acid + Misoprostol				
diclofenac + misoprostol (X)	Arthrotec®	75-150	2-3	++
fenoprofen (B/D)	Nalfon®	1200-3200	3-4	++
flurbiprofen (B)	Ansaid®	100-300	2-3	++
ibuprofen (B/D)	Advil®, Motrin®, Nuprin®	1200-3200	3-6	++
ketoprofen (B)	Actron, Orudis®, Orudis®KT, Oruvail®	100-400	3-4	++
Naphthaleneacetic acid				
naproxen (B)	Aleve®, Anaprox®, Naprelan®, Naprosyn®	250-1500	2	++
Indoleacetic acid				
etodolac (C)	Lodine®, Lodine®XL	600-1200	3-4 1	+
indomethacin (B/D)	Indocin®, Indocin®SR	50-200	2-4	+++
sulindac (B/D)	Clinoril®	300-400	2	+++

Oral NSAIDs by Classification

(Gastrointestinal Adverse Effects: + mild, ++ frequent, +++ more frequent/severe)

Generic Name	Trade Name	mg/Day	Doses per Day	GI AE
Pyrrolealkanoic acid				
tolmetin (C)	Tolectin®	800-1600	4-6	++
Pyrazolidineadiones				
phenylbutazone (D)	Azolid®, Butazolidin®	200-800	1-4	++
Oxicams				
piroxicam (C)	Feldene®	20	1	+++
meloxicam (C)	Mobic®	7.5-15	1	+
Pyrrolo-pyrroles				
ketorolac (C)	Toradol®	15-150	4	+++
Naphthylalkanone				
nabumetone (C)	Relafen®	1000-2000	1-2	+
Oxazolepropionic acids				
oxaprozin (C)	Daypro®	600-1200	1	++

Comment: NSAIDs should be taken with food to decrease gastric upset. Dosing of NSAIDs should be scheduled rather than PRN for maximal benefit. *Ibuprofen* is contraindicated in children <6 months of age. *Ibuprofen* is contraindicated in 3rd trimester pregnancy. Concomitant use of *misoprostol* (**Cytotec®**) with NSAIDs reduces gastric upset and potential for ulceration; however, *misoprostol* is pregnancy category X.

Appendix K: Topical Glucocorticosteroids by Strength

Comment: All topical glucocorticosteroids are pregnancy category C. Use with caution in children. Potency guide:
    Face: Low potency
    Ears/scalp margin: Intermediate potency
    Eyelids: Hydrocortisone in ophthalmic ointment base 1%
    Chest/back: Intermediate potency
    Skin folds: Low potency

Generic Name	Brand Name/ Frequency	Formulation Strength/Size
Low Potency		
Alclometasone dipropionate (C)	**Aclovate**®Crm bid-tid	0.05% (15,45, 60 g)
	Aclovate®Oint bid-tid	0.05% (15,45, 60 g)
Fluocinolone acetonide (C)	**Synalar**®Soln bid-qid	0.01% (20, 60 ml)
hydrocortisone base or acetate (C)	**Anusol**®-HC Crm bid-qid	2.5% (30 g)
	Hytone® Crm bid-qid	1% (1, 2 oz)
	Hytone® Oint bid-qid	1% (1 oz)
	Hytone® Lotn bid-qid	1% (2 oz)
	Hytone® Crm bid-qid	2.5% (1, 2 oz)
	Hytone® Oint bid-qid	2.5% (1 oz)
	Hytone® Lotn bid-qid	2.5% (1 oz)
	U-cort® Crm bid-qid	1% (7, 28, 35 g)
Triamcinolone acetonide (C)	**Aristocort**® Crm tid-qid	0.025 (15, 60 g)
	Aristocort®A Crm tid-qid	0.025% (15, 60 g)
	Kenalog® Crm bid-qid	0.025% (15, 80 g)
	Kenalog® Lotn bid-qid	0.025% (60 ml)
	Kenalog® Oint bid-qid	0.025% (15, 60, 80g)

Generic Name	Brand Name/ Frequency	Formulation Strength/Size
Intermediate Potency		
betamethasone valerate (C)	**Luxiq**® Foam bid	0.12% (100 g)
desonide (C)	**DesOwen**® Crm bid-tid	0.05% (15, 60 g)
	DesOwen® Lotn bid-tid	0.05% (2, 4 fl oz)
	DesOwen® Oint bid-tid	0.05% (15, 60 g)
	Tridesilon® Crm bid-qid	0.05% (15, 60 g)
	Tridesilon® Oint bid-qid	0.05% (15, 60 g)
desoximetasone (C)	**Topicort**®-LP Emol Crm bid	0.05% (15, 60 g, 4 oz)
fluocinolone acetonide (C)	**Derma-Smoothe**®/FS Oil tid	0.01% (4 oz)
	Derma-Smoothe®/FS Shampoo daily	0.01% (4 oz)
	Synalar® Crm bid-qid	0.025% (15, 30, 60 g)
	Synalar® Oint bid-qid	0.025% (15, 60 g)
flurandrenolide (C)	**Cordran**®-SP Crm bid-tid	0.025% (30, 60 g)
	Cordran® Oint bid-tid	0.025% (30, 60 g)
	Cordran®-SP Crm bid-tid	0.05% (15, 30, 60 g)
	Cordran® Lotn bid-tid	0.05% (15, 60 ml)
	Cordran® Oint bid-tid	0.05% (15, 30, 60 g)
fluticasone propionate (C)	**Cutivate**® Oint bid	0.05% (15, 30, 60 g)
	Cutivate® Crm daily-bid	0.05% (15, 30, 60 g)
hydrocortisone probutate (C)	**Pandel**® Crm daily-bid	0.1% (15, 45 g)
hydrocortisone butyrate (C)	**Locoid**® Crm bid-tid	0.1% (15, 45 g)
	Locoid® Oint bid-tid	0.1% (15, 45 g)
	Locoid® Soln bid-tid	0.1% (30, 60 ml)
hydrocortisone valerate (C)	**Westcort**® Crm bid-tid	0.2% (15, 45, 60, 120 g)
	Westcort® Oint bid-tid	0.2% (15, 45, 60 g)
mometasone furoate (C)	**Elocon**® Crm daily	0.1% (15, 45 g)
	Elocon® Lotn daily	0.1% (30, 60 ml)
	Elocon® Oint daily	0.1% (15, 45 g)
prednicarbate	**Dermatop**® Emol Crm bid	0.1% (15, 60 g)
triamcinolone acetonide (C)	**Aristocort**® Crm tid-qid	0.1% (15, 60 g)
	Aristocort®A Crm tid-qid	0.1% (15, 60 g)
	Aristocort® Oint tid-qid	0.1% (15, 60 g)
	Aristocort®A Oint tid-qid	0.1% (15, 60 g)
	Kenalog® Crm bid-tid	0.1% (15, 60, 80 g)
	Kenalog® Lotn bid-tid	0.1% (60 ml)
	Kenalog®Aerosol bid-tid	0.2% (63 g)

Generic Name	Brand Name/ Frequency	Formulation Strength/Size
High Potency		
amcinonide (C)	**Cyclocort**® Crm bid-tid	0.1% (15, 30, 60 g)
	Cyclocort® Lotn bid	0.1% (20, 60 ml)
	Cyclocort® Oint bid	0.1% (15, 30, 60 g)
betamethasone dipropionate, augmented (C)	**Diprolene**®AF Emol Crm daily-bid	0.05% (15, 50 g)
	Diprolene® Lotn daily-bid	0.05% (30, 60 ml)
Desoximetasone (C)	**Topicort**® Gel bid	0.05% (15, 60 g)
	Topicort® Emol Crm bid	0.25% (15, 60 g)
	Topicort® Oint bid	0.25% (15, 60 g)
diflorasone (C)	**Florone**® Oint daily-qid	0.05% (15, 30, 60 g)
	Psorcon® Crm bid	0.05% (15, 30, 60 g)
	Psorcon® Oint daily-tid	0.05% (15, 30, 60 g)
	Psorcon®e Crm bid	0.05% (15, 30, 60 g)
	Psorcon®e Oint daily-tid	0.05% (15, 30, 60 g)
fluocinonide (C)	**Lidex**® Crm bid-qid	0.05% (15, 30, 60, 120 g)
	Lidex® Gel bid-qid	0.05% (15, 30, 60 g)
	Lidex® Oint bid-qid	0.05% (15, 30, 60, 120 g)
	Lidex® Soln bid-qid	0.05% (20, 60 ml)
	Lidex®-E Emol Crm bid-qid	0.05% (15, 30, 60 g)
halcinonide (C)	**Halog**® Crm bid-tid	0.1% (15, 30, 60, 240 g)
	Halog® Oint bid-tid	0.1% (15, 30, 60, 120 g)
	Halog® Soln bid-tid	0.1% (20, 60 ml)
	Halog®-E Emol Crm daily-tid	0.1% (15, 30, 60 g)
triamcinolone acetonide (C)	**Aristocort**®A Crm tid-qid	0.5% (15 g)
	Aristocort® Crm tid-qid	0.5% (15 g)
	Aristocort® Oint tid-qid	0.5% (15, 240 g)
	Kenalog® Crm bid-tid	0.5% (20 g)

Generic Name	Brand Name/ Frequency	Formulation Strength/Size
Super High Potency		
betamethasone dipropionate, augmented (C)	**Diprolene®** Oint daily-bid **Diprolene®** Gel daily-bid	0.05% (15, 50 g) 0.05% (15, 50 g)
clobetasol propionate (C)	**Olux®** Foam **Temovate®** Crm bid **Temovate®** Gel bid **Temovate®** Oint bid **Temovate®** Scalp App bid **Temovate®-E** Emol Crm bid	0.05% (50, 100 g) 0.05% (15, 30, 45, 60 g) 0.05% (15, 30, 60 g) 0.05% (15, 30, 45, 60 g) 0.05% (25, 50 ml) 0.05% (15, 30, 60 g)
diflorasone (C)	**Psorcon®** Oint daily-tid	0.05% (15, 30, 60 g)
flurandrenolide (C)	**Cordran®** Tape q 12 hours	4 mcg/sq cm (roll of 3"x 80")
halobetasol propionate (C)	**Ultravate®** Crm daily-bid **Ultravate®** Oint daily-bid	0.05% (15, 45 g) 0.05% (15, 45 g)

Appendix L: Oral Glucocorticosteroids

Oral Glucocorticosteroids with Dose Form(s)

Comment: Systemic glucocorticosteroids increase glucose intolerance, reduce the action of insulin and oral hypoglycemic agents, reduce adrenal cortex activity, decrease immunity, mask signs of infection, impair wound healing, suppress growth in children, and promote osteoporosis, fluid retention, and weight gain. Use systemic steroids with caution, using the lowest possible dose to affect clinical response, and withdraw (wean) gradually in tapering doses to avoid adrenal insufficiency.

▶ *betamethasone* **(C)** initally 0.6-7.2 mg daily
    Pediatric: same as adult
  Celestone® *Tab:* 0.6 mg; *Syr:* 0.6 mg/5 ml (120 ml)

▶ *cortisone* **(D)**
    Pediatric: not recommended
  Cortone®**Acetate** initially 25-300 mg daily or every other day
    Tab: 25 mg

▶ *dexamethasone* **(C)(G)** initially 0.75-9 mg/day
    Pediatric: same as adult
  Decadron® *Syr:* 0.5 mg/5 ml (100 ml); *Tab:* 0.5*, 0.75*, 4*mg
  Decadron®**5-12 Pak** *5-12 pak:* 0.75*mg tabs (12/pck)

▶ *hydrocortisone* **(C)** 20-240 mg daily
    Pediatric: 2-8 mg/day
  Cortef® *Tab:* 5, 10, 20 mg; *Oral susp:* 10 mg/5 ml
  Hydrocortone® *Tab:* 10 mg

▶ *methylprednisolone* **(C)(G)** 4-48 mg/day
    Pediatric: same as adult
  Medrol® *Tab:* 2*, 4*, 8*, 16*, 24*, 32*mg
  Medrol®**Dosepak** *Dosepak:* 4*mg tabs (21/pck)

▶ *prednisolone* **(C)(G)** initially 5-60 mg/day in 1-2 doses x 3-5 days
    Pediatric: 0.14-2 mg/kg/day in 3-4 doses x 3-5 days
  Orapred® *Soln:* 15 mg/5 ml (grape, dye-free, alcohol 2%)
  Orapred®**ODT** *Tab:* 10, 15, 30 mg orally disintegrating (grape)
  Pediapred® *Soln:* 5 mg/5 ml (raspberry, sugar-, alcohol-, dye-free)
  Prelone® *Syr:* 15 mg/5 ml

▶ *prednisone* **(C)(G)** initially 5-60 mg/day in 1-2 doses x 3-5 days
    Pediatric: 0.14-2 mg/kg/day in 3-4 doses x 3-5 days
  Deltasone® *Tab:* 2.5*, 5*, 10*, 20*, 50*mg

▶ *triamcinolone* **(C)(G)** initially 4-48 mg/day in 1-2 doses x 3-5 days
　　Pediatric: 0.14-2 mg/kg/day in 3-4 doses x 3-5 days
Aristocort® *Tab:* 4*mg
Aristocort®Forte *Susp:* 40 mg/ml (benzoyl alcohol)
Aristocort®Aristopak *Tab:* 4*mg (16/pck)

Appendix M: Parenteral Glucocorticosteroids

Parenteral Glucocorticosteroids with Dose Form(s)

Comment: Systemic glucocorticosteroids increase glucose intolerance, reduce the action of insulin and oral hypoglycemic agents, reduce adrenal cortex activity, decrease immunity, mask signs of infection, impair wound healing, suppress growth in children, and promote osteoporosis, fluid retention, and weight gain. Use systemic steroids with caution, using the lowest possible dose to affect clinical response, and withdraw (wean) gradually in tapering doses to avoid adrenal insufficiency.

▶ *betamethasone* **(C)**
    Celestone® 0.5-9 mg IM/IV x 1 dose
        Vial: 3 mg/ml (10 ml)
    Celestone®Soluspan 0.5-9 mg IM/IV x 1 dose; usual IM dose 6 mg
        Vial: 6 mg/ml (10 ml)

▶ *cortisone* **(D)**
    Pediatric: not recommended
    Cortone®Acetate 20-300 mg IM
        Vial: 50 mg/ml (10 ml)

▶ *dexamethasone* **(C)** initially 0.5-9 mg IM/IV daily
    Dalalone D.P.®
        Vial: 16 mg/ml (1, 5 ml)
    Decadron®
        Vial: 4, 24 mg/ml for IM use (5 ml, sulfites)
    Decadron®-LA
        Vial: 8 mg/ml (1, 5 ml)

▶ *hydrocortisone* **(C)**
    Hydrocortone® initially 100-500 mg IM/IV daily
        Vial: 50 mg/ml (5 ml)
    Solu-Cortef® initially 100-500 mg IM/IV daily
        Pediatric: 2-8 mg/kg loading dose (max 250 mg); then 8 mg/kg/day
        Vial: 100 mg (2 ml); 250 mg (2 ml); 500 mg (4 ml); 1 g (8 ml)

▶ *hydrocortisone phosphate* **(C)**
    Hydrocortone® for IM, IV, and SC injection
        Vial: 50 mg/ml (2 ml)

▶ *methylprednisolone* **(C)**
    Depo-Medrol® 40-120 mg IM/week for 1-4 weeks
        Vial: 20 mg/ml (5 ml); 40 mg/ml (5, 10 ml); 80 mg/ml (5 ml)

▶ *methylprednisolone sodium succinate* **(C)**
    Solu-Medrol® 10-40 mg IV initially; then, IM <u>or</u> IV
        Pediatric: 1-2 mg/kg loading dose; then 1.6 mg/kg/day in divided doses at least 6 hours apart
        Vial: 40 mg (1 ml), 125 mg (2 ml), 500 mg (4 ml); 1 g (8 ml); 2 g (8 ml)

▶ *triamcinolone* **(C)**
    Aristocort®
        Vial: 25 mg/ml (5 ml)
    Aristocort®Forte 40 mg IM/week
        Vial: 40 mg/ml (1, 5 ml) *(do not administer IV)*
    Aristospan®
        Vial: 5 mg/ml (5 ml); 20 mg/ml (1, 5 ml)
    TAC®-3 for intralesional and intradermal use
        Vial: 3 mg/ml (5 ml)

Injectable Glucocorticosteroid/Anesthetic

▶ *dexamethasone/lidocaine* **(C)** 0.1-0.75 ml into painful area
    Decadron®Phosphate with Xylocaine®
        Vial: dexa 4 mg/*lido* 10 mg per ml (5 ml)

Appendix N: Inhalational Glucocorticosteroids

Inhalational Glucocorticosteroids with Dose Form(s)

Comment: Inhaled glucocorticosteroids are indicated for the long-term control of asthma. Inhaled glucocorticosteroids are not indicated for exercise-induced asthma or for relief of acute symptoms (i.e., "rescue"). Low-doses are indicated for mild persistent asthma, medium doses are indicated for moderate persistent asthma, and high doses are reserved for severe cases. Titrate to lowest effective dose. To reduce the potential for adverse effects with inhalers, the patient should use a spacer or holding chamber and rinse the mouth and spit after every inhalation treatment. Linear growth should be monitored in children. Consider adding a long-acting inhaled Beta-2 agonist to a low-to-medium dose of inhaled steroid rather than using a higher dose of inhaled steroid (especially for nocturnal symptoms). When inhaled doses exceed 1000 mcg/day, consider supplements of calcium (1-1.5 g/day), vitamin D (400 IU/day), and estrogen replacement therapy for postmenopausal women.

▶*beclomethasone* **(C)**
 Beclovent® 2 inhalations tid-qid or 4 inhalations bid; max 20 inhalations/day
  Pediatric: <6 years: not recommended
   6-12 years: 1-2 inhalations tid-qid <u>or</u> 4 inhalations bid; max 10 inhalations/day
  Inhaler: 42 mcg/actuation (6.7 g, 80 inh); 16.8 g (200 inh)
 Qvar®
  Pediatric: not recommended
  If previously using only bronchodilators, initiate 40-80 mcg bid; max 320 mcg/day
  If previously using an inhaled corticosteroid, initiate 40-160 mcg bid; max 320 mcg/day
  If previously taking a systemic corticosteroid, attempt to wean off the systemic drug after approximately 1 week after initiating Qvar®
  Inhaler: 40, 80 mcg/actuation (7.3g, 100 inh); 13.2 g (200 Inh; chlorofluorocarbon [CFC]-free)
 Vanceril® 2 inhalations tid-qid <u>or</u> 4 inhalations bid
  Pediatric: <6 years: not recommended
   6-12 years: 1-2 inhalations tid-qid
  Inhaler: 42 mcg/actuation (16.8 g, 200 inh)

Vanceril®Double Strength 2 inhalations bid
    Pediatric: <6 years: not recommended
                6-12 years: 1-2 inhalations bid
    Inhaler: 84 mcg/actuation (12.2 g, 120 inh)

▶ *budesonide* **(B)**
    Pulmicort®Respules use turbuhaler
        Pediatric: <12 months: not recommended
                  12 months-8 years:
                  Previously using only bronchodilators, initiate 0.5 mg/day daily <u>or</u> in 2 divided doses; may start at 0.25 mg/day
                  Previously using inhaled corticosteroids, initiate 0.5 mg/day daily <u>or</u> in 2 divided doses; max 1 mg/day
                  Previously using oral corticosteroids, initiate 1 mg/day daily <u>or</u> in 2 divided doses;
    Inhal susp: 0.25 mg/2 ml (30/box)
    Pulmicort®Turbuhaler 1-2 inhalations bid; if previously on oral corticosteroids, 2-4 inhalations bid
        Pediatric: <6 years: not recommended
                    >6 years: 1-2 inhalations bid
    Turbuhaler: 200 mcg/actuation (200 inh)

▶ *flunisolide* **(C)**
    AeroBid® and **AeroBid®M** initially 2 inhalations bid; max 8 inhalations/day
        Pediatric: <6 years: not recommended
                    6-15 years: 2 inhalations bid
    Inhaler: 250 mcg/actuation (7 g, 100 inh)

▶ *fluticasone* **(C)**
    Flovent®HFA initially 88 mcg bid; if previously using an inhaled corticosteroid, initially 88-220 mcg bid; if previously taking an oral corticosteroid, initially 880 mcg/day
        Pediatric: use **Rotadisk®**: initially 50-88 mcg inh bid
                    <4 years: not recommended
                    4-11 years: initially 50-88 mcg bid
                    >11 years: initially 100 mcg bid; if previously using an inhaled corticosteroid, initially 100-200 mcg bid; if previously taking an oral corticosteroid, initially 1000 mcg bid

Inhaler: 44 mcg/actuation (7.9 g, 60 inh; 13 g, 120 inh) 110 mcg/actuation (13 g, 120 inh); 220 mcg/actuation (13 g, 120 inh)

Rotadisk: 50 mcg/actuation (60 blisters/disk); 100 mcg/actuation (60 blisters/disk); 250 mcg/actuation (60 blisters/disk)

▶ *mometasone furoate* (**C**)

If previously using a bronchodilator or inhaled corticosteroid: 220 mcg q PM or bid; max 440 mcg q PM or 220 mcg bid

If previously using an oral corticosteroid: 440 mcg bid; max 880 mcg/day

Pediatric: <12 years: not recommended

Asmanex®Twisthaler

Inhaler: 220 mcg/actuation (6.7 g, 80 inh); 16.8 g (200 inh)

Appendix O: Systemic Antiarrhythmia Drugs

Antiarrhythmics by Classification with Dose Form(s)

Brand/*generic* Pregnancy Category	Class/Indication(s)	Dose Form(s)
Betapace® *sotalol* (B)	*Class:* Class II and III Antiarrhythmic *Indications:* Documented life-threatening ventricular arrhythmias	*Tab:* 80*, 120*, 160*, 240*mg
Betapace®**AF** *sotalol* (B)	*Class:* Class II and III Antiarrhythmic *Indications:* Maintenance of normal sinus rhythm in patients with highly symptomatic atrial fibrillation or atrial flutter who are currently in sinus rhythm	*Tab:* 80*, 120*, 160*mg
Calan® *verapamil* (C)	*Class:* Calcium Channel Blocker *Indications:* Control (with *digitalis*) of ventricular rate in patients with chronic atrial fibrillation or atrial flutter; prophylaxis of repetitive paroxysmal supraventricular tachycardia	*Tab:* 40, 80*, 120*mg
Cordarone® *amiodarone* (D)	*Class:* Class III Antiarrhythmic *Indications:* Documented life-threatening recurrent refractory ventricular fibrillation or hemodynamically unstable ventricular tachycardia	*Tab:* 200*mg
Guinidex® *quinidine sulfate* (C)	*Class:* Class I Antiarrhythmic *Indications:* Atrial and ventricular arrhythmias	*Tab:* 300 mg ext-rel
Inderal® *propranolol* (C) **Inderal**®**XL** *propranolol* (C) **InnoPran**®**XL** *propranolol* (C)	*Class:* Beta Blocker *Indications:* Atrial and ventricular arrhythmias; tachyarrhythmias due to *digitalis* intoxication; reduce mortality and risk of reinfarction in stabilized patients after myocardial infarction	*Tab:* 10*, 20*, 40*, 60*, 80*mg *Cap:* 60, 80, 120, 160 mg sust-rel *Cap:* 80, 120 mg ext-rel

Antiarrhythmics by Classification with Dose Form(s)

Brand/*generic* Pregnancy Category	Class/Indication(s)	Dose Form(s)
Mexitil® *mexiletine* (C)	*Class:* Class IB Antiarrhythmic *Indications:* Documented life-threatening ventricular arrhythmias	*Cap:* 150, 200, 250 mg
Norpace® *disoyramide* (C)	*Class:* Class I Antiarrhythmic *Indications:* Documented life-threatening ventricular arrhythmias	*Cap:* 100, 150 mg
Procanbid® *procainamide* (C)	*Class:* Class IA Antiarrhythmic *Indications:* Life-threatening ventricular arrhythmias	*Tab:* 500, 1000 mg ext rel
Quinaglute® *quinidine gluconate* (C)	*Class:* Class I Antiarrhythmic *Indications:* Atrial and ventricular arrhythmias	*Tab:* 324 mg ext-rel
Rhythmol® *propafenone* (C)	*Class:* Class IC Antiarrhythmic *Indications:* Documented life-threatening ventricular arrhythmias; prolonged recurrence of paroxysmal atrial fibrillation and/or atrial flutter or paroxysmal supraventricular tachycardia associated with disabling symptoms in patients without structural heart disease	*Tab:* 150*, 225*, 300* mg
Sectral® *acebutolol* (B)	*Class:* Beta Blocker *Indications:* Ventricular arrhythmias	*Cap:* 200, 400 mg
Tambocor® *flecainide acetate* (C)	*Class:* Class IC Antiarrhythmic *Indications:* Documented life-threatening ventricular arrhythmias; paroxysmal atrial fibrillation and/or atrial flutter or paroxysmal supraventricular tachycardia in patients without structural heart disease	*Tab:* 50, 100*, 150* mg
Tenormin® *atenolol* (C)	*Class:* Beta Blocker *Indications:* Reduce mortality and in stabilized patients after myocardial infarction	*Tab:* 25, 50, 100 mg *Inj:* 5 mg/ml (10 ml) for IV administration

Antiarrhythmics by Classification with Dose Form(s)		
Brand/*generic* **Pregnancy Category**	**Class/Indication(s)**	**Dose Form(s)**
aTikosyn® *defotilide* **(C)**	*Class:* Class III Antiarrhythmic *Indications:* Maintenance of normal sinus rhythm in patients with atrial fibrillation or atrial flutter of >1 week duration who were converted to normal sinus rhythm (only for highly symptomatic patients); conversion to normal sinus rhythm	*Cap:* 125, 250, 500 mcg
Tonocard® *tocainide* **(C)**	*Class:* Class I Antiarrhythmic *Indications:* Documented life-threatening ventricular arrhythmias	*Tab:* 400*, 600*mg
Toprol®**XL** *metoprolol* **(C)**	*Class:* Beta Blocker *Indications:* Ischemic, hypertensive, or cardiomyopathic heart failure	*Tab:* 25*, 50*, 100*, 200*mg

Appendix P: Systemic Antineoplasia Drugs

Antineoplastics by Classification with Dose Form(s)

Brand/*generic* Pregnancy Category	Class/Indication(s)	Dose Form(s)
Alkeran® *melphalan* (D)	Alkylating Agent	*Tab:* 2*mg
Arimidex® *anastrozole* (D)	Aromatase Inhibitor	*Tab:* 1 mg
Aromasin® *exemestane* (D)	Aromatase Inactivator	*Tab:* 25 mg
Arranon® *nelarabine* (D)	Nucleoside Analog	*Vial:* 250 mg for IV infusion
Casodex® *Bicalutamide*(X)	Antiandrogen	*Tab:* 50mg
Cytoxan® *cyclo-phosphamide*(D)	Alkylating Agent	*Tab:* 25, 50 mg
Eligard® *leuprolide acetate* (X)	GnRH Analogue	*Inj:* 7.5 mg ext-rel per monthly SC injection
Eulexin® *flutamide* (D)	Antiandrogen	*Cap:* 125 mg
Faslodex® *fluvestrant* (D)	Estrogen Receptor Antagonist	*Prefilled syringe for IM inj:* 50 mg/ml (2.5, 5 ml per syringe)
Femara® *letrozole* (D)	Aromatase Inhibitor	*Tab:* 2.5 mg
Gleevec® *imatinib mesylate* (D)	Signal Transduction Inhibitor	*Cap:* 100 mg
Hydrea® *hydroxyurea* (D)	Substituted Urea	*Cap:* 500 mg
Iressa® *gefitinib* (D)	Epidermal Growth Factor receptor-tyrosine kinase inhibitor	*Tab:* 250 mg
Leukeran® *chlorambucil* (D)	Alkylating Agent	*Tab:* 2 mg

Antineoplastics by Classification with Dose Form(s)

Brand/*generic* Pregnancy Category	Class/Indication(s)	Dose Form(s)
Lupron® *leuprolide* (**X**)	GnRH Analogue	*Susp for IM inj:* 1 mg (daily) 7.5 mg depot (monthly) 22.5 mg depot (every 3 months) 30 mg depot (every 4 months)
Megace®, **Megace**®**Oral Suspension**, **Megace**®**ES**, *megestrol acetate* (**D**)	Progestin	*Tab:* 20*, 40*mg; *Susp:* 40 mg/ml; ES concentrate: 125 mg/ml, 625 mg/5 ml
Nexavar® *sorafenib* (**D**)	Multikinase Inhibitor	*Tab:* 200 mg
Nolvadex® *tamoxefin citrate* (**D**)	Antiestrogen	*Tab:* 10, 20 mg
Velcade® *bortezomib* (**D**)	Proteasome Inhibitor	3.5 mg (pwd for IV injection after reconstitution
Viadur® *leuprolide acetate* (**X**)	GnRH Analogue	*SC implant:* 65 mg depot (every 12 months)
Xeloda® *capecitabine* (**D**)	Fluoropyrimidine (prodrug of *5-fluorouracil*)	*Tab:* 150, 500 mg
Zoladex® *goserelin acetate* (**D**)	GnRH Analogue	*SC implant:* 3.6 mg depot (28 days), 10.8 mg depot (3-month)
Zometa® *zoledronic acid* (**D**)	Bisphosphonate	*Inj for IV infusion:* 4 mg/vial (pwd for reconstitution)

Appendix Q: Antipsychosis Drugs

Antipsychotics with Dose Form(s)

Comment: Patients receiving an antipsychosis agent should be monitored closely for the following adverse side effects: neuroleptic malignant syndrome, extrapyramidal reactions, tardive dyskinesia, blood dyscrasias, anticholinergic effects, drowsiness, hypotension, photosensitivity, retinopathy, and lowered seizure threshhold. Use lower doses for elderly or debilitated patients. Prescriptions should be written for the smallest practical amount. Foods and beverages containing alcohol are contraindicated for patients receiving psychotropic drug therapy.

▶ *aripiprazole* **(C)**
  Abilify® *Tab:* 2, 5, 10, 15, 20, 30 mg; *Oral soln:* 1 mg/ml (150 ml; orange-crème, parabens)

▶ *chlorpromazine* **(C)**
  Thorazine® *Tab:* 10, 25, 50, 100, 200 mg; *Cap:* 30, 75, 150 mg sust-rel; *Syr:* 10 mg/5 ml (4 oz, orange-custard); *Inj:* 25 mg/ml (1, 2 ml amps, 10 ml vial, sulfites)

▶ *clozapine* **(B)**
  Clozaril® *Tab:* 25*, 100* mg

▶ *fluphenazine* **(C)**
  Prolixin® *Tab:* 1, 2.5, 5*, 10 mg (tartrazine); *Conc:* 5 mg/ml (4 oz w/cal dropper, alcohol 14%); *Syr:* 5 mg/ml (2 oz w/ cal dropper, alcohol 14%); *Inj:* 25 mg/ml (10 ml vial)

▶ *fluphenazine decanoate* **(C)**
  Prolixin®**Decanoate** *Inj:* 25 mg/ml (5 ml vial, 1 ml syringe; benzyl alcohol)

▶ *fluphenazine ethanate* **(C)**
  Prolixin®**Ethanate** *Inj:* 25 mg/vial (5 ml; benzyl alcohol)

▶ *olanzapine* **(C)**
  Zyprexa® *Tab:* 2.5, 5, 7.5, 10, 15, 20 mg
  Zyprexa®**Zydis** *Tab:* 5, 10, 15, 20 mg orally-disintegrating (phenylalanine)

▶ *perphenazine* **(C)**
  Trilafon® *Tab:* 2, 4, 8, 16 mg; *Inj:* 5 mg/ml (1 ml amp; sulfites)

▶ *prochlor-perazine* **(C)**
  Compazine® *Tab:* 5, 10 mg; *Cap:* 10, 15 mg sus-rel; *Syr:* 5 mg/5 ml (4 oz; fruit); *Supp:* 2.5, 5, 25 mg

Antipsychotics with Dose Form(s)

▶ *quetiapine* **(C)**
  Seroquel® *Tab:* 25, 100, 200, 300 mg
▶ *risperidone* **(C)**
  Risperdal® *Tab:* 0.25, 0.5, 1, 2, 3, 4 mg; *Soln:* 1 mg/ml (30 ml w. pipette); *Consta (Inj):* 25, 37.5, 50 mg
  Risperdal®**M-Tabs** *M-tab:* 0.5, 1, 2, 3, 4 mg orally disintegrating (phenylalanine)
▶ *thioridazine* **(C)**
  Mellaril® *Tab:* 10, 15, 25, 50, 100, 150, 200 mg; *Conc:* 30 mg/ml (4 oz w. cal dropper; alcohol 4.2%); *Susp:* 5, 20 mg/ml (buttermint)
▶ *trifluoperazine* **(C)**
  Stelazine® *Tab:* 1, 2, 5, 10 mg; *Conc:* 10 mg/ml; (2 oz w. cal dropper; banana-vanilla, sulfites); *Inj:* 2 mg/ml (10 ml vial)
▶ *ziprasidone* **(C)**
  Geodon® *Cap:* 20, 40, 60, 80 mg

Appendix R: Anticonvulsant Drugs

Anticonvulsants with Dose Form(s)

▶ *carbarbamazepine* **(D)**
  Carbatrol® *Cap:* 200, 300 mg ext-rel
  Equetro® *Cap:* 100, 200, 300 mg ext-rel
  Tegretol® *Tab:* 200*mg; *Chew tab:* 100*mg; *Oral susp:* 100 mg/5 ml (450 ml; citrus-vanilla)
  Tegretol®**XR** *Tab:* 100, 200, 400 mg ext-rel
▶ *clonazepam* **(D)(IV)**
  Klonopin® *Tab:* 0.5*, 1, 2 mg
▶ *diazepam* **(D)(IV)**
  Diastat®**Rectal delivery system**: *Adult:* 10, 15, 20 mg; *Ped:* 2.5, 5, 10 mg
  Valium® *Tab:* 2*, 5*, 10*mg
▶ *divalproex sodium* **(D)**
  Depakene® *Cap:* 250 mg; *Syr:* 250 mg/5 ml (16 oz)
  Depakote® *Tab:* 125, 250 mg
  Depakote®**ER** *Tab:* 250, 500 mg ext-rel
  Depakote®**Sprinkle** *Cap:* 125 mg
▶ *ethotoin* **(C)**
  Felbatol® *Tab:* 400*, 600*mg; *Oral susp:* 600 mg/5 ml (8, 32 oz)
  Peganone® *Tab:* 250, 500 mg
▶ *gabapentin* **(C)**
  Neurontin® *Cap:* 100, 300, 400 mg; *Tab:* 600*, 800*mg; *Oral soln:* 250 mg/5 ml (480 ml)(strawberry-anise)
▶ *lamotrigine* **(C)**
  Lamictal® *Tab:* 25*, 100*, 150*, 200*mg; *Chew tab:* 2*, 5*, 25*mg (black currant)
▶ *mephobarbital* **(D)(II)**
  Mebarol® *Tab:* 32, 50, 100 mg
▶ *methsuximide* **(C)**
  Celontin®**Kapseals** *Cap:* 150, 300 mg
▶ *oxcarbazepine* **(C)**
  Trileptal® *Tab:* 150, 300, 600 mg; *Oral susp:* 300 mg/5 ml (lemon, alcohol)

Anticonvulsants with Dose Form(s)

▶ *phenytoin* **(D)(G),** *primidone* **(D)(G)**
   Dilantin® *Cap:* 30, 100 mg ext-rel; *Infa tab:* 50 mg;
   Chew tab: 50*mg; *Oral susp:* 125 mg/5 ml (237 ml)
   Phenytek® *Cap:* 200, 300 mg ext-rel
▶ *pregabalin* **(C)(V)**
   Lyrica® *Cap:* 25, 50, 75, 100, 200, 225, 300 mg
▶ *primidone* **(C)**
   Mysoline® *Tab:* 50*, 250*mg; *Oral susp:* 250 mg/5 ml (8 oz)
▶ *tiagabine* **(C)**
   Gabitril® *Tab:* 2, 4, 12, 16 mg
▶ *topiramate* **(C)**
   Topamax® *Tab:* 25, 50, 100, 200 mg
   Topamax®**Sprinkle Caps** *Cap:* 15, 25, 50 mg
▶ *zonisamide* **(C)**
   Zonegran® *Cap:* 25, 50, 100 mg

Appendix S: Anti-HIV Drugs

Anti-HIV Drugs with Dose Forms

▶ *abacavir sulfate* **(C)**
   Ziagen® *Tab:* 300 mg; *Oral soln:* 20 mg/ml (240 ml; strawberry-banana, parabens, propylene glycol)
▶ *abacavir sulfate/lamivudine* **(C)**
   Epzicom® *Tab:* aba 600/*lami* 300 mg
▶ *abacavir sulfate/lamivudine/zidovudine* **(C)**
   Trizivir® *Tab:* aba 300/*lami* 150/*zido* 300 mg
▶ *adefovir dipivoxil* **(C)**
   Hepsera® *Tab:* 10 mg
▶ *amprenavir* **(C)**
   Agenerase® *Cap:* 50 mg (plus Vit E 36 IU/cap), 150 mg (plus Vit E 109 IU/cap); *Oral soln:* 15 mg/ml (*plus* Vit E 46 IU/ml) (240 ml; grape-bubble gum-peppermint, propylene glycol)
▶ *atazanavir* **(B)**
   Reyataz® *Cap:* 100, 150, 200 mg
▶ *cidofovir* **(C)**
   Vistide® *Inj:* 75 mg/ml (5 ml vials for IV infusion; preservative-free)
▶ *darunavir* **(C)**
   Prezista® *Tab:* 300 mg
▶ *delavirdine mesylate* **(C)**
   Rescriptor® *Tab:* 100, 200 mg
▶ *didanosine* **(C)**
   Videx®**EC** *Cap:* 125, 200, 250, 400 mg e-c del-rel; *Chew tab:* 25, 50, 100, 150, 200 mg (mandarin orange, buffered with calcium carbonate and magnesium hydroxide, phenylalanine); *Pwdr for oral soln:* 100, 167, 250 mg pkts (buffered with citrate-phosphate, sodium 1.38 g/pkt); *Ped pwdr for oral soln:* (2, 4 g per bottle)
▶ *efavirenz* **(C)**
   Sustiva® *Tab:* 600 mg; *Cap:* 50, 100, 200 mg
▶ *efavirenz/emtricitabine/tenofovir* **(D)**
   Atripla® *Tab:* efa 600 mg/*emtri* 200 mg/*teno DF* 300 mg
▶ *emtricitabine* **(B)**
   Emtriva® *Cap:* 200 mg

Anti-HIV Drugs with Dose Forms

▶ *emtricitabine/tenofovir disoproxil fumarate* (**B**)
  Truvada® *Cap:* 200, 300 mg
▶ *enfuvirtide* (**B**)
  Fuzeon® *Vial:* 90 mg/ml (1 ml; 60 vials/kit)
▶ *fosamprenavir* (**B**)
  Lexiva® *Tab:* 700 mg
▶ *ganciclovir* (**C**)
  Cytovene® *Cap:* 250, 500 mg; *Inj:* 500 mg
▶ *indinavir sulfate* (**C**)
  Crixivan® *Cap:* 100, 200, 333, 400 mg
▶ *lamivudine* (**C**)
  Epivir® *Tab:* 150 mg; *Oral soln:* 10 mg/ml (240 ml; strawberry-banana, alcohol 6%)
▶ *lamivudine/zidovudine* (**C**)
  Combivir® *Tab: lami* 150/*zido* 300 mg
▶ *lopinavir* plus *ritonavir* (**C**)
  Kaletra® *Cap: lopin* 133.3/*riton* 33.3 mg; *Oral soln: lopin* 80/*riton* 20 mg per ml (160 ml w. dose cup; cotton candy, alcohol 42%)
▶ *nelfinavir mesylate* (**B**)
  Viracept® *Tab:* 250 mg; *Pwdr for oral soln:* 50 mg/g (144 g; phenylalanine)
▶ *nevirapine* (**C**)
  Viramune® *Tab:* 200*mg; *Oral susp:* 50 mg/5 ml (240 ml)
▶ *ritonavir* (**B**)
  Norvir® *Soft gel cap:* 100 mg (alcohol); *Oral soln:* 80 mg/ml (8 oz; peppermint-caramel, alcohol)
▶ *saquinavir* (**B**)
  Fortovase® *Soft gel cap:* 200 mg
▶ *saquinavir mesylate* (**B**)
  Invirase® *Hard gel cap:* 200 mg
▶ *stavudine* (**C**)
  Zerit® *Cap:* 15, 20, 30, 40 mg; *Oral soln:* 1 mg/ml (200 ml; fruit, dye-free)
▶ *tenofovir disoproxil fumarate* (**C**)
  Viread® *Tab:* 300 mg
▶ *tipranavir* (**C**)
  Aptivus® *Cap:* 250 mg
▶ *valganciclovir* (**C**)
  Valcyte® *Tab:* 450 mg

Anti-HIV Drugs with Dose Forms

▶ *zalcitabine* **(C)**
　　Hivid® *Tab:* 0.375, 0.75 mg

▶ *zidovudine* **(C)**
　　Retrovir® *Tab:* 300 mg; *Cap:* 300 mg; *Syr:* 50 mg/ml (240 ml; strawberry); *Vial:* 10 mg/ml (20 ml vial for IV infusion; peservative-free)

Appendix T: Coumadin (Warfarin) Therapy

Coumadin (Warfarin) with Dose Form(s)

▶ *warfarin* **(X)(G)** dosage initially 2-5 mg/day; usual maintenance 2-10 mg/day; adjust dosage to maintain INR in therapeutic range:
> *Venous thrombosis:* 2.0-3.0
> *Atrial fibrillation*: 2.0-3.0
> *Post MI:* 2.5-3.5
> *Mechanical and bioprosthetic heart valves:* 2.0-3.0 for 12 weeks after valve insertion, then 2.5-3.5 long-term
> *Pediatric:* not recommended under 18 years
> **Coumadin**® *Tab:* 1*, 2*, 2.5*, 3*, 4*, 5*, 6*, 7.5*, 10* mg
> **Coumadin**®**for Injection** *Vial:* 2 mg/ml (2.5 ml)

Comment: **Coumadin**®**for Injection** is for peripheral IV administration only.

Coumadin Overanticoagulation

▶ *phytonadione (vitamin K)***(G)**
> **AquaMEPHYTON**® 2.5-10 mg; up to 25 mg IM
>   *Vial:* 1 mg/0.5 ml (0.5 ml); 10 mg/ml (1, 2.5, 5 ml)
> **Mephyton**® 2.5-10 mg; max 25 mg po
>   *Tab:* 5 mg

Agents that Inhibit Warfarin's Anticoagulation Effects

Increase Metabolism	Decrease Absorption	Other Mechanism(s)
azathioprine	azathioprine	coenzyme Q10
carbamazepine	cholestyramine	estrogen
dicloxacillin	cholestipol	griseofulvin
ethanol	sucralfate	oral contraceptives
griseoulvin		ritonavir
nafcillin		spironolactone
pentobarbital		trazodone
phenobarbital		vitamin C (high dose)
phenytoin		vitamin K
primidone		
rifabutin		
rifampin		

Appendix U: Low Molecular Weight Heparins

Low Molecular Weight Heparins with Dose Forms

Comment: All low molecular weight heparins are pregnancy category B. Administer by subcutaneous injection *only* and rotate sites. Avoid concommittant drugs that affect hemostasis (e.g., oral anticoagulants and platelet inhibitors, including *aspirin*, NSAIDs, *dipyridamole*, *sulfinpyrazone*, *ticlopidine*). Pediatrics not recommended.

▶*ardeparin* (**C**)
  Normiflo® *Soln for inj:* 5,000 anti-Factor Xa U/0.5 ml; 10,000 anti-Factor Xa U/0.5 ml (sulfites, parabens)

▶*dalteparin* (**B**)
  Fragmin® *Prefilled syringe:* 2500 IU/0.2 ml, 5000 IU/0.2 ml (10/box; preservative-free); *Multidose vial:* 1,000 IU/ml (95,000 IU, 9.5 ml; benzyl alcohol)

▶*danaparoid* (**B**)
  Orgaran® Amp: 750 anti-Xa units/0.6 ml (0.6 ml, 10/box); *Prefilled syringe:* 750 anti-Xa units/0.6 ml (0.6 ml, 10/box; sulfites)

▶*enoxaparin* (**B**)
  Lovenox® *Prefilled syringe:* 30 mg/0.3 ml, 40 mg/0.4 ml, 60 mg/0.6 ml, 80 mg/0.8 ml, (100 mg/ml; preservative-free); *Vial:* 100 mg/ml (3 ml)

▶*fondaparinux* (**B**)
  Arixtra® *Prefilled syringe:* 2.5 mg *Factor Xa inhibitor*/0.5 ml (0.5 ml syringes, 10/pkg)

▶*tenzaparin* (**B**)
  Innohep® *Vial:* 20,000 *anti-Factor Xa* IU/ml (2 ml; sulfites, benzyl alcohol)

Appendix V: Vitamin & Mineral Supplements

Vitamin and mineral supplements are presented, with their contents, in alphabetical order by brand name.

Comment:

- Vitamin and mineral supplements are pregnancy category A.
- The formulation varies with each brand; therefore individualize according to individual patient's needs.
- Some formulations contain herbs which may have significant potential for interaction with other drugs.
- Prenatal vitamins are indicated for nutritional supplementation during pregnancy, the prenatal period, and the postnatal period.
- Excessive vitamin A has been linked to birth defects.
- Pyridoxine and iron antagonize levodopa.
- Calcium and iron decrease *tetracycline* absorption.
- Calcium absorption is decreased by corticosteroids.
- Calcium absorption is decreased by foods such as rhubarb, spinach, and bran.
- Folic acid may mask B-12 deficiency (pernicious anemia).
- The B vitamins are: B-1 (thiamin), B-2 (riboflavin), B-3 (niacinamide), B-5 (pantothenic acid), B-6 (pyridoxine), B-9 (folic acid), B-12 (cyanocobalamin).
- Accidental overdose of iron-containing products is a leading cause of fatal poisoning in children under 6 years-of-age.
- All vitamin and mineral supplements should be kept out of the reach of children.

	Page
Appendix V.1: Vitamin & Mineral Supplements for Adults	**509**
Appendix V.2: Vitamin & Mineral Supplements for Infants and Children	**514**
Appendix V.3: Prenatal Vitamin & Mineral Supplements	**517**

Appendix V.1: Vitamin & Mineral Supplements for Adults

▶**Berocca**® 1 caplet daily
  Cplt: A (5000 IU, 40% as beta carotene)/B-1, thiamin (20 mg)/B-2, riboflavin (20 mg)/B-3, niacinamide (100 mg)/B-6, pyridoxine (25 mg)/B-9, folic acid (0.8 mg)/B-12, cyanocobalamin (50 mcg)/C (750 mg)/E (30 IU)/biotin (0.15 mg)/chromium (0.1 mg)/copper (3 mg)/iron (27 mg)/manganese (5 mg)/magnesium (50 mg)/pantothenic acid (25 mg)/zinc (22.5 mg)

▶**Cefol**®**Plus** 1 tab daily
  Tab: B-1, thiamin (15 mg)/B-2, riboflavin (10 mg)/B-6, pyridoxine (5 mg)/B-9, folic acid (0.5 mg)/B-12, cyanocobalamin (6 mcg)/(500 mg)/E (30 IU)/calcium pantothenate (20 mg)

▶**Centrum**® **(OTC)** 1 tab daily
  Tab: A (5000 IU, 40% as beta carotene)/B-1, thiamin (1.5 mg)/B-2, riboflavin (1.7 mg)/B-3, niacinamide (20 mg)/B-5, pantothenic acid (10 mg)/B-6, pyridoxine (2 mg)/B-9, folic acid (0.4 mg)/B-12, cyanocobalamin (6 mcg)/C (60 mg)/D (400 mg)/E (30 IU)/K (25 mcg)/biotin (30 mcg)/boron (150 mcg)/calcium (162 mg as phosphate and carbonate)/chloride (7.2 mg as potassium)/chromium (120 mcg as chloride)/copper (2 mg as oxide)/iodine (150 mcg as potassium)/iron (18 mg as fumarate)/ magnesium (100 mg as oxide)/manganese (2 mg)/molybdenum (75 mcg)/nickel (5 mcg)/phosphorus (109 mg as calcium)/potassium (80 mg (as chloride)/selenium (20 mcg)/zinc 15 mg (as oxide)

▶**Chromagen**® 1 cap daily
  Cap: B-12 (10 mcg)/C (250 mg)/iron (66 mg, 200 mg as fumarate)/desiccated stomach substance (100 mg)

▶**Chromagen**®**FA** 1 cap daily
  Cap: B-9, folic acid (1 mg)/B-12, cyanocobalamin (10 mcg)/C (250 mg)/iron (66 mg, 200 mg as fumarate)

▶**Chromagen**®**Forte** 1 cap daily
  Cap: B-9, folic acid (1 mg), B-12, cyanocobalamin (10 mcg)/C (60 mg)/iron (151 mg, 460 mg as fumarate) desiccated stomach substance (100 mg)

▶**Citracal**® **(OTC)** 1-2 tabs bid
  Tab: calcium, elemental (200 mg as citrate)

▶**Citracal**®**+D (OTC)** 1-2 caplets bid
  Cplt: calcium, elemental (315 mg as citrate)/D (200 IU)

▶**Citracal**®**250+D (OTC)** 1-2 tabs bid

Cplt: calcium, elemental (250 mg as citrate)/D (62.3 IU)
▶**Citracal®Liquitab (OTC)** 1 effervescent tab dissolved in water daily-bid (phenylalanine)
Liqutab: calcium, elemental (500 mg as citrate)
▶**Citracal®Plus w. Magnesium (OTC)** 1-2 tabs bid
Tab: B-6, pyridoxine (5 mg)/D (125 IU)/boron (0.5 mcg)/calcium, elemental (250 mg as citrate)/copper (0.5 mg as gluconate)/magnesium (40 mg as oxide)/manganese (0.5 mg as gluconate)/zinc (5 mg as oxide)
▶**Feosol®Tablets (OTC)** 1 tab tid-qid pc and HS
Tab: iron (65 mg, 200 mg as sulfate)
▶**Feosol®Caplets (OTC)** 1 tab tid pc
Cplt: iron (45 mg as carbonyl)
▶**Feosol®Capsules (OTC)** 1-2 caps daily
Cap: iron (50 mg, 169 mg as sulfate; sust-rel)
▶**Feosol®Elixir (OTC)** 5-10 ml tid (16 oz)
Listed component is per 5 ml
Elix: iron (44 mg, 220 mg as sulfate)
▶**Fergon® (OTC)** 1 tab daily
Tab: iron (27 mg, 240 mg as gluconate)
▶**Fer-In-Sol®Syrup (OTC)** 5 ml daily (480 ml)
Listed component is per 5 ml
Syr: iron (18 mg, 90 mg as sulfate)
▶**Fero-Folic®-500** 1 tab daily
Tab: B-9, folic acid (0.8 mg)/C (500 mg)/iron (105 mg as sulfate)
▶**Fero-Grad-500®Filmtab** 1 tab daily
Filmtab: iron (525 mg as sulfate)/C (500 mg)
▶**Folbee®** 1 tab daily
Tab: B-6, pyridoxine (25 mg)/B-9, folic acid (2.5 mg)/B-12, cyanocobalamin (1 mg)
▶**Folbee®Plus** 1 tab daily
Tab: B-1, thiamin (1.5 mg)/B-2, riboflavin (1.5 mg)/B-3, niacinamide (100 mg)/B-5, pantothenic acid (10 mg)/B-6, pyridoxine (50 mg)/B-9, folic acid (5 mg)/B-12, cyanocobalamin (1 mg)/biotin (300 mcg)/C (60 mg)
▶**Folbic®** 1 tab daily
Tab: B-6, pyridoxine (25 mg)/B-9, folic acid (2.5 mg)/B-12, cyanocobalamin (2 mg)
▶**Foltx®** 1 tab daily (dye-free)
Comment: Adjunct in hyperhomocysteinemia, homocysteinuria, dialysis, end stage renal disese (ESRD), and vascular disease.
Tab: B-6, pyridoxine (25 mg)/B-9, folic acid (2.5 mg)/B-12 (2 mg)

▶**Glutofac-ZX®** 1 tab daily
Comment: Adjunct in hyperhomocysteinemia, homocysteinuria, dialysis, end stage renal disese (ESRD), and vascular disease.
  Tab: A (5000 IU)/B-1, thiamin (20 mg)/B-2, riboflavin (20 mg)/B-3, niacinamide (100 mg)/B-5, pantothenic acid (25 mg)/B-6, pyridoxine (25 mg)/B-9, folic acid (0.8 mg)/B-12, cyanocobalamin (50 mcg)/C (500 mg)/D (400 IU)/E (30 IU)/biotin (200 mcg)/calcium (50 mg as citrate)/chromium (200 mcg as picolinate)/copper (5 mg as sulfate)/magnesium (50 mg as oxide)/manganese/(5 mg as dioxide)/selenium (50 mcg)/zinc (40 mg as oxide)

▶**Iberet®500 Filmtab** 1 tab daily
  Filmtab: iron (525 mg as sulfate, controlled-release)

▶**Iberet®-500 Liquid** 2 tsp bid (8 oz)
  Listed components are per 5 ml
  Liq: B-1, thiamin (1.5 mg)/B-2, riboflavin (1.5 mg)/B-3, niacinamide (7.5 mg)/B-6, pyridoxine/(1.25 mg)/B-12, cyanocobalamin (6.25 mcg)/C (125 mg)/dexpantenol (2.5 mg)/iron (26.25 mg as sulfate)

▶**Iberet®-Folic-500 Filmtab** 1 filmtab daily
  Filmtab: B-1, thiamin (6 mg)/B-2, riboflavin (6 mg)/B-3, niacinamide (30 mg)/B-6, pyridoxine (5 mg)/B-9, folic acid (0.8 mg)/B-12, cyanocobalamin (25 mcg)/C (500 mg)/calcium (10 mg)/iron (525 mg as sulfate)

▶**Icar®-C Plus** 1 tab daily
  Tab: B-9, folic acid (1 mg)/B-12, cyanocobalamin (5 mcg)/C (250 mg)/iron (100 mg carbonyl)

▶**Nascobal®Gel** 1 spray intranasally once per week; may increase dose if serum B-12 levels decline; adjust dose in 500 mcg increments.
Comment: For maintenance of hematologic remission following intramuscular B-12 therapy.
  Nasal spray: B-12, cyanocobalamin (500 mcg/0.1 ml actuation [2.3 ml])

▶**Niferex® (OTC)** 1-2 tabs bid
  Tab: iron (50 mg, as cell-contracted akaganeite)

▶**Niferex®Elixir (OTC)** 5-10 ml daily
  Listed component is per 5 ml
  Elix: iron (100 mg as cell-contracted akaganeite)

▶**Niferex®-150 (OTC)** 1-2 caps daily
  Cap: iron (150 mg (as cell-contracted akaganeite)

▶**Niferex®-150 Forte** 1 cap daily
  Cap: B-9, folic acid (1 mg)/ B-12, cyanocobalamin (25 mcg)/iron 150 mg (as cell-contracted akaganeite)

- **Os-Cal® (OTC)(G)** 1 chewtab bid-tid
    Chew tab: calcium, elemental (500 mg as carbonate)
- **Os-Cal®250+D (OTC)(G)** 1 tab tid with meals
    Tab: calcium, elemental (250 mg(as carbonate)/D (125 IU)
- **Os-Cal®500+D (OTC)(G)** 1 tab tid with meals
    Tab: calcium, elemental (500 mg as carbonate)/D (125 IU)
- **Renax®Caplets** 1 tab daily (gluten-free, lactose-free)

Comment: **Renax®** is formulated to meet the nutritional needs of the renal patient.

   Cplt: B-1, thiamin (3 mg)/B-2, riboflavin (2 mg)/B-3, niacinamide (20 mg)/B-5, pantothenic acid (10 mg)/B-6, pyridoxine (15 mg/B-9 folic acid (2.5 mg)/B-12 cyanocobalamin (12 mcg)/C (50 mg)/E (30 IU)/biotin (300 mcg)/chromium (200 mcg as chloride)/selenium (70 mcg)/zinc (20 mg)
- **Slow Fe® (OTC)** 1-2 tabs daily
    Tab: Iron (50 mg as 160 as sulfate, sust-rel)
- **Slow Fe®Plus Folic Acid (OTC)** 1 tab daily
    Tab: B-9, folic acid (0.4 mg)/iron (50 mg as 160 as sulfate, sust-rel)
- **Slow-Mag® (OTC)** 1-2 tabs daily
    Tab: calcium (110 mg as carbonate)/magnesium (64 mg as chloride)
- **Strovite®Advance Caplets** 1 tab daily (dye-free, iron-free, gluten-free, lactose-free)
    Tab: A (3000 IU, 40% as carotenoids)/B-1 (20 mg)/B-2, riboflavin (5 mg)/B-3, niacinamide (25 mg)/B-5 pantothenic acid (15 mg)/B-6, pyridoxine (25 mg)/B-9, folic acid (1 mg)/B-12, cyanocobalamin (50 mcg)/C (300 mg)/D (400 mg)/E (100 IU)/K (25 mcg)/alpha lipoic acid (15 mg)/biotin (15 mcg)/chromium (50 mcg as chloride)/copper (1.5 mg as sulfate)/lutein (5 mg)/magnesium (50 mg as oxide)/manganese 1.5 mg/selenium (100 mcg)/zinc 25 mg (as oxide)
- **Trinsicon®** 1 cap bid
    Cap: B-9, folic acid (0.5 mg)/B-12, cyanocobalamin (15 mcg)/C (75 mg)/iron (110 mg as fumarate)/liver-stomach concentrate (240 mg)
- **Theragran® (OTC)** 1 tab daily
    Tab: A (5000 IU)/B-1, thiamin (3 mg)/B-2, riboflavin (3.4 mg)/B-3, niacinamide (20 mg)/B-5, pantothenic acid (10 mg)/B-6, pyridoxine (3 mg)/B-9, folic acid (0.4 mg)/B-12, cyanocobalamin (9 mcg)/ C (90 mg)/D (400 IU)/E (30 IU)/biotin (30 mcg)
- **Theragran®Liquid (OTC)** 5 ml daily (4 oz)
    Listed components are per 5 ml

Liq: A (5000 IU)/B-1, thiamin (10 mg)/B-2, riboflavin (10 mg)/B-3, niacinamide (100 mg)/B-5, pantothenic acid (21.4 mg)/B-6, pyridoxine (4.1 mg)/B-12, cyanocobalamin (5 mcg)/C (200 mg)/ D (400 IU)

▶**Theragran®M (OTC)** 1 tab daily

Tab: A (5000 IU, 40% as acetate and beta carotene)/B-1, thiamin 3mg)/ B-2, riboflavin (3.4 mg)/B-3, niacinamide (20 mg)/B-5, pantothenic acid (10 mg)/B-6, pyridoxine (3 mg)/B-9, folic acid (0.4 mg)/B-12, cyanocobalamin (9 mcg)/C (90 mg)/D (400 mg)/E (30 IU)/K (28 mcg)/biotin (30 mcg)/calcium (40 mg as carbonate)/chloride (7.5 mg as potassium)/chromium (26 mcg as chloride)/copper (2 mg as oxide)/iodine (150 mcg as potassium)/iron (18 mg as fumarate)/ magnesium (100 mg as oxide)/manganese (3.5 mg)/molybdenum (32 mcg)/nickel (5 mcg)/phosphorus (31 mg as calcium)/potassium (7.5 mg (as chloride)/selenium (21 mcg)/zinc (15 mg)

▶**Theragran®Stress (OTC)** 1 tab daily

Tab: B-1, thiamin (15 mg)/B-2, riboflavin (15 mg)/B-3, niacinamide (100 mg)/B-5, pantothenic acid (20 mg)/B-6, pyridoxine (25 mg)/B-9, folic acid (0.4 mg)/B-12 (12 mcg)/C (600 mg)/D (400 mg)/E (30 IU)/biotin (45 mcg)/iron (27 mg)

▶**Vicon®C (OTC)** 1 cap bid-tid

Cap: B-1, thiamin (20 mg)/B-2, riboflavin (10 mg)/B-3, niacinamide (100 mg)/B-5, pantothenic acid (10 mg)/B-6, pyridoxine (5 mg)/C (300 mg)/magnesium (6.4 mg as sulfate)/zinc (15.9 mg as sulfate)

▶**Vicon®Forte** 1 cap daily

Cap: A (8000 IU) B-1, thiamin (10 mg)/B-2, riboflavin (3.4 mg)/B-3, niacinamide (25 mg)/B-5, pantothenic acid (10 mg)/B-6, pyridoxine (2 mg)/B-9, folic acid (1 mg)/B-12, cyanocobalamin (10 mcg)/C (150 mg)/E (50 IU)/ magnesium (100 mg as sulfate)/manganese (4 mg)/zinc (80 mg as sulfate)

▶**Vicon®Plus (OTC)** 1 cap bid; maz 8 caps/day

Cap: A (4000 IU) B-1, thiamin (10 mg)/B-2, riboflavin (5 mg)/B-3, niacinamide (25 mg)/B-5, pantothenic acid (10 mg)/B-6, pyridoxine (2 mg)/C (150 mg)/E (50 IU)/ magnesium (5 mg as sulfate)/ manganese (1 mg)/zinc (10 mg as sulfate)

Appendix V.2: Vitamin & Mineral Supplement for Infants & Children

▶**Feosol®Caplets (OTC)**
    <6 years use elixir
    6-12 years: 1 tab tid pc
    Cplt: iron (45 mg as carbonyl)

▶**Feosol®Capsules (OTC)**
    <6 years use elixir
    6-12 years: 1 cap daily
    Cap: iron (50 mg, 169 mg as sulfate, sust-rel)

▶**Feosol®Tablets (OTC)**
    <6 years use elixir
    6-12 years: 1 tab tid pc
    Tab: iron (65 mg, 200 mg as sulfate)

▶**Feosol®Elixir (OTC)** (16 oz)
    <1 year: use drops
    >1 year: 2.5-5 ml tid between meals
    Listed component is per 5 ml
    Elix: iron (44 mg, 220 mg as sulfate)

▶**Fer-In-Sol®Syrup (OTC)** (480 ml)
    <4 years, use drops
    >4 years: 5 ml daily
    Listed component is per 5 ml
    Syr: iron (18 mg, 90 mg as sulfate)

▶**Fer-In-Sol®Drops (OTC)** (50 ml)
    <4 years: 0.6 ml daily
    >4 years: use syrup
    Listed component is per 5 ml
    Drops: iron 15 mg (75 mg as sulfate)

▶**Iberet®-500 Liquid** (8 oz)
    1-3 years: 1 tsp bid
    >3 years: 2 tsp bid
    Listed components are per teaspoon
    Liq: B-1, thiamin (1.5 mg)/B-2, riboflavin (1.5 mg)/B-3, niacinamide (7.5 mg)/B-6, pyridoxine (1.25 mg)/B-12, cyanocobalamin (6.25 mcg)/C (125 mg)/dexpantenol (2.5 mg)/iron (26.25 mg (as sulfate)

▶**Niferex®**
    <6 years: not recommended
    6-12 years: 1-2 tabs daily

Tab: iron (50 mg as cell-contracted akaganeite)

▶**Niferex®Elixir**
<6 years: not recommended
6-12 years: 5 ml daily
Listed component is per 5 ml
Elix: iron (100 mg as cell-contracted akaganeite)

▶**Poly-Vi-Flor®Chewable Tabs** 1 chew tab daily; base dose on fluoride content of water; indicate fluoride content (0.25 mg or 0.5 mg or 1 mg/chew tab); <4 years use drops

       Water fluoridation 0.3-0.6 ppm:
           <3 years: not recommended
           3-6 years: 0.25 mg fluoride/day
           6-16 years: 0.5 mg fluoride/day
       Water fluoridation <0.3 ppm:
           <6 months: not recommended
           6 months-3 years: 0.25 mg fluoride/day
           3-6 years: 0.5 mg fluoride/day
           6-16 years: 1 mg fluoride/day

Chew tab: A (2500 IU)/B-1, thiamin (1.05 mg)/B-2, riboflavin (1.2 mg)/B-3, niacinamide (13.5 mg)/B-6, pyridoxine (1.05 mg)/B-9, folic acid (0.3 mg)/B-12, cyanocobalamin (4.5 mcg)/C (60 mg)/D (400 IU)/E (15 IU)/fluoride (0.25 mg or 0.5 mg or 1 mg as sodium)

▶**Poly-Vi-Flor®Drops** base dose on fluoride content of water (see **Poly-Vi-Flor®Chewable** Tab above); indicate fluoride content of drops: 0.25 mg or 0.5 mg/ml (50 ml); <4 years use drops
Chew tab: A (1500 IU)/B-1, thiamin (0.5 mg)/B-2, riboflavin (0.6 mg)/B-3, niacinamide (8 mg)/B-6, pyridoxine (0.4 mg)/B-12, cyanocobalamin (2 mcg)/C (35 mg)/D (400 IU)/E (5 IU)/fluoride (0.25 mg or 0.5 mg/ml as sodium)

▶**Poly-Vi-Flor®w. Iron Chewable Tabs** 1 chew tab daily; base dose on fluoride content of water; indicate fluoride content (0.25 mg or 0.5 mg/chew tab); <4 years use drops
Chew tab: A (2500 IU)/B-1, thiamin (1.05 mg)/B-2, riboflavin (1.2 mg)/B-3, niacinamide (13.5 mg)/B-6, pyridoxine (1.05 mg)/B-9, folic acid (0.3 mg)/B-12 cyanocobalamin (4.5 mcg)/C (60 mg)/D (400 IU)/E (15 IU)/fluoride (0.25 mg or 0.5 mg or 1 mg/ml as sodium)/iron (12 mg as fumarate)/zinc (10 mg as oxide)

▶**Poly-Vi-Flor®w. Iron Drops** base dose on fluoride content of water (see Poly-Vi-Flor® Chewable Tab® above); indicate fluoride content of drops: 0.25 mg or 0.5 mg/ml (50 ml); <4 years use drops
Drops: A (1500 IU)/B-1, thiamin (0.5 mg)/B-2, riboflavin (0.6

mg)/B-3, niacinamide (8 mg)/B-6, pyridoxine (0.45 mg)/C (35 mg)/ D (400 IU)/E (5 IU)/fluoride (0.25 mg <u>or</u> 0.5 mg/ml as sulfate heptahydrate)/iron (10 mg as fumarate)

▶ **Poly-Vi-Sol®Chewable Tabs (OTC)** >4 years, 1 chew tab daily
▶ **Poly-Vi-Sol®Drops (OTC)** <4 years, 1 ml daily
▶ **Poly-Vi-Sol®w/Iron Drops (OTC)** <4 years, 1 ml daily
▶ **Poly-Vi-Sol®with Iron & Zinc Drops (OTC)** <4 years, 1 ml daily
▶ **Poly-Vi-Sol®with Iron & Zinc Chewable Tabs (OTC)** >4 years, 1 chew tab daily
▶ **Slow Fe® (OTC)**
　　<6 years: not recommended
　　6-12 years: 1 tab daily
　　Tab: iron (50 mg, 160mg as sulfate; sust-rel)
▶ **Tri-Vi-Flor®Drops** base dose on fluoride content of water; indicate fluoride content of drops: 0.25 mg or 0.5 mg/ml (50 ml); <4 years use drops

　　　　Water fluoridation 0.3-0.6 ppm:
　　　　　　<3 years: not recommended
　　　　　　3-6 years: 0.25 mg fluoride/day
　　　　　　6-16 years: 0.5 mg fluoride/day
　　　　Water fluoridation <0.3 ppm:
　　　　　　<6 months: not recommended
　　　　　　6 months-3 years: 0.25 mg fluoride/day
　　　　　　3-6 years: 0.5 mg fluoride/day
　　　　　　6-16 years: 1 mg fluoride/day
　　Drops: A (1500 IU)/C (35 mg)/D (400 IU)/fluoride (0.25 mg or 0.5 mg/ml as sodium)
▶ **Tri-Vi-Flor®w. Iron Drops** base dose on fluoride content of water (see Tri-Vi-Flor® Drops above); indicate fluoride content of drops: 0.25 mg <u>or</u> 0.5 mg/ml (50 ml); <4 years use drops
　　Drops: A (1500 IU)/C (35 mg)/D (400 IU)/fluoride (0.25 mg <u>or</u> 0.5 mg/ml (as sodium)/iron (10 mg as sulfate heptahydrate)
▶ **Tri-Vi-Sol® (OTC)** infants, 1 ml daily
▶ **Tri-Vi-Sol®with Iron (OTC)** infants, 1 ml/day

Appendix V.3: Prenatal Vitamin & Mineral Supplements

▶**Advanced Formula Zenate®** 1 tab daily **(G)**
   Tab: A (300 IU as beta carotene)/B-1, thiamin (3mg)/B-2, riboflavin (1.5 mg)/B-3, niacinamide (17 mg)/B-6, pyridoxine (2.2 mg)/B-9, folic acid (1 mg)/B-12, cyanocobalamin (2.2 mcg)/C (70 mg)/D (400 mg)/E (10 IU)/ calcium (200 mg as carbonate)/iodine (175 mcg as potassium)/iron (65 mg as carbonyl)/magnesium (100 mg as hydroxide)/zinc (15 mg)

▶**Advanced NatalCare® (G)** 1 tab daily
   Comment: **Advanced NatalCare®** is OU kosher certified.
   Tab: A (2700 IU as beta carotene)/B-1, thiamin (3mg)/B-2, riboflavin (3.4 mg)/B-3, niacinamide (20 mg)/B-6, pyridoxine (20 mg)/B-9, folic acid (1 mg)/B-12, cyanocobalamin (12 mcg)/C (120 mg)/D (400 mg)/E (30 IU)/ calcium (200 mg as carbonate)/copper (2 mg)/docusate sodium (50 mg)/iron (90 mg as carbonyl)/zinc (25 mg)

▶**Chromagen®OB (G)** 1 cap daily
   Cap: B-1, thiamin (1.6mg)/B-2, riboflavin (1.8 mg)/B-3, niacinamide (5 mg)/B-6, pyridoxine (20 mg)/B-9, folic acid (1 mg)/B-12, cyanocobalamin (12 mcg)/C (60 mg)/D (400 mg)/E (30 IU)/calcium (200 mg as carbonate)/copper (2 mg as sulfate)/ docusate calcium (25 mg)/iron (28 mg as fumarate)/manganese (2 mg as sulfate)/zinc (25 mg)

▶**Citracal®Prenatal Rx** 1 cap daily
   Cap: A (2700 IU)/B-1, thiamin (3mg)/B-2, riboflavin (3.4 mg)/ B-3, niacinamide (20 mg)/B-6, pyridoxine (20 mg)/B-9, folic acid (1 mg)/B-12, cyanocobalamin (6 mcg)/C (120 mg)/D (400 mg)/E (30 IU)/calcium (125 mg as citrate)/copper (2 mg as xide)/docusate sodium (50 mg)/iodine (150 mcg as potassium)/iron (27 mg as carbonyl and gluconate)/zinc (25 mg as oxide)

▶**Citracal®Prenatal+DHA** 1 cap and 1 tab daily
   Tab: A (2700 IU)/B-1, thiamin (3mg)/B-2, riboflavin (3.4 mg)/B-3, niacinamide (20 mg)/B-6, pyridoxine (20 mg)/B-9, folic acid (1 mg)/C (120 mg)/D (400 mg)/D-3, cholecalciferol (400 IU)/E (30 IU)/ calcium (125 mg as citrate)/copper (2 mg as oxide)/DHA (250 mg)/docusate sodium (50 mg)/iodine (150 mcg as potassium)/iron (27 mg as carbonyl and gluconate)/zinc (25 mg as oxide)/DHA (250 mg)

▶**Duet Chewable by StuartNatal®** 1 tab daily
   Tab: same as **Duet by StuartNatal®** (except contains phenylalanine)

▶**Duet by StuartNatal®** 1 tab daily
   Tab: A (3000 IU as beta carotene)/B-1, thiamin (1.8mg)/B-2, riboflavin (4 mg)/B-3, niacinamide (20 mg)/B-6, pyridoxine (25 mg)/B-9, folic acid (1 mg)/B-12, cyanocobalamin (12 mcg)/C (120 mg)/D (400 mg)/E (30 IU)/ calcium (200 mg as carbonate)/copper (2 mg)/docusate sodium (50 mg)/magnesium (25 mg as oxide)/iron (29 mg as fumarate and bisglycinate chelate)/zinc (15 mg as oxide)

▶**Duet DHA by StuartNatal®** 1 tab daily
   Tab: A (3000 IU, 40% as beta carotene)/B-1, thiamin (1.8mg)/B-2, riboflavin (4 mg)/B-3, niacinamide (20 mg)/B-6, pyridoxine (25 mg)/B-9, folic acid (1 mg)/B-12, cyanocobalamin (12 mcg)/C (120 mg)/D (400 mg)/E (30 IU)/calcium (200 mg as carbonate)/copper (2 mg as oxide)/iron (29 mg as fumarate and bisglycinate chelate)/ magnesium (25 mg as oxide)/ zinc (15 mg as oxide)

▶**Enfamil®Natalins Rx (G)** 1 tab daily
   Tab: A (4000 IU as beta carotene)/B-1, thiamin (1.5mg)/B-2, riboflavin (1.6 mg)/B-3, niacinamide (17 mg)/B-6, pyridoxine (2.6 mg)/B-9, folic acid (0.5 mg)/B-12, cyanocobalamin (2.5 mcg)/C (70 mg)/D (400 mg)/E (15 IU)/calcium (200 mg as carbonate)/copper (1.5 mg)/magnesium (100 mg as hydroxide)/iron (27 mg as fumarate)/ zinc (15 mg as oxide)

▶**NataChew® (G)** 1 chew tab daily
   Tab: A (1000 IU as beta carotene)/B-1, thiamin (2mg)/B-2, riboflavin (3 mg)/B-3, niacinamide (20 mg)/B-6, pyridoxine (10 mg)/B-9, folic acid (0.4 mg)/B-12, cyanocobalamin (12 mcg)/C (120 mg)/D (400 mg)/E (11 IU)/iron (29 mg as fumarate)

▶**NataFort® (G)** 1 tab daily
   Tab: A (1000 IU as beta carotene)/B-1, thiamin (2mg)/B-2, riboflavin (3 mg)/B-3, niacinamide (20 mg)/B-6, pyridoxine (10 mg)/B-9, folic acid (1 mg)/B-12, cyanocobalamin (12 mcg)/C (120 mg)/D (400 mg)/E (11 IU)/iron (60 mg as carbonyl and sulfate)

▶**Natalins®Rx (G)** 1 tab daily
   Tab: A (4000 IU as beta carotene)/B-1, thiamin (1.5mg)/B-2, riboflavin (1.6 mg)/B-3, niacinamide (17 mg)/B-5, pantothenic acid (7 mg)/B-6, pyridoxine (4 mg)/B-9, folic acid (1 mg)/B-12, cyanocobalamin (2.5 mcg)/C (80 mg)/D (400 mg)/E (15 IU)/biotin (0.03 mcg)/calcium (200 mg as carbonate)/copper (3 mg as oxide)/iron (60 mg as carbonyl)/ magnesium (100 mg as hydroxide)/zinc (25 mg)

▶**Nestabs®CBF (G)** 1 tab daily
   Tab: A (4000 IU as beta carotene)/B-1, thiamin (3mg)/B-2, riboflavin (3 mg)/B-3, niacinamide (3 mg)/B-6, pyridoxine (3

mg)/B-9, folic acid (1 mg)/B-12, cyanocobalamin (8 mcg)/C (120 mg)/D (400 mg)/E (30 IU)/calcium (200 mg as carbonate)/iron (50 mg as carbonyl)/zinc (15 mg)

▶**Nestabs®FA (G)** 1 tab daily

Tab: A (4000 IU as beta carotene)/B-1, thiamin (3mg)/B-2, riboflavin (3 mg)/B-3, niacinamide (3mg)/B-6, pyridoxine (3 mg)/B-9, folic acid (1 mg)/B-12, cyanocobalamin (8 mcg)/C (120 mg)/D (400 mg)/E (30 IU)/calcium (200 mg as carbonate)/iodine (150 mcg)/iron (29 mg as carbonyl)/magnesium (100 mg as hydroxide)/zinc (15 mg)

▶**Nestabs®Rx (G)** 1 tab daily

Tab: A (4000 IU as beta carotene)/B-1, thiamin (3 mg)/B-2, riboflavin (3 mg)/B-3, niacinamide (3 mg)/B-5, pantothenic acid (7 mg)/B-6, pyridoxine (3 mg)/B-9, folic acid (1 mg)/B-12, cyanocobalamin (8 mcg)/C (120 mg)/D (400 IU)/E (30 IU)/biotin (30 mcg)/calcium (200 mg as carbonate)/copper (3 mg as oxide)/iodine (150 mgas carbonyl)/iron (29 mg as carbonyl)/magnesium (100 mg as hydroxide)/zinc (15 mg)

▶**Niferex®-PN (G)** 1 tab daily

Tab: A (4000 IU as acetate and beta carotene)/B-1, thiamin (2.43 mg)/B-2, riboflavin (3 mg)/B-3, niacinamide (10 mg)/B-6, pyridoxine (10 mg)/B-9, folic acid (1 mg)/B-12, cyanocobalamin (3 mcg)/C (50 mg)/D (400 IU)/calcium (125 mg as carbonate)/iron (60 mg as as polysaccharide-iron complex, as cell-contracted akaganeite)/zinc (15 mg)

▶**Niferex®-PN Forte (G)** 1 tab daily

Tab: A (5000 IU as acetate and beta carotene)/B-1, thiamin (3 mg)/B-2, riboflavin (3.4 mg)/B-3, niacinamide (20 mg)/B-6, pyridoxine (4 mg)/B-9, folic acid (1 mg)/B-12, cyanocobalamin (12 mcg)/C (80 mg)/D (400 IU)/E (30 IU)/calcium (250 mg as carbonate)/copper (2 mg)/iodine (0.2 mg/iron (60 mg as polysaccharide-iron complex, as cell-contracted akaganeite)/magnesium (10 mg as hydroxide)/zinc (25 mg)

▶**NutriNate®Chewable** 1 tab daily

Comment: **NutriNate®Chewable** is OU kosher certified.

Tab: A (1000 IU as beta carotene)/B-1, thiamin (2 mg)/B-2, riboflavin (3 mg)/B-3, niacinamide (20 mg)/B-6, pyridoxine (10 mg)/B-9, folic acid (0.4 mg)/B-12, cyanocobalamin (12 mcg)/C (120 mg)/D (400 IU)/E (11 IU)/iron (29 mg as fumarate)

▶**PreCare®** 1 caplet daily

Cplt: B-1, thiamin (3 mg)/B-2, riboflavin (3.4 mg)/B-3, niacinamide (20 mg)/B-6, pyridoxine (20 mg)/B-9, folic acid (1 mg)/B-12, cyanocobalamin (12 mcg)/C (50 mg)/D (6 mcg)/E (3.5 IU)/calcium (250 mg as carbonate)/copper (2 mg as sulfate)/iron (40 mg as fumarate and carbonyl)/magnesium (50 mg as oxide)/zinc (15 mg as sulfate)

▶**PreCare®Chewables** 1 chew tab daily
Tab: B-6, pyridoxine (2 mg)/B-9, folic acid (1 mg)/B-12, cyanocobalamin (12 mcg)/C (50 mg)/D (6 mcg)/E (3.5 IU)/calcium (250 mg as carbonate)/copper (2 mg as oxide)/iron (40 mg as fumarate)/ magnesium (50 mg as hydroxide)/zinc (15 mg)

▶**PreCare®Conceive** 1 tab daily
Tab: B-1, thiamin (3 mg)/B-2, riboflavin (3.4 mg)/B-3, niacinamide (20 mg)/B-6, pyridoxine (50 mg)/B-9, folic acid (1 mg)/B-12, cyanocobalamin (12 mcg)/C (60 mg)/D (6 mcg)/E (30 IU)/calcium (200 mg as carbonate)/copper (2 mg as oxide)/iron (40 mg as fumarate and carbonyl)/magnesium (100 mg as hydroxide)/zinc (15 mg)

▶**PremesisRx®** 1 tab daily
Tab: B-6, pyridoxine (75 mg)/B-9, folic acid (1 mg)/B-12, cyanocobalamin (12 mcg)/calcium (200 mg as carbonate)

▶**Prenate®90 (G)** 1 tab daily
Tab: A (4000 IU as beta carotene)/B-1, thiamin (3 mg)/B-2, riboflavin (3.4 mg)/B-3, niacinamide (20 mg)/B-6, pyridoxine (20 mg)/B-9, folic acid (1 mg)/B-12, cyanocobalamin (12 mcg)/C (120 mg)/D (400 mg)/E (30 IU)/calcium (250 mg as carbonate)/copper (2 mg as oxide)/docusate sodium (50 mg)/iodine (150 mcg)/iron (90 mg as carbonyl)/zinc 25 mg (as oxide)

▶**Prenate®Advance** 1 tab daily (dye-free)
Tab: A (2700 IU as beta carotene)/B-1, thiamin (3 mg)/B-2, riboflavin (3.4 mg)/B-3, niacinamide (20 mg)/B-6, pyridoxine (20 mg)/B-9, folic acid (1 mg)/B-12, cyanocobalamin (12 mcg)/C (120 mg)/D (400 mg)/E (30 IU)/calcium (200 mg as carbonate)/copper (2 mg)/ docusate sodium (50 mg)/iron (90 mg as carbonyl)/zinc 25 mg (as oxide)

▶**Prenate®Elite** 1 tab daily
Tab: B-1, thiamin (3 mg)/B-2, riboflavin (3.4 mg)/B-3, niacinamide (20 mg)/B-5, pantothenic acid (6 mg)/B-6, pyridoxine (20 mg)/B-9, folic acid (0.4 mg)/B-12, cyanocobalamin (12 mcg)/C (120 mg)/D (400 mg)/E (10 IU)/calcium (200 mg as carbonate)/copper (2 mg)/ docusate sodium (50 mg)/iron (90 mg as carbonyl)/L-methylfolate (0.6 mg)/magnesium (30 mg as oxide)/zinc 25 mg (as oxide)

▶**Prenate®GT** 1 geltab daily
Geltab: A (2700 IU as beta carotene)/B-1, thiamin (3 mg)/B-2,

riboflavin (3.4 mg)/B-3, niacinamide (20 mg)/B-5, pantothenic acid (6 mg)/B-6, pyridoxine (20 mg)/B-9, folic acid (1 mg)/B-12, cyanocobalamin (12 mcg)/C (120 mg)/D (400 mg)/E (10 IU)/calcium (200 mg as carbonate)/copper (2 mg)/docusate sodium (50 mg)/iron (90 mg as carbonyl)/magnesium (30 mg as oxide)/zinc 15 mg (as oxide)

▶**Prenate®Ultra** 1 tab daily **(G)**
   Tab: A (2700 IU as beta carotene)/B-1, thiamin (3 mg)/B-2, riboflavin (3.4 mg)/B-3, niacinamide (20 mg)/B-6, pyridoxine (20 mg)/B-9, folic acid (1 mg)/B-12, cyanocobalamin (12 mcg)/C (120 mg)/D (400 mg)/E (30 IU)/calcium (200 mg as carbonate)/copper (2 mg)/ docusate sodium (50 mg)/iron (90 mg as carbonyl)/zinc 25 mg

▶**PrimaCare®** 1 cap in AM and 1 tab in PM (dye-free)
   Cap: D (170 IU)/E (30 IU)/calcium (150 mg as carbonate)/ linoleic acid (25 mg)/linolenic acid (25 mg)/omega-3 fatty acids (150mg)
   Tab: B-1, thiamin 3mg)/B-2, riboflavin (3.4 mg)/B-3, niacinamide (20 mg)/B-5, pantothenic acid (7 mg)/B-6, pyridoxine (10 mg)/B-9, folic acid (1 mg)/B-12, cyanocobalamin (12 mcg)/C (100 mg)/D (230 mg)/K (90 mcg)/biotin (35 mcg)/calcium (200 mg as carbonate)/chromium (45 mcg as chloride)/copper (1.3 mg as oxide)/iron (30 mg as fumarate)/molybdenum (50 mcg)/selenium (75 mcg as oxide)/zinc (11 mg as oxide)

▶**StrongStart®Caplets** 1 cap daily
   Cap: A (1000 IU as beta carotene)/B-1, thiamin (3mg)/ B-2, riboflavin (3 mg)/B-3, niacinamide (15 mg)/B-5, pantothenic acid (7 mg)/B-6, pyridoxine (20 mg)/B-9, folic acid (1 mg)/B-12, cyanocobalamin (12 mcg)/C (100 mg)/D (400 mg)/E (30 IU)/calcium (200 mg as carbonate)/docusate sodium (25 mg)/iron (29 mg as fumarate)/zinc (20 mg)

▶**StrongStart®Chewables (G)** 1 chew tab daily
   Chew tab: A (1000 IU as beta carotene)/B-1, thiamin (3mg)/ B-2, riboflavin (3 mg)/B-3, niacinamide (15 mg)/B-5, pantothenic acid (7 mg)/B-6, pyridoxine (20 mg)/B-9, folic acid (1 mg)/B-12, cyanocobalamin (12 mcg)/C (100 mg)/D (400 mg)/E (30 IU)/ calcium (200 mg as carbonate)/iron (29 mg as fumarate)/zinc (15 mg)

▶**Stuartnatal®Plus (G)** 1 tab daily
   Tab: A (4000 IU as beta carotene)/B-1, thiamin (1.84 mg)/B-2, riboflavin (3 mg)/B-3, niacinamide (20 mg)/B-6, pyridoxine (10 mg)/B-9, folic acid (1 mg)/B-12, cyanocobalamin (12 mcg)/C (120 mg)/D (400 mg)/E (22 IU)/calcium (200 mg as carbonate)/copper (2 mg)/iron (27 mg as fumarate)/zinc (25 mg)

▶**Stuartnatal®Plus 3 (G)** 1 tab daily (dye-free)
   Tab: A (3000 IU as beta carotene)/B-1, thiamin (1.8 mg)/B-2, riboflavin (4 mg)/B-3, niacinamide (20 mg)/B-6, pyridoxine (25 mg)/B-9, folic acid (1 mg)/B-12, cyanocobalamin (12 mcg)/C (120 mg)/D (400 mg)/E (22 IU)/calcium (200 mg as carbonate)/copper (2 mg)/iron (28 mg as fumarate)/magnesium (25 mg as oxide)/zinc (25 mg)

▶**Ultra NatalCare®Chewable (G)** 1 chew tab daily
Comment: **Ultra NatalCare®** is OU-dairy kosher certified.
   Chew tab: A (2700 IU as beta carotene)/B-1, thiamin (3mg)/B-2, riboflavin (3.4 mg)/B-3, niacinamide (20 mg)/B-6, pyridoxine (20 mg)/B-9, folic acid (1 mg)/B-12, cyanocobalamin (12 mcg)/C (120 mg)/D (400 mg)/E (30 IU)/calcium (200 mg as carbonate)/copper (2 mg)/ docusate sodium (50 mg)/iron (90 mg as carbonyl)/zinc (25 mg)

▶**Vinate®GT** 1 tab daily
   Tab: A (2700 IU as beta carotene)/B-1, thiamin (3 mg)/B-2, riboflavin (3.4 mg)/B-6, pyridoxine (20 mg)/B-9, folic acid (1 mg)/B-12, cyanocobalamin (12 mcg)/C (120 mg)/D-3, cholecalciferol (400 IU)/E (10 IU)/biotin (30 mcg)/calcium (200 mg as carbonate)/ copper (2 mg)/docusate sodium (50 mg)/iron (90 mg as carbonyl)/ magnesium (30 mg as oxide)/pantothenic acid (6 mg)/zinc 15 mg (as oxide)

Appendix W: Oral Drugs for the Management of Common Respiratory Symptoms

Oral drugs for the management of common respiratory symptoms are presented, with generic components and additives in alphabetical order by brand name.

		Page
Single Agents		
Appendix W.1:	1st Generation Antihistamines	525
Appendix W.2:	2nd Generation Antihistamines	527
Appendix W.3:	Decongestants	528
Appendix W.4:	Expectorants	529
Appendix W.5:	Antitussives	530
Combination Agents		
Appendix W.6:	Antihistamine/Decongestant	531
Appendix W.7:	Decongestant/Expectorant	537
Appendix W.8:	Decongestant/Analgesic	540
Appendix W.9:	Decongestant/Antihistamine/Analgesic	540
Appendix W.10:	Antitussive/Antihistamine	541
Appendix W.11:	Antitussive/Decongestant	542
Appendix W.12:	Antitussive/Expectorant	543
Appendix W.13:	Antitussive/Decongestant/Antihistamine	546
Appendix W.14:	Antitussive/Decongestant/Expectorant	551
Appendix W.15:	Antitussive/Decongestant/Expectorant/ Antihistamine	553
Appendix W.16:	Antitussive/Decongestant/Analgesic	553
Appendix W.17:	Antitussive/Decongestant/Expectorant/ Analgesic	554
Appendix W.18:	Antitussive/Antihistamine/Decongestant/ Analgesic	554
Appendix W.19:	Antitussive/Antihistamine/Decongestant/ Analgesic/Caffeine	554

Legend:

	acet	acetaminophen
	acriv	acrivastine
	atro	atropine
	azat	azatadine
	benzo	aenzonatate
	brom	brompheniramine
	caf	caffeine
	carb	carbinoxamine
	carbet	carbetapentane
	carbeta	carbetaplex
	chlor	chlorpheniramine
	citir	citirizine
	clem	clemastine
	cod	codeine
	cypro	cyproheptadine
	des	desloratadine
	dex	dexbrompheniramine
	dexchlor	dexchlorpheniramine
	dextro	dextromethorphan
	diph	diphenhydramine
	ephed	ephedrine
	fexo	fexofenadine
	guaiac	potassium guaiacolsolfonate
	guaif	guaifenesin
	hom	homatropine
	hydro	hydrocodone
	hydrox	hydroxyzine pamoate
	hyo	hyoscyamine
	ibup	ibuprofen
	lorat	loratadine
	meth	methscopolamine
	phen	phenindamine
	pheni	pheniramine
	phenyl	phenylephedrine
	phenyle	phenylephrine
	phenylt	phenyltoloxamine
	pot	potassium iodine
	prom	promethazine
	pseud	pseudoephedrine
	pyr	pyrilamine
	scop	scopolomine
	trip	triprolidine

Appendix W.1: 1st Generation Antihistamines

▶**Atarax® (B)** 25 mg tid-qid prn
  Pediatric: <2 years: not recommended
  2-6 years: 6.25 mg q 4-6 hours prn
  6-12 years: 12.5-25 mg q 4-6 hours prn
  Tab: hydrox 10, 25, 50, 100 mg; *Syr:* 10 mg/5 ml (alcohol 0.5%)

▶**Benadryl®Allergy (B)(OTC)** 25-50 mg q 4-6 hours prn
  Pediatric: <2 years: not recommended
  2-6 years: 6.25 mg q 4-6 hours prn
  6-12 years: 12.5-25 mg q 4-6 hours prn
  Chew tab: diph 12.5 mg (grape, phenylalanine); *Liq:* diph 12.5 mg per 5 ml (4, 8 oz); *Tab, Cap:* diph 25 mg; *Dye-free liq:* diph 12.5 mg per 5 ml (4 oz); *Dye-free softgel:* diph 25 mg

▶**Chlor-Trimeton®4 Hour Allergy Tablets (B)(OTC)** 1 tab q 4-6 hours prn; max 6 tabs/day
  Pediatric: <6 years: not recommended
  6-12 years: 1/2 tab q 4-6 hours prn; max 3 tabs/day
  Tab: chlor 4*mg

▶**Chlor-Trimeton®8 Hour Allergy Tablets (C)(OTC)** 1 tab q 8 hours prn
  Pediatric: <12 years: not recommended
  Tab: chlor 8 mg

▶**Chlor-Trimeton®12 Hour Allergy (C)(OTC)** 1 tab q 12 hours prn
  Pediatric: <12 years: not recommended
  Tab: chlor 12 mg

▶**Dimetapp®Allergy (C)(OTC)** 1 tab or cap q 4-6 hours prn
  Pediatric: <6 years: not recommended
  6-12 years: 2 mg q 4-6 hours prn
  Tab, Cap: brom 4 mg

▶**Histex®-Pd (C)** 2 tsp qid hours prn
  Pediatric: <1 month: not recommended
  1-3 months: 1/4 tsp qid hours prn
  3-6 months: 1/2 tsp qid hours prn
  6-9 months: 3/4 tsp qid hours prn
  9-18 months: ¾ -1 tsp qid hours prn
  18 months-6 years: 1tsp qid hours prn
  >6 years: same as adult
  Oral drops: carb 2 mg per 5 ml (4 oz; dye-free, sugar-free, alcohol-free)

▶**Lodrane®12 Hours (C)(OTC)(G)** 1-2 tabs q 12 hours prn

Pediatric: <6 years: not recommended
6-12 years: 1 tab q 12 hours prn
Tab: brom 6 mg ext-rel (dye-free)

▶**Lodrane®24 Hours (C)(OTC)(G)** 1-2 tabs q 24 hours prn
Pediatric: <12 years: not recommended
Tab: brom 12 mg ext-rel (dye-free)

▶**PBZ® (B)** 25-50 mg q 4-6 hours prn; max 600 mg/day
Pediatric: 5 mg/kg/day in 4-6 doses; max 300 mg/day
Tab: trip 25, 50 mg; *Elix:* trip 37.5 mg per 5 ml

▶**PBZ®-SR (B)** 100 mg bid-tid prn; max 300 mg/day
Pediatric: not recommended
Tab: trip 100 mg sust-rel

▶**Palgic® (C)** 4 mg daily prn; max 24 mg/day in divided doses 6-8 hours apart
Pediatric: <1 year: not recommended
1-6 years: 2 mg daily prn; max 0.2-0.4 mg/kg per day in divided doses 6-8 hours apart
>6 years: same as adult
Tab: carb 4*mg; *Syr:* carb 4 mg per 5 ml (bubble gum)

▶**Pediatex® (C)** 2 tsp q 4-6 hours prn
Pediatric: 1-3 months: 1/4 tsp qid prn
3-6 months: 1/2 tsp qid prn
6-9 months: 3/4 tsp qid prn
9-18 months: ¾-1 tsp qid prn
18 months-6 years: 1 tsp qid prn
>6 years: same as adult
Syr: carb 2 mg per 5 ml

▶**Pediox® (C)** 1 tsp qid prn
Pediatric: <3 months: not recommended
3-9 months: 1/4 tsp qid prn
9-18 months: 1/4-1/2 tsp qid prn
18 months-6 years: 1 tsp q qid prn
>6 years: same as adult
Syr: carb 4 mg per 5 ml

▶**Periactin® (B)** initially 4 mg tid prn, then adjust as needed; usual range 12-16 mg/day; max 32 mg/day
Pediatric: <2 years: not recommended
2-6 years: 2 mg bid-tid prn; max 12 mg/day
7-14 years: 4 mg bid-tid prn; max 16 mg/day
>14 years: same as adult
Tab: cypro 4*mg; *Syr:* cypro 2 mg per 5 ml

▶**Phenergan® (C)(G)** 25 mg po or rectally tid ac and HS prn

Pediatric: <2 years: not recommended
>2 years: 0.5 mg/lb or 6.25-25 mg po or rectally tid ac and HS prn

Tab: 12.5*, 25*, 50 mg; *Syr: prom* 6.25 mg per 5 ml; *Syr fortis: prom* 25 mg per 5 ml; *Rectal supp: prom* 12.5, 25, 50 mg

▶**Ryneze® (C)** 1 tab q 12 hours prn
Pediatric: <6 years: not recommended
6-12 years: 1/2 tab q 12 hours prn

Tab: chlor 8 mg/*meth* 2.5 mg

▶**Tavist®24 Hour Allergy (C)(OTC)** 1 tab q 12 hours prn; max 2 tabs/day
Pediatric: <6 years: not recommended
6-12 years: ½-1 tab bid prn; max 2 tabs/day

Tab: clem 1*mg

▶**Vistaril® (C)(G)** 25 mg tid-qid prn
Pediatric: <6 years: 50 mg/day prn
6-12 years: 50-100 mg daily prn

Cap: hydrox 25, 50, 100 mg; *Susp: hydrox* 25 mg/5 ml (lemon)

Appendix W.2: 2nd Generation Antihistamines

▶**Alavert® (B)(OTC)(G)** 10 mg daily prn
Pediatric: <6 years: not recommended
>6 years: same as adult

Tab: lor 10 mg; *ODT: lor* 10 mg orally disintegrating (phenylalanine)

▶**Allegra® (C)** 60 mg bid or 180 mg daily prn
Pediatric: <6 years: not recommended
6-12 years: 30 mg bid prn

Tab: fexo 30, 60, 180 mg; *Cap: fexo* 60 mg

▶**Clarinex® (C)** 1 tab daily prn
Pediatric: <6 years: not recommended

Tab: des 5 mg

▶**Clarinex®RediTabs (C)** 1 tab daily prn
Pediatric: <2 years: not recommended

Tab: des 2.5, 5 mg orally-disintegrating (tutti-frutti, phenylalanine)

▶**Clarinex®Syrup (C)** 1 tab daily prn
Pediatric: <6 months: not recommended
6-11 months: 1 mg (2 ml) daily prn
1-5 years: 1.25 mg (2.5 ml) daily prn
6-11 years: 2.5 mg (5 ml) daily prn
>12 years: 5 mg (10 ml) daily prn

Tab: des 0.5 mg per ml (4 oz) (tutti-frutti, phenylalanine)
▶**Claritin® (B)(OTC)(G)** 10 mg daily prn
Pediatric: <2 years: not recommended
2-5 years: 1 tsp daily prn
>6 years: same as adult

Tab: lor 10 mg; Redi*Tab: lor* 10 mg rapidly disintegrating (mint);
Syr: lor 1 mg/ml (16 oz) (fruit, dye-free, alcohol-free)
▶**Zyrtec® (B)** 5-10 mg daily prn; max 10 mg/day
Pediatric: <2 years: not recommended
2-5 years: 2.5 mg daily or 2.5 mg bid or 5 mg daily prn; max 5 mg/day
6-12 years: 5 mg daily or 5 mg bid or 10 mg daily prn; max 10 mg/day

Tab: cet 5 mg, 10 mg; *Syr: cet* 1 mg per ml (4, 16 oz) (banana-grape, dye-free, alcohol-free)

Appendix W.3: Decongestants

▶**PediaCare®Infant' Decongestant (C)(OTC)(G)**
Pediatric: <3 months: not recommended
3 months (6-11 lb): 0.4 ml q 4-6 hours
4-11 months (12-17 lb): 0.8 ml q 4-6 hours
12-23 months (18-23 lb): 1.2 ml q 4-6 hours
2-3 years: (24-35 lb): 1.6 ml q 4-6 hours
All max 4 doses/day

Oral drops: pseud 7.5 mg per 0.8 ml (15 ml) (alcohol-free)
▶**Children's Sudafed®Chewables (C)(OTC)(G)**
Pediatric: 2-6 years: 1 tab q 4-6 hours prn; max 4 doses/day
6-12 years: 2 tabs q 4-6 hours prn; max 4 doses/day

Chew tab: pseud 15 mg
▶**Children's Sudafed®Liquid (C)(OTC)(G)** 4 tsp q 4-6 hours prn
Pediatric: < 2 years: titrate individually
2-6 years: 1 tsp q 4-6 hours prn
6-12 years: 2 tsp q 4-6 hours prn

Liq: pseud 15 mg per 5 ml (4 oz; sugar-free, alcohol-free)
▶**Dimetapp®Infant Drops Decongestant (C)(OTC)(G)**
Pediatric: 2-3 years: 2 dropperfull (1.6 ml) q 4-6 hours prn; max 4 doses/day

Oral drops: pseud 7.5 mg/0.8 ml (1/4 oz)
▶**Sudafed® (C)(OTC)(G)** 2 tabs q 4-6 hours prn; max 240 mg/day
Pediatric: <2 years: not recommended
2-6 years: use liquid

6-12 years: 30 mg q 4-6 hours prn; max 120 mg/day
Tab: pseud 30 mg
▶**Sudafed®12 Hour (C)(OTC)(G)** 1 tab q 12 hours prn
Pediatric: <12 years: not recommended
Cplt: pseud 120 mg sust-rel
▶**Sudafed®24 Hour (C)(OTC)(G)** 1 tab q 24 hours prn
Pediatric: <12 years: not recommended
Tab: pseud 240 mg sust-rel
▶**Sudafed®Pediatric Nasal Decongestant Oral Drops (C)(OTC)(G)**
Pediatric: <2 years: not recommended
2-6 years: 1.6 ml q 4-6 hours prn; max 4 doses/day
Oral drops: pseud 7.5 mg/0.8 ml (1/2 oz)
▶**Triaminic®Allergy Decongestant (C)(OTC)(G)** 4 tsp q 6 hours prn
Pediatric: <4 months: not recommended
4-12 months (12-17 lb): 1/4 tsp q 4-6 hours prn
12-24 months (18-23 lb): 1/2 tsp q 4-6 hours prn
2-6 years (24-47 lb): 1 tsp q 4-6 hours prn
6-12 years (48-95 lb): 2 tsp q 4-6 hours prn
Liq: pseud 15 mg per 5 ml (4, 8 oz) (alcohol-free)
▶**Triaminic®Infant Oral Decongestant Drops (C)(OTC)(G)**
Pediatric: <4 months: not recommended
4-11 months (12-17 lb): 0.8 ml q 4-6 hours prn
12-23 months (18-23 lb): 1.2 ml q 4-6 hours prn
2-3 years (24-35 lb): 1.6 ml q 4-6 hours prn
Oral drops: pseud 7.5 mg per 0.8 ml (15 ml) (dye-free, alcohol-free)

Appendix W.4: Expectorants

▶**Allfen® (C)** 1 tab q 12 hours prn
Pediatric: <6 years: not recommended
6-12 years: 1/2 tab q 12 hours prn
Tab: guaif 1000 mg sust-rel
▶**Duratuss®G (C)** 1 tab q 12 hours prn
Pediatric: <6 years: not recommended
6-12 years: 1/2 tab q 12 hours prn
Tab: guaif 1200*mg sust-rel (dye-free)
▶**Humibid®LA (C)** 1-2 tabs q 12 hours prn
Pediatric: <2 years: not recommended
2-6 years: 1/2 tab q 12 hours prn
6-12 years: 1 tab q 12 hours prn
Tab: guaif 600*mg sust-rel
▶**Humibid®Pediatric (C)** 2-4 caps q 12 hours prn

    Pediatric: <2 years: not recommended
               2-6 years: 1 cap q 12 hours prn
               6-12 years: 2 caps q 12 hours prn
    Cap: guaif 300 mg sust-rel

▶**Humibid®Sprinkle (C)** 2-4 caps q 12 hours prn; max 8 caps/day
    Pediatric: <2 years: not recommended
               2-6 years: 1 cap q 12 hours prn
               6-12 years: 2 caps q 12 hours prn
    Cap: guaif 300 mg sust-rel

▶**Liquibid® (C)** 1 tab bid prn
    Pediatric: <6 years: not recommended
               6-12 years: 1/2 tab q 12 hours prn
    Tab: guaif 1200*mg sust-rel

▶**Mucinex® (C)(OTC)** 1-2 tabs q 12 hours prn
    Pediatric: <12 years: not recommended
    Tab: guaif 600 mg ext-rel (gluten- and sugar-free)

▶**Organidin®NR (C)** 200-400 mg q 4 hours prn
    Pediatric: <6 months: not recommended
               6 months-2 years: 25-50 mg q 4 hours prn
               2-6 years: 50-100 mg q 4 hours prn
               6-12 years: 100-200 mg q 4 hours prn
    Tab: guaif 200*mg; *Liq:* guaif 100 mg/5 ml

▶**Robitussin® (C)(OTC)(G)** 2-4 tsp q 4 hours prn
    Pediatric: <6 months: not recommended
               6-11 months (14-17 lb): 1/4 tsp q 4 hours prn
               12-23 months (18-23 lb): 1/2 tsp q 4 hours prn
               2-6 years (24-47 lb): ½-1 tsp q 4 hours prn
               6-12 years: 1-2 tsp q 4 hours prn
    Syr: guaif 100 mg/5 ml (4, 8, 16 oz)

Appendix W.5: Antitussives

▶**Benylin®DM Adult (C)(OTC)** 2 tsp q 6-8 hours prn
    Pediatric: <2 years: not recommended
               2-6 years: 1/2 tsp 6-8 hours prn
               6-12 years: 1 tsp q 6-8 hours prn
    Liq: dextro 15 mg/5 ml (4 oz; sugar-free, alcohol-free)

▶**Delsym® (C)(OTC)** 2 tsp q 12 hours prn
    Pediatric: <2 years: not recommended
               2-5 years: 1/2 tsp q 12 hours prn
               6-12 years: 1 tsp q 12 hours prn
    Liq: dextro 30 mg/5 ml (3 oz)

▶**Robitussin®Pediatric Cough Suppressant (C)(OTC)** 4 tsp q 6-8 hours prn
   Pediatric: <6 months: not recommended
   6-11 months (14-17 lb): 1/4 tsp q 6-8 hours prn
   12-23 months (18-23 lb): 1/2 tsp q 6-8 hours prn
   2-6 years (24-47 lb): 1 tsp q 6-8 hours prn
   6-12 years: 10 ml q 6-8 hours prn
   Liq: dextro 7.5 mg/5 ml (4, 8 oz)
▶**Tessalon® (C)** 100-200 mg tid prn; max 600 mg/day
   Pediatric: <10 years: not recommended
   >10 years: same as adult
   Cap: benzo 200 mg; *Perles:* benzo 100 mg
▶**Triaminic Softchew®Cough (C)(OTC)**
   Pediatric: <2 years: not recommended
   2-5 years: 1 tab q 6-8 hours prn
   6-12 years: 2 tabs q 6-8 hours prn
   Tab: dex 7.5 mg

Appendix W.6: Antihistamine/Decongestant

▶**AccuHist®LA (C)(OTC)** 1 tab q 12 hours prn
   Pediatric: <12 years: not recommended
   Tab: chlor 8 mg/phenyle 20 mg/scop 0.01 mg/atro 0.04 mg/ hyo 0.19 mg sust-rel (dye-free)
▶**Actifed®Cold & Allergy Tabs (C)(OTC)** 1 tab q 4-6 hours prn
   Pediatric: <6 years: not recommended
   6-12 years: 1/2 tab q 4-6 hours prn; max 4 doses/day
   Tab: trip 2.5 mg/pseud 60 mg*
▶**Allegra®-D (C)** 1 tab bid prn
   Pediatric: <12 years: not recommended
   Cap: fexo 60 mg/pseud 120 mg ext-rel
▶**Astrohist®Pediatric (C)** 2 caps q 12 hours prn
   Pediatric: <6 years: not recommended
   6-12 years: 1 cap q 12 hours prn
   Cap: chlor 4 mg/pseud 60 mg
▶**Astrohist®Pediatric (C) Suspension**
   Pediatric: 2-6 years: ½-1 tsp q 12 hours prn
   6-12 years: 1-2 tsp q 12 hours prn
   Susp: chlor 2 mg/pyr 12.5 mg/phenyle 5 mg per 5 ml
▶**Benadryl®Allergy/Congestion (C)(OTC)** 1 tab q 4-6 hours prn
   Pediatric: <12 years: titrate individually
   Tab: diph 25 mg/pseud 60 mg

▶**Bromfed®Capsules (C)** 1 cap q 12 hours prn
  Pediatric: <12 years: not recommended
  Cap: brom 12 mg/*pseud* 120 mg ext-rel
▶**Bromfed®-PD (C)** 1-2 caps q 12 hours prn
  Pediatric: <6 years: not recommended
      6-12 years: 1 cap q 12 hours prn
  Cap: brom 6 mg/*pseud* 60 mg sust-rel
▶**Bromfed® Syrup(C)(OTC)** 2 tsp q 4-6 hours prn; max 4 doses/day
  Pediatric: <6 years: not recommended
      6-12 years: 1 tsp q 4-6 hours prn; max 4 doses/day
  Syr: brom 2 mg/*pseud* 30 mg per 5 ml (4, 16 oz) (alcohol-free)
▶**Bromfed®Tabs (C)** 1 tab q 4 hours prn
  Pediatric: <6 years: not recommended
      6-12 years: 1/2 tab q 4 hours prn
  Tab: brom 4 mg/*pseud* 60mg*
▶**Children's Dimetapp®Cold & Allergy (C)(OTC)(G)** 2 tsp q 4 hours prn; max 4 doses/day
  Pediatric: <6 months (14 lb): not recommended
      6-11 months: (14-17 lb) 1/4 tsp q 4 hours prn
      12-23 months: (18-23 lb) 1/4-1/2 tsp q 4 hours prn
      2-5 years: 1/2 tsp q 4 hours prn
      6-12 years: 1 tsp q 4 hours prn
      All max 4 doses/day
  Syr: brom 1 mg/*pseud* 15 mg per 5 ml (4, 8, 12 oz) (alcohol-free)
▶**Chlor-Trimeton®4 Hour Allergy Decongestant Tablets (B)(OTC)(G)** 1 tab q 4-6 hours prn; max 4 tabs/day
  Pediatric: <6 years: not recommended
      6-12 years: 1/2 tab q 4-6 hours prn; max 2 tabs/day
  Tab: chlor 4 mg/*pseud* 60 mg*
▶**Chlor-Trimeton®12 Hour Allergy Decongestant Tablets (C)(OTC)(G)** 1tab q 12 hours prn; max 2 tabs/day
  Pediatric: <12 years: not recommended
  Tab: chlor 8 mg/*pseud* 120 mg sust-rel
▶**Clarinex®-D (C) 12 Hour** 1 tab bid prn
  Pediatric: not recommended
  Tab: des 5 mg/*pseud* 120 mg ext-rel
▶**Clarinex®-D (C) 24 Hour** 1 tab daily prn
  Pediatric: <12 years: not recommended
  Tab: des 5 mg/*pseud* 240 mg ext-rel
▶**Claritin-D®12 Hour (B)(OTC)(G)** 1 tab q 12 hours prn
  Pediatric: not recommended
  Tab: lorat 5 mg/*pseud* 120 mg sust-rel

- **Claritin-D®24 Hour (B)(OTC)(G)** 1 tab daily prn
  Pediatric: not recommended
  Tab: lorat 10 mg/*pseud* 240 mg sust-rel
- **D.A.®Chewables (C)** 1-2 tabs q 4 hours prn
  Pediatric: 6-12 years: 1 tab q 4 hours prn
  Chew tab: chlor 2 mg/*meth* 1.25 mg/*phenyle* 10 mg
- **Deconamine® (C)** 1 tab tid-qid prn
  Pediatric: <12 years: use syrup
  Tab: chlor 4 mg/*pseud* 60 mg
- **Deconamine®SR (C)** 1 cap q 12 hours prn
  Pediatric: <12 years: use syrup
  Cap: chlor 8 mg/*pseud* 120 mg sust-rel
- **Deconamine®Syrup (C)** 1-2 tsp tid-qid prn
  Pediatric: <2 years: not recommended
  2-6 years: 1/2 tsp tid-qid prn; max 2 tsp/day
  6-12 years: ½-1 tsp tid-qid prn; max 4 tsp/day
  Syr: chlor 2 mg/*pseud* 30 mg per 5 ml (dye-free, alcohol-free)
- **Dimetapp®Elixir (C)(OTC)(G)** 2 tsp q 4 hours prn; max 4 doses/day
  Pediatric: <6 years: titrate individually
  6-12 years: 2 tsp q 4 hours prn; max 4 doses/day
  Liq: dextro 5 mg/*pseud* 15 mg per 5 ml (4, 8, 12 oz) (alcohol-free)
- **Drixoral®Cold & Allergy (C)(OTC)** 1 tab q 12 hours prn
  Pediatric: not recommended
  Tab: dex 6 mg/ *pseud* 120 mg sust-rel
- **Duradryl®Syrup (C)** 1-2 tsp q 3-4 hours prn
  Pediatric: <6 years: titrate dosage individually
  6-12 years: ½-1 tsp q 4 hours prn
  Syr: chlor 2 mg/*meth* 1.25 mg/*phenyle* 10 mg per 5 ml (cherry)
- **Dura-Tap®/PD (C)** 2 caps q 12 hours prn
  Pediatric: <6 years: not recommended
  6-12 years: 1 cap q 12 hours prn
  Cap: chlor 4 mg/*pseud* 60 mg
- **Dura-Vent®/DA (C)** 1 tab q 12 hours prn
  Pediatric: <6 years: not recommended
  6-12 years: 1/2 tab q 12 hours prn
  Tab: chlor 8 mg/*meth* 2.5 mg/*phenyle* 20 mg sust-rel
- **Extendryl®Chewable Tabs (C)** 2 tabs <u>or</u> 2 tsp q 4 hours prn
  Pediatric: <6 years: not recommended
  6-12 years: 1 chew tab q 4 hours prn
  Chew tab: chlor 2 mg/*meth* 1.25 mg/*phenyle* 10*mg
- **Extendryl®JR (C)**
  Pediatric: 6-12 years: 1 cap q 12 hours prn

Cap: chlor 4 mg/*meth* 1.25 mg/*phenyle* 10 mg sust-rel; *Syr: chlor* 4 mg/*meth* 1.25/*phenyle* 10 mg mg per 5 ml

▶**Extendryl®SR (C)** 1 cap q 12 hours prn
  Pediatric: <12 years: not recommended
  Cap: chlor 8 mg/*meth* 2.5 mg/*phenyle* 20 mg sust-rel

▶**Extendryl®Syrup (C)** 10 ml q 4-6 hours prn
  Pediatric: <6 years: not recommended
       6-12 years: 5 ml q 4-6 hours prn
  Syr: chlor 2 mg/*meth* 1.25 mg/*phenyle* 10 mg per 5 ml (root beer)

▶**Kronofed®-A (C)** 1 cap q 12 hours prn
  Pediatric: <12 years: not recommended
  Cap: chlor 8 mg/*pseud* 120 mg sust-rel

▶**Kronofed®-A-Jr (C)** 1-2 caps q 12 hours prn
  Pediatric: <6 years: not recommended
       6-12 years: 1 cap q 12 hours prn
  Cap: chlor 4 mg/*pseud* 60 mg

▶**Lodrane®Decongestant (C)(OTC)** 1 tsp q 4-6 hours prn
  Pediatric: <12years: not recommended
  Liq: brom 4 mg/*pseud* 60 mg per 5 ml (dye-free, sugar-free, alcohol-free)

▶**Lodrane®LD (C)(OTC)** 1 tab q 12 hours prn
  Pediatric: <12years: not recommended
  Cap: brom 6 mg/*pseud* 60 mg sust-rel (dye-free)

▶**Mescolor®Tabs (C)** 1 tab q 12 hours prn
  Pediatric: <6 years: not recommended
        6-12 years: 1/2 tab q 12 hours prn
  Tab: chlor 2 mg/*meth* 2.5 m/*pseud* 120 mg*

▶**Nalex®-A (C)** 1 tab bid-tid prn
  Pediatric: <6 years: not recommended
       6-12 years: 1/2 tab bid-tid prn
  Tab: chlor 8 mg/*phenylt* 40 mg/*phenyle* 20 mg*

▶**Nalex®-A Liquid (C)** 2 tsp q 4-6 hours prn
  Pediatric: <6 years: not recommended
       2-6 years: 1/4-1/2 tsp q 4-6 hours prn
       6-12 years: 1 tsp q 4-6 hours prn
  Liq: chlor 2.5 mg/*phenylt* 7.5 mg/*phenyle* 5 mg per 5 ml

▶**Novafed®A (C)** 1 cap q 12 hours prn
  Pediatric: <12 years: not recommended
  Cap: chlor 8 mg/*pseud* 120 mg sust-rel

▶**Palgic®-DS (C)** 4 tsp qid prn
  Pediatric: <18 months: not recommended
       18 months-6 years: 1 tsp qid prn

>6 years: 2 tsp qid prn
Syr: chlor 2 mg/*pseud* 15 mg

▶**Pediatex®-D Liquid (C)** 2 tsp q 4-6 hours prn
Pediatric: 1-3 months: 1/4 tsp qid hours prn
3-6 months: 1/2 tsp qid hours prn
6-9 months: 3/4 tsp qid hours prn
9-18 months: ¾-1 tsp qid hours prn
18 months-6 years: 1 tsp qid hours prn
>6 years: same as adult
Syr: carb 2 mg/*pseud* 15 mg per 5 ml (dye-free, sugar-free, alcohol-free)

▶**Phenergan®VC (C)** 1 tsp q 4-6 hours prn
Pediatric: <2 years: not recommended
2-6 years: 1/4-1/2 tsp q 4-6 hours prn
6-12 years: 1 tsp q 4-6 hours prn
Syr: prom 6.25 mg/*phenyle* 5 mg per 5 ml

▶**Rescon Mx® (C)** 1 tab q 12 hours prn
Pediatric: <6 years: not recommended
6-12 years years: 1/2 tab q 12 hours prn
Tab: chlor 8 mg/*pseud* 120 mg/*meth* 2.5 mg*

▶**Respahist®Chewable (C)** 1-2 capsules q 12 hours prn
Pediatric: <6 years: not recommended
6-12 years: 1 cap q 12 hours prn
Cap: brom 6 mg/*pseud* 60 mg sust-rel

▶**Rondec® (C)** 1 tab qid prn
Pediatric: <6 years: not recommended
>6 years: 1 tab qid prn
Tab: carb 4 mg/*pseud* 60 mg

▶**Rondec®Chewable (C)** 1 tab q 4 hours prn
Pediatric: <6 years: not recommended
6-12 years: 1/2 tab q 4 hours prn
Chew tab: brom 4 mg/*pseud* 60 mg

▶**Rondec®Oral Drops (C)**
Pediatric: 1-3 months: 0.25 ml qid prn
3-6 months: 0.5 ml qid prn
6-9 months: 0.75 ml qid prn
9-18 months: 1 ml qid prn
Oral drops: carb 2 mg/*pseud* 25 mg per ml (30 ml)

▶**Rondec®Syrup (C)** 1 tsp qid prn
Pediatric: <18 months: not recommended
18 months-6 years: 1/2 tsp qid prn
>6 years: same as adult

Syr: carb 4 mg/*pseud* 60 mg per 5 ml (4 oz)
- **Rondec®TR (C)** 1 tab q 12 hours prn
    Pediatric: <12 years: not recommended
    Tab: carb 8 mg/*pseud* 120 mg sust-rel
- **Ryna® (C)(OTC)** 2 tsp q 4-6 hours prn; max 8 tsp/day
    Pediatric: <6 years: not recommended
    6-12 years: 1 tsp q 4-6 hours prn; max 4 tsp/day
    Liq: chlor 2 mg/*pseud* 30 mg per 5 ml
- **Ryna®-12 Suspension (C)** 2 tsp q 12 hours prn
    Pediatric: <2 titrate individually
    2-6 years: ½-1 tsp q 12 hours prn
    6-12 years: 1-2 tsp q 12 hours prn
    Oral susp: pyr 30 mg/*phenyle* 5 mg per 5 ml
- **Rynatan® (C)** 1-2 tabs q 12 hours prn
    Pediatric: <12 years: not recommended
    Tab: azat 1 mg/*phenyle* 120 mg
- **Rynatan®Pediatric Suspension (C)**
    Pediatric: <2 years: not recommended
    2-6 years: ½-1 tsp q 12 hours prn
    >6 years: 1-2 tsp q 12 hours prn
    Susp: chlor 4.5 mg/*pyr* 12.5 mg/*phenyle* 5 mg per 5 ml
- **Rynatuss® (C)(OTC)** 1-2 tabs q 12 hours prn
    Pediatric: not recommended
    Tab: carbet 60 mg/*chlor* 5 mg/*ephed* 10 mg/*phenyle* 10 mg
- **Rynatuss®Pediatric Suspension (C)**
    Pediatric: <2 years: titrate individually
    2-6 years: ½-1 tsp q 12 hours prn
    6-12 years: 1-2 tsp q 12 hours prn
    Susp: carbet 30 mg/*chlor* 4 mg/*ephed* 5 mg/*phenyle* 5 mg per 5 ml
- **Semprex®-D (B)** 1 cap q 4-6 hours prn; max 4 doses/day
    Pediatric: <12 years: not recommended
    6-12 years: same as adult
    Cap: acriv 8 mg/*pseud* 60 mg
- **Sudafed®Suspension (C)(OTC)(G)** 2-4 tsp q 12 hours prn
    Pediatric: <12 years: not recommended
    Oral susp: chlor 4.5 mg/*pseud* 75 mg per 5 ml (4, 16 oz)
- **Tanafed®Suspension (C)** 2-4 tsp q 12 hours prn
    Pediatric: <3 years: not recommended
    3-6 years: 1/4-1/2 tsp q 12 hours prn
    6-12 years: 1-2 tsp q 12 hours prn
    Oral susp: chlor 4.5 mg/*pseud* 75 mg per 5 ml
- **Triaminic®Cold & Allergy (C)(OTC)(G)** 4 tsp q 4-6 hours prn

Pediatric: <4 months: not recommended
4-12 months (12-17 lb): 1/4 tsp q 4-6 hours prn
12-24 months (18-23 lb): 1/2 tsp q 4-6 hours prn
2-6 years (24-47 lb): 1 tsp q 4-6 hours prn
6-12 years (48-95 lb): 2 tsp q 4-6 hours prn
Liq: chlor 1 mg/*pseud* 15 mg per 5 ml (4, 8 oz) (alcohol-free)
▶**Triaminic®Softchews Cold & Allergy (C)(OTC)** 4 chew tabs q 4 hours prn
Pediatric: <6 years: not recommended
6-12 years: 2 chewtabs q 4 hours prn
Chew tab: chlor 1 mg/*pseud* 15 mg (dissolve or chew)
▶**Trinalin® (C)** 1 tab q 12 hours prn
Pediatric: <12 years: not recommended
Tab: azat 1 mg/*pseud* 120 mg sust-rel
▶**Zyrtec®-D 12 Hour (C)** 1 tab q 12 hours prn
Pediatric: <12 years: not recommended
Tab: citri 5 mg/*pseud* 120 mg ext-rel

Appendix W.7: Decongestant/Expectorant

▶**Aquatab®D (C)** 1tab q 12 hours prn
Pediatric: <12 years: not recommended
Tab: pseud 60 mg/*guaif* 1200 mg
▶**Crantex®Liquid (C)** 1-2 tsp q 4-6 hours prn; max 8 tsp/day
Pediatric: <2 years: not recommended
2-6 years: 1/2 tsp q 4-6 hours prn
6-12 years: 1 tsp q 4-6 hours prn
Liq: phenyle 7.5/*guaif* 100 mg mg per 5 ml (dye-free, sugar-free, alcohol-free)
▶**Crantex®LA Tablets (C)** 1 tab q 12 hours prn; max 2 tabs/day
Pediatric: <6 years: not recommended
6-12 years: 1/2 tab q 12 hours prn; max 1 tab/day
Tab: phenyle 30/*guaif* 600 mg sust-rel
▶**Deconsal®II (C)** 1-2 tabs q 12 hours prn
Pediatric: <2 years: not recommended
2-6 years: 1/2 tab q 12 hours prn
6-12 years: 1 tab q 12 hours prn
Tab: phenyle 20 mg/*guaif* 375 mg ext-rel (tartrazine)
▶**Defen®-LA (C)** 1-2 tabs q 12 hours prn
Pediatric: <3 years: not recommended
3-6 years: 1/2 tab q 12 hours prn
6-12 years: 1 tab q 12 hours prn

Tab: pseud 60 mg/*guaif* 600 mg
- ▶**Duratuss® (C)** 1 tab q 12 hours prn
    Pediatric: <6 years: not recommended
    6-12 years: 1/2 tab q 12 hours prn
    Tab: pseud 120 mg/*guaif* 600 mg* sust-rel (dye-free)
- ▶**Duratuss®GP (C)** 1 tab q 12 hours prn
    Pediatric: <12 years: not recommended
    Tab: pseud 120 mg/*guaif* 1200 mg sust-rel (dye-free)
- ▶**Entex®LA (C)(G)** 1 tab q 12 hours prn
    Pediatric: <6 years: not recommended
    >6 years: 1/2 tab q 12 hours prn
    Cap: phenyle 30 mg/*guaif* 400 mg* sust-rel (black-cherry, dye-free, alcohol-free)
- ▶**Entex®Liquid (C)(G)** 1-2 tsp q 4-6 hours prn; max 8 tsp/day
    Pediatric: <2 years: not recommended
    2-6 years: 1/2 tsp q 4-6 hours prn; max 2 tsp/day
    6-12 years: 1 tsp q 4-6 hours prn; max 4 tsp/day
    Liq: phenyle 7.5 mg/*guaif* 100 mg per 5 ml (8 oz)(punch, dye-free, sugar-free, alcohol-free)
- ▶**Entex®PSE (C)(G)** 1 tab q 12 hours prn
    Pediatric: <6 years: not recommended
    6-12 years: 1/2 tab q 12 hours prn
    Cap: pseud 120 mg/*guaif* 400 mg* immed- and sust-rel
- ▶**Guai-Vent®/PSE (C)** 1 tab q 12 hours prn
    Pediatric: <6 years: not recommended
    6-12 years: 1/2 tab q 12 hours prn
    Tab: pseud 120 mg/*guaif* 600 mg
- ▶**Maxifed®G (C)** 1-2 tabs q 12 hours prn
    Pediatric: <6 years: not recommended
    6-12 years: ½-1 tab q 12 hours prn
    Tab: pseud 60 mg/*guaif* 550 mg sust-rel
- ▶**Maxifed®G Tab 100's (C)** 1-2 tabs bid prn
    Pediatric: <2 years: not recommended
    2-6 years: 1/4-1/2 tab bid prn
    6-12 years: 1/2 tab bid prn
    Tab: pseud 60 mg/*guaif* 550 mg* sust-rel
- ▶**Maxifed®Tab 100's (C)** 1-1½ tabs bid <u>or</u> 1 tab tid, prn
    Pediatric: <6 years: not recommended
    6-12 years: ½-1 tab bid prn
    Tab: pseud 80 mg/*guaif* 700 mg* sust-rel
- ▶**Mucinex®-D (C)(OTC)** 1-2 tabs q 12 hours prn
    Pediatric: <12 years: not recommended

Tab: pseud 60 mg/*guaif* 600 mg ext-rel

▶**Nalex® (C)** 1 cap q 12 hours prn
  Pediatric: <12 years: not recommended
  Cap: pseud 120 mg/*guaif* 250 mg

▶**Nalex®Jr. (C)** 1 cap q 12 hours prn
  Pediatric: <6 years: not recommended
  >6 years: same as adult
  Cap: pseud 60 mg/*guaif* 300 mg

▶**Nasatab®LA (C)** 1 tab q 12 hours prn
  Pediatric: <6 years: not recommended
  6-12 years: 1/2 tab q 12 hours prn
  Tab: pseud 120 mg/*guaif* 500 mg* sust-rel (dye-free)

▶**Panmist®LA (C)** 1 tab bid prn
  Pediatric: not recommended
  Tab: pseud 90 mg/*guaif* 600 mg

▶**Prolex®D (C)** 1-2 tabs bid prn
  Pediatric: <6 years: not recommended
  6-12 years: ½-1 tab bid prn
  Tab: phenyle 10 mg/*guaif* 600 mg (dye-free)

▶**Prolex®PD (C)** 1-2 tabs bid prn
  Pediatric: <6 years: not recommended
  6-12 years: ½-1 tab bid prn
  Tab: phenyle 10 mg/*guaif* 600 mg* (dye-free)

▶**Robitussin®PE (C)(OTC)(G)** 2 tsp q 4 hours prn; max 4 doses/day
  Pediatric: <6 months, 14 lbs: not recommended
  6-11 months, 14-17 lbs: 1/4 tsp q 4 hours prn
  12-23 months, 18-23 lbs: 1/4-1/2 tsp q 4 hours prn
  2-6 years, 24-47 lbs: 1/2 tsp q 4 hours prn; max 4 doses/day
  6-12 years, 48-95 lbs: 5 ml q 4 hours prn; max 4 doses/day
  Syr: pseud 30 mg/*guaif* 100 mg per 5 ml (4, 8 oz)

▶**Ru-Tuss®DE (C)** 1 tab q 12 hours prn
  Pediatric: <6 years: not recommended
  6-12 years: 1/2 tab q 12 hours prn
  Tab: pseud 120 mg/*guaif* 600 mg* sust-rel

▶**Sudal®60/500 (C)(G)** 1-2 tabs q 12 hours prn
  Pediatric: <6 years: not recommended
  6-12 years: 1/2 tab q 12 hours prn
  Tab: pseud 60 mg/*guaif* 500 mg*

▶**Sudal®120/600 (C)(G)** 1 tab q 12 hours prn
  Pediatric: <6 years: not recommended

6-12 years: 1/2 tab q 12 hours prn
Tab: pseud 120 mg/*guaif* 600 mg*

▶**Zephrex® (C)(G)** 1 tab q 12 hours prn
Pediatric: <6 years: not recommended
6-12 years: 1/2 tab q 12 hours prn
Tab: pseud 60 mg/*guaif* 400 mg*

Appendix W.8: Decongestant/Analgesic

▶**Children's Motrin®Cold (C)(OTC)**
Pediatric: <2 years: not recommended
2-5 years: 1 tsp q 6 hours prn; max 4 doses/day
6-11 years: 2 tsp q 6 hours prn; max 4 doses/day
Oral susp: pseud 15 mg/*ibup* 100 mg per 5 ml (4 oz)

▶**Maximum Strength Tylenol®Sinus (C)(OTC)** 2 caplets q 4-6 hours prn; max 8 caplets/day
Pediatric: <12 years: not recommended
Cplt: pseud 30 mg/*acet* 500 mg

▶**Ornex® (C)(OTC)** 2 caps q 4-6 hours prn; max 8 caps/day
Pediatric: <6 years: not recommended
6-12 years: 1 cap q 4-6 hours prn; max 4 caps/day
Cap: pseud 30 mg/*acet* 325 mg

▶**Tavist®Sinus (C)(OTC)** 1-2 caplets q 6 hours prn; max 8 caplets/day
Pediatric: not recommended
Cplt: pseud 30 mg/*acet* 500 mg

Appendix W.9: Decongestant/Antihistamine

▶**Benadryl®Allergy/Cold Tablets (C)(OTC)(G)** 2 tabs q 6 hours prn; max 8 tabs/day
Pediatric: <12 years: not recommended
Tab: pseud 30 mg/*diphen* 12.5/*acet* 500 mg

▶**Dimetapp®Cold and Fever Suspension (C)** 4 tsp q 4 hours prn; max 4 doses/day
Pediatric: <6 years: not recommended
6-12 years: 2 tsp q 4 hours prn; max 4 doses/day
Oral susp: pseud 15 mg/*brom* 1 mg/*acet* 160 mg per 5 ml (4 oz)

▶**Pannaz® (C) 2** tsp qid prn
max 4 doses/day
Pediatric: <2 years: 1/4 tsp qid prn
2-6 years: 1/2 tsp qid prn

6-12 years: 1 tsp qid prn

Oral susp: pseud 15 mg/*carb* 2 mg/*meth* 1.25 mg per 5 ml (sugar, alcohol-free)

▶**Tanafed®DMX (C)** 2-4 tsp q 12 hours prn

Pediatric: <2 years: not recommended
2-6 years: ½-1 tsp q 12 hours prn
6-12 years: 1-2 tsp q 12 hours prn

Oral susp: dexchlor 2.5 mg/*pseud* 75 mg/dextro 25 mg per 5 ml (cotton candy, alcohol-free)

▶**Tanafed®DP (C)** 2-4 tsp q 12 hours prn

Pediatric: <2 years: not recommended
2-6 years: ½-1 tsp q 12 hours prn
6-12 years: 1-2 tsp q 12 hours prn

Oral susp: dexchlor 2.5 mg/*pseud* 75 mg/dextro 25 mg per 5 ml (strawberry banana, alcohol-free)

Appendix W.10: Antitussive/Antihistamine

▶**Hycodan® (C)(III)** 1 tab q 4-6 hours prn; max 6 tabs/day

Pediatric: <6 years: not recommended
6-12 years: 1/2 tab q 4-6 hours prn; max 3 tabs/day

Tab: hydro 5 mg/*hom* 1.5 mg*

▶**Hycodan®Syrup (C)(III)** 5 ml q 4-6 hours prn; max 6 tsp/day

Pediatric: <6 years: not recommended
6-12 years: 2.5 ml q 4-6 hours prn; max 15 ml/day

Syr: hydro 5 mg/*hom* 1.5 mg per 5 ml

▶**Phenergan®w. Codeine (C)(III)** 1 tsp q 4-6 hours prn; max 30 ml/day

Pediatric: <2 years: not recommended
2-6 years: 1/4-1/2 tsp q 4-6 hours prn
6-12 years: ½-1 tsp q 4-6 hours prn
25 lb max 6 ml/day
30 lb max 7 ml/day
35 lb max 8 ml/day
40 lb max 9 ml/day

Syr: cod 10 mg/*prom* 6.25 mg per 5 ml

▶**Phenergan®w. Dextromethorphan (C)** 1 tsp q 4-6 hours prn; max 4 tsp/day

Pediatric: <2 years: not recommended
2-6 years: 1/4-1/2 tsp q 4-6 hours prn; max 2 tsp /day
6-12 years: 1/2-1 tsp q 4-6 hours prn; max 4 tsp/day

Syr: dextro 15 mg/*prom* 6.25 mg per 5 ml (4, 16 oz)

▶**Tussi-12®Suspension (C)** 1-2 tsp q 12 hours prn
   Pediatric: <2 years: ½ tsp q 12 hours prn
              2-6 years: ½-1 tsp q 12 hours prn
              6-11 years: 1 tsp q 12 hours prn
   Susp: carbeta 30 mg/*chlor* 4 mg per 5 ml (strawberry currant, tartrazine)
▶**Tussi-12®Tablets (C)** 1-2 tabs q 12 hours prn
   Pediatric: <2 years: use susp
              2-6 years: ½-1 tab q 12 hours prn
              6-11 years: 1 tab q 12 hours prn
   Tab: carbeta 60 mg/*chlor* 5*mg
▶**Tussionex® (C)(III)** 5 ml q 12 hours prn
   Pediatric: <6 years: not recommended
              6-12 years: 2.5 ml q 12 hours prn
   Oral susp: hydro 10 mg/*chlor* 8 mg per 5 ml ext-rel

Appendix W.11: Antitussive/Decongestant

▶**Dimetapp®Infant Drops Decongestant Plus Cough (C)(OTC)**
   Pediatric: 2-3 years: 2 dropperful q 4 hours prn; max 4 doses/day
   Oral drops: dex 2.5 mg/*pseud* 7.5 mg per dropperful (0.8 ml) (8ml)
▶**Dimetapp®Non-Drowsy Flu Suspension (C)(OTC)** 4 tsp q 4 hours prn
   Pediatric: <2 years: titrate individually
              2-6 years: 1 tsp q 4 hours prn
              6-12 years: 2 tsp q 4 hours prn
   Oral susp: dextro 5 mg/*pseud* 15 mg per 5 ml (4 oz) (alcohol-free)
▶**Histussin®D (C)(III)** 1 tsp qid prn
   Pediatric: 25-49 lb: 1.25 tsp qid prn
              50-90 lb: 1.5 tsp qid prn
              >90 lb: same as adult
   Liq: hydro 5 mg/*pseud* 60 mg per 5 ml
▶**Nalex®DH (C)(III)** 2 tsp q 4-6 hours prn; max 4 doses/day
   Pediatric: <2 years: not recommended
              2-6 years: ½ -1 tsp q 4-6 hours prn
              6-12 years: 1 tsp q 4-6 hours prn
   Liq: hydro 2.5 mg/*phenyle* 5 mg per 5 ml
▶**PediaCare®Infants' Decongestant & Cough (C)(OTC)**
   Pediatric: 0-4 months (6-11 lb): 0.4 ml q 4-6 hours prn
              4-11 months (12-17 lb): 0.8 ml q 4-6 hours prn
              12-23 months (18-23 lb): 1.2 ml q 4-6 hours prn
              2-3 years (24-35 lb): 1.6 ml q 4-6 hours prn

All: max 4 doses/day
Oral drops: dextro 2.5 mg/*pseud* 7.5 mg per 0.8 ml (15 ml) (alcohol-free)

▶**Triaminic®Cough/Congestion (C)(OTC)(G)** 4 tsp q 4-6 hours prn; max 4 doses/day
Pediatric: <4 months: not recommended
4-12 months (12-17 lb): 1/4 tsp q 4-6 hours prn
1-2 years (18-23 lb): 1/2 tsp q 4-6 hours prn
2-6 years (24-47 lb): 1 tsp q 4-6 hours prn
6-12 years (48-95 lb): 2 tsp q 4-6 hours prn
All max 4 doses/day
Liq: dextro 7.5 mg/*pseud* 15 mg per 5 ml (4, 8 oz)

▶**Triaminic®Cough (C)(OTC)(G)**
Pediatric: <2 years: not recommended
2-5 years: 1 tsp q 4-6 hours prn; max 4 doses/day
6-12 years: 2 tsp q 4-6 hours prn; max 4 doses/day
Liq: dextro 5 mg/*pseud* 15 mg per 5 ml (4 oz) (alcohol-free)

▶**Triaminic®Cough & Congestion (C)(OTC)(G)** 4 tsp q 4-6 hours prn; max 4 doses/day
Pediatric: <4 months: not recommended
4-12 months (12-17 lb): 1/4 tsp q 4-6 hours prn
1-2 years (18-23 lb): 1/2 tsp q 4-6 hours prn
2-6 years (24-47 lb): 1 tsp q 4-6 hours prn
6-12 years (48-95 lb): 2 tsp q 4-6 hours prn
Liq: dextro 7.5 mg/*pseud* 15 mg per 5 ml (4 oz)

Appendix W.12: Antitussive/Expectorant

▶**Aquatab®DM** 1 tab q 12 hours prn
Pediatric: <12 years: not recommended
Tab: dextro 60 mg/*guaif* 1200*mg sust-rel

▶**Allfen®DM** 1 tab q 12 hours prn
Pediatric: <6 years: not recommended
6-12 years: 1/2 tab q 12 hours prn
Tab: dextro 50 mg/*guaif* 1000 mg* sust-rel

▶**Atuss®EX (C)(III)** 2-3 tsp q 4-6 hours prn; max 4 doses/day
Pediatric: <2 years: not recommended
2-6 years: ½ -1 tsp q 4-6 hours prn; max 4 doses/day
6-12 years: 1-2 tsp q 4-6 hours prn; max 4 doses/day
Liq: hydro 2.5 mg/*guaiac* 120 mg per 5 ml (dye-free)

▶**Bidex®DM** 1-2 tabs q 12 hours prn
Pediatric: <2 years: not recommended

    2-6 years: 1/2 tab q 12 hours prn
    6-12 years: 1 tab q 12 hours prn
  Tab: dextro 30 mg/*guaif* 800*mg sust-rel
▶**Brontex® (C)(III)** 1 tab q 4 hours prn
  Pediatric: <6 years: not recommended
    6-12 years: use liquid
  Tab: cod 10 mg/*guaif* 300 mg
▶**Brontex®Liquid (C)(III)** 4 tsp q 4 hours prn
  Pediatric: <6 years: not recommended
    6-12 years: 2 tsp q 4 hours prn
  Liq: cod 10 mg/*guaif* 300 mg per 20 ml
▶**Codiclear®DH (C)(III)** 1 tsp pc and HS prn, at least 4 hours apart; max 6 tsp/day
  Pediatric: <6 years: not recommended
    6-12 years: 1½ tsp pc and HS prn, at least 4 hours apart; max 3 tsp/day
  Syr: hydro 5 mg/*guaif* 100 mg per 5 ml
▶**Duratuss®DM (C)** 1 tsp q 4 hours prn; max 6 doses/day
  Pediatric: 2-6 years: 1/4 tsp q 4 hours prn; max 6 doses/day
    6-12 years: 1/2 tsp q 4 hours prn; max 6 doses/day
  Elix: dextro 20 mg/*guaif* 200 mg per 5 ml
▶**Humibid®DM (C)** 1-2 tabs q 12 hours prn
  Pediatric: <2 years: not recommended
    2-6 years: 1/2 tab q 12 hours prn
    6-12 years: 1 tab q 12 hours prn
  Tab: dextro 30 mg/*guaif* 600 mg* sust-rel
▶**Hycotuss® (C)(III)** 5 ml pc and HS prn at least 4 hours apart; max 30 ml/day
  Pediatric: <6 years: not recommended
    6-12 years: 2.5 ml, at least 4 hours apart, prn; max 30 ml/day
  Syr: hydro 5 mg/*guaif* 100 mg per 5 ml (butterscotch, alcohol 10%)
▶**Maxi-Tuss®DM (C)** 1 tsp q 4 hours prn
  Pediatric: 2-6 years: 1/4 tsp q 4 hours prn
    6-12 years: 1/2 tsp q 4 hours prn
  Liq: dextro 20 mg/*guaif* 200 mg per 5 ml
▶**Mucinex®DM (C)(OTC)** 1 tab q 12 hours prn
  Pediatric: not recommended
  Tab: dextro 30 mg/*guaif* 600 mg ext-rel
▶**Pneumotussin®2.5 Cough Syrup (C)(III)** 2-3 tsp q 4-6 hours prn; max 4 doses/day
  Pediatric: <2 years: not recommended

2-6 years: ½-1 tsp q 4-6 hours prn; max 4 doses/day
6-12 years: 1-2 tsp q 4-6 hours prn; max 4 doses/day
Liq: hydro 2.5 mg/*guaiac* 200 mg per 5 ml (dye-free)

▶**Pneumotussin®Tablets (C)(III)** 1 tab q 4 hours prn
Pediatric: <6 years: not recommended
6-12 years: use liquid
Tab: hydro 2.5 mg/*guaif* 300 mg

▶**Prolex®DH (C)(III)** 1-1½ tsp q 6 hours prn
Pediatric: <3 years: not recommended
3-6 years: 1/4-1/2 tsp q 6 hours prn
6-12 years: ½-1 tsp q 6 hours prn
Liq: hydro 5 mg/*guaiac* 300 mg per 5 ml

▶**Prolex®DM (C)** 1-1½ tsp q 6 hours prn
Pediatric: <3 years: not recommended
3-6 years: 1/4-1/2 tsp q 6 hours prn
6-12 years: ½-1 tsp q 6 hours prn
Liq: dextro 15 mg/*guaiac* 300 mg per 5 ml

▶**Protuss® (C)(III)** 1-2 tsp q 6 hours prn
Pediatric: <3 years: not recommended
3-6 years: 1/4-1/2 tsp q 6 hours prn
6-12 years: ½-1 tsp q 6 hours prn
Liq: hydro 5 mg/*guaiac* 300 mg per 5 ml (4, 16 oz)

▶**Robitussin®A-C (C)(III)** 2 tsp q 4 hours prn; max 60 ml/day
Pediatric: <2 years: not recommended
2-6 years: 1/4-1/2 tsp q 4 hours prn
6-12 years: 1 tsp q 4 hours prn
Liq: cod 10 mg/*guaif* 100 mg per 5 ml

▶**Robitussin®DM (C)(OTC)** 2 tsp q 4 hours prn; max 6 doses/day
Pediatric: <6 months: not recommended
6-11 months (14-17 lb): 1.25 ml q 4 hours prn
12-23 months (18-23 lb): 2.5 ml q 4 hours prn
2-6 years (24-47 lb): 2.5 ml q 4 hours prn
6-12 years (48-95 lb): 5 ml q 4 hours prn
Liq: dextro 10 mg/*guaif* 100 mg per 5 ml (4, 8, 12, 16 oz) (alcohol-free)

▶**Robitussin®Sugar-Free (C)(OTC)** 2 tsp q 4 hours prn; max 6 doses/day
Pediatric: <6 months: not recommended
6-11 months (14-17 lb): 1.25 ml q 4 hours prn
12-23 months (18-23 lb): 2.5 ml q 4 hours prn
2-6 years (24-47 lb): 2.5 ml q 4 hours prn
6-12 years (48-95 lb): 5 ml q 4 hours prn

Liq: dextro 10 mg/*guaif* 100 mg per 5 ml (4 oz; sugar-free, alcohol-free)

▶**Sudal®DM (C)** 1-2 tabs q 12 hours prn
  Pediatric: <2 years: not recommended
    2-6 years: 1/2 tab q 12 hours prn
    6-12 years: ½-1 tab q 12 hours prn
  Liq: dextro 30 mg/*guaif* 500 mg*

▶**Tussi-Organidin®DM NR Liquid (C)(III)** 2 tsp q 4 hours prn; max 60 ml/day
  Pediatric: <2 years: not recommended
    2-6 years: 1 mg/kg/day codeine in 4 divided doses prn
    6-12 years: 1 tsp q 4 hours prn; max 30 ml/day
  Liq: dextro 10 mg/*guaif* 100 mg per 5 ml (raspberry)

▶**Tussi-Organidin®NR (C)** 2 tsp q 4 hours prn; max 60 ml/day
  Pediatric: <2 years: not recommended
    2-6 years: 1 mg/kg/day codeine in 4 divided doses prn
    6-12 years: 1 tsp q 4 hours prn; max 30 ml/day
  Liq: cod 10 mg/*guaif* 100 mg per 5 ml (raspberry)

▶**Vicodin®Tuss (C)(III)** 1 tsp pc and HS prn at least 4 hours apart; max 30 ml/day
  Pediatric: <6 years: not recommended
    6-12 years: 1/2 tsp pc and HS prn at least 4 hours apart; max 5 ml/dose
  Syr: hydro 5 mg/*guaif* 100 mg per 5 ml (dye-free, sugar-free)

Appendix W.13: Antitussive/Decongestant/Antihistamine

▶**Anaplex®DH (C)(III)** 1-2 tsp q 4 hours prn
  Pediatric: <2 years: not recommended
    2-6 years: 1/2 tsp q 4 hours prn
    6-12 years: 1 tsp q 4 hours prn
  Syr: hydro 1.66 mg/*phenyle* 5 mg/*pyr* 8.33 mg/ per 5 ml

▶**Anaplex®HD Cough (C)(III)** 1-2 tsp q 4-6 hours prn; max 4 tsp/day
  Pediatric: 2-6 years: 1/2 tsp q 4-6 hours prn; max 4 doses/day
    6-12 years: 1 tsp q 4-6 hours prn; max 4 dose/day
  Syr: hydro 2.5 mg/*pseud* 30 mg/*chlor* 2 mg per 5 ml

▶**Atuss®HD (C)(III)** 2 tsp q 4 hours prn; max 8 tsp/day
  Pediatric: <3 years: titrate individually
    3-6 years: 1/2 tsp q 4 hours prn; max 2 tsp/day
    6-12 years: 1 tsp q 4 hours prn; max 4 tsp/day
  Liq: hydro 2.5 mg/*phenyle* 10 mg/ *chlor* 4 mg per 5 ml

▶**Atuss®-DM (C)** 1-2 tsp q 6 hours prn

Pediatric: <2 years: not recommended
2-6 years: 1/2 tsp q 6 hours prn
6-12 years: ½-1 tsp q 6 hours prn
Syr: dextro 15 mg/*phenyle* 10 mg/*chlor* 2 mg per 5 ml

▶**Atuss®-MS (C)(III)** 2 tsp q 6 hours prn; max 8 tsp/day.
Pediatric: <6 years: not recommended
6-12 years: 1 tsp q 6 hours prn; max 4 tsp/day
Syr: hydro 5 mg/*phenyle* 10 mg/*chlor* 2 mg per 5 ml

▶**Children's Dimetapp®DM Cold & Cough (C)(OTC)**
Pediatric: <6 months: not recommended
6-11 months (14-17 lb): 1/2 tsp q 6-8 hours prn
12-23 months (18-23 lb): 3/4 tsp q 6-8 hours prn
2-5 years (24-47 lb): 1 tsp q 6-8 hours prn
6-11 years (48-95 lb): 2 tsp q 6-8 hours prn
All max 4 doses/day
Liq: dextro 10 mg/*pseud* 15 mg/*brom* 1 mg per 5 ml (4, 8 oz) (alcohol-free)

▶**Codimal®DH (C)(III)** 1-2 tsp q 4 hours prn
Pediatric: <2 years: not recommended
2-6 years: 1/2 tsp q 4 hours prn
6-12 years: 1 tsp q 4 hours prn
Syr: hydro 1.66 mg/*phenyle* 5 mg/*pyr* 8.33 mg/ per 5 ml

▶**Codimal®DM (C)** 2 tsp q 4 hours prn; max 12 tsp/day
Pediatric: <6 years: not recommended
6-12 years: 1 tsp q 4 hours prn; max 6 tsp/day
Syr: dextro 10 mg/*phenyle* 5 mg/*pyr* 8.33 mg per 5 ml

▶**Dimetane®DX (C)** 10 ml q 4 hours prn
Pediatric: <2 years: not recommended
2-6 years: 2.5 ml q 4 hours prn
6-12 years: 5 ml q 4 hours prn
Liq: dextro 10 mg/*pseud* 30 mg/*brom* 2 mg per 5 ml (sugar-free)

▶**Dimetapp®DM Cough & Cold (C)** 10 ml q 4 hours prn
Pediatric: <2 years: not recommended
2-6 years: 2.5 ml q 4 hours prn; max 6 doses/day
6-12 years: 5 ml q 4 hours prn; max 6 doses/day
Liq: dextro 5 mg/*phenyle* 15 mg/*brom* 1 mg per 5 ml (4, 8 oz)

▶**Endal®HD (C)(III)** 2 tsp q 4 hours prn; max 8 tsp/day
Pediatric: <6 years: not recommended
6-12 years: 1 tsp q 4 hours prn; max 4 tsp/day
Liq: hydro 2 mg/*phenyle* 5 mg/*chlor* 2 mg per 5 ml (cherry, alcohol-free)

▶**Endal®HD Plus (C)(III)** 2 tsp q 4 hours prn; max 8 tsp/day

Pediatric: <6 years: not recommended
6-12 years: 1 tsp q 4 hours prn; max 4 tsp/day

Liq: hydro 3.5 mg/*phenyle* 5 mg/*chlor* 2 mg per 5 ml (black raspberry, alcohol-free)

▶**Histacol®DM Pediatric Drops (C)**
Pediatric: <1 month: not recommended
1-3 months: 1/4 dropperful (1/4 ml) qid prn
3-6 months: 1/2 dropperful (1/2 ml) qid prn
6-9 months: 3/4 dropperful (3/4 ml) qid prn
9-18 months: 1 dropperful (1 ml) qid prn
>18 months: may use syrup

Drops: dextro 4 mg/*pseud* 15 mg/*brom* 1 mg per dropperful (30 ml; grape, sugar-free, alcohol-free)

▶**Histex®HC (C)(III)** 2 tsp q 4-6 hours prn
Pediatric: <2 years: 0.6 mg/kg/day; equally divided doses
2-4 years: 1/2 tsp q 4-6 hours prn
4-10 years: 1 tsp q 4-6 hours prn
>10 years: same as adult

Liq: hydro 2.5 mg/*pseud* 30 mg/*carb* 2 mg per 5 ml

▶**Histussin®HC (C)(III)** 2 tsp q 4 hours prn; max 8 tsp/day
Pediatric: <6 years: not recommended
6-12 years: 1 tsp q 4 hours prn

Syr: hydro 2.5 mg/*phenyle* 5 mg/*chlor* 2 mg per 5 ml

▶**Maxi-Tuss®DH (C)(III)** 1 tsp q 4 hours prn; max 6 tsp/day
Pediatric: <6 years: not recommended
6-12 years: 1/2 tsp q 4 hours prn; max 3 tsp/day

Syr: hydro 2.5 mg/*phenyle* 10 mg/*chlor* 4 mg per 5 ml

▶**Novahistine®DH (C)(III)** 10 ml q 4-6 hours prn; max 40 ml/day
Pediatric: <25 lb: not recommended
24-50 lb: 1.25-2.5 ml q 4-6 hours prn; max 10 ml/day
50-90 lb: 2.5-5 ml q 4-6 hours prn; max 20 ml/day
>90 lb: same as adult

Liq: cod 10 mg/*pseud* 30 mg/*chlor* 2 mg per 5 ml

▶**PediaCare®Cough-Cold (C)(OTC)(G)**
Pediatric: <2 years: not recommended
2-3 years (24-35 lb): 5 ml q 4-6 hours prn
4-5 years (36-47 lb): 7.5 ml q 4-6 hours prn
6-8 years (48-59 lb): 10 ml q 4-6 hours prn
9-10 years (60-71 lb): 12.5 ml q 4-6 hours prn
11-12 years (72-95 lb): 15 ml q 4-6 hours prn
All: max 4 doses/day

Liq: dextro 5 mg/*pseud* 15 mg/*chlor* 1 mg per 5 ml (4 oz) (alcohol-free)

▶ **PediaCare®Cough-Cold Chewable Tabs (C)(OTC)(G)**

Pediatric: <2 years: not recommended
                2-3 years (24-35 lb): 1 tab q 4-6 hours prn
                4-5 years (36-47 lb): 1½ tab q 4-6 hours prn
                6-8 years (48-59 lb): 2 tabs q 4-6 hours prn
                9-10 years (60-71 lb): 2½ tabs q 4-6 hours prn
                11-12 years (72-95 lb): 3 tabs q 4-6 hours prn
                All: max 4 doses/day

Chew tab: dextro 5 mg/*pseud* 15 mg/*chlor* 1 mg*

▶ **PediaCare®Nightrest (C)(OTC)**

Pediatric: <2 years: not recommended
                2-3 years (24-35 lb): 5 ml q 6-8 hours prn
                4-5 years (36-47 lb): 7.5 ml q 6-8 hours prn
                6-8 years (48-59 lb): 10 ml q 6-8 hours prn
                9-10 years (60-71 lb): 12.5 ml q 6-8 hours prn
                11-12 years (72-95 lb): 15 ml q 6-8 hours prn
                All: max 4 doses/day

Liq: dextro 7.5 mg/*pseud* 15 mg/*chlor* 1 mg per 5 ml (4 oz) (alcohol-free)

▶ **Pediatex®DM (C)** 2 tsp qid

Pediatric: <18 months: not recommended
                18 months-6 years: 1/2 tsp qid
                6-12 years: 1 tsp qid

Syr: dextro 15 mg/*pseud* 15 mg/*carb* 2 mg per 5 ml (dye-free, sugar-free, alcohol-free)

▶ **Phenergan®VC with Codeine (C)(III)(G)** 5 ml q 4-6 hours prn

Pediatric: <2 years: not recommended
                2-6 years: 1.25-2.5 ml q 4-6 hours prn;
                   25 lb: max 6 ml/day
                   30 lb: max 7 ml/day
                   35 lb: max 8 ml/day
                   40 lb: max 9 ml/day
                6-12 years: 2.5-5 ml q 4-6 hours prn
                >6 years: max 30 ml/day

Syr: cod 10 mg/*phenyle* 5 mg/*prom* 6.25 mg per 5 ml (alcohol 7%)

▶ **Promethazine®w. Codeine (C)(G)** 1 tsp q 4-6 hours prn; max 30 ml/day

Pediatric: <2 years: not recommended
                2-6 years: 1.25-2.5 ml q 4-6 hours prn
                6-12 years: 2.5-5 ml q 4-6 hours prn

Syr: dextro 5 mg/*pseud* 15 mg/*chlor* 1 mg per 5 ml (cherry,

alcohol-free)
- **P-V-Tussin® (C)(III)** 1-2 tsp q 4-6 hours prn; max 4 tsp/day
    Pediatric: 2-6 years: 1/2 tsp q 4-6 hours prn; max 4 doses/day
    6-12 years: 1 tsp q 4-6 hours prn; max 4 dose/day
    Syr: hydro 2.5 mg/*pseud* 30 mg/*chlor* 2 mg per 5 ml
- **Ryna®-C (C)(III)** 2 tsp q 4-6 hours prn; max 8 tsp/day
    Pediatric: <6 years: not recommended
    6-12 years: 1 tsp q 4-6 hours prn; max 4 tsp/day
    Liq: cod 10 mg/*pseud* 30 mg/*chlor* 2 mg per 5 ml
- **Rondec®-DM (C)** 1 tsp qid prn
    Pediatric: <18 months: use drops
    18 months-6 years: 1/2 tsp qid prn
    >6 years: same as adult
    Syr: dextro 15 mg/*pseud* 60 mg/*carb* 4 mg per 5 ml (4 oz)
- **Rondec®-DM Drops (C)**
    Pediatric: 1-3 months: 0.25 ml qid prn
    3-6 months: 0.5 ml qid prn
    6-9 months: 0.75 ml qid prn
    9-18 months: 1 ml qid prn
    Oral drops: dextro 4 mg/*pseud* 25 mg/*carb* 2 mg per 1 ml (30 ml)
- **Tanafed®DMX (C)** 2-4 tsp q 12 hours prn
    Pediatric: <2 years: not recommended
    2-6 years: ½-1 tsp q 12 hours prn
    6-12 years: 1-2 tsp q 12 hours prn
    Oral susp: dexchlor 2.5 mg/*pseud* 75 mg/*dextro* 25 mg per 5 ml (cotton candy, alcohol-free)
- **Triaminic®Cold & Cough (C)(OTC)** 4 tsp q 4-6 hours prn max 4 doses/day
    Pediatric: <4 months: not recommended
    4-12 months (12-17 lb): 1/4 tsp q 4-6 hours prn
    1-2 years (18-23 lb): 1/2 tsp q 4-6 hours prn
    2-6 years (24-47 lb): 1 tsp q 4-6 hours prn
    6-12 years (48-95 lb): 2 tsp q 4-6 hours prn
    Liq: dextro 5 mg/*pseud* 15 mg/*chlor* 1 mg per 5 ml (4, 8 oz)
- **Triaminic®Cold & Night Time Cough (C)(OTC)** 4 tsp q 6 hours prn; max 4 doses/day
    Pediatric: <6 years: not recommended
    6-12 years: 2 tsp q 6 hours prn
    Liq: dextro 7.5 mg/*pseud* 15 mg/*chlor* 1 mg per 5 ml (4, 8 oz)
- **Triaminic®Soft Chew Cold & Cough (C)(OTC)** 4 tabs q 4-6 hours prn
    Pediatric: <6 years: not recommended

6-11 years: 2 tabs q 4-6 hours prn
Chew tab: dextro 5 mg/*pseud* 15 mg/*chlor* 1 mg (dissolve in mouth or chew)

▶**Trital®DM Liquid (C)** 1 tsp q 4 hours prn; max 6 doses/day
Pediatric: <6 years: not recommended
6-12 years: 1/2 tsp q 4 hours prn; max 6 doses/day
Liq: dextro 15 mg/*phenyle* 10 mg/*chlor* 4 mg per 5 ml (grape, dye-free, sugar-free, alcohol-free)

▶**Tussi-12®D Tablets (C)** 1-2 tabs q 12 hours prn
Pediatric: <2 years: use susp
2-6 years: ½-1 tab q 12 hours prn
6-11 years: 1 tab q 12 hours prn
Tab: carbeta 60 mg/*pyr* 40 mg/*phenyle* 10*mg

▶**Tussi-12®D S (C)** 1-2 tsp q 12 hours prn
Pediatric: <2 years: not recommended
2-6 years: ½-1 tsp q 12 hours prn
6-12 years: 1 tsp q 12 hours prn
Liq: carbeta 30 mg/*pyr* 30 mg/*phenyle* 5 mg per 5 ml (strawberry currant, tartrazine)

Appendix W.14: Antitussive/Decongestant/Expectorant

▶**Atuss®G (C)(III)** 2 tsp q 4 hours prn; max 8 tsp/day
Pediatric: <6 years: not recommended
6-12 years: 1 tsp q 4 hours prn; max 4 tsp/day
Syr: hydro 2 mg/*phenyle* 10 mg/*guaif* 100 mg per 5 ml

▶**Aquatab®C (C)** 1 tab q 12 hours prn
Pediatric: <12 years: not recommended
Tab: dextro 60 mg/*pseud* 120 mg/*guaif* 1200*mg

▶**Carbetaplex®Liquid (C)** 1 tsp q 4-6 hours prn; max 4 doses/day
Pediatric: <2 years: not recommended
2-6 years: 1/4 tsp q 4-6 hours prn; max 1 tsp/day
6-12 years: 1/2 tsp q 4-6 hours prn; max 2 tsp/day
Liq: carbeta 20 mg/*phenyle* 15 mg/*guaif* 100 mg per 5 ml (strawberry, dye-free, sugar-free, alcohol-free)

▶**Duratuss®HD (C)(III)** 2 tsp q 4 hours prn; max 8 tsp/day
Pediatric: <6 years: not recommended
6-12 years: 1 tsp q 4 hours prn; max 4 tsp/day
Elix: hydro 2.5 mg/*pseud* 30 mg/*guaif* 100 mg per 5 ml (fruit punch, alcohol 5%)

▶**Entex®HC (C)(III)** 2 tsp q 4 hours prn; max 8 tsp/day

Pediatric: <6 years: not recommended
6-12 years: 1 tsp q 4 hours prn; max 4 tsp/day
Liq: hydro 5 mg/*phenle* 7.5 mg/*guaif* 100 mg per 5 ml (black-cherry, dye-free, alcohol-free)

▶**Novahistine®DMX (C)** 2 tsp q 4 hours prn; max 8 tsp/day
Pediatric: <2 years: not recommended
2-6 years: 1/2 tsp q 4 hours prn; max 2 tsp/day
6-12 years: 1 tsp q 4 hours prn; max 4 tsp/day
Liq: dextro 10 mg/*pseud* 30 mg/*guaif* 100 mg per 5 ml (alcohol 10%)

▶**Nucofed®Expectorant (C)(III)** 5 ml q 6 hours prn; max 20 ml/day
Pediatric: <2 years: not recommended
2-5 years: 1.25 ml q 6 hours prn; max 5 ml/day
6-11 years: 2.5 ml q 6 hours prn; max 10 ml/day
>11 years: same as adult
Elix: cod 20 mg/*pseud* 60 mg/*guaif* 200 mg per 5 ml

▶**Panmist®DM (C)** 2 tsp tid-qid prn
Pediatric: <2 years: not recommended
2-6 years: 1/2 tsp tid-qid prn
6-12 years: 1 tsp tid-qid prn
Liq: dextro 15 mg/*pseud* 40 mg/*guaif* 100 mg per 5 ml (dye-free, sugar-free, alcohol-free)

▶**Protuss®D (C)(III)** 1-1½ tsp q 6 hours prn
Pediatric: <3 years: not recommended
3-6 years: 1/4-1/2 tsp q 6 hours prn
6-12 years: ½-1 tsp q 6 hours prn
Liq: hydro 5 mg/*pseud* 30/*guaiac* 300 mg per 5 ml

▶**Protuss®DM (C)** 1-2 tabs q 12 hours prn
Pediatric: <3 years: not recommended
3-6 years: 1/2 tab q 12 hours prn
6-12 years: 1 tab q 12 hours prn
Tab: dextro 30 mg/*pseud* 60 mg/*guaif* 600 mg

▶**Robitussin®-CF (C)(OTC)** 10 ml q 4 hours prn
Pediatric: <6 months (14 lb): not recommended
6-11 months (14-17 lb): 1.25 ml q 4 hours prn
12-23 months (18-23 lb): 2.5 ml q 4 hours prn
2-6 years (24-47 lb): 2.5 ml q 4 hours prn
6-12 years (48-95 lb): 5 ml q 4 hours prn
Liq: dextro 10 mg/*pseud* 30 mg/*guaif* 100 mg per 5 ml (4, 8, 12 oz) (alcohol-free)

▶**Robitussin®Cold & Congestion (C)(OTC)** 2 softgel or caplets q 4 hours prn

Pediatric: <6 years: not recommended
    6-12 years: 1 softgel or caplet q 4 hours prn
Cplt: dextro 10 mg/*pseud* 30 mg/*guaif* 200 mg; *Softgel: dextro* 10 mg/*pseud* 30 mg/*guaif* 200 mg

▶**Robitussin®-DAC (C)(III)** 10 ml q 4 hours prn; max 40 ml/day
Pediatric: <6 years: not recommended
    6-12 years: 5 ml q 4 hours prn; max 20 ml/day
Syr: cod 10 mg/*pseud* 30 mg/*guaif* 100 ml per 5 ml

▶**Z-Cof®-DM (C)** 1-2 tsp bid-tid prn
Pediatric: 2-6 years: 1/2 tsp bid-tid prn
    6-12 years: 1 tsp bid-tid prn
Syr: dextro 15 mg/*pseud* 40 mg/*guaif* 200 mg per 5 ml (sugar-free, alcohol-free)

Appendix W.15: Antitussive/Decongestant/Expectorant/Antihistamine

▶**Histacol®DM Pediatric Syrup (C)**
Pediatric: <2 years: not recommended
    2-6 years: 1/2 tsp q 6 hours prn
    6-12 years: 1 tsp q 6 hours prn
    >12 years: may use syrup
Syr: dextro 5 mg/*pseud* 30 mg/*guaif* 50 mg/*brom* 2 mg per 5 ml (16 oz; grape, alcohol-free)

Appendix W.16: Antitussive/Decongestant/Analgesic

▶**Dimetapp®Non-Drowsy Flu Syrup(C)(OTC)** 4 tsp q 4 hours prn; max 4 doses/day
Pediatric: <2 years: titrate individually
    2-6 years: 1 tsp q 4 hours prn; max 4 doses/day
    6-12 years: 2 tsp q 4 hours prn; max 4 doses/day
Liq: dextro 5 mg/*pseud* 15 mg/*acet* 160 mg per 5 ml (4 oz) (alcohol-free)

▶**Triaminic®Cold, Cough & Fever (C)(OTC)** 4 tsp q 6 hours prn; max 4 doses/day
Pediatric: <4 months: not recommended
    4-12 months (12-17 lb): 1/4 tsp q 6 hours prn
    1-2 years (18-23 lb): 1/2 tsp q 6 hours prn
    2-6 years (24-47 lb): 1 tsp q 6 hours prn
    6-12 years (48-95 lb): 2 tsp q 6 hours prn

Liq: dextro 7.5 mg/*pseud* 15 mg/*acet* 160 mg per 5 ml (4 oz)

▶**Triaminic®Cough & Sore Throat (C)(OTC)** 4 tsp q 6 hours prn max 4 doses/day

Pediatric: <4 months: not recommended
4-12 months (12-17 lb): 1/4 tsp q 6 hours prn
1-2 years (18-23 lb): 1/2 tsp q 6 hours prn
2-6 years (24-47 lb): 1 tsp q 6 hours prn
6-12 years (48-95 lb): 2 tsp q 6 hours prn

Liq: dextro 7.5 mg/*pseud* 15 mg/*acet* 160 mg per 5 ml (4, 8 oz)

Appendix W.17: Antitussive/Decongestant/Expectorant/Analgesic

▶**Robitussin®Cold & Multisystem Cold & Flu (C)(OTC)** 2 softgel or caplets q 4 hours prn

Pediatric: <6 years: not recommended
6-12 years: 1 softgel or caplet q 4 hours prn

Cplt: dextro 10 mg/*pseud* 30 mg/*guaif* 200 mg/*acet* 250;
Softgel: dextro 10 mg/*pseud* 30 mg/*guaif* 100 mg/*acet* 325

Appendix W.18: Antitussive/Antihistamine/Decongestant/Analgesic

▶**Dimetapp®Nighttime Flu Syrup (C)(OTC)** 4 tsp q 4 hours prn; max 4 doses/day

Pediatric: <6 years: titrate individually
6-12 years: 2 tsp q 4 hours prn; max 4 doses/day

Syr: dextro 5 mg/*pseud* 15 mg/*brom* 1 mg/*acet* 160 mg per 5 ml (4 oz; alcohol-free)

Appendix W.19: Antitussive/Antihistamine/Decongestant/Analgesic/Caffeine

▶**Hycomine®Compound (C)(III)** 1 tab qid prn; max 4 dose/day

Pediatric: <6 years: not recommended
6-12 years: 1/2 tab qid prn; max 4 doses/day

Tab: hydro 5 mg/*chlor* 2 mg/*phenyle* 10 mg/*acet* 250 mg/*caf* 30 mg*

Appendix X: Systemic Antiinfective Drugs

Comment:

- Adverse effects of aminoglycosides include nephrotoxicity and ototoxicity.
- Use cephalosporins with caution in persons with penicillin allergy.
- *Erythromycin* should be taken with food to avoid gastric upset.
- Sulfonamides are contraindicated with sulfa allergy and G6PD deficiency. A high fluid intake is indicated during sulfonamide therapy.
- Tetracyclines should be taken on an empty stomach to facilitate absorption. Tetracyclines should not be taken with milk.
- Tetracyclines are contraindicated during pregnancy and in children <8 years of age due to the risk of tooth enamel discoloration.
- Systemic quinolones and fluoroquinolones are contraindicated in pregnancy and children <8 years of age due to the risk of joint dysplasia.

Antiinfectives by Class with Dose Forms

Generic Name	Brand Name	Dose Form(s)
		Amebicide
chloroquine phosphate (C)	Aralen®	*Tab:* 500 mg; *Inj:* 50 mg/ml (5 ml)
iodoquinol (C)	Yodoxin®	*Tab:* 210, 650 mg
metronidazole (not for use in 1st; B in 2nd, 3rd)(G)	Flagyl®, Protostat®	*Tab:* 250*, 500* mg
	Flagyl®375	*Cap:* 375 mg
	Flagyl®ER	*Tab:* 750 mg ext-rel
		Anthelmintic
albendazole (C)	Albenza®	*Tab:* 200 mg
mebendazole (C)	Vermox®	*Chew tab:* 100 mg

Antiinfectives by Class with Dose Forms

Generic Name	Brand Name	Dose Form(s)
pyrantel pamoate (C)(OTC)	Antiminth®	*Cap:* 180 mg; *Liq:* 50 mg/ml (30 ml); *Oral susp:* 50 mg/ml (60 ml)
	Pin-X®	*Cap:* 180 mg; *Liq:* 50 mg/ml (30 ml); *Oral susp:* 50 mg/ml (30 ml)
thiabendazole(C)	Mintezol®	*Chew tab:* 500*mg (orange); *Oral susp:* 500 mg/5 ml (120 ml; orange)
Antifungal		
atovaquone (C)	Mepron®	*Susp:* 750 mg/5ml (210 ml)
clotrimazole (B)	Mycelex Troche®	10 mg (70, 40/bottle)
fluconazole (C)	Diflucan®	*Tab:* 50, 100, 150, 200 mg; *Oral susp:* 10, 40 mg/ml (35 ml; orange)
griseofulvin, microsize (C)	Grifulvin®V	*Tab:* 250, 500 mg; *Oral susp:* 125 mg/5 ml (120 ml; alcohol 0.02%)
griseofulvin, ultramicrosize (C)	Fulvicin®P/G	*Tab:* 125, 165, 250, 330 mg
	Grisactin®	*Tab:* 250, 330 mg
	Grisactin® Ultra	*Cap:* 250 mg
	Gris-PEG®	*Tab:* 125, 250 mg
itraconazole (C)	Sporanox®	*Cap:* 100 mg; *Soln:* 10 mg/ml (150 ml): **Pulse Pack**®: 100 mg caps (7/pck)
ketoconazole (C)	Nizoral®	*Tab:* 200 mg
nystatin (C)	Mycostatin®	*Pastille:* 200,000 units/pastille (30 pastilles/pck); *Oral susp:* 100,000 units/ml (60 ml w. dropper)
terbinafine (B)	Lamisil®	*Tab:* 250 mg
voriconazole (D)	Vfend®	*Tab:* 50, 200 mg
Antimalarial		

Antiinfectives by Class with Dose Forms

Generic Name	Brand Name	Dose Form(s)
atovaquone/proquanil (C)	Malarone®	*Tab*: atov 250 mg/proq 100 mg
	Malarone®Pediatric	*Tab*: atov 62.5 mg/proq 25 mg
chloroquine (C)(G)	Aralen®	*Tab*: 500 mg; *Amp*: 50 mg/ml (5 ml)
doxycycline (D)(G)	Adoxa®	*Tab*: 50, 100 mg enteric-coated
	Doryx®	*Cap*: 100 mg
	Monodox®	*Cap*: 50, 100 mg
	Oracea®	*Cap*: 40 mg
	Vibramycin®	*Cap*: 50, 100 mg; *Syr*: 50 mg/5 ml (1, 16 oz); *Oral susp*: 25 mg/5 ml (2 oz)
	Vibra-Tab®	*Tab*: 100 mg film-coat
hydroxychloroquine(C)(G)	Plaquenil®	*Tab*: 200 mg
mefloquine	Lariam®	*Tab*: 250 mg
Antiprotozoal/Antibacterial		
metronidazole (not for use in 1st; B in 2nd, 3rd)(G)	Flagyl®, Protostat®	*Tab*: 250*, 500* mg
	Flagyl® 375	*Cap*: 375 mg
	Flagyl® ER	*Tab*: 750 mg ext-rel
tinidazole (C)	Tindamax®	*Tab*: 250*, 500*mg
Antiviral (for HIV-specific antiviral drugs see page)		
acyclovir (C)	Zovirax®	*Cap*: 200 mg; *Tab*: 400, 800 mg; *Oral susp*: 200 mg/5 ml (banana)
amantadine (C)	Symmetrel®	*Tab*: 100 mg; *Syr*: 50 mg/5ml
famciclovir (B)	Famvir®	*Tab*: 125, 250, 500 mg

Antiinfectives by Class with Dose Forms

Generic Name	Brand Name	Dose Form(s)
lamivudine (C)	Epivir®-HBV	*Tab:* 100 mg; *Oral soln:* 5 mg/ml (240 ml)
oseltamivir (C)	Tamiflu®	*Cap:* 75 mg
rimantadine (C)	Flumadine®	*Tab:* 100 mg
valacyclovir (B)	Valtrex®	*Tab:* 500 mg; 1 g
zanamivir	Relenza®	*Tab: lami* 150/*zido* 300 mg
		Antitubercular
ethambutol (EMB) (B)(G)	Myambutol®	*Tab:* 100, 400*mg
isoniazid (INH)	generic only	*Tab:* 100, 300*mg; *Syr:* 50 mg/5 ml; *Inj:* 100 mg/ml
pyrazinamide (PZA) (C)	generic only	*Tab:* 500*mg
rifampin (C)(G)	Priftin®	*Tab:* 150 mg
	Rifadin®,	*Cap:* 150, 300 mg
	Rimactane®	*Cap:* 300 mg
rifampin/isoniazid (C)	Rifamate®	*Cap: rif* 300 mg/*iso* 150 mg
rifampin/isoniazid/ pyrazinamide (C)	Rifater®	*Tab: rif* 120 mg/*iso* 50 mg/*pyr* 300 mg
		Aminoglycoside
amikacin (C)	Amikin®	*Vial:* 500 mg, 1 g (2 ml)
gentamicin (C)	Garamycin®	*Vial:* 20, 80 mg/2 ml
spectinomycin (B)	Trobicin®	*Vial:* 2.4 g
streptomycin (D)	Streptomycin®	*Amp:* 1 g/2.5 ml or 400 mg/ml (2.5 ml)
		Cephalosporin

Antiinfectives by Class with Dose Forms

Generic Name	Brand Name	Dose Form(s)
First Generation Cephalosporin		
cefadroxil (B)	Duricef®	*Cap*: 500 mg; *Tab*: 1 g; *Oral susp*: 250 mg/5 ml (100 ml); 500 mg/5 ml (75, 100 ml) (orange-pineapple)
cefazolin (B)	Ancef®, Zolicef®	*Vial*: 500 mg; 1, 10 g
cephalexin (B)	Keflex®	*Cap*: 250, 500, 750 mg; *Oral susp*: 125, 250 mg/5 ml (100, 200 ml)
	Keftab®	*Tab*: 500 mg
	Keftab® K-pak	*Tab*: 20-500 mg tabs/pck
cephradine (B)	Velosef®	*Cap*: 250, 500 mg; *Oral susp*: 125, 250 mg/5 ml (100, 200 ml)
Second Generation Cephalosporin		
Cefaclor (B)	Ceclor® (G)	*Pulvule*: 250, 500 mg; *Oral susp*: 125, 250 mg/5 ml (75, 150 ml); 187, 375 mg/5 ml (50, 100 ml; strawberry)
	Ceclor®CD	*Tab*: 375, 500 mg ext-rel
	Ceclor®CDpak	*Tab*: 500 mg (14 tabs/CDpak)
	Raniclor® (G)	*Chew tab*: 125, 187, 250, 375 mg
cefamandole (B)	Mandol®	*Vial*: 1, 2 g
cefotetan (B)	Cefotan®	*Vial*: 1, 2 g
cefoxitin (B)	Mefoxin®	*Vial*: 1,2 g
cefprozil (B)	Cefzil®	*Tab*: 250, 500 mg; *Oral susp*: 125, 250 mg/5 ml (50, 75, 100 ml; bubble gum, phenylalanine)
cefuroxime axetil (B)	Ceftin®	*Tab*: 125, 250, 500 mg; *Oral susp*: 125, 250 mg/5 ml (50, 100 ml; tutti-frutti)
cefuroxime sodium (B)	Zinacef®	*Vial*: 750 mg; 1.5 g

Antiinfectives by Class with Dose Forms

Generic Name	Brand Name	Dose Form(s)
loracarbef (B)	Lorabid®	*Pulvule:* 200, 400 mg; *Oral susp:* 100 mg/5 ml (50, 100 ml); 200 mg/5 ml (50, 75, 100 ml) (strawberry bubble gum)
Third Generation Cephalosporin		
cefoperazone (B)	Cefobid®	*Vial:* 1, 2 g pwdr for reconstitution
cefotaxime (B)	Claforan®	*Vial:* 500 mg; 1, 2 g pwdr for reconstitution
cefpodoxime (B)	Vantin®	*Tab:* 100, 200 mg; *Oral susp:* 50, 100 mg/5 ml (50, 75, 100 ml; lemon-creme)
ceftazidime (B)	Ceptaz®	*Vial:* 1, 2 g pwdr for reconstitution
	Fortaz®	*Vial:* 500 mg; 1, 2 g pwdr for reconstitution
	Tazicef®	*Vial:* 1, 2 g pwdr for reconstitution
	Tazidime®	*Vial:* 1, 2 g pwdr for reconstitution
ceftibuten (B)	Cedax®	*Cap:* 400 mg; *Oral susp:* 90 mg/5 ml (30, 60, 90, 120 ml); 180 mg/5 ml (30, 60, 120 ml; cherry)
Fourth Generation Cephalosporin		
cefdinir (B)	Omnicef®	*Cap:* 300 mg; *Oral susp:* 125 mg/5 ml (60, 100 ml; strawberry)
cefditoren pivoxil (C)	Spectracef®	*Tab:* 200 mg
cefepime (B)	Maxipime®	*Vial:* 1 g pwdr for reconstitution
cefixime (B)	Suprax®	*Oral Susp:* 100 mg/5 ml (50, 75, 100 ml) (strawberry)
ceftriaxone (B)	Rocephin®	*Vial:* 250, 500 mg; 1, 2 g
Fluoroquinolone & Quinolone		
First Generation Quinolone		
enoxacin (C)	Penetrex®	*Tab:* 200, 400 mg

Antiinfectives by Class with Dose Forms

Generic Name	Brand Name	Dose Form(s)
Second Generation Fluoroquinolone		
ciprofloxacin (C)	**Cipro®**	*Tab:* 100, 250, 500, 750 mg; *Oral susp:* 250 mg/5 ml (100 ml; (strawberry)
lomefloxacin (C)	**Maxaquin®**	*Tab:* 400 mg
norfloxacin (C)	**Noroxin®**	*Tab:* 400 mg
ofloxacin (C)	**Floxin®**	*Tab:* 200, 300, 400 mg
Third Generation Fluoroquinolone		
levofloxacin (C)	**Levaquin®**	*Tab:* 250, 500 mg
sparfloxacin (C)	**Zagam®**	*Tab:* 200 mg
Fourth Generation Fluoroquinolone		
moxifloxacin (C)	**Avelox®**	*Tab:* 400 mg
trovafloxacin (C)	**Trovan®**	*Tab:* 100, 200 mg
Ketolide		
telithromycin (C)	**Ketek®**	*Tab:* 400 mg
Macrolide		
azithromycin (B)	**Zithromax®**	*Tab:* 250, 500 mg
	ZithPed®Syr	*Oral susp:* 100 mg/5 ml, (15 ml); 200 mg/5 ml (15, 22.5, 30 ml) (cherry-vanilla-banana)
	Zithromax®Tri-Pak	*Tab:* 3-500 mg
	Zithromax®Z-pak	*Tab:* 6-250 mg tabs/pck
	Zmax®	*Pkt:* 2 g for reconstitution (cherry-banana)
clarithromycin (C)	**Biaxin®**	*Tab:* 250, 500 mg; *Oral susp:* 125, 250 mg/5 ml (50, 100 ml; fruit-punch)

Antiinfectives by Class with Dose Forms

Generic Name	Brand Name	Dose Form(s)
dirithromycin (C)	Biaxin®XL	*Tab:* 500 mg ext-rel
	Dynabac®	*Tab:* 250 mg
erythromycin base (B)	PCE®	*Tab:* 333, 500 mg
	E-Mycin®	*Tab:* 250, 333 mg
	Eryc®	*Cap:* 250 mg ent-coat pellets
	Ery-Tab®	*Tab:* 250, 333, 500 mg ent-coat
	PCE®	*Tab:* 333, 500 mg
erythromycin ethylsuccinate (B)	E.E.S.®	*Tab:* 400 mg; *Oral susp:* 200 mg/5 ml (100, 200 ml; cherry); 200, 400 mg/5 ml (100 ml; fruit)
	EryPed®	*Oral susp:* 200 mg/5 ml (100, 200 ml; fruit); 400 mg/5 ml (60, 100, 200 ml; banana); *Oral drops:* 200, 400 mg/5 ml (50 ml; fruit); *Chew tab:* 200 mg wafer (fruit)
erythromycin estolate (B)	Ilosone®	*Pulvule:* 250 mg; *Tab:* 500 mg; *Liq:* 125, 250 mg/5 ml (100 ml)
erythromycin stearate (B)	Erythrocin®	*Filmtab:* 250, 500 mg
Penicillin		
amoxicillin (B)(G)	Amoxil®	*Cap:* 250, 500 mg; *Tab:* 500, 875* mg; *Chewtab:* 125 , 200, 250, 400 mg (cherry-banana-peppermint; phenylanine); *Oral susp:* 125, 250 mg/ml (80, 100, 150 ml; bubble gum); 200, 400 mg/5ml (50, 75, 100 ml; bubble gum flvor); *Oral drops:* 50 mg/ml (130 ml; bubble gum)
	Trimox	*Cap:* 250, 500 mg; *Oral susp:* 125, 250 mg/5ml (80, 100, 150 ml; raspberry-strawberry)

Antiinfectives by Class with Dose Forms

Generic Name	Brand Name	Dose Form(s)
amoxicillin/clavulanate (B)(G)	Augmentin®	*Tab*: 250, 500, 875 mg; *Chewtab*: 125, 200, 250, 400 mg; *Oral susp*: 125, 250 mg/ml (80, 100, 150 ml); 200, 400 mg/5ml (50, 75, 100 ml)
	Augmentin®ES-600	*Oral susp*: 600 mg/5 ml (50, 75, 100, 150 ml)
	Augmentin®XR	*Tab*: 1000 mg ext rel
ampicillin (B)(G)	Omnipen®	*Cap*: 250, 500 mg; *Oral susp*: 125, 250 mg/ml (100, 150, 200 ml)
	Principen®	*Cap*: 250, 500 mg; *Syr*: 125, 250 mg/5 ml
ampicillin/sulbactam (B)	Unasyn®	*Vial*: 1.5, 3 g
carbenicillin (B)	Geocillin®	*Tab (film-coat)*: 382 mg
cloxacillin (B)	Tegopen®	*Tab*: 250, 500 mg; *Liq*: 125 mg/5 ml (100, 200 ml)
dicloxacillin (B)	Dynapen®	*Cap*: 125, 250, 500 mg; *Oral susp*: 62.5 mg/5 ml (80, 100, 200 ml)
ertapenem (B)	Ivanz®	*Vial*: 1 g pwdr for reconstitution
meropenem (B)	Merrem®	*Vial*: 500 mg; 1 g pwdr for reconstitution (sodium 3.92 mEq/g)
penicillin G benzathine (B)	Bicillin®LA, Bicillin®C-R	*Cartridge-needle unit*: 600,000 million units (1 ml); 1.2 million units (2 ml); 2.4 million units (4 ml)
penicillin G procaine (B)	Permapen®	*Prefilled syringe*: 1.2 million units
	Wycillin®	*Prefilled syringe*: 1.2 million units
penicillin V potassium (B)	Pen-Vee K®	*Tab*: 250, 500 mg; *Oral soln*: 125 mg/5 ml (100, 200 ml); 250 mg/5 ml (100, 150, 200 ml)
	Veetids®	*Tab*: 250, 500 mg; *Oral soln*: 125, 250 mg/5 ml (100, 200 ml)
piperacillin/tazobactam (B)	Zosyn®	*Vial*: 2, 3, 4 g pwdr for reconstitution
Sulfonamide		
sulfamethoxazole (B/D)	Gantrisin®Pediatric	*Oral susp*: 500 mg/5 ml (4, 16 oz); *Syr*: 500 mg/5 ml (16 oz)

Antiinfectives by Class with Dose Forms

Generic Name	Brand Name	Dose Form(s)
trimethoprim (C)	Primsol®	*Oral soln:* 50 mg/5 ml (bubble gum, dye-free, alcohol-free)
	Trimpex®	*Tab:* 100 mg
	Proloprim®	*Tab:* 100, 200 mg
trimethoprim/sulfamethoxazole (C)	Bactrim®, Septra®	*Tab:* trim 80 mg/sulfa 400 mg*
	Bactrim®DS, Septra®DS	*Tab:* trim 160 mg/sulfa 800 mg*; *Oral susp:* trim 40 mg/sulfa 200 mg per 5 ml (100 ml; cherry, alcohol 0.3%)
Tetracycline		
demeclocycline (D)	Declomycin®	*Tab:* 300 mg
doxycycline (D)	Adoxa®	*Tab:* 50, 100 mg ent-coat
	Doryx®	*Cap:* 100 mg
	Monodox®	*Cap:* 50, 100 mg
	Vibramycin®	*Cap:* 50, 100 mg; *Syr:* 50 mg/5 ml (raspberry, sulfites); *Oral susp:* 25 mg/5 ml (raspberry-apple); *IV conc:* doxy 100 mg/asc acid 480 mg after dilution; doxy 200 mg/asc acid 960 mg after dilution
	Vibra-Tab®	*Tab:* 100 mg film-coat
minocycline (D)	Minocin®	*Cap:* 100 mg
tetracycline (D)	Achromycin®V	*Cap:* 250, 500 mg
	Sumycin®	*Tab:* 250, 500 mg; *Oral susp:* 125 mg/5 ml (fruit, sulfites)
Macrolide/Sulfasoxazole		
erythromycin ethylsuccinate/ sulfasoxazole (C)	Pediazole®	*Oral susp:* eryth 200 mg/sulf 600 mg per 5 ml (100, 150, 200 ml; strawberry-banana)
Miscellaneous		

Antiinfectives by Class with Dose Forms

Generic Name	Brand Name	Dose Form(s)
chloramphenicol (C)	Chloromycetin®	*Vial*: 1 g
clindamycin (B)	Cleocin®	*Cap*: 75 (tartrazine), 150 (tartrazine), 300 mg; *Oral susp*: 5 mg/5 ml (100 ml; cherry)
lincomycin (B)	Lincocin®	*Vial*: 300 mg/ml (10 ml)
meropenem (B)	Merrem®	*Vial*: 500 mg; 1 g pwdr for reconstitution (sodium 3.92 mEq/g)
nitrofurantoin (B)	Furadantin®	*Oral susp*: 25 mg/5 ml (60 ml)
	Macrobid®	*Cap*: 100 mg
	Macrodantin®	*Cap*: 25, 50, 100 mg
vancomycin (C)	Vancocin®	*Cap*: 125, 250 mg

AppendiY Y: Antiinfectives: Dose by Weight for Liquid Forms

		Page
Appendix Y.1	*acyclovir* (Zovirax®)	568
Appendix Y.2	*amantadine* (Symmetrel®)	568
Appendix Y.3	*amoxicillin* (Amoxil®, Trimox®)	569
Appendix Y.4	*ampicillin* (Omnipen®, Principen®)	570
Appendix Y.5	*amoxicillin+clavulanate* (Augmenten®)	571
Appendix Y.6	*amoxicillin+clavulanate* (Augmentin®ES 600)	572
Appendix Y.7	*azithromycin* (Zithromax®, Zmax®)	573
Appendix Y.8	*cefdinir* (Omnicef®)	574
Appendix Y.9	*cefaclor* (Ceclor®)	575
Appendix Y.10	*cefadroxil* (Duricef®)	576
Appendix Y.11	cefixime (Suprax®)	577
Appendix Y.12	*cefpodoxime proxetil* (Vantin®)	578
Appendix Y.13	*cefprozil* (Cefzil®)	579
Appendix Y.14	*ceftibuten* (Cedax®)	580
Appendix Y.15	*cefuroxime axetil* (Ceftin®)	581
Appendix Y.16	*cephalexin* (Keflex®)	582
Appendix Y.17	*cephradine* (Velosef®)	583
Appendix Y.18	*clarithromycin* (Biaxin®)	584
Appendix Y.19	*clindamycin* (Cleocin®)	585
Appendix Y.20	*dicloxacillin* (Dynapen®)	586
Appendix Y.21	*doxycycline* (Vibramycin®)	587
Appendix Y.22	*erythromycin estolate* (Ilosone®)	588
Appendix Y.23	*erythromycin ethylsuccinate* (E.E.S.®, Ery-Ped®)	589
Appendix Y.24	erythromycin+sulfamethoxazole (Eryzole®, Pediazole®)	590
Appendix Y.25	*fluconazole* (Diflucan®)	591
Appendix Y.26	*furazolidone* (Furoxone®)	591
Appendix Y.27	*griseofulvin, microsize* (Grifulvin V®)	592
Appendix Y.28	*itraconazole* (Sporanox®)	592
Appendix Y.29	*loracarbef* (Lorabid®)	593
Appendix Y.30	*nitrofurantoin* (Furadantin®)	593
Appendix Y.31	*penicillin v* (Pen-Vee®K, Veetids®)	594
Appendix Y.32	*rimantidine* (Flumadine®)	595
Appendix Y.33	*tetracycline* (Sumycin®)	595
Appendix Y.34	*trimethoprim* (Primsol®)	596

Appendix Y.35	*trimethoprim+sulfamethoxazole* (Bactrim®, Septra®)	597
Appendix Y.36	*vancomycin* (Vancocin®)	598

Appendix Y.1: *acyclovir*, Zovirax®Suspension

Weight													
Pounds (lb)	15	20	25	30	35	40	45	50	55	60	65	70
Kilograms (kg)	6.8	9	11.4	13.6	15.9	18.2	20.5	22.7	25	27.3	29.5	31.8
Dose/Volume (5 days) in ml													
20 mg/kg qid	3.5	4.5	5.5	6.5	8	9	10	11.5	12.5	13.5	14.5	16
mg/5ml	200	200	200	200	200	200	200	200	200	200	200	200
Vol	70	90	110	130	160	180	200	230	250	270	290	320

Zovirax®Suspension (B)(G) >2 years: not recommended; 250 mg/5 ml; banana

Appendix Y.2: *amantadine*, Symmetrel®Syrup

Weight													
Pounds (lb)	15	20	25	30	35	40	45	50	55	60	65	70
Kilograms (kg)	6.8	9	11.4	13.6	15.9	18.2	20.5	22.7	25	27.3	29.5	31.8
Dose/Volume (10 days) in ml													
2 mg/lb/day	3	4	5	6	7	8	9	10	11	12	13	14
mg/5ml	50	50	50	50	50	50	50	50	50	50	50	50
Vol	30	40	50	60	70	80	90	100	110	120	130	140
4 mg/lb/day	6	8	10	12				9-12 years: 2 tsp bid				
mg/5ml	50	50	50	50				>12 years: same as adult				
Vol	60	80	100	60								

Symmetrel®Suspension (C)(G) <1 year: not recommended; 1-8 yrs: max 150 mg/day; 50 mg/5 ml; raspberry

Appendix Y.3: *amoxicillin*, Amoxil®Suspension, Trimox®Suspension

Weight												
Pounds (lb)	15	20	25	30	35	40	45	50	55	60	65	70
Kilograms (kg)	6.8	9	11.4	13.6	15.9	18.2	20.5	22.7	25	27.3	29.5	31.8
Dose/Volume (10 days) in ml												
20 mg/kg÷tid	2	2.5	3	3.5	4	5	5.5	6	7	7.5	8	9
mg/5ml	125	125	125	125	125	125	125	125	125	125	125	125
Vol	60	75	90	105	120	150	165	180	210	225	240	270
30 mg/kg÷tid	3	3.5	2.5	3	3	3.5	4	4.5	5	5.5	6	6.5
mg/5ml	125	125	250	250	250	250	250	250	250	250	250	250
Vol	90	105	75	90	90	105	120	135	150	165	180	195
40 mg/kg÷bid	5	7	4.5	5	6	7	8	9	10	11	12	13
mg/5ml	125	125	250	250	250	250	250	250	250	250	250	250
Vol	100	140	90	100	120	140	160	180	200	220	240	250
45 mg/kg÷bid	4	2.5	3	4	4.5	5	6	6.5	7	7.5	8.5	9
mg/5ml	200	400	400	400	400	400	400	400	400	400	400	400
Vol	80	50	60	80	90	100	120	130	140	150	170	180
90 mg/kg÷bid	8	5	6	7	9	10	12	13	14	15	17	18
mg/5ml	200	400	400	400	400	400	400	400	400	400	400	400
Vol	160	100	120	140	180	200	240	260	280	300	340	360

Amoxil®Suspension (B)(G) 125, 250 mg/5ml (80, 100, 150 ml; strawberry); 200, 400 mg/5 ml (50, 75, 100 ml; bubble gum)
Trimox® Suspension (B)(G) 125, 250 mg/ml (80, 100, 150 ml; raspberry-strawberry)

Appendix Y.4: *ampicillin*, Omnipen®Suspension, Principen®Suspension

Weight													
Pounds (lb)	15	20	25	30	35	40	45	50	55	60	65	70
Kilograms (kg)	6.8	9	11.4	13.6	15.9	18.2	20.5	22.7	25	27.3	29.5	31.8
Dose/Volume (10 days) in ml													
50 mg/kg÷q6h	3.5	4.5	3	3.5	4	4.5						
mg/5ml	125	125	250	250	250	250			>20 kg: same as adult			
Vol	140	180	120	140	160	180						
100 mg/kg÷q6h	3.5	4.5	6	7	8	9						
mg/5ml	250	250	250	250	250	250						
Vol	140	180	240	280	320	360						

Omnipen®Suspension, Principen®Suspension (B)(G) 125, 250 mg/5 ml (100, 150, 200 ml; fruit)

Appendix Y.5: *amoxicillin+clavulanate*, Augmentin®Suspension

Weight													
Pounds (lb)	15	20	25	30	35	40	45	50	55	60	65	70
Kilograms (kg)	6.8	9	11.4	13.6	15.9	18.2	20.5	22.7	25	27.3	29.5	31.8
Dose/Volume (10 days) in ml													
40 mg/kg÷bid	5.5	7	4.5	5.5	6.5	7	8	9	10	11	12	13
mg/5ml	125	125	250	250	250	250	250	250	250	250	250	250
Vol	110	140	90	110	130	140	160	180	200	220	240	260
45 mg/kg÷bid	3	4	5	6	7	8	9	10	11.5	12.5	13.5	14.5
mg/5ml	250	250	250	250	250	250	250	250	250	250	250	250
Vol	60	80	100	120	140	160	180	200	230	250	270	290
45 mg/kg÷bid	4	2.5	3	4	4.5	5	6	6.5	7	7.5	8.5	9
mg/5ml	200	400	400	400	400	400	400	400	400	400	400	400
Vol	80	50	60	80	90	100	120	130	140	150	170	180
90 mg/kg÷bid	4	5	6.5	8	9	10	11.5	13	14	15.5	16.5	18
mg/5ml	400	400	400	400	400	400	400	400	400	400	400	400
Vol	80	100	130	160	180	200	240	260	280	300	340	360

Augmentin®Suspension (B)(G) 125mg/5 ml (75, 100, 150 ml; banana), 250 mg/5 ml (75, 100, 150 ml; orange); 200, 400 mg/5 ml (50, 75, 100 ml; orange-raspberry, phenylalanine)

Appendix Y.6: *amoxicillin+clavulanate*, Augmentin®ES 600 Suspension

Weight												
Pounds (lb)	15	20	25	30	35	40	45	50	55	60	65	70
Kilograms (kg)	6.8	9	11.4	13.6	15.9	18.2	20.5	22.7	25	27.3	29.5	31.8
Dose/Volume (10 days) in ml												
40 mg/kg÷bid	1	1.5	2	2	2.5	3	3.5	4	4	4.5	5	5
mg/5ml	600	600	600	600	600	600	600	600	600	600	600	600
Vol	30	40	40	40	50	60	70	80	80	90	100	100
45 mg/kg÷bid	1.25	1.5	2	2.5	3	3.5	4	4.5	5	5	5.5	6
mg/5ml	600	600	600	600	600	600	600	600	600	600	600	600
Vol	25	30	40	50	60	70	80	90	100	100	110	120
90 mg/kg÷bid	2.5	3.5	4	5	6	7	8	8.5	9.5	10	11	12
mg/5ml	600	600	600	600	600	600	600	600	600	600	600	600
Vol	50	70	80	100	120	140	160	170	190	200	220	240

Augmentin®ES 600 Suspension (B) 600 mg/5 ml (50, 75, 100, 150 ml; orange-raspberry, phenylalanine)

Appendix Y.7: *azithromycin*, Zithromax®Suspension, Zmax®Suspension

Weight								
Pounds (lb)	11	22	33	44	55	66	77	88
Kilograms (kg)	5	10	15	20	25	30	35	40
Dose/Volume in ml								
3 Day Regimen								
10 mg/kg qd	2.5	5	7.5					
mg/5ml	100	100	100					
Vol	7.5	15	22.5					
10 mg/kg qd				5	6	7.5	9	10
mg/5ml				200	200	200	200	200
Vol				15	18	22.5	27	30
5 Day Regimen								
10 mg/kg qd								
Day 1	2.5	5	7.5	5	6	7.5	7.5	10
Days 2-5	1.25	2.5	4	2.5	3	4	4	5
mg/5ml	100	100	100	200	200	200	200	200
Vol	10	15	23.5	15	18	23.5	23.5	30

Zithromax®ES 600 Suspension (B) 100 mg/5 ml (15 ml), 200 mg/5 ml (15, 22.5, 30 ml); cherry-vanilla-banana flavor

Appendix Y.8: *cefdinir*, Omnicef®Suspension

Weight												
Pounds (lb)	15	20	25	30	35	40	45	50	55	60	65	70
Kilograms (kg)	6.8	9	11.4	13.6	15.9	18.2	20.5	22.7	25	27.3	29.5	31.8
Dose/Volume (10 days) in ml												
7 mg/kg bid	2	2.5	3	4	4.5	5	6	6.5	7	7.5	8	9
mg/5ml	125	125	125	125	125	125	125	125	125	125	125	125
Vol	40	50	60	80	90	100	120	130	140	150	160	180
14 mg/kg qd	4	5	6	8	9	10	12	13	14	15	16	18
mg/5ml	125	125	125	125	125	125	125	125	125	125	125	125
Vol	40	50	60	80	90	100	120	130	140	150	160	180

Omnicef®Suspension (B) <6 months: not recommended; 125 mg/5 ml (60, 100 ml; strawberry)

Appendix Y.9: *cefaclor*, Ceclor®Suspension

Weight												
Pounds (lb)	15	20	25	30	35	40	45	50	55	60	65	70
Kilograms (kg)	6.8	9	11.4	13.6	15.9	18.2	20.5	22.7	25	27.3	29.5	31.8
Dose/Volume (10 days) in ml												
20 mg/kg tid	2	2.5	3	3.5	4	5	5.5	6	7	7.5	8	8.5
mg/5ml	125	125	125	125	125	125	125	125	125	125	125	125
Vol	60	75	90	105	120	150	165	180	210	225	240	255
20 mg/kg tid	1.5	1.5	2	2.5	3	3	4	4	4.5	5	5.5	6
mg/5ml	187	187	187	187	187	187	187	187	187	187	187	187
Vol	45	45	60	75	90	90	105	120	135	150	165	180
40 mg/kg tid	2	2.5	3	3.5	4	5	5.5	6	6.5	7	8	8.5
mg/5ml	250	250	250	250	250	250	250	250	250	250	250	250
Vol	60	75	90	105	120	150	165	180	195	210	240	255
40 mg/kg tid	1.5	1.5	2	2.5	3	3	3.5	4	4.5	5	5	5.5
mg/5ml	375	375	375	375	375	375	375	375	375	375	375	375
Vol	45	45	60	75	90	90	105	120	135	150	150	165

Ceclor®Suspension **(B)** <6 months: not recommended; 125, 250 mg/5 ml (75, 150 ml) 187, 375 mg/5ml (50, 100 ml); strawberry

Appendix Y.10: *cefadroxil*, Duricef®Suspension

Weight													
Pounds (lb)	15	20	25	30	35	40	45	50	55	60	65	70
Kilograms (kg)	6.8	9	11.4	13.6	15.9	18.2	20.5	22.7	25	27.3	29.5	31.8
Dose/Volume (10 days) in ml													
30 mg/kg bid	2	3	3.5	4	5	5.5	6	7	7.5	8	9	9.5
mg/5ml	250	250	250	250	250	250	250	250	250	250	250	250
Vol	40	60	75	80	100	110	120	140	150	160	180	190
30 mg/kg qd	2	3	3.5	4	5	5.5	6	7	7.5	8	9	9.5
mg/5ml	500	500	500	500	500	500	500	500	500	500	500	500
Vol	20	30	35	40	50	55	60	70	75	80	90	95

Duricef®Suspension (B) 250 mg/5 ml (100 ml), 500 mg/5ml (75, 100 ml); orange-pineapple

Appendix Y.11: *cefixime*, Suprax®Oral Suspension

Weight												
Pounds (lb)	15	20	25	30	35	40	45	50	55	60	65	70
Kilograms (kg)	6.8	9	11.4	13.6	15.9	18.2	20.5	22.7	25	27.3	29.5	31.8
Dose/Volume (10 days) in ml												
8 mg/kg qd	2.7	3.6	4.5	5.5	6.3	7.2	8.2	9	10ml	11	12	13
mg/5ml	100	100	100	100	100	100	100	100	100	100	100	100
Vol	27	36	45	55	65	70	80	90	100	110	120	130
8 mg/kg÷bid	1.3	1.8	2.2	2.5	3.1	3.5	4	4.5	5	5.5	6	6.5
mg/5ml	100	100	100	100	100	100	100	100	100	100	100	100
Vol	27	36	45	55	65	70	80	90	100	110	120	130

Suprax®Oral Suspension (B)(G) <6 months: not recommended; 100 mg/5 ml (50, 75, 100 ml; strawberry)

Appendix Y.12: *cefpodoxime proxetil*, Vantin®Suspension

Weight												
Pounds (lb)	15	20	25	30	35	40	45	50	55	60	65	70
Kilograms (kg)	6.8	9	11.4	13.6	15.9	18.2	20.5	22.7	25	27.3	29.5	31.8
Dose/Volume (10 days) in ml												
5 mg/kg bid	3.5	4.5	5.5	7	8	9	10	11	12.5	13.5	15	16
mg/5ml	50	50	50	50	50	50	50	50	50	50	50	50
Vol	70	90	110	140	160	180	200	220	250	270	300	320
5 mg/kg bid	2	2	3	3.5	4	4.5	5	5.5	6	7	7.5	8
mg/5ml	100	100	100	100	100	100	100	100	100	100	100	100
Vol	40	40	60	70	80	90	100	110	120	140	150	160

Vantin®Suspension (B) <2 months: not recommended; 50, 100 mg/5 ml (50, 75, 100 ml; lemon-crème)

Appendix Y.13: *cefprozil*, Cefzil®Suspension

Weight													
Pounds (lb)	15	20	25	30	35	40	45	50	55	60	65	70
Kilograms (kg)	6.8	9	11.4	13.6	15.9	18.2	20.5	22.7	25	27.3	29.5	31.8
Dose/Volume (10 days) in ml													
7.5 mg/kg bid	2	3	3.5	4	5	5.5	6	7	7.5	4	4.5	5
mg/5ml	125	125	125	125	125	125	125	125	125	250	250	250
Vol	40	60	70	80	100	110	120	140	150	80	90	100
15 mg/kg bid	2	3	3.5	4	5	5	6	7	7.5	8	9	9.5
mg/5ml	250	250	250	250	250	250	250	250	250	250	250	250
Vol	40	60	70	80	100	100	120	140	150	160	180	190
20 mg/kg qd	3	3.5	4.5	5.5	6.5	7	8	9	10	11	12	13
mg/5ml	250	250	250	250	250	250	250	250	250	250	250	250
Vol	60	70	90	110	130	140	160	180	200	220	240	260

Cefzil®Suspension (B) >12 years: same as adult; 125, 250 mg/5 ml (50, 75, 100 ml; bubble gum flavor, phenylalanine)

Appendix Y.14: *ceftibuten*, Cedax®Suspension

Weight												
Pounds (lb)	15	20	25	30	35	40	45	50	55	60	65	70
Kilograms (kg)	6.8	9	11.4	13.6	15.9	18.2	20.5	22.7	25	27.3	29.5	31.8
Dose/Volume (10 days) in ml												
9 mg/kg/day	3.5	4.5	6	7	8	9	10	11.5	12.5	13.5	15	16
mg/5ml	90	90	90	90	90	90	90	90	90	90	90	90
Vol	35	45	60	70	80	90	100	115	125	135	150	160
9 mg/kg/day	1.75	2.3	3	3.5	4	4.5	5	5.4	6.2	6.6	7.5	8
mg/5ml	180	180	180	180	180	180	180	180	180	180	180	180
Vol	20	25	30	35	40	45	50	55	60	65	70	80

Cefzil®Suspension (B) 90 mg/5 ml (30, 60, 90, 120 ml), 180 mg/5ml (30, 60, 120 ml) (cherry flavor)

Appendix Y.15: *cefuroxime axetil* Ceftin®Suspension

Weight												
Pounds (lb)	15	20	25	30	35	40	45	50	55	60	65	70
Kilograms (kg)	6.8	9	11.4	13.6	15.9	18.2	20.5	22.7	25	27.3	29.5	31.8
Dose/Volume (10 days) in ml												
20 mg/kg÷bid	2.5	3.5	4.5	3	3	3.5	4	4.5	5	5.5	6	6.5
mg/5ml	125	125	125	250	250	250	250	250	250	250	250	250
Vol	50	70	90	60	60	70	80	90	100	110	120	130
30 mg/kg÷bid	2	3	3.5	4	5	5.5	6	7	7.5	8	9	9.5
mg/5ml	250	250	250	250	250	250	250	250	250	250	250	250
Vol	40	60	70	80	100	110	120	140	150	160	180	190

Ceftin®Suspension (B) 125, 250 mg/5 ml (50, 100 ml; tutti-frutti)

Appendix Y.16: *cephalexin* (Keflex®Suspension)

Weight													
Pounds (lb)	15	20	25	30	35	40	45	50	55	60	65	70
Kilograms (kg)	6.8	9	11.4	13.6	15.9	18.2	20.5	22.7	25	27.3	29.5	31.8
Dose/Volume (10 days) in ml													
25 mg/kg÷tid	1	1.5	2	2	3	3	3.5	4	4	4.5	5	5
mg/5ml	125	125	125	125	125	125	125	125	125	125	125	125
Vol	30	45	60	60	90	90	105	120	120	135	150	150
25 mg/kg÷qid	1	1	1.5	2	2	2.5	2.5	3	3	3.5	4	4
mg/5ml	250	250	250	250	250	250	250	250	250	250	250	250
Vol	40	40	60	80	80	100	100	120	120	140	160	160
50 mg/kg÷tid	2	3	4	4.5	5	6	7	7.5	8	9	10	10.5
mg/5ml	250	250	250	250	250	250	250	250	250	250	250	250
Vol	60	90	120	135	150	180	210	225	240	270	300	315
50 mg/kg÷qid	2	2	3	3.5	4	4.5	5	6	6	7	7.5	8
mg/5ml	250	250	250	250	250	250	250	250	250	250	250	250
Vol	80	80	120	140	160	180	200	240	240	280	300	320

Keflex®Suspension (B)(G) <2 months: not recommended; 125, 250 mg/5 ml (100, 200 ml; lemon-crème)

Appendix Y.17: *cephradine* (Velosef®Suspension)

Weight												
Pounds (lb)	15	20	25	30	35	40	45	50	55	60	65	70
Kilograms (kg)	6.8	9	11.4	13.6	15.9	18.2	20.5	22.7	25	27.3	29.5	31.8
Dose/Volume (10 days) in ml												
25 mg/kg÷q12h	2	2	3	3.5	4	4.5	5	6	6	7	7.5	8
mg/5ml	250	250	250	250	250	250	250	250	250	250	250	250
Vol	40	40	60	70	80	90	100	120	120	140	150	160
50 mg/kg÷q12h	3.5	4.5	6	7	8	9	10	11.5	12.5	14	15	16
mg/5ml	250	250	250	250	250	250	250	250	250	250	250	250
Vol	70	90	120	140	160	180	200	230	250	280	300	320
75 mg/kg÷q12h	5	7	8.5	10	12	14	16					
mg/5ml	250	250	250	250	250	250	250					
Vol	100	140	170	200	240	280	320					
100mg/kg÷q12h	7	9	11.5	13.5	16							
mg/5ml	250	250	250	250	250							
Vol	140	180	230	270	320							

Velosef®Suspension **(B)** <9 months: not recommended; 125, 250 mg/5 ml (100, 200 ml; lemon-crème)

Appendix Y.18: *clarithromycin* (Biaxin®Suspension)

Weight												
Pounds (lb)	15	20	25	30	35	40	45	50	55	60	65	70
Kilograms (kg)	6.8	9	11.4	13.6	15.9	18.2	20.5	22.7	25	27.3	29.5	31.8
Dose/Volume (10 days) in ml												
7.5 mg/kg bid	2	3	3.5	4	5	5.5	6	7	7.5	8	9	10
mg/5ml	125	125	125	125	125	125	125	125	125	125	125	125
Vol	40	60	70	80	100	110	120	140	150	160	180	200
7.5 mg/kg bid	1	1.5	2	2	2.5	3	3	3.5	4	4	4.5	5
mg/5ml	250	250	250	250	250	250	250	250	250	250	250	250
Vol	20	30	40	40	50	60	60	70	80	80	90	100

Biaxin®Suspension (B) <6 months: not recommended; 125, 250 mg/5 ml (50, 100 ml; fruit-punch

Appendix Y.19: *clindamycin* (Cleocin®Pediatric Granules)

Weight												
Pounds (lb)	15	20	25	30	35	40	45	50	55	60	65	70
Kilograms (kg)	6.8	9	11.4	13.6	15.9	18.2	20.5	22.7	25	27.3	29.5	31.8
Dose/Volume (10 days) in ml												
8 mg/kg÷tid	1	1.5	2	2.5	3	3	3.5	4	4.5	5	5	5.5
mg/5ml	75	75	75	75	75	75	75	75	75	75	75	75
Vol	30	45	60	75	90	90	105	120	135	150	150	165
16 mg/kg÷tid	2.5	3	4	5	5.5	6.5	7	8	9	9.5	10.5	11
mg/5ml	75	75	75	75	75	75	75	75	75	75	75	75
Vol	75	90	120	150	165	105	210	240	270	285	315	330

Cleocin®Pediatric Granules (B)(G) 75 mg/5 ml (100 ml; cherry)

Appendix Y.20: *dicloxacillin* Dynapen®Suspension

Weight												
Pounds (lb)	15	20	25	30	35	40	45	50	55	60	65	70
Kilograms (kg)	6.8	9	11.4	13.6	15.9	18.2	20.5	22.7	25	27.3	29.5	31.8
Dose/Volume (10 days) in ml												
12.5 mg/kg÷qid	2	2.5	3	3.5	4	4.5	5	6	6	7	7.5	8
mg/5ml	62.5	62.5	62.5	62.5	62.5	62.5	62.5	62.5	62.5	62.5	62.5	62.5
Vol	80	100	120	140	160	180	200	240	240	280	300	320
25 mg/kg÷qid	3.5	4.5	6	7	8	9	10	11.5	12.5	13.5	15	16
mg/5ml	62.5	62.5	62.5	62.5	62.5	62.5	62.5	62.5	62.5	62.5	62.5	62.5
Vol	140	180	240	280	320	360	400	460	500	540	600	640

Dynapen®Suspension (B)(G) 6.25 mg/5 ml (80, 100 ml; raspberry-strawberry)

Appendix Y.21: *doxycycline* (Vibramycin®Syrup/Suspension)

Weight												
Pounds (lb)	15	20	25	30	35	40	45	50	55	60	65	70
Kilograms (kg)	6.8	9	11.4	13.6	15.9	18.2	20.5	22.7	25	27.3	29.5	31.8
Dose/Volume												
1 mg/lb daily	1.5	2	2.5	3	3.5	4	4.5	5	5.5	6	6.5	7
50 mg/5ml	50	50	50	50	50	50	50	50	50	50	50	50
Vol	15	20	25	30	35	40	45	50	55	60	65	70
1 mg/lb daily	3	4	5	6	7	8	9	10	11	12	13	14
25 mg/5ml	25	25	25	25	25	25	25	25	25	25	25	25
Vol	30	40	50	60	70	80	90	100	110	120	130	140

Vibramycin®Syrup (B)(G) <8 years: not recommended; double dose first day; 50 mg/5 ml (80, 100, ml; raspberry-apple; sulfites)
Vibramycin®Suspension (B)(G) <8 years: not recommended; double dose first day; 25 mg/5 ml (80, 100, ml; raspberry)

Appendix Y.22: *erythromycin estolate* (Ilosone®Suspension)

Weight												
Pounds (lb)	15	20	25	30	35	40	45	50	55	60	65	70
Kilograms (kg)	6.8	9	11.4	13.6	15.9	18.2	20.5	22.7	25	27.3	29.5	31.8
Dose/Volume (10 days) in ml												
10 mg/kg bid	3	3.5	4.5	5.5	6	7	8	9	10	5.5	6	6.5
mg/5ml	125	125	125	125	125	125	125	125	125	250	250	250
Vol	60	70	90	110	120	140	160	180	200	110	120	130
15 mg/kg bid	4	5.5	7	8	9.5	5.5	6	7	7.5	8	9	9.5
mg/5ml	125	125	125	125	125	250	250	250	250	250	250	250
Vol	80	110	140	160	190	110	120	140	150	160	180	190
20 mg/kg bid	3	3.5	4.5	5.5	6.5	7	8	9	10	11	12	13
mg/5ml	250	250	250	250	250	250	250	250	250	250	250	250
Vol	60	70	90	110	120	140	160	180	200	220	240	260
25 mg/kg bid	3.5	4.5	5.5	7	8	9	10	11.5	12.5	13.5	15	16
mg/5ml	250	250	250	250	250	250	250	250	250	250	250	250
Vol	70	90	110	140	160	180	200	230	250	280	300	320

Ilosone®Suspension (B)(G) 125, 250 mg/5 ml (100 ml)

Appendix Y.23: *erythromycin ethylsuccinate*, E.E.S.®Suspension, Ery-Ped®Drops/Suspension

Weight													
Pounds (lb)	15	20	25	30	35	40	45	50	55	60	65	70
Kilograms (kg)	6.8	9	11.4	13.6	15.9	18.2	20.5	22.7	25	27.3	29.5	31.8
Dose/Volume (10 days) in ml												
30 mg/kg÷qid	1.5	2	2	2.5	3	3.5	4	4	4.5	5	5.5	6
mg/5ml	200	200	200	200	200	200	200	200	200	200	200	200
Vol	60	80	80	100	120	140	160	160	180	200	220	240
30 mg/kg÷qid			1	1.5	1.5	2	2	2	2.5	2.5	3	3
mg/5ml			400	400	400	400	400	400	400	400	400	400
Vol			40	60	60	80	80	80	100	100	120	120
50 mg/kg÷qid	2	3	3.5	4.5	5	5.5	6.5	7	8	8.5	9	10
mg/5ml	200	200	200	200	200	200	200	200	200	200	200	200
Vol	80	120	140	180	200	220	260	280	320	340	360	400
50mg/kg÷qid	1	1.5	2	2	2.5	3	3	3.5	4	4.5	4.5	5
mg/5ml	400	400	400	400	400	400	400	400	400	400	400	400
Vol	40	60	80	80	100	120	140	140	160	180	180	200

Ery-Ped®Drops/Suspension **(B)(G)** 200 mg/5 ml (100, 200 ml; fruit); 400 mg/5 ml (60, 100, 200 ml; banana); Oral drops: 200, 400 mg/5 ml (50 ml; fruit)

E.E.S.®Suspension **(B)(G)** 200 mg/5 ml, 400 mg/5 ml (100 ml; fruit)

E.E.S. ®Granules **(B)(G)** 200 mg/5 ml (100, 200 ml; cherry)

Appendix Y.24: *erythromycin+sulfamethoxazole*, Eryzole®, Pediazole®

Weight												
Pounds (lb)	15	20	25	30	35	40	45	50	55	60	65	70
Kilograms (kg)	6.8	9	11.4	13.6	15.9	18.2	20.5	22.7	25	27.3	29.5	31.8
Dose/Volume (10 days) in ml												
10 mg/kg bid	3	4	5	6	6.5	7.5	8.5	9.5	10	11	12	13.5
mg/5ml	200	200	200	200	200	200	200	200	200	200	200	200
Vol	90	120	150	180	200	225	255	285	300	330	360	400

Eryzole® (C)(G) <2 months: not recommended; *eryth* 200 mg/*sulf* 600 mg/5 ml (100, 150, 200, 250 ml)
Pediazole® (C)(G) <2 months: not recommended; *eryth* 200 mg/*sulf* 600 mg/5 ml (100, 150, 200 ml; strawberry-banana)

Appendix Y.25: *fluconazole* (Diflucan®Suspension)

Weight												
Pounds (lb)	15	20	25	30	35	40	45	50	55	60	65	70
Kilograms (kg)	6.8	9	11.4	13.6	15.9	18.2	20.5	22.7	25	27.3	29.5	31.8
Dose/Volume (21 days) in ml												
3 mg/kg/day	2	3	3.5	4	5	5.5	6	7	7.5	8	9	9.5
mg/ml	10	10	10	10	10	10	10	10	10	10	10	10
Vol	44	66	77	88	110	121	132	154	165	176	198	209
6 mg/kg/day	4	5.5	2	2	2.5	3	3	3.5	4	4	4.5	5
mg/ml	10	10	40	40	40	40	40	40	40	40	40	40
Vol	88	121	44	44	55	66	66	77	88	88	99	110

Diflucan®Suspension **(B)(G)** double-dose first day; 10, 40 mg/5 ml (35 ml); orange)

Appendix Y.26: *furazolidone*, Furoxone®Liquid

Weight												
Pounds (lb)	15	20	25	30	35	40	45	50	55	60	65	70
Kilograms (kg)	6.8	9	11.4	13.6	15.9	18.2	20.5	22.7	25	27.3	29.5	31.8
Dose/Volume (7 days) in ml												
5 mg/kg÷qid	2.5	3.5	4	5	6	7	8	8.5	9.5	10	11	12
mg/15 ml	50	50	50	50	50	50	50	50	50	50	50	50
Vol	100	140	160	200	240	280	320	340	380	400	440	480

Furoxone®Liquid **(C)(G)** double-dose first day; 50 mg/15 ml (35 ml)

Appendix Y.27: *griseofulvin, microsize*, Grifulvin V®Suspension

Weight												
Pounds (lb)	15	20	25	30	35	40	45	50	55	60	65	70
Kilograms (kg)	6.8	9	11.4	13.6	15.9	18.2	20.5	22.7	25	27.3	29.5	31.8
Dose/Volume (30 days) in ml												
5 mg/lb/day	3	4	5	6	7	8	9	10	11	12	13	14
mg/5ml	125	125	125	125	125	125	125	125	125	125	125	125
Vol	90	120	150	180	210	240	270	300	330	360	390	420

Grifulvin V®Suspension (C)(G) double-dose first day; 125 mg/5 ml (120 ml; orange, alcohol 0.02%))

Appendix Y.28: *itraconazole*, Sporanox®Solution

Weight												
Pounds (lb)	15	20	25	30	35	40	45	50	55	60	65	70
Kilograms (kg)	6.8	9	11.4	13.6	15.9	18.2	20.5	22.7	25	27.3	29.5	31.8
Dose/Volume (7 days) in ml												
5 mg/kg/day	3.5	4.5	6	7	8	9	10	11.5	12.5	14	15	16
mg/ml	10	10	10	10	10	10	10	10	10	10	10	10
Vol	25	32	42	49	56	63	70	71	88	98	105	112

SporanoxV®Solution (C)(G) double-dose first day; 10 mg/ml (150 ml; cherry-caramel flavor)

Appendix Y.29: *loracarbef*, Lorabid®Suspension

Weight												
Pounds (lb)	15	20	25	30	35	40	45	50	55	60	65	70
Kilograms (kg)	6.8	9	11.4	13.6	15.9	18.2	20.5	22.7	25	27.3	29.5	31.8
Dose/Volume (10 days) in ml												
15 mg/kg bid	2.5	3.5	4	5	3	3.5	4	4	5	5	5.5	6
mg/5ml	100	100	100	100	200	200	200	200	200	200	200	200
Vol	50	70	80	100	60	70	80	80	100	100	110	120
30 mg/kg bid	2.5	3.5	4	5	6	7	8	8.5	9.5	10	11	12
mg/5ml	200	200	200	200	200	200	200	200	200	200	200	200
Vol	50	70	80	100	120	140	160	170	190	200	220	240

Lorabid®Suspension (B) 100 mg/5 ml (50, 100 ml); 200 mg/5 ml (50, 75, 100 ml) (strawberry bubble gum flavor)

Appendix Y.30: *nitrofurantoin*, Furadantin®Suspension

Weight												
Pounds (lb)	15	20	25	30	35	40	45	50	55	60	65	70
Kilograms (kg)	6.8	9	11.4	13.6	15.9	18.2	20.5	22.7	25	27.3	29.5	31.8
Dose/Volume (10 days) in ml												
5 mg/kg÷qid	1.5	2.5	3	3.5	4	4.5	5	5.5	6	7	7.5	8
mg/5 ml	25	25	25	25	25	25	25	25	25	25	25	25
Vol	60	100	120	140	160	190	200	220	240	280	300	320

Furadantin®Suspension (B)(G) 25 mg/5 ml (60 ml)

Appendix Y.31: *penicillin v* (Pen-Vee®K Solution, Veetids®Solution)

Weight												
Pounds (lb)	15	20	25	30	35	40	45	50	55	60	65	70
Kilograms (kg)	6.8	9	11.4	13.6	15.9	18.2	20.5	22.7	25	27.3	29.5	31.8
Dose & Volume (10 days) in ml												
25 mg/kg÷qid	2	2.5	3	3.5	4	4.5	5	5.5	6	7	7.5	8
mg/5ml	125	125	125	125	125	125	125	125	125	125	125	125
Vol	80	90	120	140	160	180	200	220	240	280	300	320
25 mg/kg÷qid	1	1	1.5	2	2	2.5	2.5	3	3	3.5	4	4
mg/5ml	250	250	250	250	250	250	250	250	250	250	250	250
Vol	40	40	60	80	80	100	100	120	120	140	160	160
50 mg/kg÷qid	2	2.5	3	3.5	4	4.5	5	6	6.5	7	7.5	8
mg/5ml	250	250	250	250	250	250	250	250	250	250	250	250
Vol	80	100	120	140	160	180	200	240	260	280	300	320

Pen-Vee®K Solution (B)(G) 125 mg/5 ml (100, 200 ml), 250 mg/5 ml (100, 150, 200 ml)
Veetids®Solution (B)(G) 125, 250 mg/5 ml (100, 200 ml)

Appendix Y.32: *rimantidine*, Flumadine®Syrup

Weight												
Pounds (lb)	15	20	25	30	35	40	45	50	55	60	65	70
Kilograms (kg)	6.8	9	11.4	13.6	15.9	18.2	20.5	22.7	25	27.3	29.5	31.8
Dose/Volume (10 days) in ml												
5 mg/kg/day	3.5	4.5	6	7	8	9	10	11.5	12.5	13.5	15	16
mg/5ml	50	50	50	50	50	50	50	50	50	50	50	50
Vol	35	45	60	70	80	90	100	115	125	135	150	160

Flumadine®Syrup (B) >10 years: same as adult; 50 mg/5 ml (2, 8, 16 oz; raspberry)

Appendix Y.33: *tetracycline*, Sumycin®Suspension

Weight												
Pounds (lb)	15	20	25	30	35	40	45	50	55	60	65	70
Kilograms (kg)	6.8	9	11.4	13.6	15.9	18.2	20.5	22.7	25	27.3	29.5	31.8
Dose/Volume (10 days) in ml												
25 mg/kg÷qid	1.5	2.5	3	3.5	4	4.5	5	6	6.5	7	7.5	8
mg/5ml	125	125	125	125	125	125	125	125	125	125	125	125
Vol	60	100	120	140	160	180	200	240	260	280	300	320
50 mg/kg÷qid	3.5	4.5	6	7	8	9	10	11.5	12.5	13.5	15	16
mg/5ml	125	125	125	125	125	125	125	125	125	125	125	125
Vol	140	180	240	280	320	360	400	460	500	540	600	640

Sumycin®Suspension (D)(G) <8 years: not recommended; 125 mg/5 ml (100, 200 ml; fruit, sulfites)

Appendix Y.34: *trimethoprim*, Primsol®Suspension

Weight												
Pounds (lb)	15	20	25	30	35	40	45	50	55	60	65	70
Kilograms (kg)	6.8	9	11.4	13.6	15.9	18.2	20.5	22.7	25	27.3	29.5	31.8
Dose/Volume (10 days) in ml												
5 mg/kg bid	3.5	4.5	6	7	8	9	10	11.5	12.5	13.5	15	16
mg/5ml	50	50	50	50	50	50	50	50	50	50	50	50
Vol	70	90	120	140	160	180	200	230	250	270	300	320

Primsol®Suspension (C)(G) 50 mg/5 ml (50 mg/5 ml; bubble gum, dye-free, alcohol-free)

Appendix Y.35: *trimethoprim+sulfamethoxazole*, Bactrim®Suspension, Septra®Suspension

Weight												
Pounds (lb)	15	20	25	30	35	40	45	50	55	60	65	70
Kilograms (kg)	6.8	9	11.4	13.6	15.9	18.2	20.5	22.7	25	27.3	29.5	31.8
Dose/Volume (10 days) in ml												
10 mg/kg bid	2	2	3	3.5	4	4.5	5	5.5	6	7	7.5	8
mg/5ml	200	200	200	200	200	200	200	200	200	200	200	200
Vol	40	40	60	70	80	90	100	110	120	140	150	160
20 mg/kg bid	4	4	6	7	8	9	10	11	12	14	15	16
mg/5ml	200	200	200	200	200	200	200	200	200	200	200	200
Vol	80	80	120	140	160	180	200	220	240	280	300	320

Bactrim®Pediatric Suspension, Septra®Pediatric Suspension (C)(G) *trim* 40 mg/*sulfa* 200 mg/5 ml (100 ml; cherry, alcohol 0.3%)

Appendix Y.36: *vancomycin*, Vancocin®Suspension)

Weight												
Pounds (lb)	15	20	25	30	35	40	45	50	55	60	65	70
Kilograms (kg)	6.8	9	11.4	13.6	15.9	18.2	20.5	22.7	25	27.3	29.5	31.8
Dose/Volume (10 days) in ml												
40 mg/kg÷tid	2	2.5	3	3.5	4.5	5	5.5	6	7	7.5	8	8.5
mg/5ml	250	250	250	250	250	250	250	250	250	250	250	250
Vol	60	75	90	105	135	150	165	180	210	225	240	255
40 mg/kg÷qid	1.5	2	2.5	3	3	3.5	4	4.5	5	5.5	6	6.5
mg/5ml	250	250	250	250	250	250	250	250	250	250	250	250
Vol	60	80	100	100	120	140	160	180	200	220	240	260
40 mg/kg÷tid	1	1	1.5	2	2	2.5	3	3	3.5	3.5	4	4
mg/6ml	500	500	500	500	500	500	500	500	500	500	500	500
Vol	30	30	45	60	60	75	75	90	105	105	120	135
40 mg/kg÷qid	1	1	1.5	1.5	1.5	2	2	2.5	2.5	3	3	3.5
mg/6ml	500	500	500	500	500	500	500	500	500	500	500	500
Vol	40	40	60	60	60	80	80	100	100	120	120	140

Vancomycin®Suspension, (C)(G)

Appendix Z: Brand/Generic Drug Cross Reference with FDA Pregnancy Category & Controlled Drug Category

Comment: See **Appendix A** for descriptions of FDA pregnancy categories.
See **Appendix B** for descriptions of controlled drug categories.
NR=not rated.

C	*abacavir,* **Ziagen**®
C	*abacavir/lamivudine,* **Epzicom**®
C	*abacavir/lidovudine/zidovudine,* **Trizivir**®
C	**A/B Otic**®, *antipyrine/benzocaine, glycerin*
X	*abarelix,* **Plenaxis**®
C	*abatacept,* **Orencia**®
C	**Abilify**®, *aripiprazole*
NR	**Abreva**®, *docosanol*
C	*acamprosate,* **Campral**®
B	*acarbos,* **Precose**®
B	**Accolate**®, *zafirlukast*
C	**AccuHist**®**LA**, *chlorpheniramine/phenylephrine/scopolamine/ atropine/hyoscyamine*
C	**Accuneb**®, *albuterol*
C/D	**Accupril**®, *quinapril*
C/D	**Accuretic**®, *quinapril/hydrochlorothiazide*
X	**Accutane**®, *isotretinoin, retinoic acid*
B	*acebutolol,* **Sectral**®
C	**Acel-Imune**®, *diphtheria/tetanus toxoids/acellular pertussis vaccine*
C/D	**Aceon**®, *perindopril*
B	*acetaminophen,* **Anacin**®**-3, Datril**®, **Panadol**®, **Phenaphen**®, **Tempra**®, **Tylenol**®, **Valadol**®
C	*acetazolamide,* **Diamox**®, **Diamox**® Sequels
NR	*acetic acid,* **Domeboro**®**Otic, Vosol**®
C	*acetohexamide,* **Dymelor**®
B	*acetylcysteine,* **Mucomyst**®
D	*acetylsalicylic acid, aspirin,* **Bayer**®, **Easprin**®, **Ecotrin**®
D	**Achromycin**®, **Achromycin**®**V**, *tetracycline*
B	**AcipHex**®, *rabeprazole*
X	*acitretin,* **Soriatane**®
C	**Aclovate**®, *alclometasone dipropionate*
C	**ActHIB**®, *haemophilus b conjugate vaccine (tetanus toxoid conjugate)*
C	**ActHIB-DTP**®, *haemophilus b conjugate vaccine (tetanus toxoid conjugate) with DPT vaccine*
B	**Acticin**®, *permethrin*
C	**Actifed**®, *pseudoephedrine/triprolidine*
C	**Actifed**®**Cold & Allergy**, *triprolidine/pseudoephedrine*

C	III	**Actifed®with Codeine,** *triprolidine/pseudoephedrine/codeine*
B		**Actigall®,** *ursodiol*
C		**Actinex®,** *masoprocol cream*
C	II	**Actiq®,** *fentanyl transmucosal unit*
X		**Activella®,** *estradiol/norethindrone*
C		**Actoplus Met®,** *pioglitazone/metformin*
C		**Actonel®,** *risedronate*
C		**Actos®,** *pioglitazone*
B		**Actron®,** *ketoprofen*
C		**Acular®, Acular®PF,** *ketorolac tromethamine*
C		*acyclovir,* **Zovirax®**
C		**Adalat®, Adalat®CC,** *nifedipine*
B		*adalimubab,* **Humira®**
C		*adapalene,* **Differin®**
C		**Adapin®TCA,** *doxepin*
C	II	**Adderall®, Adderall®XR,** *dextroamphetamine saccharate/ dextroamphetamine sulfate/amphetamine aspartate/amphetamine sulfate*
C		*adenovir dipivoxil,* **Hepsera®**
C	IV	**Adipex-P®,** *phentermine*
C		**Adipra®,** *insulin glulisine (rDNA origin)*
D		**Adoxa®,** *doxycycline*
C		**Adrenalin®,** *epinephrine*
D		**Adrucil®,** *fluorouracil, 5-fluorouracil, 5-FU*
C		**Advair®DisKus,** *fluticasone propionate/salmeterol*
A		**Advanced NatalCare®,** *prenatal vitamin*
NR		**Advanced Relief Visine®,** *tetrahydrozoline/polyethylene glycol, povidone/dextran*
X		**Advicor®,** *niacin/lovastatin*
B/D		**Advil®,** *ibuprofen*
C		**AeroBid®, Aerobid®M,** *flunisolide*
C		**Aerolate®,** *theophylline*
B		**Aerosporin®,** *polymixin b*
C		**Afrin®,** *oxymetazoline*
C		**Aftate®,** *tolnaftate*
C		**Agenerase®,** *amprenavir*
D		**Aggrenox®,** *dipyridamole/aspirin*
C		**Agrylin®,** *anagrelide*
C		**Akineton®,** *biperiden hydrochloride, biperiden lactate*
C		**Alamast®,** *pemirolast*
C		**Ala-Scalp®,** *hydrocortisone*
C		*alatrofloxacin,* **Trovan®IV**
C		*albendazole,* **Albenza®**
C		**Albenza®,** *albendazole*
C		*albuterol,* **Accuneb, Proventil®, Proventil®HFA, Salbutamol®, Ventolin®, Volmax®, Vospire®ER**
C		*alclometasone,* **Aclovate®**

D		**Aldactazide®**, *spironolactone/hydrochlorothiazide*
D		**Aldactone®**, *spironolactone*
B		**Aldara®**, *imiquinod*
C		**Aldoclor®**, *methyldopa/chlorothiazide*
B		**Aldomet®**, *methyldopa*
C		**Aldoril®**, *methyldopa/hydrochlorothiazide*
B		*alefacept*, **Amevive**
B		*alfuzosin*, **UroXatral®**
C		*alendronate*, **Fosamax®**
X		**Alesse®-21, Alesse®-28**, *ethinyl estradiol/levonorgestrel*
B		**Aleve®**, *naproxen*
C		**Alferon N®**, *interferon alfa-n3 (human leukocyte derived)*
B		**Alinia®**, *nitazoxanide*
D		**Alkeran®**, *melphalan*
C		**Allegra®**, *fexofenadine*
C		**Allegra® D 24 Hour**, *fexofenadine/pseudoephedrine*
C		**Allfen®**, *guaifenesin*
C		**Allfen®DM**, *dextromethorphan, guaifenesin*
C		*allopurinol*, **Aloprim®, Lopurin®, Zyloprim®**
B		**Alocril®**, *nedocromil*
B		**Alomide®**, *lodoxamide tromethamine*
C		*almotriptan*, **Axert®**
C		**Aloprim®**, *allopurinol*
X		**Alora®**, *estradiol*
B		**Aloxi®**, *palonosetron*
B		**Alphagan®**, *brimonidine*
C		**Alphatrex®**, *betamethasone dipropionate*
B		*alosetron*, **Lotronex®**
D	IV	*alprazolam*, **Niravam®, Xanax®, Xanax®XR**
X		*alprostadil for injection*, **Edex®**
X		*alprostadil urethral suppository*, **Muse®**
C		**Alrex®**, *loteprednol etabonate*
C/D		**Altace®**, *ramipril*
C		**ALTernaGEL®**, *aluminum hydroxide*
X		**Altoprev®**, *lovastatin*
C		*aluminum hydroxide*, **ALTernaGEL®, Amphojel®**
C		**Alupent®**, *metaproterenol*
C		*amantadine*, **Symmetrel®**
C		**Amaryl®**, *glimepiride*
C	III	**Ambenyl®**, *codeine/bromodiphenhydramine*
B	IV	**Ambien®**, *zolpidem*
B		**Amcill®**, *ampicillin*
C		*amcinonide*, **Cyclocort®**
X		**Amen®**, *medroxyprogesterone*
C		**Amerge®**, *naratriptan*
C		**Americaine®, Americaine®Otic**, *benzocaine*
B		**Amevive®**, *alefacept*

C		*amikacin*, **Amikin®**
C		**Amikin®**, *amikacin*
B		*amiloride*, **Midamor®**
B		*amiloride/hydrochlorothiazide*, **Moduretic®**
D		*aminoglutethimide*, **Cytadren®**
C		*aminophylline*, **Somophyllin®, Somophyllin®DF**
D		*amiodarone*, **Cordarone®**
C		**Amitryl®**, *amitriptyline*
C		*amitriptyline*, **Amitryl®, Endep®**
C		**Amitiza®**, *lubiprostone*
B		*amlexanox*, **Aphthasol®, OraDisc A®**
C		*amlodipine*, **Norvasc®**
X		*amlodipine/atorvastatin*, **Caduet®**
C/D		*amlodipine/benazepril*, **Lotrel®**
D	II	*amobarbital*, **Amytal®**
D	II	*amobarbital/secobarbital*, **Tuinal®**
C		*amoxapine*, **Asendin®**
B		*amoxicillin*, **Amoxil®, Larotid®, Novamoxin®, Polymox®, Sumox®, Trimox®, Utimox®, Wymox®**
B		*amoxicillin/clavulanate potassium (clavulanic acid)*, **Augmentin®, Augmentin®ES-600, Augmentin®XR**
B		**Amoxil®**, *amoxicillin*
C		**Amphojel**, *aluminum hydroxide*
C		*amphotericin b*, **Fungizone®**
B		*ampicillin*, **Amcill®, Omnipen®, Omnipen®-N, Polycillin®, Principen®, Totacillin®, Totacillin®-N**
B		*ampicillin/sulbactam*, **Unasyn®**
C		*amprenavir*, **Agenerase®**
D	II	**Amytal®**, *amobarbital*
B		**Anacin®-3**, *acetaminophen*
C		**Anafranil®**, *clomipramine*
C		*anagrelide*, **Agrylin®**
B		*anakinra*, **Kinert®**
C		**Ana-Kit®**, *epinephrine/chlorpheniramine*
C		**Anaprox®, Anaprox®DS**, *naproxen*
D		*anastrozole*, **Arimidex®**
C		**Anbesol®**, *benzocaine*
B		**Ancef®**, *cefazolin*
X	III	**Androderm®**, *testosterone*
X	III	**AndroGel®**, *testosterone*
X	III	**Android®**, *methyltestosterone*
C	III	**Anexsia®**, *hydrocodone bitartate/acetaminophen*
C		**Animet®**, *carbidopa/levodopa*
B		**Ansaid®**, *flurbiprofen*
B		**Anspor®**, *cephradine*
X		**Antabuse®**, *disulfiram*
C		**Antara®**, *fenofibrate*

C		*anthralin,* **Drithocreme®, Dritho-Scalp®, Micanol®**
C		**Antiminth®,** *pyrantel pamoate*
B		**Antispas®,** *dicyclomine*
B		**Antivert®,** *meclizine*
C		**Anturane®,** *sulfinpyrazone*
C		**Anusol®,** *pramoxine/zinc oxide*
C		**Anusol®HC,** *hydrocortisone*
B		**Anzimet®,** *dolasetron*
B		**Aphthasol®,** *amlexanox*
B		**Apidra®,** *insulin glulisine (rDNA origin)*
C		**Aplisol®,** *purified protein derivative for tuberculin skin test*
C	II	**Apokyn®,** *apomorphine*
C	II	*apomorphine,* **Apokyn®**
C		*apraclonidine,* **Iopidine®**
B		*aprepitant,* **Emend®**
C		**Apresazide®,** *hydralazine/hydrochlorothiazide*
C		**Apresoline®,** *hydralazine*
X		**Apri®,** *ethinyl estradiol/desogestrel*
C		**Aptivus®,** *tipranavir*
C		**AquaMEPHYTON®,** *phytonadione, vitamin k*
A		**Aquasol®A,** *vitamin a palmitate*
A		**Aquasol®E,** *tocopherol, vitamin e*
C		**Aquatab®C,** *guaifenesin/pseudoephedrine/dextromethorphan*
C		**Aquatab®D,** *guaifenesin/pseudoephedrine*
C		**Aralen®,** *chloroquine*
X		**Aranelle®,** *ethinyl estradiol/norethindrone*
C		**Aranesp®,** *darbepoetin alpha*
X		**Arava®,** *leflunomide*
C		*ardeparin,* **Normiflo®**
D		**Arestin®,** *minocycline*
C		**Aricept®,** *donepezil*
D		**Arimidex®,** *anastrozole*
C		*aripiprazole,* **Abilify®**
C		**Aristocort®,** *triamcinolone*
C		**Aristocort®A,** *triamcinolone acetonide*
C		**Aristocort®Forte,** *triamcinolone diacetate*
B		**Arixtra®,** *fondaparinex sodium*
A		**Armour Thyroid®,** *liothyronine/levothyroxine*
D		**Aromasin®,** *exemestane*
D		**Arranon®,** *nelarabine*
C		**Artane®,** *trihexyphenidyl*
X		**Arthrotec®,** *diclofenac/misoprostol*
B		**Asacol®,** *mesalamine*
C		*ascorbic acid,* **Ce-Vi-Sol®**
D		**Ascriptin®,** *aspirin/magnesium hydroxide/aluminum*
C		**Asendin®,** *amoxapine*
C		**Asmanex®,** *mometasone furoate*

D		*aspirin*, *acetylsalicylic acid*, **Bayer®**, **Easprin®**, **Ecotrin®**
D	III	*aspirin/codeine*, **Empirin®with Codeine #2, #3, #4**
D		**Aspirin Regimen Bayer®**, *aspirin*
C		**Astelin®Ready Spray**, *azelastine*
C		*astemizole*, **Hismanal®**
C	II	**Astramorph/PF®**, *morphine sulfate*
C		**Astrohist®, Astrohist®Pediatric Suspension**, *chlorpheniramine/pseudoephedrine*
C		**Atabrine®**, *quinacrine*
C/D		**Atacand®**, *candesartan*
C/D		**Atacand®HCT**, *candesartan/hydrochlorothiazide*
C		**Atapryl®**, *selegiline*
C		**Atarax®**, *hydroxyzine*
B		*atazanavir*, **Reytaz®**
D		*atenolol*, **Tenormin®**
D		*atenolol/chlorthalidone*, **Tenoretic®**
D	IV	**Ativan®**, *lorazepam*
X		*atorvastatin*, **Lipitor®**
C		*atovaquone/proquanil*, **Malarone®, Malarone®Pediatric**
D		**Atripla®**, *efavirenz/emtricitabine/tenofovir*
C		**Atrofen®**, *baclofen*
C		**Atromid-S®**, *clofibrate*
NR		**Atropen®**, *atropine*
NR		*atropine*, **Atropen®**
B		**Atrovent®**, *ipratropium bromide*
NR		*attapulgite*, **Donnagel®**
C		**Atuss®DM**, *dextromethorphan/phenylephrine/chlorpheniramine*
C	III	**Atuss®EX**, *hydrocodone/potassium guaiacosulfonate*
C	III	**Atuss®G**, *hydrocodone/phenylephrine/guaifenesin*
C	III	**Atuss®HD**, *hydrocodone/phenylephrine/chlorpheniramine*
C	III	**Atuss®MS**, *hydrocodone/phenylephrine/chlorpheniramine*
B		**Augmentin®, Augmentin®ES-600, Augmentin®XR**, *amoxicillin/clavulanate potassium(clavulanic acid)*
C		**Auralgan®Otic**, *antipyrine/benzocaine/glycerin*
C		*auranofin*, **Ridaura®**
D		**Aureomycin®**, *chlortetracycline*
C		**Auroto®**, *antipyrine/benzocaine/glycerin*
X		**Avage®**, *tazarotene*
C/D		**Avalide®**, *irbesartan/hydrochlorothiazide*
C		**Avandamet®**, *rosiglitazone/metformin*
C		**Avandaryl®**, *rosiglitazone/glimepiride*
C		**Avandia®**, *rosiglitazone*
C/D		**Avapro®**, *irbesartan*
C		**Avastin®**, *bevacizumab*
A		**Aveeno®**, *oatmeal colloid*
C		**Avelox®**, *moxifloxacin*
D		**Aventyl®**, *nortriptyline*

X		**Aviane®**, *ethinyl estradiol/levonorgestrel*
C	II	**Avinza®**, *morphine sulfate*
C		**Avita®**, *tretinoin*
X		**Avodart®**, *dutasteride*
C		**Avonex®**, *interferon beta-1a*
C		**AVC®**, *sulfanilamide*
C		**Axert®**, *almotriptan*
C		**Axid®, Axid®AR**, *nizatidine*
C	II	**Axocet®**, *butalbital/acetaminophen*
NR		**Axsain®**, *capsaicin*
X		**Aygestin®**, *norethindrone*
B		**Azactam®**, *aztreonam*
D		*azactidine*, **Vidaza®**
D		**Azasan®**, *azathioprine*
B		*azatadine*, **Optimine®**
D		*azathioprine*, **Azasan®, Imuran®**
B		*azelaic acid*, **Azelex®, Finacea®, Finevin®, Optivar®**
C		*azelastine*, **Astelin® Ready Spray**
B		**Azelex®**, *azelaic acid*
C		*azidothymidine, zidovudine, azt*, **Retrovir®**
B		*azithromycin*, **ZithPed®Syr, Zithromax®, Zithromax®Tri-Pak, Zmax®**
C		**Azmacort®**, *triamcinolone acetonide*
B/D		**Azo-Gantanol®, Azo-Gantrisin®**, *sulfisoxazole/phenazopyridine*
D		**Azolid®**, *phenylbutazone*
C		**Azopt®**, *brinzolamide*
C		*azt, azidothymidine, zidovudine*, **Retrovir®**
B		*aztreonam*, **Azactam®**
B/D		**Azulfidine®, Azulfidine®EN**, *sulfasalazine*
C		**Babylax®**, *glycerin suppository*
B		*bacampicillin*, **Spectrobid®**
C		*bacitracin*, **Bacitin®, Bacitracin®Ophthalmic**
C		**Bacitracin®Ophthalmic**, *bacitracin*
C		*baclofen*, **Atrofen®, Kemstro®, Lioresal®, Lioresal®DS**
C		**Bactine®**, *bacitracin*
B		**Bactocill®**, *oxacillin*
C		**Bactrim®, Bactrim®DS**, *sulfamethoxazole/trimethoprim*
B		**Bactroban®**, *mupirocin*
C	IV	**Balacet®**, *propoxyphene napsalate/acetaminophen*
NR		**Balmex®**, *aloe/vitamin e, zinc oxide*
B		*balsalazide*, **Colazal®**
C		**Banflex®**, *orphenadrine*
C		**Baraclude®**, *entecavir*
D		**Bayer®**, *aspirin*
C		**Bayrab®**, *rabies immune globulin (human)*
C		**Baytet®**, *tetanus immune globulin (human)*
C		*becaplermin*, **Regranex®Gel**

C		*beclomethasone dipropionate*, **Beclovent®, Beconase®AQ, Beconex®, Qvar®, Vancenase®, Vancenase®AQ, Vanceril®, Vanceril®DS**
C		**Beclovent®**, *beclomethasone dipropionate*
C		**Beconase®AQ**, *beclomethasone dipropionate*
C		**Beconex®**, *beclomethasone dipropionate*
A		**Beesix®**, *pyridoxine, vitamin b₆*
D	IV	*benactyzine/meprobamate*, **Deprol®**
B		**Benadryl®**, *diphenhydramine*
B		**Benadryl®Allergy/Congestion**, *diphenhydramine/pseudoephedrine*
C/D		*benazepril*, **Lotensin®**
C/D		*benazepril/hydrochlorothiazide*, **Lotensin®HCT**
B		**Benemid®**, *probenecid*
C/D		**Benicar®**, *olmesartan*
C/D		**Benicar®HCT**, *olmesartan medoxomil/hydrochlorothiazide*
C		**Benoquin®**, *monobenzone*
NR		*bentoquantam*, **IvyBlock®**
B		**Bentyl®**, *dicyclomine*
C		**Benylin®DM**, *dextromethorphan*
C		**Benzac®**, *benzoyl peroxide*
C		**BenzaClin®**, *clindamycin/benzoyl peroxide*
C		**Benzagel®**, *benzoyl peroxide*
C		**Benzamycin®**, *benzoyl peroxide/erythromycin*
C		**Benzamycin®Topical Gel**, *erythromycin/benzoyl peroxide*
C		*benzocaine*, **Americaine®, Americaine®Otic® Anbesol®, Hurricaine®, Orajel®, Solarcaine®**
C		*benzonatate*, **Tessalon®Perles**
C		**Benzotic®**, *antipyrine/benzocaine/glycerin*
C		**Benzoyl®**, *benzoyl peroxide*
C		*benzoyl peroxide*, **Benzac®, Benzac®Wash, Benzagel®, Benziq®, Benziq®Gel, Benziq®Wash, Benzoyl®, Brevoxyl®, Clearasil®, Desquam-X®, Fostex®, Persa-Gel®, Topex Oxy®, Triaz®, ZoDerm®**
C		*benzoyl peroxide/erythromycin*, **Benzamycin®**
C		*benzoyl peroxide/hydrocortisone*, **Vanoxide®HC**
X	III	*benzphetamine*, **Didrex®**
C		*benztropine*, **Cogentin®**
C		*bepridil*, **Vascor®**
A		**Berocca®**, *multivitamin*
A		**Berocca®Plus**, *multivitamin with minerals*
B		**Betadine®**, *povidone-iodine*
C		**Betagan®**, *levobunolol*
A/C		**Betalin®12**, *cyanocobalamin, vitamin b₁₂*
A		**Betalins**, *thiamine*
C		*betamethasone*, **Celestone®**
C		*betamethasone dipropionate*, **Alphatrex®, Diprolene®, Diprolene® AF, Diprosone®, Maxivate®**
C		*betamethasone sodium phosphate*, **Celestone® Phosphate**
C		*betamethasone sodium phosphate/betamethasone acetate*, **Celestone®**

		Soluspan
C		*betamethasone valerate*, **Betatrex®**, **Beta-Val®**, **Luxiq®**, **Valisone®**
C		**Betapace®**, **Betapace®-AF**, *sotalol*
B		**Betapen®-VK**, *penicillin v potassium*
C		**Betaseron®**, *interferon beta-1b*
C		**Betatrex®**, *betamethasone valerate*
C		**Beta-Val®**, *betamethasone valerate*
C		*betaxolol*, **Betoptic®**, **Betoptic®S**, **Kerlone®**
C		*bethanechol*, **Urecholine®**
C		**Betimol®**, *timolol*
C		**Betoptic®**, **Betoptic®S**, *betaxolol*
C		*bevacizumab*, **Avastin®**
C/D		**Bextra®**, *valdecoxib*
C		**Biaxin®**, *clarithromycin*
X		*bicalutamide*, **Casodex®**
B		**Bicillin®**, **Bicillin®L-A**, *penicillin g benzathine*
B		**Bicillin®C-R**, *penicillin g benzathine/penicillin g procaine*
C		**BiDil®**, *hydralazine/isosorbide dinitrate*
C		*bimatoprost*, **Lumigan®**
NR		**Bion®Tears**, *hydroxypropyl methylcellulose*
C		**Biohist®-LA**, *carbinoxamine/pseudoephedrine*
C		*biperiden hydrochloride, biperiden lactate*, **Akineton®**
B		*bisacodyl*, **Dulcolax®**, **Gentlax®**
C/D		*bismuth subsalicylate*, **Pepto-Bismol®**
C		*bisoprolol*, **Zebeta®**
C		*bisoprolol/hydrochlorothiazide*, **Ziac®**
C		*bitolterol*, **Tornalate®**
C		**Black Draught®**, *senna*
D		**Blenoxane®**, *bleomycin*
D		*bleomycin*, **Blenoxane®**
C		**Bleph-10®**, *sulfacetamide*
C		**Blephamide®Liquifilm**, *sulfacetamide/prednisolone*
C		**Blocadren®**, *timolol*
B		**Bonine®**, *meclizine*
C	III	**Bontril®**, *phendimetrazine*
D		*bortezomib*, **Velcade®**
NR		**Botox®**, *botulinum toxin type A*
NR		*botulinum toxin type A*, **Botox®**
B		**Brethaire®**, *terbutaline*
B		**Brethine®**, *terbutaline*
C		**Brevibloc®**, *esmolol*
X		**Brevicon®-21**, **Brevicon®-28**, *ethinyl estradiol/norethindrone*
C		**Brevoxyl®**, *benzoyl peroxide*
B		**Bricanyl®**, *terbutaline*
B		*brimonidine*, **Alphagan®**
C		*brinzolamide*, **Azopt®**
C		*brofenac*, **Xibrom®**

C		**Bromfed®, Bromfed®Cap, Bromfed®PD, Bromfed®Syr, Bromfed®Tab, Respahist®**, *brompheniramine/ pseudoephedrine*
C		*bromfenac*, **Xibrom®**
B		*bromocriptine*, **Parlodel®**
C		*brompheniramine*, **Dimetapp®Allergy, Lodrane®24**
C		**Broncholate®**, *pseudoephedrine/guaifenesin*
C		**Bronkosol®**, *isoetharine*
C	III	**Brontex®, Brontex®Liquid**, *guaifenesin/codeine*
B		*budesonide*, **Entocort®EC, Pulmicort®Respules, Pulmicort® Turbuhaler, Rhinocort, Rhinocort® Aqua**
C/D		**Bufferin®**, *aspirin/magnesium carbonate/magnesium oxide*
C		*bumetanide*, **Bumex®**
C		**Bumex®**, *bumetanide*
C	II	**Bupap®**, *butalbital/acetaminophen*
C		*bupivacaine*, **Sensorcaine®**
C	II	**Buprenex®**, *buprenorphine*
C	III	*buprenorphine*, **Buprenex®, Subutex®**
C	III	*buprenorphine/naloxone*, **Suboxone®**
B		*bupropion*, **Wellbutrin®, Wellbutrin®SR, Wellbutrin®XL, Zyban®**
B		**BuSpar®**, *buspirone*
B		*buspirone*, **BuSpar®**
B	II	*butabarbital*, **Butalan®, Butisol®Na**
B	II	**Butalan®**, *butabarbital*
C	II	*butalbital/acetaminophen*, **Axocet®, Bupap®, Cephadyn®, Dolgic®, Phrenilin®, Phrenilin®Forte, Promacet®, Prominol®**
C	II	*butalbital/acetaminophen/caffeine*, **Esgic®, Esgic®Plus, Fioricet®, Zebutal®**
C	III	*butalbital/acetaminophen/caffeine/codeine*, **Fioricet®with Codeine**
C	II	*butalbital/aspirin/caffeine*, **Fiorinal®**
C	III	*butalbital/aspirin/caffeine/codeine*, **Fiorinal®with Codeine**
D		**Butazolidin®**, *phenylbutazone*
B		*butenafine*, **Mentax®**
D	II	**Butisol®Na**, *butabarbital*
C		*butoconazole*, **Femstat®-3, Gynazole®-1**
C	IV	*butorphanol*, **Stadol®**
C		*bupivacaine*, **Marcaine®**
C		**Byetta®**, *exenatide*
B		*cabergoline*, **Dostinex®**
X		**Cafergot®**, *ergotamine/caffeine*
X		**Caduet®**, *amlodipine/atorvastatin*
C		**Calan®, Calan®SR**, *verapamil*
C		**Calcibind®**, *cellulose sodium phosphate*
C		**Calciferol®**, *ergocalciferol, vitamin d*
NR		**Calcilac®**, *calcium carbonate*
C		**Calcimar®**, *calcitonin-salmon*
C		*calcipotriene*, **Dovonex®**
C		*calcipotriene/betamethsone dipropionate*, **Taclonex®**

C	*calcitonin-salmon*, **Calcimar®, Fortical®, Miacalcin®Injectable, Miacalcin® Nasal Spray**
C	*calcitriol*, **Rocaltrol®**
C	*calcium acetate*, **Phos-Ex®, PhosLo®**
NR	*calcium carbonate*, **Calcilac®, Os-Cal®, Oystercal®, Rolaids®Extra Strength, Titralac®, Tums®, Tums®E-X**
B	*calcium carbonate/magnesium hydroxide*, **Rolaids® Sodium Free**
C	*calcium citrate*, **Citrucel®**
C	**Calcium Folinate®**, *leucovorin calcium*
C	*calcium polycarbophil*, **Fibercon®**
X	**Camila®**, *norethindrone*
B/D III	*camphorated tincture of opium*, **Paregoric®**
C	**Campral®**, *acamprosate*
B	**Canasa®**, *mesalamine*
C/D	*candesartan*, **Atacand®**
C/D	*candesartan/hydrochlorothiazide*, **Atacand®HCT**
NR	*cantharidin*, **Cantherone®, Verrusol®**
NR	**Cantherone®**, *cantharidin*
B	**Cantil®**, *mepenzolate*
C	**Capastat®**, *capreomycin*
D	*capecitabine*, **Xeloda®**
C	**Capex®Shampoo**, *fluocinolone acetonide*
C	**Capitrol®**, *chloroxine*
C/D	**Capoten®**, *captopril*
C/D	**Capozide®**, *captopril/hydrochlorothiazide*
C	*capreomycin*, **Capastat®**
NR	*capsaicin*, **Axsain®, Capzasin®-P, Dolorac®, DoubleCap®, Zostrix®, Zostrix®HP**
C/D	*captopril*, **Capoten®**
C/D	*captopril/hydrochlorothiazide*, **Capozid®e**
X	**Carac®**, *fluorouracil*
B	**Carafate®**, *sucralfate*
C	*carbachol*, **Isopto Carbachol®**
D	*carbamazepine*, **Carbatrol®, Equetro®, Equitrol®, Tegretol®, Tegretol®XR**
A	*carbamide peroxide*, **Debrox®, Gly-Oxide®**
D	**Carbatrol®**, *carbamazepine*
B	*carbenicillin*, **Geocillin®, Geopen®**
C	**Carbetaplex®Liquid**, *phenylephrine, carbetapentane, guaifenesin*
C	**Carbex®**, *selegiline*
C	*carbidopa/levodopa*, **Animet®, Parcopa®, Sinemet®, Sinemet®CR**
C	*carbidopa/levodopa/entacapone*, **Stalevo®**
C	*carbinoxamine*, **Biohist®-LA, Carbiset®, Carbodec®, Carbodec® Syr, Carbodec®TR, Cardec®-S Syr, Histex®Pd, Palgic®, Rondec® Filmtab**
C	**Carbiset®**, *carbinoxamine/pseudoephedrine*
C	**Carbocaine®**, *mepivacaine*

C		**Carbodec®, Carbodec®Syr, Carbodec®-S Syr,** *carbinoxamine/ pseudoephedrine*
C		**Cardec®,** *carbinoxamine/pseudoephedrine*
C		**Cardene®, Cardene®SR,** *nicardipine*
C		**Cardizem®, Cardizem®CD, Cardizem®LA, Cardizem®SR,** *diltiazem*
C		**Cardura®, Cardura®XL,** *doxazosin*
C		*carisoprodol,* **Soma®**
C		*carisoprodol/aspirin,* **Soma®Compound**
C	III	*carisoprodol/aspirin/codeine,* **Soma®Compound with Codeine**
C		**Carmol®40,** *urea cream*
C		*carteolol,* **Cartrol®, Ocupress®**
C		**Cartia®XT,** *diltiazem*
C		**Cartrol®,** *carteolol*
C		*carvedilol,* **Coreg®**
C		**Cascara Sagrada®,** *casanthranol, cascara sagrada*
X		**Casodex®,** *bicalutamide*
X		*castor oil,* **Neoloid®**
B		**Cataflam®,** *diclofenac potassium*
C		**Catapres®, Catapres®-TTS,** *clonidine*
B		**Ceclor®, Ceclor®CD,** *cefaclor*
B		**Cedax®,** *ceftibuten*
B		*cefaclor,* **Ceclor®, Ceclor®CD**
B		*cefadroxil,* **Duricef®, Ultracef®**
B		**Cefadyl®,** *cephapirin*
B		*cefamandole,* **Mandol®**
B		*cefazolin,* **Ancef®, Kefzol®, Zolicef®**
B		*cefdinir,* **Omnicef®**
C		*cefditoren pivoxil,* **Spectracef®**
B		*cefepime,* **Maxipime®**
B		*cefixime,* **Suprax®for Oral Suspension**
B		**Cefizox®,** *ceftizoxime*
B		**Cefobid®,** *cefoperazone*
A		**Cefol®,** *multivitamin*
B		*cefonicid,* **Monocid®**
B		*cefoperazone,* **Cefobid®**
B		*ceforanide,* **Precef®**
B		**Cefotan®,** *cefotetan*
B		*cefotaxime,* **Claforan®**
B		*cefotetan,* **Cefotan®**
B		*cefoxitin,* **Mefoxinv**
B		*cefpodoxime proxetil,* **Vantin®**
B		*cefprozil,* **Cefzil®**
B		*ceftazidime,* **Ceptaz®, Fortaz®, Tazicef®, Tazidime®**
B		*ceftibuten,* **Cedax®**
B		**Ceftin®,** *cefuroxime axetil*
B		*ceftizoxime,* **Cefizox®**

B		*ceftriaxone*, **Rocephin**®
B		*cefuroxime axetil*, **Ceftin**®
B		*cefuroxime*, **Kefurox**®
B		**Cefzil**®, *cefprozil*
C		**Celebrex**®, *celecoxib*
C		*celecoxib*, **Celebrex**®
C		**Celestone**®, *betamethasone acetate*
C		**Celestone**® **Phosphate**, *betamethasone sodium phosphate*
C		**Celestone**® **Soluspan**, *betamethasone sodium phosphate/ betamethasone acetate*
C		**Celexa**®, *citalopram*
C		*cellulose sodium phosphate*, **Calcibind**®
C		**Celontin**®**Kapseals**, *methsuximide*
X		**Cenestin**®, *conjugated estrogens*
B		**Centany**®, *mupirocin*
D	IV	**Centrax**®, *prazepam*
C	II	**Cephadyn**®, *butalbital/acetaminophen*
B		*cephalexin*, **Keflet**®, **Keflex**®, **Keftab**®, **Keftab**®**K Pak**, **Novolexin**®
B		*cephalothin*, **Keflin**®
B		*cephapirin*, **Cefadyl**®
B		*cephradine*, **Anspor**®, **Velosef**®
C		**Cephulac**®, *lactulose*
B		**Ceptaz**®, *ceftazidime*
NR		**CeraLyte**®, *oral rehydration formula*
A		**Cerumenex**®, *triethanolamine*
C		**Cervita**®, *diphtheria/tetanus toxoid/acellular pertussis vaccine*
C		**Cesamet**®, *nabilone*
C		**Cetacort**®, *hydrocortisone*
C		**Cetamide**®, *sulfacetamide*
B		*cetirizine*, **Zyrtec**®, **Zyrtec**®**Chewable Tablets**
C		*cetirizine/pseudoephedrine*, **Zyrtec**®**-D 12 Hour**
C		*cetuximab*, **Erbitux**®
C		*cevimeline*, **Evoxac**®
C		**Ce-Vi-Sol**®, *ascorbic acid*
C		**Chantix**®, *varenicline*
C		**Chemet**®, *succimer*
C		**Chibroxin**®, *norfloxacin*
C		**Children's Motrin**®**Cold**, *pseudoephedrine/ibuprofen*
B		**Children's NasalCrom**®, *cromolyn sodium*
C		*chloral hydrate*, **Noctec**®
D		*chlorambucil*, **Leukeran**®
C		*chloramphenicol*, **Chloromycetin**®, **Chloroptic**®, **Ophthochlor**®
D	IV	*chlordiazepoxide*, **Libritabs**®, **Librium**®
D	IV	*chlordiazepoxide/amitriptyline*, **Limbitrol**®
D	IV	*chlordiazepoxide/clidinium*, **Librax**®
B		*chlorhexidine gluconate*, **Hibiclens**®, **Hibistat**®, **Peridex**®, **PerioGard**®

C	**Chloromycetin®**, *chloramphenicol*
C	*chloroprocaine*, **Nesacaine®, Nesacaine®-CE**
C	**Chloroptic®**, *chloramphenicol*
C	*chloroquine*, **Aralen®**
C	*chlorothiazide*, **Diuril®**
X	*chlorotrianisene*, **Tace®**
C	*chloroxine*, **Capitrol®**
C	*chloroxylenol/premoxine*, **PramOtic®**
C	*chloroxylenol/pramoxine/hydrocortisone*, **Zoto®-AC**
B	*chlorpheniramine*, **Chlor-Trimeton®, Contac®**
C	*chlorpromazine*, **Thorazine®**
C	*chlorpropamide*, **Diabinese®**
C	*chlorprothixene*, **Taractan®**
D	*chlortetracycline*, **Aureomycin®**
B	*chlorthalidone*, **Hygroton®, Hylidon®, Novothalidone®, Thalitone®**
D	*chlorthalidone/reserpine*, **Regroton®**
B	**Chlor-Trimeton®**, *chlorpheniramine*
C	*chlorzoxazone*, **Paraflex®, Parafon Forte®**
C	**Choledyl®SA**, *oxtriphylline*
C	*cholestyramine*, **Questran®, Questran®Light**
C	*choline magnesium trisalicylate*, **Trilisate®**
C	**Choloxin®**, *dextrothyroxine*
C	**Cholybar®**, *cholestyramine resin*
C	*chorionic gonadotropin*, **Pregnyl®, Profasi®HP**
A	**Chromagen®, Chromagen®FA, Chromagen®Forte**, *iron supplement*
A	**Chromagen®OB**, *prenatal vitamin*
C	**Chronulac®**, *lactulose*
B	**Cialis®**, *tadalafil*
B	*ciclopirox*, **Loprox®**
NR	*ciclopirox topical solution*, **Penlac®Nail Laquer**
B	**Cidecin®**, *daptomycin*
C	*cidofovir*, **Vistide®**
C	*cilostazol*, **Pletal®**
C	**Ciloxan®**, *ciprofloxacin ophthalmic*
B	*cimetidine*, **Tagamet®, Tagamet®HB**
C	*cinacalcet*, **Sensipar®**
B	**Cinobac®**, *cinoxacin*
B	*cinoxacin*, **Cinobac®**
C	**Cipro®**, *ciprofloxacin*
C	**Ciprodex®**, *ciprofloxacin/dexamethasone*
C	*ciprofloxacin*, **Cipro®**
C	*ciprofloxacin/dexamethasone*, **Ciprodex®**
C	*ciprofloxacin/hydrocortisone*, **Cipro®HC Otic**
C	*ciprofloxacin ophthalmic*, **Ciloxan®**
C	**Cipro®HC Otic**, *ciprofloxacin/hydrocortisone*
D	*cisplatin*, **Platinol®**

C		*citalopram*, **Celexa**®
A		**Citracal**®**Prenatal Rx, Citracal**® **Prenatal+DHA**, *prenatal vitamin*
B		**Citrate of Magnesia**®, *magnesium citrate*
B		**Citroma**®, *magnesium citrate*
C		**Citrucel**®, *calcium citrate*
B		**Claforan**®, *cefotaxime*
C		**Clarinex**®**, Clarinex**®**RediTab, Clarinex**®**Syrup**, *desloratadine*
C		*clarithromycin*, **Biaxin**®
B		**Claritin**®, *loratadine*
B		**Claritin**®**-D 12 Hour, Claritin**®**-D 24 Hour**, *loratadine/ pseudoephedrine*
B		**Clavulin**®, *amoxicillin/clavulanate potassium (clavulanic acid)*
C		**Clearasil**®, *benzoyl peroxide*
B		*clemastine*, **Tavist**®**, Tavist**®**-1**
C		*clemastine/pseudoephedrine*, **Tavist**®**D**
C		**Clenia**®, *sulfacetamide/sulfur*
B		**Cleocin**®**, Cleocin**®**T, Cleocin**®**Vaginal Cream, Cleocin**®**Vaginal Ovules**, *clindamycin*
X		**Climara**®, *estradiol transdermal system*
X		**Climara**®**Pro**, *estradiol/levonorgestrel*
B		*clindamycin*, **Clindets**®**, Cleocin**®**, Cleocin**®**T, Cleocin**®**Vaginal Cream, Cleocin**®**Vaginal Ovules, Evoclin**®**Foam**
C		*clindamycin/benzoyl peroxide*, **BenzaClin**®**, Duac**®
B		**Clindets**®, *clindamycin*
B/D		**Clinoril**®, *sulindac*
C		*clobetasol propionate*, **Clobex**®**Shampoo, Clobex**®**Spray, Cormax**®**, Olux**®**, Temovate**®
C		**Clobex**®**Shampoo, Clobex**®**Spray**, *clobetasol propionate*
C		*clofazimine*, **Lamprene**®
C		*clofibrate*, **Atromid**®**-S**
X		**Clomid**®, *clomiphene*
X		*clomiphene*, **Clomid**®**, Serophene**®
C		*clomipramine*, **Anafranil**®
C	IV	*clonazepam*, **Klonopin**®
C		*clonidine*, **Catapres**®**, Catapres**®**-TTS**
C		*clonidine/chlorthalidone*, **Clorpres**®
C		*clonidine/chlorthalidone/polysorbate/acetic acid*, **Combipres**®
B		*clopidogrel*, **Plavix**®
C	IV	*clorazepate*, **Tranxene**®**, Tranxene**®**-SD, Tranxene**®**-SD Half Strength**
C		**Clorpres**®, *clonidine/chlorthalidone*
B		*clotrimazole*, **Fungoid**®**, Gyne-Lotrimin**®**, Gyne-Lotrimin**®**-3, Lotrimin**®**, Mycelex**®**G, Mycelex**®**G Vaginal, Mycelex**®**Troche**
C		*clotrimazole/betamethasone dipropionate*, **Lotrisone**®
B		*cloxacillin*, **Tegopen**®
B		**Cloxapen**®, *cloxapen*
B		*cloxapen*, **Cloxapen**®

B		*clozapine*, **Clozaril®**, **Fazaclo®**
B		**Clozaril®**, *clozapine*
C		*coal tar*, **DHS®Zinc Shampoo**, **Fototar®**, **Zetar®**, **Zetar®Shampoo**
A/C		**Cobex®**, *cyanocobalamin*, *vitamin b₁₂*
C	III	**Codeine®**, *codeine*
C	III	*codeine*, **Codeine®**
C	III	**Codeprex®**, *codeine polistirex/chlorpheneramine*
C	III	**Codiclear®DH**, *guaifenesin/hydrocodone*
C	III	**Codimal®DH**, *hydrocodone/phenylephrine/pyrilamine*
C		**Codimal®DM**, *dextromethorphan/phenylephrine/pyrilamine*
C		**Cogentin®**, *benztropine*
C		**Cognex®**, *tacrine*
C		**Colace®**, **Colace®Enema**, *docusate*
B		**Colazal®**, *balsalazide*
C		**ColBENEMID®**, *colchicine/probenecid*
C		**Colchicine®**, *colchicine*
C		*colchicine*, **Colchicine®**, **Novocolchine®**
C		*colchicine/probenecid*, **ColBENEMID®**
B		*colesevelam*, **Welchol®**
C		**Colestid®**, *colestipol*
C		*colestipol*, **Colestid®**, **Lestid®**
C		*colistimethate*, **Coly-Mycin®M**
C	III	**Colrex®Compound**, *codeine/chlorpheniramine/phenylephrine/ acetaminophen*
C		**Coly-Mycin®M**, *colistimethate*
C		**Coly-Mycin®S Otic**, *colistin/neomycin/hydrocortisone/thonzonium*
X		**CombiPatch®**, *estradiol/norethindrone transdermal system*
C		**Combipres®**, *clonidine/chlorthalidone/polysorbate/acetic acid/ sodium*
C		**Combivent®**, *ipratropium/albuterol*
C		**Combivir®**, *lamivudine/zidovudine*
C	II	**Combunox®**, *oxycodone/ibuprofen*
C		**Compazine®**, *prochlorperazine*
C		**Comtan®**, *entocapone*
C		**Comvax®**, *haemophilus b conjugate/hepatitis b (recombinant) vaccine*
C		**Concerta®**, *methyphenidate*
C		**Condylox®**, *podofilox*
X		*conjugated estrogens*, **Cenestin®**, **Enjuvia®**, **Premarin®**, **Premarin® Vaginal Cream®**
X		*conjugated estrogens/medroxyprogesterone*, **Premphase®**, **Prempro®**
B		**Contac®**, *chlorpheniramine*
X		**Copegus®**, *ribavirin*
D		**Cordarone®**, *amiodarone*
C		**Cordran®**, **Cordran®SP**, *flurandrenolide*
C		**Coreg®**, *carvedilol*
C		**Corgard®**, *nadolol*
C		**Cormax®**, *clobetasol propionate*

C	**Correctol®**, *phenolphalein*	
C	**Cortaid®**, *hydrocortisone*	
C	**Cortane®-B Otic**, *hydrocortisone/chloroxylenol/pramoxine*	
C	**Cortef®**, *hydrocortisone*	
C	**Cortenema®**, *hydrocortisone*	
C	**Cortifoam®**, *hydrocortisone*	
C	*cortisone*, **Cortistan®**, **Cortone®Acetate**	
C	**Cortisporin®Cream, Cortisporin®Ophthalmic, Cortisporin®Otic**, *polymixin b/neomycin/hydrocortisone*	
C	**Cortisporin®Ointment**, *polymixin b/bacitracin zinc/neomycin/ hydrocortisone*	
C	**Cortisporin®TC**, *colistin/neomycin/hydrocortisone/thonzonium*	
D	**Cortistan®**, *cortisone*	
D	**Cortone®Acetate**, *cortisone*	
C	**Corzide®**, *nadolol/bendroflumethiazide*	
C	**Cosmegen®**, *dactinomycin*	
C	**Cosopt®**, *dorzolamide/timolol*	
C	**Cotazym®, Cotazym® S**, *pancrelipase*	
D	**Coumadin®**, *warfarin*	
C	**Covera®-HS**, *verapamil*	
C/D	**Cozaar®**, *losartan*	
C	**Crantex®LA Tablets, Crantex®Liquid**, *phenylephrine/guafenesin*	
C	**Creon®**, *pancrelipase*	
X	**Crestor®**, *rosuvastatin*	
X	**Crinone®**, *progesterone*	
C	**Crixivan®**, *indinavir*	
B	**Crolom®**, *cromolyn sodium*	
B	*cromolyn sodium*, **Children's NasalCrom®, Crolom®, Intal®, NasalCrom®, Opticrom®**	
C	*crotamiton*, **Eurax®**	
X	**Cryselle®**, *ethinyl estradiol/norgestrel*	
A/C	**Crystamine®**, *cyanocobalamin, vitamin b₁₂*	
A/C	**Crysti®12**, *cyanocobalamin, vitamin b₁₂*	
B	**Crysticillin®AS**, *penicillin g procaine*	
C	**Crystodigin®**, *digitoxin*	
B	**Cubicin®**, *daptomycin*	
D	**Cuprimine®**, *penicillamine*	
X	**Curretab®**, *medroxyprogesterone*	
C	**Cutivate®**, *fluticasone propionate*	
A/C	**Cyanabin®**, *cyanocobalamin, vitamin b₁₂*	
A/C	*cyanocobalamin, vitamin b₁₂*, **Betalin®12, Cobex®, Crystamin®e, Crysti®12, Cyanabin®, Nascobal®, Redisol®, Rubesol®, Rubramin®PC**	
NR	*cyclacillin*, **Cyclapen®**	
NR	*cyclandelate*, **Cyclospasmol®**	
NR	**Cyclapen®**, *cyclacillin*	
X	**Cyclessa®**, *ethinyl estradiol/desogestrel*	

B		*cyclizine lactate*, **Marzine**®, **Merezine**®**Lactate**
B		*cyclobenzaprine*, **Flexeril**®
C		**Cyclocort**®, *amcinonide*
D		*cyclophosphamide*, **Cytoxan**®
C		*cycloserine*, **Seromycin**®
NR		**Cyclospasmol**®, *cyclandelate*
C		*cyclosporine*, **Neoral**®, **Restasis**®
X		**Cycrin**®, *medroxyprogesterone*
B		**Cylert**®, *pemoline*
C		**Cymbalta**®, *duloxetine*
B		*cyproheptadine*, **Periactin**®
C		**Cystospaz**®, *hyoscyamine*
D		**Cytadren**®, *aminoglutethimide*
A		**Cytomel**®, *liothyronine*
X		**Cytotec**®, *misoprostol*
D		**Cytoxan**®, *cyclophosphamide*
C		**D.A.**®**II, D.A.**®**Chewables**, *chlorpheniramine, phenylephrine/ methscopolomine*
C		*dactinomycin*, **Cosmegen**®
C		**Dalalone**®, **Dalalone**®**DP, Dalalone**®**LA**, *dexamethasone*
B		**Dalcaine**®, *lidocaine*
C		**Dalgan**®, *dezocine*
X	IV	**Dalmane**®, *flurazepam*
C		*dalteparin*, **Fragmin**®
C		*danaparoid*, **Orgaran**®
X		*danazol*, **Danocrine**®
X		**Danocrine**®, *danazol*
C		**Dantrium**®, *dantrolene*
C		*dantrolene*, **Dantrium**®
B		*daptomycin*, **Cubicin**®
C		**Daranide**®, *dichlorphenamide*
C		**Daraprim**, *pyrimethamine*
C		*darbepoetin alpha*, **Aranesp**®
C		*darifenacin*, **Enablex**®
B		*darunavir*, **Prezista**®
C		**Darvocet**®**A500, Darvocet**®**-N50, Darvocet**®**-N100**, *propoxyphene/ acetaminophen*
D	IV	**Darvon**®**Compound-65**, *propoxyphene/aspirin/caffeine*
C	II	**Daytrana**®, *methylphenidate*
B		**Datril**®, *acetaminophen*
C		**Daypro**®, *oxaprozin*
B		**DDAVP**®**Nasal Spray**, *desmopressin*
A		**Debrox**®, *carbamide peroxide*
C		**Decaderm**, *dexamethasone*
C		**Decadron**®, **Decadron**®**LA**, *dexamethasone*
C		**Decadron**®**Phosphate Injectable, Decadron**®**Phosphate Ophthalmic Solution**, *dexamethasone sodium phosphate*

C		**Decaject®, Decaject®-LA**, *dexamethasone*
D		**Declomycin®**, *demeclocycline*
C		**Deconamine®, Deconamine®SR, Deconamine®Syr**, *chlorpheniramine/pseudoephedrine*
C		**Deconsal®II**, *guaifenesin/pseudoephedrine*
C		**Defen®-LA**, *guaifenesin, pseudoephedrine*
B		*deferasirox*, **Exjade®**
X	III	**Delatestryl®**, *testosterone enthanate*
C		*delavirdine mesylate*, **Rescriptor®**
X		**Delestrogen®**, *estradiol valerate*
C		**Delsym®**, *dextromethorphan*
C		**Delta Cortef®**, *prednisolone*
C		**Deltasone®**, *prednisone*
B		**Demadex®**, *torsemide*
X		*demecarium ophthalmic solution*, **Humorsol®**
D		*demeclocycline*, **Declomycin®**
B/D	II	**Demerol®**, *meperidine*
X		**Demulen®1/35-21, Demulen®1/50-21, Demulen®1/35-28, Demulen®1/50-28**, *ethinyl estradiol/ethynodiol diacetate*
B		**Denavir®**, *penciclovir*
D		**Depakene®**, *valproic acid*
D		**Depakote®**, *divalproex*
D		**Depen®**, *penicillamine*
X		**Depo-Estradiol Cypionate®**, *estradiol*
X		**Depogen®**, *estradiol*
C		**Depo-Medrol®**, *methylprednisolone*
C		**Deponit®**, *nitroglycerin*
X		**Depo-Provera®, Depo-SubQ®**, *medroxyprogesterone*
X	III	**Depo-Testosterone®**, *testosterone*
D	IV	**Deprol®**, *benactyzine/meprobamate*
C		**Derma-Smoothe®/FS**, *fluocinolone acetonide*
C		**Dermatop®**, *prednicarbate*
X		*des, diethylstilbestrol*, **Stilbestrol®**
C		*desloratadine*, **Clarinex®, Clarinex®RediTab, Clarinex®Syrup**
NR		**Desenex®**, *undecylenic acid*
C		*desipramine*, **Norpramin®, Pertofrane®**
B		*desmopressin*, **DDAVP®Nasal Spray, DDAVP®Rhinal Tube, Stimate®**
X		**Desogen®-28**, *ethinyl estradiol/desogestrel diacetate*
C		*desonide*, **DesOwen®, Tridesilon®**
C		**DesOwen®**, *desonide*
C		*desoximetasone*, **Topicort®**
C	II	**Desoxyn®**, *methamphetamine*
C		**Desquam®-X**, *benzoyl peroxide*
C		**Desyrel®**, *trazodone*
C		**Detrol®, Detrol®LA**, *tolterodine*
C		**Dexacort®Turbinaire**, *dexamethasone sodium phosphate*

C		**Dexameth®**, *dexamethasone*
C		*dexamethasone*, **Dalalone®, Dalalone®DP, Dalalone®LA, Decaderm®, Decadron®, Decadron®LA, Decaject®, Decaject®-LA, Dexameth®, Hexadrol®, Maxidex®, Turbinaire®**
C		*dexamethasone sodium phosphate*, **Decadron®Phosphate Injectable, Decadron®Phosphate Ophthalmic Solution, Dexacort® Turbinaire**
B		**Dexchlor®**, *dexchlorpheniramine*
B		*dexchlorpheniramine*, **Dexchlor®, Polaramine®**
C	II	**Dexedrine®**, *dextroamphetamine sulfate*
C	II	*dexmethylphenidate*, **Focalin®, Focalin®XR**
C	II	*dextroamphetamine saccharate/dextroamphetamine sulfate/ amphetamine aspartate/amphetamine sulfate* **Adderall®, Adderall®XR**
C	II	*dextroamphetamine sulfate*, **Dexedrine®, Dextrostat®**
C		*dextromethasone phosphate*, **Maxidex®Ophthalmic**
C		*dextromethorphan*, **Benylin®DM**
C		**Dextrostat®**, *dextroamphetamine sulfate*
C		*dextrothyroxine*, **Choloxin®**
C		*dezocine*, **Dalgan®**
C	III	**DHC®Plus**, *dihydrocodeine/acetaminophen/caffeine*
X		**DHE®45**, *dihydroergotamine*
C		**DHS®Zinc Shampoo**, *coal tar*
B		**DiaBeta®**, *glyburide*
C		**Diabinese®**, *chlorpropamide*
C		**Dialose®**, *docusate potassium*
C		**Diamox®, Diamox®Sequels**, *acetazolamide*
NR		**Dianabol®**, *methandrostenolone*
B		**Diapid®**, *lypressin*
D	IV	**Diastat®**, *diazepam*
D	IV	*diazepam*, **Diastat®, Valium®**
C		*diazoxide*, **Proglycem®**
C		**Dibenzyline®**, *phenoxybenzamine*
C		*dibucaine*, **Nupercainal®**
C		*dichlorphenamide*, **Daranide®**
B		*diclofenac*, **Solaraze®, Voltaren®, Voltaren®Ophthalmic Solution, Voltaren®-XR**
X		*diclofenac/misoprostol*, **Arthrotec®**
B		*diclofenac potassium*, **Cataflam®**
B		*dicloxacillin*, **Dycill®, Dynapen®, Pathocil®**
B		*dicyclomine*, **Antispas®, Benty®l**
B		*didanosine*, **Videx®, Videx®EC**
X	III	**Didrex®**, *benzphetamine*
C		**Didronel®**, *etidronate disodium*
X		*dienestrol*, **Ortho®Dienestrol**
B	IV	*diethylpropion*, **Tenuate®, Tepanil®**
X		*diethylstilbestrol*, **Stilbestrol®, Stilphostrol®**
C		*difenoxin/atropine*, **Motofen®**

C		**Differin®**, *adapalene*
C		*diflorasone*, **Florone®, Florone®E, Maxiflor, Psorcon®**
C		**Diflucan®**, *fluconazole*
C		*diflunisal*, **Dolobid®**
C		*digitoxin*, **Crystodigin®**
C		*digoxin*, **Lanoxicaps®, Lanoxin®**
D	III	*dihydrocodeine*, **Synalgos®-DC**
X		*dihydroergotamine*, **DHE®45, Migranal®**
NR		*dihydroxyaluminum sodium carbonate*, **Rolaids®**
C		*diiodohydroxyquin, iodoquinol*, **Yodoxin®**
C		**Dilacor®**, *diltiazem*
D		**Dilantin®**, *phenytoin*
C		**Dilatrate®-SR**, *isosorbide dinitrate*
C	II	**Dilaudid®, Dilaudid®HP**, *hydromorphone*
C	II	**Dilaudid®Cough Syr**, *guaifenesin/hydromorphone*
C		**Dilor®**, *dyphylline*
C		**Dilor®-G**, *guaifenesin/dyphylline*
C		*diltiazem*, **Cardizem®, Cardizem®CD, Cardizem®LA, Cardizem® SR, Cartia®XT, Dilacor®, Tiazac®**
C		*diltiazem maleate*, **Tiamate®**
B		*dimenhydrinate*, **Dramamine®**
C	III	**Dimetane®-DC**, *codeine/brompheniramine*
C		**Dimetane®Decongestant**, *phenylephrine/brompheniramine*
C		**Dimetane®-DM**, *dextromethorphan/brompheniramine/*
C		**Dimetane®-DX**, *dextromethorphan/brompheniramine/ pseudoephedrine*
C		**Dimetapp®, Dimetapp®Syr, Dimetapp®Extentabs, Dimetapp® Quick Dissolve**, *brompheniramine/phenylephrine*
C		**Dimetapp®Allergy**, *brompheniramine*
C		**Diocto-K®**, *docusate*
C/D		**Diovan®**, *valsartan*
C/D		**Diovan®HCT**, *valsartan/hydrochlorothiazide*
C		**Dipentum®**, *olsalazine*
B		*diphenhydramine*, **Benadryl®, Nytol®Quipcaps, Nytol®Quiptabs, Sominex®, Sominex® Max Str, Unisom®Sleepgels, Unisom® Sleeptabs**
C		*diphenidol*, **Vontrol®**
C	V	*diphenoxylate/atropine*, **Lomotil®**
C		*diphtheria/tetanus toxoid/acellular pertussis vaccine (absorbed)*, **Acel-Imune®, Certiva®, Tripedia®**
C		*diphtheria/tetanus toxoid/pertussis/haemophilus b conjugate vaccine*, **Tetramune®**
B		*dipivefrin*, **Propine®**
C		**Diprolene®, Diprolene®AF**, *betamethasone dipropionate*
C		**Diprosone®**, *betamethasone dipropionate*
B		*dipyridamole*, **Persantine®**
D		*dipyridamole/aspirin*, **Aggrenox®**

C		*dirithromycin*, **Dynabac®**
C		**Disalcid®**, *salsalate*
C		*disopyramide*, **Napramide®, Norpace®, Norpace®CR**
X		*disulfiram*, **Antabuse®, Ro-sulfiram®**
B		**Ditropan®, Ditropan®XL**, *oxybutynin*
B		**Diucardin®**, *hydroflumethiazide*
C		**Diupres®**, *reserpine/chlorothiazide*
B		**Diurese®**, *trichlormethiazide*
C		**Diuril®**, *chlorothiazide*
D		*divalproex*, **Depakote®**
NR		*docosanol*, **Abreva®**
C		*docusate/dioctyl calcium sulfosuccinate*, **Surfak®**
C		*docusate/phenolphthalein*, **Doxidan®**
C		*docusate*, **Colace®, Colace® Enema**
C		*docusate casanthranol*, **Peri-Colace®**
C		*docusate potassium*, **Dialose®, Diocto-K®**
B		*dolasetron*, **Anzimet®**
C	II	**Dolgic®**, *butalbital/acetaminophen*
C		**Dolobid®**, *diflunisal*
B		**Dolophine®**, *methadone*
NR		**Domeboro®Otic**, *acetic acid in aluminum sulfate*
C		*donepezil*, **Aricept®**
NR		**Donnagel®**, *attapulgite*
C	II	**Donnatal®**, *phenobarbital/hyoscyamine/atropine/scopolamine*
C		**Donnazyme®**, *pancrelipase*
C		**Dopar®**, *levodopa, l-dopa*
B		**Dopram®**, *doxapram*
X	IV	**Doral®**, *quazepam*
X		**Doriden®**, *glutethimide*
B		**Dostinex®**, *cabergoline*
D		**Doryx®**, *doxycycline*
C		*dorzolamide*, **Trusopt®**
C		*dorzolamide/timolol*, **Cosopt®**
NR		**DoubleCap®**, *capsaicin*
C		**Dovonex®**, *calcipotriene*
B		*doxapram*, **Dopram®**
C		*doxazosin*, **Cardura®, Cardura®XL**
C		*doxecalciferol*, **Hectoral®**
C		*doxepin*, **Adapin®TCA, Prudoxin®, Sinequan®, Zonalon®**
C		**Doxidan®**, *docusate/phenolphthalein*
D		**Doxy®, Doxy®-C, Doxy®-Cap**, *doxycycline*
D		**Doxychel®**, *doxycycline*
D		**Doxycin®**, *doxycycline*
D		*doxycycline*, Adoxa, **Doryx®, Doxy®, Doxy®-C, Doxy®-Cap, Doxychel®, Doxycin®, Monodox®, Oracea®, Vibramycin®, Vibra-Tab®, Vivox®**
B		**Dramamine®**, *dimenhydrinate*

B		**Dramamine®** II, *meclizine*
C		**Drithocreme®, Dritho-Scalp®,** *anthralin*
C		**Drixoral®Cold & Allergy,** *dexbrompheniramine/pseudoephedrine*
C	III	*dronabinol,* **Marinol®**
C		**Dryvax®,** *vaccina virus vaccine (dried calf lymph type)*
C		**Duac®,** *clindamycin/benzoyl peroxide*
A		**Duet by StuartNatal®,** *prenatal vitamin*
C		**Duetact®,** *pioglitazone/glimepiride*
B		**Dulcolax®,** *bisacodyl*
C		*duloxetine,* **Cymbalta®**
NR		**DuoFilm®,** *salicylic acid*
C		**DuoNeb®,** *ipratropium/albuterol*
NR		**DuoPlant®,** *salicylic acid*
B		**Duphalac®,** *lactulose*
B		**Duracillin®,** *penicillin g procaine*
C		**Duradryl®,** *phenylephrine/chlorpheniramine/methscopolamine*
C	II	**Duragesic®,** *fentanyl transdermal system*
C		**Dura-Gest®,** *guaifenesin/phenylephrine/pseudoephedrine*
C		**Duralone®,** *methylprednisolone*
C	II	**Duramorph®PF,** *morphine sulfate*
C		**Duraquin®,** *quinidine gluconate*
C		**Dura®-Tap/PD,** *chlorpheniramine/pseudoephedrine*
NR		**Duratears®Naturale,** *petrolatum/lanolin, mineral oil*
C		**Duratuss®,** *guaifenesin/pseudoephedrine*
C		**Duratuss®DM,** *guaifenesin/dextromethorphan*
C		**Duratuss®G,** *guaifenesin*
C	III	**Duratuss®HD,** *guaifenesin/hydrocodone/pseudoephedrine*
C		**Dura-Vent®,** *guaifenesin/pseudoephedrine*
C		**Dura-Vent®/DA,** *chlorpheniramine/phenylephrine/methscopolamine*
B		**Duricef®,** *cefadroxil*
X		*dutasteride,* **Avodart®**
B		**Dyazide®,** *triamterene/hydrochlorothiazide*
B		**Dycill®,** *dicloxacillin*
C		**Dyclone®,** *dyclonine*
C		*dyclonine,* **Dyclone®**
C		**Dymelor®,** *acetohexamide*
C		**Dynabac®,** *dirithromycin*
D		**Dynacin®,** *minocycline*
C		**DynaCirc®, DynaCirc®CR,** *isradipine*
B		**Dynapen®,** *dicloxacillin*
C		**Dynex®,** *guaifenesin/phenylephrine*
C		*dyphylline,* **Dilor®, Lufyllin®**
B		**Dyrenium®,** *triamterene*
D		**Easprin®,** *aspirin, acetylsalicylic acid, asa*
C		*echothiophate,* **Phospholine Iodide®**
B		**EC-Naprosyn®,** *naproxen*
C		*econazole,* **Spectazole®**

C		**Econopred®**, *prenisolone acetate*
D		**Ecotrin®**, *enteric-coated aspirin*
B		**Edecrin®**, *ethacrynic acid*
X		**Edex®**, *alprostadil for injection*
B		**E.E.S.®**, *erythromycin ethylsuccinate*
C		*efalizumab*, **Raptiva®**
C		*efavirenz*, **Sustiva®**
B		**Effer-Syllium®**, *psyllium hydrophilic mucilloid*
C		**Effexor®, Effexor®XR**, *venlafaxine*
C		*eflornithine*, **Vaniqa®**
D		**Efudex®**, *fluorouracil, 5-fluorouracil, 5-FU*
C		**Eldepryl®**, *selegiline*
C		**Eldopaque®Forte**, *hydroquinone*
C		**Eldoquin®Forte**, *hydroquinone*
A		*electrolyte supplement*, **KaoLectrolyte®, Pedialyte®**
C		**Elestat®**, *epinastine*
C		*eletriptan*, **Relpax®**
C		**Elidel®**, *pimecrolimus*
X		**Eligard®**, *leuprolide acetate*
B		**Elimite®**, *permethrin*
B		**Elmiron®**, *pentosan polysulfate sodium*
C		**Elocon®**, *mometasone furoate*
C		**Emadine®**, *emedastine difumarate*
C		*emedastine difumarate*, **Emadine®**
B		**Emend®**, *aprepitant*
NR		**Emetrol®**, *phosphorated carbohydrated solution*
B		**Emgel®**, *erythromycin base*
D	III	**Empirin®with Codeine #2, #3, #4**, *aspirin/codeine*
C		**Emsam®**, *selegiline*
B		*emtricitabine*, **Emtriva®**
B		**Emtriva®**, *emtricitabine*
B		**E-Mycin®, E-Mycin®333**, *erythromycin base*
C		**Enablex®**, *darifenacin*
C/D		*enalapril*, **Vasotec®**
C/D		*enalapril/diltiazem*, **Teczem®**
C/D		*enalapril/felodipine*, **Lexxel®**
C/D		*enalapril/hydrochlorothiazide*, **Vaseretic®**
B		**Enbrel®**, *etanercept*
C	III	**Endal®HD, Endal®HD Plus**, *hydrocodone/phenylephrine/chlorpheniramine*
C		**Endep®**, *amitriptyline*
B		**Enduron®**, *methyclothiazide*
B		**Enduronyl®**, *methyclothiazide/deserpidine*
A		**Enfamil®Natalins Rx**, *prenatal vitamin*
B		*enfuvirtide*, **Fuzeon**
C		**Engerix-B®**, *hepatitis b vaccine (recombinant)*
X		**Enjuvia®**, *conjugated estrogens*

C		*enoxacin*, **Penetrex**®
B		*enoxaparin*, **Lovenox**®
X		**Enpresse**®, *ethinyl estradiol/levonorgestrel*
C		*entacapone*, **Comtan**®
C		*entecavir*, **Baraclude**®
C		**Entex**®, **Entex**®**LA**, **Entex**®**PSE**, *guaifenesin/pseudoephedrine*
C		**Entex**®**HC**, *guaifenesin/hydrocodone bitartrate/phenylephrine*
C		**Entocort**®**EC**, *budesonide*
X		**Enpresse**®, *ethinyl estradiol/levonorgestrel*
C		**Epi-E-Zpen**®, *epinephrine*
C		*epinastine*, **Elestat**®
C		*epinephrine*, **Adrenalin**®, **Epi-E-Zpen**®, **EpiPen**®, **EpiPen**®**Jr**, **Sus-Phrine**®
C		*epinephrine/chlorpheniramine*, **Ana-Kit**®
C		*epinephrine (racemic)*, **Vaponefrin**®
C		**EpiPen**®, **EpiPen**®**Jr**, *epinephrine*
C		**Epivir**®, **Epivir**®**-HBV**, *lamivudine, 3TC*
B		*eplerenone*, **Inspra**®
C		**Epogen**®, *epoetin alpha*
C		*epoetin alpha*, **Epogen**®, **Procrit**®
C/D		*eprosartan*, **Teveten**®
C/D		*eprosartan/hydrochlorothiazide*, **Teveten**®
A		**Epsom Salt**®, *magnesium sulfate*
C		**Epzicom**®, *abacavir/lamivudine*
D	IV	**Equagesic**®, *meprobamate/aspirin*
D		**Equanil**®, *meprobamate*
D		**Equetro**®, *carbamazepine*
D		**Equitrol**®, *carbamazepine*
C		**Erbitux**®, *cetuximab*
C		*ergocalciferol, vitamin d*, **Calciferol**®
C		*ergoloid*, **Hydergine**®**LC**, **Hydergine**®**Liquid**
X		**Ergomar**®, **Ergomar**®**Sublingual**, *ergotamine*
X		**Ergostat**®, *ergotamine*
X		*ergotamine*, **Ergomar**®, **Ergomar**®**Sublingual**, **Ergostat**®
X		*ergotamine/caffeine*, **Cafergot**®, **Wigraine**®
X		**Errin**®, *norethindrone*
C		**Ertaczo**®, *sertaconazole*
B		*ertapenem*, **Ivanz**®
B		**ERYC**®, *erythromycin base*
C		**Erycette**®, *erythromycin base*
B		**Erycream**®, *erythromycin base*
B		**EryDerm**®, *erythromycin base*
B		**Erygel**®, *erythromycin base*
C		**Erymax**®, *erythromycin base*
B		**Erypar**®, *erythromycin stearate*
B		**EryPed**®, *erythromycin ethylsuccinate*
B		**Ery-Tab**®, *erythromycin base*

B		**Erythrocin®**, *erythromycin stearate*
B		*erythromycin base*, **Emgel®, E-Mycin®, E-Mycin®333, ERYC®, Erycette®, Erycream®, EryDerm®, Erygel®, Erymax®, Ery-Tab®, Erythromycin Base®, PCE®, Robimycin®, Theramycin®Z**
B		**Erythromycin Base®**, *erythromycin base*
C		*erythromycin/benzoyl peroxide*, **Benzamycin®Topical Gel**
B		*erythromycin estolate*, **Ilosone®**
B		*erythromycin ethylsuccinate*, **E.E.S.®, EryPed®, Pediamycin®**
C		*erythromycin ethylsuccinate/sulfasoxazole*, **Eryzole®, Pediazole®**
B		*erythromycin glucptate*, **Ilotycin Gluceptate®**
B		*erythromycin stearate*, **Erypar®, Erythrocin®**
C		**Eryzole®**, *erythromycin ethylsuccinate/sulfisoxazole*
C		*escitalopram*, **Lexapro®**
X		**Esclim®**, *estradiol transdermal system*
C	II	**Esgic®, Esgic®Plus**, *butalbital/acetaminophen/caffeine*
B		**Esidrix®**, *hydrochlorothiazide*
D		**Eskalith®, Eskalith®CR**, *lithium carbonate*
B		**Esmil®**, *guanethidine monosulfate/hydrochlorothiazide*
C		*esmolol*, **Brevibloc®**
B		*esomeprazole*, **Nexium®**
X	IV	*estazolam*, **ProSom®**
X		*esterified estrogen*, **Estratab®, Menest®**
X		*esterified estrogen/methyltestosterone*, **Estratest®, Estratest® HS, Syntest®D.S., Syntest®H.S.**
X		**Estinyl®**, *ethinyl estradiol*
X		**Estrace®, Estrace® Vaginal Cream**, *estradiol*
X		**Estraderm®**, *estradiol*
X		*estradiol*, **Alora®, Climara®, Esclim®, Estraderm®, Estrace®, Estrace®Vaginal Cream, Estrasorb®, Estratab®, Estring®, Femring®, Femtrace®, Gynodiol®, Menostar®, Vagifem®, Vivelle®, Vivelle®-Dot**
X		*estradiol cypionate*, **Depo-Estradiol Cypionate®, Depogen®**
X		*estradiol/levonorgestrel*, **Climara®Pro**
X		*estradiol/norethindrone*, **Activella®, FemHRT®1/5**
X		*estradiol/norethindrone transdermal system*, **CombiPatch®**
X		*estradiol/norgestimate*, **Ortho-Prefest®**
X		*estradiol valerate*, **Delestrogen®**
X		**Estrasorb®**, *estradiol*
X		**Estratab®**, *esterified estrogens*
X		**Estratest®, Estratest®HS**, *esterified estrogens/methyltestosterone*
X		**Estring®**, *estradiol vaginal ring*
X		*estropipate*, **Ogen®, Ogen®Vaginal Cream, Ortho-Est®**
X		**Estrostep®21**, *ethinyl estradiol/norethindrone*
X		**Estrostep®FE**, *ethinyl estradiol/norethindrone/ferrous fumarate*
C	IV	*eszopiclone*, **Lunesta®**
B		*etanercept*, **Enbrel®**
B		*ethacrynic acid*, **Edecrin®**
B		*ethambutol*, **Myambutol®**

C	*ethchlorvynol*, **Placidyl®**
X	*ethinyl estradiol*, **Estinyl®**
X	*ethinyl estradiol/desogestrel diacetate*, **Apri®, Cyclessa®, Desogen®-28, Kariva®, Mircette®, Ortho-Cept®-21, Ortho-Cept®-28, Velivet®**
X	*ethinyl estradiol/drospirenone*, **Yasmin®, Yaz®**
X	*ethinyl estradiol/ethynodiol diacetate*, **Demulen®1/35, Demulen®1/50, Kelnor®1/35, Zovia®1/50-21, Zovia®1/50-28**
X	*ethinyl estradiol/levonorgestrel*, **Alesse®, Alesse®-28, Aviane®, Enpresse®, Lessina®, Levlen®-21, Levlen®-28, Levlite®-28, Levora®-21, Levora®-28, Nordette®-21, Nordette®-28, Portia®, Preven®, Quasense®, Seasonale®, Seasonique®, Tri-Levlen®-21, Tri-Levlen®-28, Triphasil®-21, Triphasil®-28, Trivora®-21, Trivora®-28, Zovia®/35-21, Zovia®1/35-28**
X	*ethinyl estradiol/mestranol*, **Nelova®1/50 M-21, Nelova®1/50M-28, Norinyl®1+50-21, Norinyl®1+50-28**
X	*ethinyl estradiol/norethindrone*, **Aranelle®, Brevicon®-21, Brevicon® 28, Estrostep®21, Jenest®-28, Junel®1/20, Junel®1.5/30, Loestrin®-21 1/20, Loestrin®-21 1.5/30, Modicon®-21, Modicon®-28, Necon®0.5/35-21, Necon®0.5/35-28, Necon®1/35-21, Necon®1/35-28, Necon®10/11-21, Necon®10/11-28, Nelova®0.5/35-21, Nelova®0.5/35-28, Nelova®1/35-21, Nelova®1/35-28, Nelova®10/11-21, Nelova®10/11-28, Nelova®1/50-21, Nelova®1/50-28, Norethin®1/35-21, Norethin®1/35-28, Norinyl®1+35-21, Norinyl®1+35-28, Norinyl®1+50-21, Norinyl®1+50-28, Nortrel®-21 0.5/35, Nortrel®-28 1/35, Nortrel®7/7/7-28, Ortho-Cyclen®, Ortho-Novum®1/35-21, Ortho-Novum®1/35-28, Ortho-Novum®1/50-28, Ortho-Novum®777-28, Ortho-Novum®10/11-21, Ortho-Novum® 10/11-28, Ovcon®35 Chewable, Ovcon®35-21, Ovcon®35-28, Ovcon®50-21, Ovcon®50-28, Tri-Norinyl®-21, Tri-Norinyl®-28**
X	*ethinyl estradiol/norethindrone/ferrous fumarate*, **Estrostep®FE, Junel®Fe 1/20, Junel®Fe 1.5/30, Loestrin®Fe-28 1/20, Loestrin®Fe-28 1.5/30, Microgestin®Fe 1/20, Microgestin®Fe 1.5/30,**
X	*ethinyl estradiol/norgestimate*, **Ortho-Cyclen®-21, Ortho-Cyclen®-28, Ortho Tri-Cyclen®-21, Ortho Tri-Cyclen®-28, Ortho Tri-Cyclen®Lo, Sprintec®28, Tri-Sprintec®28**
X	*ethinyl estradiol/norgestrel*, **Cryselle®, Lo-Ogestrel®-21, Lo-Ogestrel®-28, Lo/Ovral®-21, Lo/Ovral®-28, Ovral®-21, Ovral®-28**
D	*ethosuximide*, **Zarontin®**
C	*etidronate disodium*, **Didronel®**
C	*ethotoin*, **Peganone®**
C	*etodolac*, **Lodine®, Lodine®XL**
C	**Etrafon®**, *perphenazine/amitriptyline*
X	*etretinate*, **Tegison®**
NR	**Euflexxa®**, *hyaluronin*
D	**Eulexin®**, *flutamide*
C	**Eurax®**, *crotamiton*
A	**Euthroid®**, *levothyroxine/liothyronine (liotrix)*

X		**Evista®**, *raloxifene*
B		**Evoclin®Foam**, *clindamycin*
C		**Evoxac®**, *cevimeline*
D		**Excedrin®Migraine**, *acetaminophen/aspirin/caffeine*
B		**Excedrin®PM**, *acetaminophen/diphenhydramine*
C		**Exelderm®**, *sulconazole nitrate*
B		**Exelon®**, *rivastigmine*
D		*exemestane*, **Aromasin®**
C		*exenatide*, **Byetta®**
B		**Exjade®**, *deferasirox*
C		**Ex-Lax®**, *phenolphalein*
C		**Exsel®**, *selenium sulfide*
C		**Extendryl®, Extendryl®JR, Extendryl®SR**, *chlorpheniramine/phenylephrine/methscopolamine*
C		**Exubera®**, *insulin human (rDNA origin) pwdr for inhalation*
C		*ezetimibe*, **Zetia®**
X		*ezetimibe/simvastatin*, **Vytorin®**
C		**Factive®**, *gemifloxacin*
B		*famciclovir*, **Famvir®**
B		*famotidine*, **Pepcid®, Pepcid®AC, Pepcid®RPD**
B		*famotidine/CaCO$_3$/Mg hydroxide*, **Pepcid®Complete**
B		**Famvir®**, *famciclovir*
D		**Fareston®**, *toremifene*
D		**Faslodex®**, *fluvestrant*
C	IV	**Fastin®**, *phentermine*
B		**Fazaclo®**, *clozapine*
C		**Fedahist®**, *pseudoephedrine/chlorpheniramine*
C		**Feen-A-Mint®**, *phenolphthalein*
C		*felbamate*, **Felbatol®**
C		**Felbatol®**, *felbamate*
C		**Feldene®**, *piroxicam*
C		*felodipine*, **Plendil®**
D		**Femara®**, *letrozole*
X		**FemHRT®1/5**, *estradiol/norethindrone*
A		**Femiron®**, *ferrous fumarate*
X		**Femring®**, *estradiol*
C		**Femstat®-3**, butoconazole
X		**Femtrace®**, *estradiol*
C		*fenofibrate*, **Antara®, TriCor®, Lofibra®**
B/D		*fenoprofen*, **Nalfon®**
C	II	*fentanyl transdermal system*, **Duragesic®**
C	II	*fentanyl transmucosal unit*, **Actiq®, Fentora®**
C	II	**Fentora®**, *fentanyl transmucosal unit*
A		**Feosol®**, *ferrous sulfate*
A		**Fergon®**, *ferrous gluconate*
A		**Fer-In-Sol®**, *ferrous sulfate*
A		**Fero-Folic®-500**, *ferrous sulfate/folic acid/vitamin c*

A		*ferrous fumarate*, **Femiron®, Hemocyte®**
A		*ferrous gluconate*, **Fergon®**
A		*ferrous sulfate*, **Feosol®, Fer-In-Sol®, FeSO₄, Slow Fe®**
A		*ferrous sulfate/folic acid*, **Slow Fe®Plus Folic Acid**
A		*ferrous sulfate/folic acid/vitamin c*, **Fero-Folic®-500**
C		*feuocinolone acetonide*, **Synemol®**
C		*fexofenadine*, **Allegra®**
C		**Fiberall®**, *psyllium*
C		**Fibercon®**, *calcium polycarbophil*
B		**Finacea®**, *azelaic acid*
X		*finasteride*, **Propecia®, Proscar®**
B		**Finevin®**, *azelaic acid*
C	II	**Fioricet®**, *butalbital/acetaminophen/caffeine*
C	III	**Fioricet®with Codeine**, *butalbital/acetaminophen/caffeine/codeine*
C	II	**Fiorinal®**, *butalbital/aspirin/caffeine*
C	III	**Fiorinal®with Codeine**, *butalbital/aspirin/caffeine/codeine*
D/B		**Flagyl®, Flagyl®375, Flagyl®ER**, *metronidazole*
C		**Flarex®**, flourometholone acetate
C		**Flatulex®**, *simethicone/activated charcoal*
C		*flavoxate*, **Urised®, Urispas®**
C		**Fleet®Enema**, *sodium phosphate/sodium biphosphate*
B		**Flexeril®**, *cyclobenzaprine*
C		**Flexon®**, *orphenadrine*
B		**Flomax®**, *tamulosin*
C		**Flonase®**, *fluticasone*
C		**Florinef®**, *fludrocortisone*
C		**Florone®, Florone®E**, *diflorasone diacetate*
C		**Floropryl®**, *isoflurophate*
C		**Flovent®HFA**, *fluticasone propionate*
C		**Floxin®, Floxin®Otic Solution**, *ofloxacin*
C		*fluconazole*, **Diflucan®**
C		*fludrocortisone*, **Florinef®**
C		**Flu-Immune®**, *influenza virus vaccine*
C		**Flumadine®**, *rimantadine*
C		**FluMist®**, *influenza vaccine (trivalent, live attenuated, virus types A and B)*
C		*flunisolide*, **AeroBid®, AeroBid®M, Nasalide®, Nasarel®**
C		*fluocinonide*, **Lidemol®, Lidex®, Lidex-E®, Lyderm®, Topsyn®, Vanos®**
C		*fluocinolone acetonide*, **Capex®Shampoo, Derma-Smoothe®/FS, Synalar®**
NR		*fluoride*, **Luride®**
C		*fluorometholone*, **FML®, FML®Forte, FML®S.O.P. Ointment**
C		*fluorometholone acetate*, **Flarex®**
D		**Fluoroplex®**, *fluorouracil, 5-fluorouracil, 5-FU*
D		*fluorouracil, 5-fluorouracil, 5-FU*, **Adrucil®, Efudex®, Fluoroplex®**
C		*fluoxetine*, **Prozac®, Prozac®Weekly, Sarafem®**

X		*fluoxymesterone,* **Halotestin**®
C		*fluphenazine,* **Prolixin**®
C		*fluphenazine decanoate,* **Prolixin**®**Decanoate**
C		*flurandrenolide,* **Cordran**®, **Cordran**®**SP**
X	IV	*flurazepam,* **Dalmane**®
B		*flurbiprofen,* **Ansaid**®
C		**Flushield**®, *influenza virus vaccine*
D		*flutamide,* **Eulexin**®
C		*fluticasone,* **Flonase**®
C		*fluticasone propionate,* **Cutivate**®, **Flovent**®**HFA**
C		*fluticasone propionate/salmeterol,* **Advair**®**DisKus**
X		*fluvastatin,* **Lescol**®
D		*fluvestrant,* **Faslodex**®
C		**Fluzone**®, **Fluzone**®**Preservative-Free: Adult Dose, Fluzone**® **Preservative-Free: Pediatric Dose**, *trivalent inactivated influenza vaccine*
C		**FML**®**Liquifilm**, *fluorometholone*
C	II	**Focalin**®, **Focalin**®**XR** *dexmethylphenidate*
A		*folic acid, vitamin b₉,* **Folvite**®
C		**Folinic**®**Acid**, *leucovorin ca*
A		**Folbee**®, **Folbee**®**Plus**, *multivitamin*
A		**Folbic**®, *multivitamin*
A		**Folvite**®, *folic acid, vitamin b₉*
B		*fondaparinux,* **Arixtra**®
C		**Foradil**®**Aerolizer**, *formoterol fumarate*
C		**Forensol**®, *lanthanum*
C		*formoterol,* **Foradil**®**Aerolizer**
B		**Fortovase**®, *saquinavir*
B		**Fortamet**®, *metformin*
B		**Fortaz**®, *ceftazidime*
C		**Forteo**®, *teriparatide*
C		**Fortical**®, *calcitonin-salmon*
C		**Fosamax**®, *alendronate*
C		*fosfanprenavir,* **Luxiva**®
C		*fosfomycin tromethamine,* **Monurol**®
C/D		*fosinopril,* **Monopril**®
C/D		*fosinopril/hydrochlorothiazide,* **Monopril**®**HCT**
C		**Fosrenol**®, *lanthanum*
C		**Fostex**®, *benzoyl peroxide*
C		**Fototar**®, *coal tar*
C		**Fragmin**®, *dalteparin*
C		**Frova**®, *frovatriptan succinate*
C		*frovatriptan succinate,* **Frova**®
C		**Fulvicin**®**P/G**, *griseofulvin ultramicrosized*
C		**Fulvicin**®**U/F**, *griseofulvin microsized*
C		**Fungizone**®, *amphotericin b*
B		**Fungoid**®, *clotrimazole*

B	**Furadantin®**, *nitrofurantoin*
C	*furazolidone*, **Furoxone®**
C	*furosemide*, **Lasix®**
C	**Furoxone®**, *furazolidone*
B	**Fuzeon®**, *enfuvirtide*
C	*gabapentin*, **Neurontin®**
C	**Gabitril®**, *tiazabine*
B	*galantamine*, **Razadyne®, Reminyl®**
C	**Gamimune®**, *immune globulin*
C	*gamma globulin, immune serum globulin*, **Gammar®**
C	**Gamma®**, *gamma globulin, immune serum globulin*
C	**Gantanol®, Gantanol®DS**, *sulfamethoxazole*
B/D	**Gantrisin®, Gantrisin®Ophthalmic Solution**, *sulfisoxazole*
C	**Garamycin®, Garamycin®Ophthalmic, Garamycin®Topical**, *gentamycin*
C	**Gas-X®**, *simethicone*
C	**Gaviscon®, Gaviscon®ES**, *aluminum hydroxide/magnesium trisilicate*
D	*gefitinib*, **Iressa®**
C	**Gelusil®, Gelusil®II, Gelusil®M**, *magnesium hydroxide/aluminum/hydroxide/simethicone*
C	*gemfibrozil*, **Lopid®**
C	*gemifloxacin*, **Factive®**
C	**Genoptic®**, *gentamicin*
C	**Gentacidin®**, *gentamicin ophthalmic ointment*
C	*gentamicin*, **Garamycin®, Garamycin®Ophthalmic, Garamycin® Topical®Genoptic, Gentacidin®**
NR	**GenTeal®Mild**, *hydroxypropyl methylcellulose*
B	**Gentlax®**, *bisocodyl*
B	**Geocillin®**, *carbenicillin*
C	**Geodon®**, *ziprasidone*
C	**Geref®**, *sermorelin*
D	**Gleevec®**, *imatinib mesylate*
B	**Geopen®**, *carbenicillin*
C	**GI Cocktail®**, *belladonna/xylocaine viscous/aluminu hydroxide/magnesium hydroxide*
C	*glimepiride*, **Amaryl®**
C	*glipizide*, **Glucotrol®, Glucotrol® XL**
C	*glipizide/meformin*, **Metaglip®**
B	*glucagon*, **Glucagon®**
B	**Glucagon®**, *glucagon*
B	**Glucophage®, Glucophage®XR**, *metformin*
C	**Glucotrol®, Glucotrol®XL**, *glipizide*
B	**Glucovance®**, *glyburide/metforman*
B	**Glumetza®**, *metformin*
X	*glutethimide*, **Doriden®**
A	**Glutofac®-ZX**, *multivitamin*

B		*glyburide*, **DiaBeta®, Glynase®, Micronase®**
B		*glyburide/metforman*, **Glucovance®**
B		*glyburide micronized*, **Glycron®**
C		*glycerin suppository*, **Babylax®**
C		**Glyceryl®Guaiacolate**, *guaifenesin*
B		**Glycet®**, *miglitol*
B		*glycopyrrolate*, **Robinul®**
C		**Glycotuss®**, *guaifenesin*
B		**Glycron®**, *glyburide micronized*
B		**Glynase®**, *glyburide*
NR		**Gly-Oxide®**, *carbamide peroxide*
C		**Glyquin®**, *hydroquinone/padinate O/oxybenzone/octyl methoxycinnamate*
C		**Glytuss®**, *guaifenesin*
X		*goserelin*, **Zoladex®**
B		*granisetron*, **Kytril®**
C		**Grifulvin®V**, *griseofulvin microsized*
C		**Grisactin®**, *griseofulvin microsized*
C		**Grisactin®Ultra**, *griseofulvin ultramicrosized*
C		*griseofulvin microsized*, **Fulvicin®U/F, Grisactin®, Grisovin®FP, Gris-PEG®, Grifulvin®V,**
C		*griseofulvin ultramicrosized*, **Fulvicin®P/G, Grisactin®Ultra**
C		**Grisovin®FP**, *griseofulvin microsized*
C		**Gris-PEG®**, *griseofulvin microsized*
C		*guaifenesin*, **Allfen®, Duratuss®G, Glyceryl®Guaiacolate, Glycotuss®, Glytuss®, Guaituss®, Humibid®LA, Humibid®Sprinkle, Hytuss®, Liquibid®1200, Mucinex®, Robitussin®, Tussi-Organidin®**
C		**Guaituss®**, *guaifenesin*
C	III	**Guaituss®AC**, *codeine/guaifenesin*
C		**Guai-Vent®PSE**, *guaifenesin/pseudoephedrine*
C		*guanabenz*, **Wytensin®**
C		*guanethidine*, **Ismelin®**
C		*guanethidine/hydrochlorothiazide*, **Esmil®**
B		*guanfacine*, **Tenex®**
B		**Gynazole®-1**, *butoconazole*
B		**Gyne-Lotrimin®, Gyne-Lotrimin®-3**, *clotrimazole*
X		*gynodiol*, **micronized estradiol**
D		**Habitrol®**, *nicotine transdermal system*
C		*haemophilus b conjugated vaccine*, **Hibtiter®, PedvaxHIB®**
C		*haemophilus b conjugate/hepatitis b (recombinant) vaccine*, **Comvax®**
C		*haemophilus b conjugated vaccine (diphtheria toxoid conjugate)*, **Prohibit®**
C		*haemophilus b conjugate vaccine/tetanus toxoid conjugate*, **Omnihib®**
D	IV	*halazepam*, **Paxipam®**
C		*halcinonide*, **Halog®, Halog®E**
X	IV	**Halcion®**, *triazolam*
C		**Haldol®**, *haloperidol*

C		**Haldol®Decanoate,** *haloperidol decanoate*
C		**Haldrone®,** *paramethasone*
C		*halobetasol propionate,* **Ultravate®**
C		**Halog®, Halog®E,** *halcinonide*
C		*haloperidol,* **Haldol, Peridol**
C		*haloperidol decanoate,* **Haldol®Decanoate**
X		**Halotestin®,** *fluoxymesterone*
C		**Havrix®,** *hepatitis a vaccine*
C		**H-BIG®,** *hepatitis b immune globulin*
B		*hctz, hydrochlorothiazide,* **Esidrix®, Hydrodiuril®, Microzide®, Oretic**
C		**HDCV®,** *rabies vaccine (human diploid cell)*
C		**Hectoral®,** *doxecalciferol*
D		**Helidac®Therapy,** *bismuth subsalicylate/metronidazole/tetracycline*
A		**Hemocyte®,** *ferrous fumarate*
C		**Heparin®,** *heparin*
C		*heparin,* **Heparin®, Liquaemin®**
C		*hepatitis a vaccine,* **Havrix®, Vaqta®**
C		*hepatitis a inactivated/hepatitis b surface antigen (recombinant) vaccine,* **Twinrix®**
C		*hepatitis b immune globulin,* **H-BIG®**
C		*hepatitis b immune globulin (human),* **Hyper Hep®**
C		*hepatitis b vaccine (recombinant),* **Engerix®-B, Recombivax®HB**
C		**Hepsera®,** *adenovir dipivoxil*
C		**Herplex®,** *idoxuridine*
A		**Hexa-Betalin®,** *pyridoxine, vitamin b_6*
C		*hexachlorophene,* **PhisoHex®**
C		**Hexadrol®,** *dexamethasone*
B		**Hibiclens®,** *chlorhexidine gluconate*
B		**Hibistat®,** *chlorhexidine gluconate*
C		**Hibtiter®,** *haemophilus b conjugate vaccine*
C		**Hiprex®,** *methenamine hippurate*
C		**Hismanal®,** *astemizole*
C		**Histacol®DM Pediatric Drops,** *pseudoephedrine/dextromethorphan/brompheniramine*
C		**Histacol®DM Pediatric Syrup,** *pseudoephedrine/dextromethorphan/brompheniramine/guafenesin*
C		**Histalet®Forte,** *pseudoephedrine/phenylephrine/chlorpheniramine/pyrilamine*
C		**Histatapp®,** *brompheniramine/phenylephrine/pseudoephedrine*
C	III	**Histussin®HC,** *hydrocodone/phenylephrine/chlorpheniramine*
C	III	**Histex®HC,** *hydrocodone/pseudoephedrine/carbinoxamine*
C		**Histex® Pd,** *carbinoxamine*
C		**Hivid®,** *zalcitabine*
C		**HMS®,** *medrysone*
C		**Homatrocel®,** *homatropine*
C		*homatropine,* **Homatrocel®**

C		**HRIG®**, *rabies immune globulin (human)*
B		**Humalog®**, *insulin lispro*
B		**Humalog®Mix 75/25, Humalog®Mix 50/50**, *insulin lispro protamine/ insulin lispro*
C		**Humatin®**, *paromomycin*
C		**Humatrope®**, *somatropin*
C		**Humibid®DM**, *guaifenesin/dextromethorphan*
C		**Humibid®LA, Humibid® Sprinkles**, *guaifenesin*
B		**Humira®**, *adalimumab*
B		**Humulin®70/30, Humulin®50/50**, *insulin insophane suspension/ insulin regular*
B		**Humulin®L, Iletin®II Lente**, *insulin zinc suspension (lente)*
B		**Humulin®N**, *insulin zinc isophane suspension*
B		**Humulin®R, Humulin®R U-500**, *insulin regular*
B		**Humulin®U**, *insulin extended zinc suspension (ultralente)*
X		**Humorsol®**, *demecarium bromide ophthalmic solution*
C		**Hurricaine®**, *benzocaine*
B		**Hyalgan®**, *sodium hyaluronate*
C		*hyaluronic acid*, **Restylane®**
NR		*hyaluronin*, **Euflexxa®**
C	III	**Hycodan®**, *hydrocodone/homatropine/methylbromide*
C	III	**Hycomine®, Hycomine®Pediatric**, *hydrocodone*
C	III	**Hycomine® Compound**, *hydrocodone/chlorpheniramin/ phenylephrine/acetaminophen/caffeine*
C	III	**Hycotuss®**, *guaifenesin/hydrocodone*
C		**Hydeltrasol®**, *prednisolone sodium phosphate*
C		**Hydeltra®-TBA**, *prednisolone tebutate*
C		**Hydergine®LC, Hydergine®Liquid**, *ergoloid*
C		*hydralazine*, **Apresoline®**
C		*hydralazine/hydrochlorothiazide*, **Apresazide®**
C		*hydralazine/isosorbide dinitrate*, **BiDil®**
D		**Hydrea®**, *hydroxyurea*
C	III	**Hydrocet®**, *hydrocodone/acetaminophen*
B		**Hydrocil®**, *psyllium hydrophilic mucilloid*
B		*hydrochlorothiazide*, **Esidrix®, Hydrodiuril®, Microzide®, Oretic®**
C		**Hydrocort®**, *hydrocortisone*
C		*hydrocortisone*, **Ala-Scalp®, Anusol®-HC, Cetacort®, Cortaid®, Cortef®, Cortifoam®, Hydrocort®, Hydrocortone®, Hytone®, Nutracort®, Proctocort®, Rectocort®, Synacort®, Texacort®**
C		*hydrocortisone acetate*, **U-Cort®**
C		*hydrocortisone butyrate*, **Locoid®**
C		*hydrocortisone/chlorcyclizine*, **Mantadil®**
C		*hydrocortisone/iodoquinol*, **Vytone®**
C		*hydrocortisone/lidocaine*, **Rectacreme®**
C		*hydrocortisone phosphate*, **Hydrocotone®Phosphate**
C		*hydrocortisone/pramoxine*, **Proctocream®-HC, Proctofoam®-HC**
C		*hydrocortisone probutate*, **Pandel®**

C		*hydrocortisone retention enema*, **Cortenema®**
C		*hydrocortisone sodium succinate*, **Solu-Cortef®**
C		*hydrocortisone valerate*, **Westcort®**
C		**Hydrocortone®**, *hydrocortisone*
C		**Hydrocotone®Phosphate**, *hydrocortisone phosphate*
B		**Hydrodiuril®**, *hydrochlorothiazide*
B		*hydroflumethiazide*, **Diucardin®**, **Saluron®**
C	II	*hydromorphone*, **Dilaudid®**, **Dilaudid®HP**, **Paladone®**
C		**Hydromox®R**, *quinethazone/reserpine*
C		**Hydropres®**, *reserpine/hydrochlorothiazide*
C		*hydroquinone*, **Eldopaque®Forte**, **Eldoquin®Forte**, **Lustra®**, **Solaquin®**, **Solaquin® Forte**, **Solaquin®Forte Gel**
C		*hydroquinone/fluocinolone/tretinoin*, **Tri-Luma®**
C		*hydroxychloroquine*, **Plaquenil®**
NR		*hydroxypropyl cellulose*, **Lacrisert®**
NR		hydroxypropyl methylcellulose, **Bion®Tears**, **GenTeal®Mild**
D		*hydroxyurea*, **Hydrea®**, **Mylocel®**
C		*hydroxyzine*, **Atarax®**, **Vistaril®**
B		**Hygroton®**, *chlorthalidone*
B		**Hylidon®**, *chlorthalidone*
B		**Hylorel®**, *qualadrel*
C		*hyoscyamine*, **Cystospaz®**, **Levbid®**, **Levsin®**, **Levsinex®Timecaps**, **NuLev®**, **Symax®SL**, **Symax®SR**
C		**Hyperab®**, *rabies immune globulin (human)*
C		**Hyper Hep®**, *hepatitis b immune globulin (human)*
C		**Hyper-Tet®**, *tetanus immune globulin (human)*
C	III	**Hy-Phen®**, *hydrocodone/acetaminophen*
NR		**Hypotears®**, *polyvinyl alcohol*
NR		**Hypotears®Ophthalmic Ointment**, *petrolatum/mineral oil*
C		**Hytone®**, *hydrocortisone*
C		**Hytrin®**, *terazosin*
C		**Hytuss®**, *guaifenesin*
C/D		**Hyzaar®**, *losartan/hydrochlorothiazide*
A		**Iberet®-Folic-500 Filmtab**, *multivitamin*
B/D		*ibuprofen*, **Advil®**, **Medipren®**, **Motrin®**, **Motrin®Migraine Pain**, **Nuprin®**, **Pamprin®-IB**, **PediaCare® Fever Drops**, **PediaProfen®**, **Rufen®**
C		*idoxuridine*, **Herplex®**, **Liquifilm®**
B		**Iletin®II Lente**, *insulin zinc suspension (lente)*
B		**Iletin®II NPH**, *insulin isophane suspension*
B		**Iletin®II Regular**, *insulin regular*
B		**Ilosone®**, *erythromycin estolate*
B		**Ilotycin®Gluceptate**, *erythromycin gluceptate*
D		*imatamib mesylate*, **Gleevec®**
B		**Imdur®**, *isosorbide mononitrate*
C		**Imferon®**, *iron dextran*
C		*imipenem/cilastatin*, **Primaxin®**

C	*imipramine,* **Janimine, Tofranil®, Tofranil®PM**
B	*imiquinod,* **Aldara®**
C	**Imitrex®, Imitrex®Injectable, Imitrex®Nasal Spray,** *sumatriptan*
C	*immune globulin,* **Gamimune®**
B	**Imodium®,** *loperamide*
B	**Imodium®AD,** *loperamide/simethicone*
C	**Imogam Rabies®,** *rabies immune globulin (human)*
C	**Imovax®, Imovax® I.D.,** *rabies vaccine (human diploid cell)*
D	**Imuran®,** *azathioprine*
B	**Increlex®,** *mecaserlin*
B	*indapamide,* **Lozol®**
C	**Inderal®, Inderal®LA,** *propranolol*
C	**Inderide®, Inderide®LA,** *propranolol/hydrochlorothiazide*
C	*indinavir,* **Crixivan®**
B/D	**Indocin®, Indocin®SR,** *indomethacin*
B/D	*indomethacin,* **Indocin®, Indocin®SR**
C	**Infergen®,** *interferon alfacon-1*
C	**Inflamase®Forte, Inflamase®Mild,** *prednisolone sodium phosphate*
C	*infliximab,* **Remicade®**
C	*influenza vaccine (trivalent, live attenuated, virus types A and B),* **Flu-Immune®, FluMist®, Flushield®**
C	**INH,** *isoniazid, isonicotinic acid hydrazide*
C	**InnoPran®XL,** *propranolol*
B	**Inspra®,** *eplernone*
C	*insulin aspart,* **NovoLog®**
C	*insulin detemir,* **Levemir®**
B	*insulin extened zinc suspension (ultralente),* **Humulin®U**
C	*insulin glargine,* **Lantus®**
B	*insulin glulisine (rDNA origin),* **Apidra®**
C	*insulin human (rDNA origin) pwdr for inhalation,* **Exubera®**
B	*insulin isophane suspension,* **Humulin®N, Iletin®II NPH, Novolin®N**
B	*insulin insophane suspension/insulin regular (***Humulin®70/30, Humulin®50/50, Novolin®70/30**)
B	*insulin lispro,* **Humalog®**
B	*insulin lispro protamine/insulin lispro,* **Humalog®Mix 75/25, Humalog®Mix 50/50**
B	*insulin regular,* **Humulin®R, Humulin®R U-500, Iletin®II Regular, Novolin®R**
B	*insulin zinc suspension (lente),* **Humulin®L, Iletin®II Lente®, Novolin®L**
B	**Intal®,** *cromolyn sodium*
C	*interferon alfa-2a,* **Roferon®-A**
C	*interferon alfa-2b,* **Intron® A**
C	*interferon alfacon-1,* **Infergen®**
C	*interferon alfa-n1,* **Wellferon®**
C	*interferon alfa-n3 (human leukocyte derived),* **Alferon®N**

C		*interferon beta-1a*, **Avonex**®
C		*interferon beta-1b*, **Betaseron**®
C		**Intron**® **A**, *interferon alfa-2b*
B		**Invanz**®, *ertapenem*
B		**Invirase**®, *saquinavir mesylate*
C		*iodoquinol, diiodohydroxyquin*, **Yodoxin**®
C	IV	**Ionamin**®, *phentermine*
C		**Iopidine**®, *apraclonidine*
C		**IPOL**®, *poliovirus vaccine*
B		*ipratropium bromide*, **Atrovent**®
C		*ipratropium/albuterol*, **Combivent**®, **DuoNeb**®
C/D		*irbesartan*, **Avapro**®
C/D		*irbesartan/hydrochlorothiazide*, **Avalide**®
D		**Iressa**®, *gefitinib*
C		*iron dextran*, **Imferon**®
C		**Ismelin**®, *guanethidine*
B		**Ismo**®, *isosorbide mononitrate*
C		**Iso-Bid**®, *isosorbide dinitrate*
C		*isocarboxazid*, **Marplan**®
C		*isoetharine*, **Bronkosol**®
C		*isoflurophate*, **Floropryl**®
C		*isometheptene/dichloralphenazone/acetaminophen*, **Midrin**®
C		*isoniazid, isonicotinic acid hydrazide*, **INH**, **Nydrazid**®
C		*isonicotinic acid, isoniazid*, **INH**, **Nydrazid**®
C		*isoproterenol,* **Isuprel**®
B		*isoproterenol*, **Medihaler**®**-ISO**
C		**Isoptin**®, **Isoptin**®**SR**, *verapamil*
C		**Isopto**®**Carbachol**, *carbachol*
C		**Isopto**®**Carpine**, *pilocarpine*
C		**Isopto**®**Eserine**, *physostigmine*
C		**Isordil**®**Sublingual, Isordil**®**Tembids, Isordil**®**Titradose**, *isosorbide dinitrate*
C		*isosorbide dinitrate*, **Dilatrate**®**-SR, Iso-Bid**®**, Isordil**® **Sublingual, Isordil**®**Tembids, Isordil**®**Titradose**, *Isotrate*®, **Novosorbide**®**, Sorbitrate**®**, Sorbitrate**®**SR**
B		*isosorbide mononitrate*, **Imdur**®**, Ismo**®**, Monoket**®
X		*isotretinoin, retinoic acid*, **Accutane**®
C		*isradipine*, **DynaCirc**®**, DynaCirc**®**CR**
C		**Istalol**®, *timolol*
C		**Isuprel**®, *isoproterenol*
C		*itraconazole*, **Sporanox**®
NR		**IvyBlock**®, *bentoquatam*
C		**Janimine**®, *imipramine*
B		**Januvia**®, *sitagliptin*
C		*Japanese encephalitis virus vaccine*, **JE-VAX**®
X		**Jenest**®**-21, Jenest**®**-28**, *ethinyl estradiol/norethindrone*
C		**JE-VAX**®, *Japanese encephalitis virus vaccine*

X		**Jolessa®**, *ethinyl estradiol/levonorgestrel*
X		**Junel®1/20, Junel®1.5/30**, *ethinyl estradiol/norethindrone*
X		**Junel®Fe 1/20, Junel®Fe 1.5/30**, *ethinyl estradiol/norethindrone*
C	II	**Kadian®**, *morphine sulfate*
D		*kanamycin*, **Kantrex®**
C		**Kaletra®**, *lopinavir/ritonavir*
D		**Kantrex®**, *kanamycin*
A		**Kaochlor®**, *potassium chloride*
A		**KaoLectrolyte®**, *electrolyte supplement*
C		*kaolin/pectin*, **Kaopectate®**
A		**Kaon®**, *potassium gluconate*
C		**Kaopectate®**, *kaolin/pectin*
X		**Kariva®**, *ethinyl estradiol*
C		**Kayexalate®**, *sodium polystyrene sulfonate*
C		**K-Dur®**, *potassium chloride*
B		**Keflet®**, *cephalexin*
B		**Keflex®**, *cephalexin*
B		**Keflin®**, *cephalothin*
B		**Keftab®, Keftab®K Pak**, *cephalexin*
B		**Kefurox®**, *cefuroxime*
B		**Kefzol®**, *cefazolin*
X		**Kelnor®**, *ethinyl estradiol/ethynodial diacetate*
C		**Kemadrin®**, *procyclidine*
C		**Kemstro®**, *baclofen*
C		**Kenacort®**, *triamcinolone acetonide*
C		**Kenalog®, Kenalog®E**, *triamcinolone*
C		**Kenalog®Injectable, Kenalog®Lotion, Kenalog®Ointment, Kenalog®Spray**, *triamcinolone acetonide*
C		**Keppra®**, *levetiracetam*
NR		**Keralyt®Gel**, *salicylic acid*
C		**Keratol®40**, *urea cream*
C		**Kerlone®**, *betaxolol*
C		**Ketek®**, *telithromycin*
C		*ketoconazole*, **Nizoral®**
B		*ketoprofen*, **Actron®, Orudis®, Orudis®KT, Oruvail®**
C		*ketorolac tromethamine*, **Acular®, Acular®PF, Toradol®**
C		*ketotifen fumarate*, **Zaditor®**
B		**Kineret®**, *anakinra*
C		**Klaron®**, *sulfacetamide*
C	IV	**Klonopin®**, *clonazepam*
A		**K-Lor®**, *potassium chloride*
A		**Klorvess®**, *potassium chloride*
A		**Klotrix®**, *potassium chloride*
A		**K-Lyte®/Cl**, *potassium chloride*
A		**K-Lyte®DS**, *potassium bicarbonate/potassium citrate*
C		**K-Norm®**, *potassium chloride*
C		**Kondremul®**, *mineral oil*

B	**Kristalose®**, *lactulose*
C	**Kronofed®-A, Kronofed®-A Jr,** *chlorpheniramine/pseudoephedrine*
C	**K-Tab®**, *potassium chloride*
C	**Kwell®Lotion, Kwell®Shampoo,** *lindane/benzene hexachloride*
B	**Kytril®**, *granisetron*
C	*labetalol*, **Normodyne®, Trandate®**
NR	**Lacri-Lube®, Lacri-Lube®NP,** *petrolatum/mineral oil*
NR	**Lacrisert®**, *hydroxypropyl cellulose*
NR	**Lactaid®**, *lactase*
NR	*lactase*, **Lactaid®**
B	*lactulose*, **Cephulac®, Chronulac®, Duphalac®, Kristalose®**
C	**Lamictal®**, *lamotrigine*
B	**Lamisil®, Lamisil®AT,** *terbinafine*
C	*lamivudine, 3TC,* **Epivir®, Epivir®-HBV**
C	*lamivudine/zidovudine,* **Combivir®**
C	*lamotrigine,* **Lamictal®**
C	**Lamprene®,** *clofazimine*
A	**Lanoxicaps®,** *digoxin*
A	**Lanoxin®,** *digoxin*
B	*lansoprazole,* **Prevacid®, Prevacid®Suspension, Prevacid®SoluTab**
B	*lansoprazole/naproxen sodium,* **Prevacid®NapraPAC,**
C	*lanthanum,* **Fosrenol®**
C	**Lantus®**, *insulin glargine*
C	**Lariam®,** *mefloquine*
C	**Larodopa®,** *levodopa, l-dopa*
B	**Larotid®,** *amoxicillin*
C	**Lasix®,** *furosemide*
C	*latanoprost,* **Xalatan®**
B	**Ledercillin®VK,** *penicillin v potassium*
X	*leflunomide,* **Arava®**
C	**Leosin®Drops, Leosin®Syrir, Leosin®S/L, Leosin®Timecaps,** *hyoscyamine*
X	**Lescol®, Lescol®XL** *fluvastatin*
X	**Jolessa®, Lessina®,** *ethinyl estradiol/levonorgestrel*
C	**Lestid®,** *colestipol*
D	*letrozole,* **Femara®**
C	*leucovorin calcium,* **Ca Folinate®, Folinic Acid®, Wellcovorin®**
D	**Leukeran®,** *chlorambucil*
X	*leuprolide,* **Viadur®**
X	*leuprolid acetate,* **Eligard®, Lupron Depot®**
C	*levalbuterol,* **Xopenex®**
C	**Levaquin®,** *levofloxacin*
C	**Levatol®,** *penbutolol*
C	**Levbid®,** *hyoscyamine*
C	**Levemir®,** *insulin detemir*
C	*levetiracetam,* **Keppra®**
B	**Levitra®,** *vardenafil*

X		**Levlen®-21, Levlen®-28**, *ethinyl estradiol/levonorgestrel*
X		**Levlite®-28**, *ethinyl estradiol/levonorgestrel*
C		*levobunolol*, **Betagan®**
C		*levocabastine*, **Livostin®**
C		*levodopa, l-dopa*, **Dopar®, Larodopa®**
B		**Levo-Dromoran®**, *levorphanol tartrate*
C		*levofloxacin*, **Levaquin®**
C		*levofloxacin ophthalmic solution*, **Quixin®**
X		*levonorgestrel*, **Nordette®, Norplant®**
X		**Levora®-21, Levora®-28**, *ethinyl estradiol/levonorgestrel*
B		*levorphanol tartrate*, **Levo-Dromoran®**
A		*levothyroxine*, **Levoxyl®, Synthroid®**
A		*levothyroxine/liothyronine (liotrix)*, **Euthroid®**
C		**Levsin®, Levsinex® Timecaps**, *hyoscyamine*
X		*levonorgestrel IUD*, **Mirena®**
A		**Levoxyl®**, *levothyroxine*
C		**Lexapro®**, *escitalopram*
C		**Lexiva®**, *fosfamprenavir*
C/D		**Lexxel®**, *enalapril/felodipine*
D	IV	**Librax®**, *chlordiazepoxide/clidinium*
D	IV	**Libritabs®, Librium®**, *chlordiazepoxide*
B		**LidaMantle®**, *lidocaine*
C		**Lidemol®**, *fluocinonide*
C		**Lidex®, Lidex-E®**, *fluocinonide*
B		*lidocaine*, **Dalcaine®, LidaMantle®, Lidoderm®, Xylocaine® Injectable, Xylocaine®Viscous Solution**
C		*lidocaine/tetracaine*, **Synera®**
B		*lidocaine/prilocaine*, **Emla® Cream, Emla® Disc**
B		**Lidoderm®**, *lidocaine*
D	IV	**Limbitrol®**, *chlordiazepoxide/amitriptyline*
B		**Lincocin®**, *lincomycin*
B		*lincomycin*, **Lincocin®**
C		*lindane/benzene hexachloride*, **Kwell®Lotion, Kwell®Shampoo, Scabene®**
C		*linezolid*, **Zyvox®**
C		**Lioresal®, Lioresal®DS**, *baclofen*
A		*liothyronine*, **Cytomel®**
A		*liothyronine/levothyroxine*, **Armour Thyroid®, Thyrolar®**
X		**Lipitor,®** *atorvastatin*
C		**Lipo-Nicin®**, *niacin, nicotinic acid, vitamin b$_3$*
C		**Liquaemin®**, *heparin*
C		**Liquibid®**, *guaifenesin*
C		**Liquibid®D**, *guaifenesin/phenylephrine*
C		**Liquifilm®**, *idoxuridine*
C/D		*lisinopril*, **Prinivil®, Zestril®**
C/D		*lisinopril/hydrochlorothiazide*, **Prinzide®, Zestoretic®**
D		**Lithane®**, *lithium carbonate*

D		*lithium carbonate*, **Eskalith®, Eskalith®CR, Lithane®, Lithobid®, Lithonate®, Lithotabs®**
D		**Lithobid®**, *lithium carbonate*
D		**Lithonate®**, *lithium carbonate*
D		**Lithotabs®**, *lithium carbonate*
C		**Livostin®**, *levocabastine*
C		**Locoid®**, *hydrocortisone butyrate*
C		**Lodine®, Lodine®XL**, *etodolac*
B		*lodoxamide tromethamine*, **Alomide®**
C		**Lodrane®24**, *brompheniramine*
X		**Loestrin®1/20, Loestrin®1.5/30**, *ethinyl estradioll/norethindrone*
X		**Loestrin®Fe 1/20, Loestrin®Fe 1.5/30, Loestrin®24 Fe**, *ethinyl estradiol/norethindrone ferrous fumarate*
C		**Lofibra®**, *fenofibrate*
C		*lomefloxacin*, **Maxaquin®**
C	V	**Lomotil®**, *diphenoxylate/atropine*
C		**Loniten®**, *minoxidil*
X		**Lo-Ogestrel®-21, Lo-Ogestrel®-28**, *ethinyl estradiol/norgestrel*
X		**Lo/Ovral®-21, Lo/Ovral®-28**, *ethinyl estradiol/norgestrel*
B		*loperamide*, **Imodium®**
B		*loperamide/simethicone*, **Imodium®AD**
C		**Lopid®**, *gemfibrozil*
C		*lopinavir/ritonavir*, **Kaletra®**
C		**Lopressor®**, *metoprolol tartrate*
C		**Lopressor®HCT**, *metoprolol tartrate/hydrochlorothiazide*
B		**Loprox®**, *ciclopirox*
C		**Lopurin®**, *allopurinol*
B		**Lorabid®**, *loracarbef*
B		*loracarbef*, **Lorabid®**
B		*loratadine*, **Claritin®**
B		*loratadine/pseudoephedrine*, **Claritin®-D 12 Hour, Claritin®-D 24 Hour**
D	IV	*lorazepam*, **Ativan®**
C	III	**Lorcet®, Lorcet®HD, Lorcet®Plus**, *hydrocodone/acetaminophen*
C	III	**Lortab®**, *hydrocodone/acetaminophen*
C	III	**Lortab®ASA**, *hydrocodone/aspirin*
C/D		*losartan*, **Cozaar®**
C/D		*losartan/hydrochlorothiazide*, **Hyzaar®**
C		**Lotemax®**, *loteprednol etabonate*
C/D		**Lotensin®**, *benazepril*
C/D		**Lotensi®HCT**, *benazepril/hydrochlorothiazide*
C		*loteprednol etabonate*, **Alrex®, Lotemax®**
C		*loteprednol/tobramycin*, **Zylet®**
C/D		**Lotrel®**, *amlodipine/benazepril*
B		**Lotrimin®**, *clotrimazole*
C		**Lotrisone®**, *clotrimazole/betamethasone dipropionate*

X		*lovastatin*, **Altoprev**®, **Mevacor**®
B		**Lovenox**®, *enoxaparin*
B		**Lozol**®, *indapamide*
C		*lubiprostone*, **Amitiza**®
B		**Ludiomil**®, *maprotiline*
C		**Lufyllin**®, *dyphylline*
C		**Lufyllin**®-**GG**, *guaifenesin/dyphylline*
C		**Lumigan**®, *bimatoprost*
D	II	**Luminal**®, *phenobarbital*
C	IV	**Lunesta**®, *eszopiclone*
X		*luprolide*, **Lupron**®**Depot**
X		**Lupron**®**Depot**, *luprolide acetate*
NR		**Luride**®, *fluoride*
C		**Lustra**®, *hydroquinone*
		lutropin alfa, **Luveris**®
		Luveris®, *lutropin alfa*
C		**Luxiq**®, *betamethasone valerate*
C		**Luxiva**®, *fosfanprenavir*
C		**Lyderm**®, *fluocinonide*
B		*lypressin*, **Diapid**®
C	V	**Lyrica**®, *pregabalin*
C		**Maalox**®, **Maalox**®**HRF**, *aluminum hydroxide/magnesium hydroxide*
C		**Maalox**®**Plus**, *aluminum hydroxide/magnesium hydroxide/ simethicone*
B		**Macrobid**®, **Macrodantin**®, *nitrofurantoin*
C		*magaldrate*, **Riopan**®
C		**Magan**®, *magnesium salicylate*
B		*magnesium citrate*, **Citrate of Magnesia**®, **Citroma**®
B		*magnesium hydroxide*, **Milk of Magnesia**®
B		*magnesium hydroxide/aluminum hydroxide/simethicone*, **Gelusil**®, **Gelusil**®**II**, **Gelusil**®**M**
B		*magnesium oxide*, **Mag-Ox**®
C		*magnesium salicylate*, **Magan**®
A		*magnesium sulfate*, **Epsom Salt**®
B		**Mag-Ox**®, *magnesium oxide*
C		**Malarone**®, **Malarone**®**Pediatric**, *atovaquone/proquanil*
B		**Mandol**®, *cefamandole*
C		**Mantadil**®, *hydrocortisone/chlorcyclizine*
B		*maprotiline*, **Ludiomil**®
C		**Marax**®, *theophylline /hydroxyzine/ephedrine*
C		**Marcaine**®, *bupivacaine*
C	III	**Marinol**®, *dronabinol*
C		**Marplan**®, *isocarboxazid*
B		**Marzine**®, *cyclizine lactate*
C		*masoprocol*, **Actinex**®
C/D		**Mavik**®, *trandolapril*
C		**Maxair**®, **Maxair**®**Autohaler**, *pirbuterol*

C		**Maxalt®, Maxalt®-MLT,** *rizatriptan*
C		**Maxaquin®,** *lomefloxacin*
C		**Maxidex®Ophthalmic,** *dexamethasone*
C	III	**Maxidone®,** *hydrocodone/acetaminophen*
C		**Maxifed®, Maxifed®-G, Maxifed®G Tab 100's, Maxifed®Tab 100's,** *guaifenesin/pseudoephedrine*
C		**Maxifed®DM, Maxifed®DM 100's** *guaifenesin/pseudoephedrine/dextromethorphan*
C		**Maxiflor®,** *diflorasone*
B		**Maxipime®,** *cefepime*
C		**Maxitrol®,** *neomycin/polymixin b/dexamethasone sodium phosphate*
C	III	**Maxi-Tuss®HC,** *hydrocodone/phenylephrine/chlorphenirimine*
C		**Maxi-Tuss®DM,** *guaifenesin/dextromethorphan*
C		**Maxivate®,** *betamethasone dipropionate*
C		**Maxzide®,** *triamterene/hydrochlorothiazide*
C		*mazindol,* **Mazanor®, Sanorex®**
C		*measles/mumps/rubella virus vaccine (live),* **M-M-R II®, M-R Vax II®**
D	II	**Mebaral®,** *mephobarbital*
C		*mebendazole,* **Vermox®**
B		*mecaserlin,* **Increlex®**
B		*meclizine,* **Antivert®, Bonine®, Dramamine®II**
B/D		**Meclofen®,** *meclofenamate*
B/D		*meclofenamate,* **Meclofen®**
B		**Medihaler®-ISO,** *isoproterenol*
B		**Medipren®,** *ibuprofen*
C		**Medrol®, Medrol® Dosepak,** *methylprednisolone*
X		*medroxyprogesterone,* **Amen®, Curretab®, Cycrin®, Depo-Provera®, DepoSubQ®, Provera®**
C		*medrysone,* **HMS®**
C		*mefenamic acid,* **Ponstan®, Ponstel®**
C		*mefloquine,* **Lariam®**
B		**Mefoxin®,** *cefoxitin*
D		**Megace®,** *megestrol*
D		**Megace®ER,** *megestrol acetate*
B		**Megacillin®,** *penicillin g potassium*
D		*megestrol,* **Megace®**
D		*megestrol acetate,* **Megace®ER**
C		*meglitimide,* **Prandin®**
D		*melphalan,* **Alkeran®**
C		**Mellaril®, Mellaril®-S,** *thioridazine*
C		*meloxicam,* **Mobic®**
C		**Menactra®,** *neisseria meningitides polysaccharides*
B		*menmantine,* **Namenda®**
X		**Menest®,** *esterified estrogens*
C		**Menomune-A/C/Y/W-135®,** *neisseria meningitis polysaccharides*
X		**Menostar®,** *estradiol*

B		**Mentax®**, *butenafine*
B		*mepenzolate*, **Cantil®**
C		*meperdine/promethazine*, **Mepergan®**, **Mepergan®Fortis**,
B/D	II	*meperidine*, **Demerol®**
C		**Mepergan®**, **Mepergan®Fortis** *meperdine/promethazine*
D		*mephenytoin*, **Mesantoin®**
D	II	*mephobarbital*, **Mebaral®**, **Methylphenobarbital®**
C		**Mephyton®**, *phytonadione*, *vitamin k*
C		*mepivacaine*, **Carbocaine®**
D		*meprobamate*, **Equanil®**, **Miltown®**
D	IV	*meprobamate/aspirin*, **Equagesic®**
B		**Merezine®Lactate**, *cyclizine lactate*
C	IV	**Meridia®**, *sibutramine*
B		*meropenem*, **Merrem®**
B		**Merrem®**, *meropenem*
C		**Meruvax®II**, *rubella virus vaccine (live)*
B		*mesalamine*, **Asacol®**, **Canasa®**, **Pentasa®**, **Rowasa®**
D		**Mesantoin®**, *mephenytoin*
C		**Mescolor®Tab**, *chlorpheniramine/pseudoephedrine/methscopolomine*
C		*mesoridazine*, **Serentil®**
X		*mestranol/norethindrone*, **Necon® 1/50-21**, **Necon® 1/50-28**, **Norethin®1/50M**, **Noriny®l 1+50-21**, **Norinyl®1+50-28**, **Ortho-Novum®1/50-21**, **Ortho-Novum®1/50-28**
C	II	**Metadate®CD**, **Metadate®ER**, *methylphenidate*
C		**Metaglip®**, *glipizide/metformin*
B		**Metahydrin®**, *trichlormethiazide*
C		**Metamucil®**, *psyllium*
C		**Metaprel®**, *metaproterenol*
C		*metaproterenol*, **Alupent®**, **Metaprel®**
B		*metaxalone*, **Skelaxin®**
B		*metformin*, **Fortamet®**, **Glucophage®**, **Glucophage®XR**, **Glumetza®**, **Riomet®**
B		*methadone*, **Dolophine®**
C	II	*methamphetamine*, **Desoxyn®**
C		*methazolamide*, **Neptazane®**
C		*methenamine hippurate*, **Hiprex®**, **Urex®**
C		**Methergine®**, *methylergonovine*
B		*methicillin*, **Staphcillin®**
D		*methimazole*, **Tapazole®**
C		*methocarbamol*, **Robaxin®**
D		*methocarbamol/aspirin*, **Robaxisal®**
D		*methotrexate*, **Mexate®**, **Rheumatrex®**, **Trexall®**
C		*methoxsalen*, **Oxsoralen®**, **Oxsoralen®Ultra**
C		*methscopolamine bromide*, **Pamine®**, **Pamine®Forte**
B		*methyclothiazide*, **Enduron®**,
B		*methyclothiazide/deserpidine*, **Enduronyl®**

B		*methyldopa*, **Aldomet**®
C		*methyldopa/chlorothiazide*, **Aldoclor**®
C		*methyldopa/hydrochlorothiazide*, **Aldoril**®
C		*methylergonovine*, **Methergine**®
C	II	**Methylin**®, **Methylin**®**ER**, *methylphenidate*
C	II	*methylphenidate*, **Concerta**®, **Daytrana**®, **Metadate**®**CD**, **Metadate**®**ER**, **Methylin**®, **Methylin**®**ER Ritalin**®, **Ritalin**®**SR**
D	II	**Methylphenobarbital**®, *mephobarbital*
C		*methylprednisolone*, **Depo-Medrol**®, **Duralone**®, **Medrol**®
C		*methylprednisolone sodium succinate*, **Solu-Medrol**®
B		*methyprylon*, **Noludar**®
C		*methsuximide*, **Celontin**®**Kapseals**
X	III	*methyltestosterone*, **Android**®, **Oreton-Methyl**®, **Testred**®, **Virilon**®
C		*methysergide*, **Sansert**®
C		**Meticorten**®, *prednisone*
C		**Metimyd**®, *sulfacetamide/prednisolone*
C		*metipranolol*, **OptiPranolol**®
B		*metoclopramide*, **Reglan**®
B		*metolazone*, **Mykrox**®, **Zaroxolyn**®
C		*metoprolol succinate*, **Toprol**®**-XL**
C		*metoprolol tartrate*, **Lopressor**®
C		*metoprolol tartrate/hydrochlorothiazide*, **Lopressor**®**HCT**
B		**MetroGel**®, **MetroGel**®**-Vaginal**, **Metrolotion**®, **Noritate**®, **Protostat**®, **Vandazole**®, *metronidazole*
D/B		*metronidazole*, **Flagyl**®, **Flagyl**®**375**, **Flagyl**®**ER**,
B		*metronidazole*, **MetroGel**®, **MetroGel**®**-Vaginal**, **Metrolotion**®, **Noritate**®, **Protostat**®, **Vandazole**®
X		**Mevacor**®, *lovastatin*
D		**Mexate**®, *methotrexate*
C		**Mezanor**®, *mazindol*
B		**Mezlin**®, *mezlocillin*
B		*mezlocillin*, **Mezlin**®
C		**Miacalcin**®**Injectable**, **Miacalcin**®**Nasal Spray**, *calcitonin-salmon*
C		**Micanol**®, *anthralin*
C/D		**Micardis**®, *telmisartan*
C/D		**Micardis**®**HCT**, *telmisartan/hydrochlorothiazide*
B		**Micatin**®, *miconazole*
B		*miconazole*, **Micatin**®, **Monistat**®, **Monistat® 3**, **Monistat®7**, **Monistat**®**Derm**, **Monistat**®**Dual-Pak**
C		**Micostatin**®, *nystatin*
X		**Microgestin**®**Fe 1/20**, **Microgestin**®**Fe 1.5/30**, *norethindrone acetate/ethinylestradiol/ferrous fumarate*
C		**Micro-K**®, *potassium chloride*
B		**Micronase**®, *glyburide*
X		**Micronor**®, *norethindrone*
B		**Microsulfon**®, *sulfadiazine*
B		**Microzide**®, *hydrochlorothiazide*

B		**Midamo®**, *amiloride*
C		*midodrine*, **ProAmatine®**
C		**Midrin®**, *isometheptene mucate/dichloralphenazone/acetaminophen*
X		**Mifeprex®**, *mifepristone*
X		*mifepristone*, **Mifeprex®**
B		*miglitol*, **Glycet®**
X		**Migranal®**, *dihydroergotamine*
B		**Milk of Magnesia®**, *magnesium hydroxide*
D	IV	**Miltown®**, *meprobamate*
A		**Mimyx®**, *olive oil, glycerin, pentylene, glycol, glycerides, vegetable oil, hydrogenated lecithin, squaline, betaine, palmitamide, MEA, sarcosine, acetamide MEA, Hydroxyethel cellulose, sodium carbomer, xanthan gum*
C		*mineral oil*, **Kondremul®**
C		**Minipress®**, *prazosin*
C		**Minitran®**, *nitroglycerin*
C		**Minizide®**, *prazosin/polythiazide*
D		**Minocin®**, *minocycline*
D		*minocycline*, **Arestin®**, **Dynacin®**, **Minocin®**
C		*minoxidil*, **Loniten®**, **Rogaine®**
C		**Mintezol®**, *thiabendazole*
C		**MiraLax®**, *polyethylene glycol*
C		**Mirapex®**, *pramipexole dihydrochloride*
X		**Mircette®**, *ethinyl estradiol/desogestrel diacetate*
X		**Mirena®**, *levonorgestrel IUD*
C		*mirtazepine*, **Remeron®**, **Remeron®Soltab**
X		*misoprostol*, **Cytotec®**
X		**Mithracin®**, *plicamycin*
D		*mitomycin*, **Mutamycin®**
C		**M-M-R II®**, *measles/mumps/rubella virus vaccine (live)*
C		**M-R Vax II®**, *measles/mumps/rubella virus vaccine (live)*
C		**Moban®**, *molindone*
C		**Mobic®**, *meloxicam*
C		*modafinil*, **Provigil®**
X		**Modicon®**, *ethinyl estradiol/norethindrone*
B		**Moduretic®**, *amiloride/hydrochlorothiazide*
C/D		*moexipril*, **Univasc®**
C/D		*moexipril/hydrochlorothiazide*, **Uniretic®**
D		**Mogadon®**, *nitrazepam*
C		*molindone*, **Moban®**
C		*mometasone furoate*, **Elocon®**, **Asmanex®**
C		*mometasone furoate monohydrate*, **Nasonex®**
B		**Monistat®, Monistat®3, Monistat®7, Monistat®Derm, Monistat® Dual Pak**, *miconazole*
C		*monobenzone*, **Benoquin®**
B		**Monocid®**, *cefonicid*
D		**Monodox®**, *doxycycline*

C		**Mono-gesic®**, *salsalate*
B		**Monoket®**, *isosorbide mononitrate*
C/D		**Monopril®**, *fosinopril*
C/D		**Monopril®HCT**, *fosinopril/hydrochlorothiazide*
B		*montelukast*, **Singulair®**, **Singulair®Chewable**
B		**Monurol®**, *fosfomycin*
C	II	*morphine sulfate*, **Astramorph®/PF, Avinza®, Duramorph®, Kadian®, MS Contin®, MSIR, Oramorph® SR, Roxanol®, Roxanol®Rescudose**
B/D		**Motrin®, Motrin® Migraine Pain**, *ibuprofen*
C		**Motofen®**, *difenoxin/atropine*
C		*moxifloxacin*, **Avelox®, Vigamox®**
C	II	**MS Contin®**, *morphine sulfate*
C	II	**MSIR®**, *morphine sulfate*
C		**Mucinex®**, *guaifenesin*
C		**Mucinex-D®**, *quaifinesin extended-relese/pseudoephedrine*
C		**Mucinex®-DM**, *guaifenesin/dextromethorphan*
B		**Mucomyst**, *acetylcysteine*
A		*multivitamin*, **Berocca®, Cefol®, Chromagen, Chromagen®FA, Chromagen®Forte, Glutofac®-ZX, Folbee®, Folbee®Plus, Folbic®, Iberet®-Folic-500 Filmtab, Theragran®, Trinsicon®, Tri-Vi-Flor®, Uni-Cap®, Vicon Forte®, Zenate®**
A		*vitamin with minerals*, **Berocca® Plus, Theragran®-M**
C		**Mumpsvax®**, *mumps virus vaccine (live)*
C		*mumps virus vaccine (live)*, **Mumpsvax®**
B		*mupirocin*, **Bactroban®, Centany®**
NR		**Muro®128, Muro®128 Ophthalmic Ointment**, *sodium chloride*
X		**Muse®**, *alprostadil urethral suppository*
D		**Mutamycin®**, *mitomycin*
B		**Myambutol®**, *ethambutol*
B		**Mybrox®**, *metolazone*
B		**Mycelex®7, Mycelex®G, Mycelex®G Vaginal Tablets, Mycelex® Troche**, *clotrimazole*
D		**Mycifradin®**, *neomycin*
C		**Mycitracin®**, *neomycin/polymixin-b/bacitracin zinc*
B		**Mycobutin®**, *rifabutin*
A		*mycofolic acid*, **Myfortic®**
C		**Mycogen®II, Mycolog®II**, *nystatin/triamcinolone acetonide*
C		**Mycostatin®**, *nystatin*
A		**Myfortic®**, *mycofolic acid*
B		**MyKrox®**, *metolazone*
C		**Mylanta®, Mylanta®DS**, *aluminum hydroxide/magnesium hydroxide/simethicone*
C		**Mylicon®**, *simethicone*
D		**Mylocel®**, *hydroxyurea*
D		**Mysoline®**, *primidone*
C		*nabilone*, **Cesamet®**

C		*nabumetone,* **Relafen**®
C		*nadolol,* **Corgard**®
C		*nadolol/bendroflumethiazide,* **Corzide**®
X		*nafarelin,* **Synarel**®
B		**Nafcil**®, *nafcillin*
B		*nafcillin,* **Nafcil**®, **Nallpen**®, **Unipen**®
B		*naftifine,* **Naftin**®
B		**Naftin**®, *naftifine*
B		*nalbuphine,* **Nubain**®
C		**Naldecon**®**Senior DX**, *guaifenesin/dextromethorphan*
C		**Nalex**®, **Nalex**®**Jr**, *guaifenesin/pseudoephedrine*
C		**Nalex**®**-A, Nalex**®**-A Liquid**, *chlorpheniramine/phenylephrine/ phenyltoloxamine*
C	III	**Nalex**®**DH**, *phenylephrine/hydrocodone*
B/D		**Nalfon**®, *fenoprofen*
B		*nalidixic acid,* **NegGram**®
B		**Nallpen**®, *nafcillin*
B		*nalmefene,* **Revex**®
B		*naloxone,* **Narcan**®
C		*naltrexone,* **ReVia**®, **Vivitrol**®
B		**Namenda**®, *mamantine*
C		*naphazoline,* **Vasocon**®**-A**
C		**Naphcon**®**A**, *naphazoline/pheniramine*
C		**Napramide**®, *disopyramide phosphate*
B		**Naprelan**®, *naproxen*
B		**Naprosyn**®, *naproxen*
B		*naproxen,* **Aleve**®, **Anaprox**®, **Anaprox**®**DS, EC-Naprosyn**®, **Naprelan**®, **Naprosyn**®
B		**Naqua**®, *trichlormethiazide*
C		*naratriptan,* **Amerge**®
B		**Narcan**®, *naloxone*
C		**Nardil**®, *phenelzine*
C		**Nasacort**®, **Nasacort**®**AQ**, *triamcinolone acetonide*
B		**NasalCrom**®, *cromolyn sodium*
C		**Nasalide**®, *flunisolide*
C		**Nasarel**®, *flunisolide*
C		**Nasatab**®**LA**, *guaifenesin/pseudoephedrine*
C		**Nascobal**®, *cyanocobalamin, vitamin b_{12}*
C		**Nasonex**®, *mometasone furoate monohydrate*
C		**Natacyn**®, *natamycin*
A		**NataChew**®, *prenatal vitamin*
A		**Natafort**®, *prenatal vitamin*
A		**Natalins**®, *prenatal vitamin*
C		*natalizumab,* **Tysabri**®
C		*natamycin,* **Natacyn**®
C		*nateglinide,* **Starlix**®
C		**Natrecor**®, *nesiritide*

C		**Navane®**, *thiothixene*
D		**Nebcin®**, *tobramycin*
C		**Nebupent®**, *pentamidine isethionate*
X		**Necon®0.5/35-21, Necon®0.5/35-28, Necon®1/35-21, Necon®1/35-28, Necon®10/11-21, Necon®10/11-28**, *ethinyl estradiol/norethindrone*
X		**Necon® 1/50-21, Necon® 1/50-28**, *mestranol/norethindrone*
B		*nedocromil*, **Alocril®, Tilade®**
B		**NegGram®**, *nalidixic acid*
C		*neisseria meningitides polysaccharides*, **Menactra®, Menomune®-A/C/Y/W-135**
D		*nelarabine*, **Arranon®**
B		*nelfinavir*, **Viracept®**
X		**Nelova®1/50-21, Nelova®1/50-28**, *ethinyl estradiol/mestranol*
X		**Nelova®0.5/35-21, Nelova®0.5/35-28, Nelova®1/35-21, Nelova®1/35-28, Nelova®10/11-21, Nelova®10/11-28**, *ethinyl estradiol/norethindrone*
D	II	**Nembutal®**, *pentobarbital*
C		*nesiritide*, **Natrecor®**
C		**NeoDecadron®Ophthalmic, NeoDecadron®Topical Cream**, *neomycin/dexamethasone sodium phosphate*
X		**Neoloid®**, *castor oil*
C		**Neomycin®**, *polymixin b/bacitracin zinc*
C		*neomycin*, **Mycifradin®**
C		*neomycin/dexamethasone sodium phosphate*, **NeoDecadron® Ophthalmic, NeoDecadron®Topical Cream**
C		*neomycin/polymixin-b/bacitracin zinc*, **Mycitracin®, Neosporin® Ointment, Neosporin®Ophthalmic Ointment**
C		*neomycin/polymixin b/dexamethasone sodium phosphate*, **Maxitrol®**
C		*neomycin/polymixin b/hydrocortisone*, **PediOtic®**
C		**Neoral®**, *cyclosporine*
C		**Neosporin®Ointment, Neosporin®Ophthalmic Ointment**, *neomycin/polymixin b/bacitracin zinc*
C		**Neo-Synephrine®**, *phenylephrine*
C		**Neptazane®**, *methazolamide*
B		**Nervocaine®**, *lidocaine*
C		**Nesacaine®, Nesacaine®-CE**, *chloroprocaine*
C		**Neurontin®**, *gabapentin*
C		*nevirapine*, **Viramune®**
B		**Nexium®**, *esomperazole*
C		*niacin, nicotinic acid, vitamin b_3*, **Lipo-Nicin®, Niacinol®, Niacor®, Niaspan®, Nicloside®, Nicolar®, Nicotinex®, Slo-Niacin®**
X		*niacin/lovostatin*, **Advicor®**
C		**Niacinol®**, *niacin, nicotinic acid, vitamin b_3*
C		**Niacor®**, *niacin, nicotinic acid, vitamin b_3*
C		**Niaspan®**, *niacin, nicotinic acid, vitamin b_3*
B		**Niazide®**, *trichlormethiazide*
C		*nicardipine*, **Cardene®, Cardene®SR**

D		**Nicoderm®, Nicoderm®CQ,** *nicotine transdermal system*
C		**Nicolar®,** *niacin, nicotinic acid, vitamin b₃*
X		**Nicorette®Gum,** *nicotine polacrilex*
D		*nicotine nasal spray,* **Nicotrol®NS**
D		*nicotine transdermal system,* **Habitrol®, Nicoderm®, Nicoderm®CQ, Nicotrol®, Nicotrol®Step-down Patch, ProStep®**
X		*nicotine polacrilex,* **Nicorette®Gum**
C		**Nicotinex®,** *niacin, nicotinic acid, vitamin b₃*
D		**Nicotrol®, Nicotrol® Step-down Patch** *nicotine transdermal system*
D		**Nicotrol®NS,** *nicotine nasal spray*
C		*nifedipine,* **Adalat®, Adalat®CC, Procardia®, Procardia®XL**
A		**Niferex®PN, Niferex®PN Forte,** *prenatal vitamin*
C		**Nilstat®,** *nystatin*
C		**Nilandron®,** *nilutamide*
C		*nilutamide,* **Nilandron®**
C		*nimodipine,* **Nimotop®**
C		**Nimotop®,** *nimodipine*
D	IV	**Niravam®,** *alprazolam*
C		*nisoldipine,* **Sular®,**
B		*nitazoxamide,* **Alinia®**
D		*nitrazepam,* **Mogadon®**
C		**Nitro-Bid®,** *nitroglycerin*
C		**Nitrodisc®,** *nitroglycerin*
C		**Nitro-Dur,** *nitroglycerin*
B		*nitrofurantoin,* **Furadantin®, Macrobid®, Macrodantin®**
C		**Nitrogard®, Nitrogard®-SR,** *nitroglycerin*
C		*nitroglycerin,* **Deponit®, Minitran®, Nitro-Bid®, Nitrodisc®, Nitro-Dur®, Nitrogard®, Nitrogard®-SR, Nitrol®, Nitrolingual®, Nitropaste®, Nitrostat®, Norto-TD®, Transderm-Nitro®**
C		**Nitrol®,** *nitroglycerin*
C		**Nitrolingual®,** *nitroglycerin*
C		**Nitropaste®,** *nitroglycerin*
C		**Nitrosta®t,** *nitroglycerin*
B		**NIX®,** *permethrin*
C		*nizatidine,* **Axid®, Axid®AR**
C		**Nizoral®,** *ketoconazole*
C		**Noctec®,** *chloral hydrate*
C		**Nolamine®,** *chlorpheniramine/pseudoephedrine/phenindamine*
B		**Noludar®,** *methyprylon*
D		**Nolvadex®,** *tamoxifen*
C	III	**Norco®,** *hydrocodone/acetaminophen*
X		**Nordette®-21, Nordette®-28,** *ethinyl estradiol/levonorgestrel*
C		**NordiFlex®,** *somatropin*
C		**Norditropin®, Norditropin®AQ, Norditropin®NordiFlex,** *somatropin*
X		*norelgestromin/ethinyl estradiol,* **Ortho Evra®**
X		**Norethin®1/35-21, Norethin®1/35-28,** *ethinyl estradiol/norethindrone*

X		**Norethin®1/50-21, Norethin®1/50-28,** *mestranol/norethindrone*
X		*norethindrone,* **Aygestin®, Camila®, Errin®, Micronor®-28, Norlutate®, Norlutin®, Nor-QD®**
X		*norethindrone acetate/ethinyl estradiol/ferrous fumarate,* **Microgestin®Fe 1/20, Microgestin®Fe 1.5/30**
C		**Norflex®,** *orphenadrine*
C		*norfloxacin,* **Chibroxin®, Noroxin®**
C		**Norgesic®,** *orphenadrine/aspirin*
C		**Norgesic®Forte,** *orphenadrine/aspirin/caffeine*
X		*norgestrel,* **Ovrette®**
X		**Norinyl®1+35-21, Norinyl®1+35-28,** *ethinyl estradiol/ norethindrone*
X		**Norinyl®1+50-21, Norinyl®1+50-28,** *mestranol/norethindrone*
D/B		**Noritate®,** *metronidazole*
X		**Norlutate®,** *norethindrone*
X		**Norlutin®,** *norethindrone*
C		**Normiflo®,** *ardeparin*
C		**Normodyne®,** *labetalol*
C		**Noroxin®,** *norfloxacin*
C		**Norpace®, Norpace®CR,** *disopyramide*
X		**Norplant®,** *levonorgestrel*
C		**Norpramin®,** *desipramine*
X		**Nor-QD®,** *norethindrone*
C		**Norto-TD®,** *nitroglycerin*
X		**Nortrel® 0.5/35, Nortrel® 1/35,** *ethinyl estradiol, norethindrone*
D		*nortriptyline,* **Aventyl®, Pamelor®**
C		**Norvasc®,** *amlodipine*
B		**Norvir®,** *ritonavir*
C		**Novacet®Lotion,** *sulfacetamide/sulfur*
C		**Novafed®,** *pseudoephedrine*
C		**Novahistine®DMX,** *guaifenesin/dextromethorphan/pseudoephedrine*
B		**Novamoxin®,** *amoxicillin*
C		**Novocolchine®,** *colchicine*
B		**Novolexin®,** *cephalexin*
B		**Novolin®70/30,** *insulin isophane suspension/insulin regular*
B		**Novolin®L,** *insulin zinc suspension (lente)*
B		**Novolin®N,** *insulin isophane suspension (lente)*
B		**Novolin®R,** *insulin regular*
C		**NovoLog®,** *insulin aspart*
C		**Novoquinine®,** *quinine*
C		**Novosorbide®,** *isosorbide dinitrate*
B		**Novothalidone®,** *chlorthalidone*
C		**Noxafil®,** *posaconazole*
B		**Nubain®,** *nalbuphine*
C	III	**Nucofed®,** *codeine/pseudoephedrine*
C	III	**Nucofed®Expectorant,** *codeine/pseudoephedrine/quaifenesin*
C		**NuLev®,** *hyoscyamine*

C	II	**Numorphan®, Opana®, Opana®ER,** *oxymorphone*
C		**Nupercainal®,** *dibucaine*
B/D		**Nuprin®,** *ibuprofen*
C		**Nutracort®,** *hydrocortisone*
C		**Nutropin®, Nutropin®AQ,** *somatropin*
C		**Nydrazid®,** *isoniazid, isonicotinic acid hydrazide*
C		*nystatin,* **Micostatin®, Mycostatin®, Nilstat®, Nystop®**
C		*nystatin/triamcinolone,* **Mycogen®II, Mycolog®II**
C		**Nystop®,** *nystatin*
B		**Nytol®Quipcaps, Nytol®Quiptabs,** *diphenhydramine*
A		*oatmeal colloid,* **Aveeno®**
NR		**Occlusal-HP®,** *salicylic acid*
C		**Ocuflox®,** *ofloxacin*
C		**Ocuhist®,** *naphazoline/pheniramine*
C		**Ocupress®,** *carteolol*
C		*ofloxacin,* **Floxin®, Floxin®Otic Solution®, Ocuflox®**
X		**Ogen®, Ogen®Vaginal Cream,** *estropipate*
C		*olanzapine,* **Zyprexa®, Zyprexa®Zudis**
C		*olanzapine/fluoxetine,* **Symbyax®**
C/D		*olmesartan medoxomil,* **Benicar®**
C/D		*olmesartan medoxomil/hydrochlorothiazide,* **Benicar®HCT**
C		*olopatadine,* **Patanol®**
C		*olsalazine,* **Dipentum®**
C		**Olux®,** *clobetasol propionate foam*
B		*omalizumab,* **Xolair®**
B		*omeprazole,* **Prilosec®, Repinex®**
B		*omeprazole/na bicarbonate,* **Zegerid®**
B		**Omnicef®,** *cefdinir*
C		**Omnihib®,** *haemophilus b conjugate vaccine/tetanus toxoid conjugate*
B		**Omnipen®, Omnipen-N®,** *ampicillin*
C	II	**Opana®, Opana®ER,** *oxymorphone*
C		**Ophthaine®,** *proparacaine*
C		**Ophthochlor®,** *chloramphenicol*
C		*opium alkaloids hydrochloride,* **Pantopon®**
B		**Opticrom®,** *cromolyn sodium*
B		**Optimine®,** *azatadine*
C		**OptiPranolol®,** *metipranolol*
C		**Optivar®,** *azelastine*
D		**Oracea®,** *doxycycline*
B		**OraDisc A®,** *amlexanox*
C		**Orajel®,** *benzocaine*
C	II	**Oramorph®SR,** *morphine sulfate*
C		**Orap®,** *pimozide*
C		**Orapred®, Orapred®ODT,** *prednisolone sodium phosphate*
C		**Orasone®,** *prednisone*
C		**Orencia®,** *abatacept*
B		**Oretic®,** *hydrochlorothiazide*

X	III	**Oreton-Methyl®,** *methyltestosterone*
C		**Organidin®-NR,** *guaifenesin/dextromethorphan*
C		**Orimune®,** *trivalent oral polio vaccine*
C		**Orinase®,** *tolbutamide*
B		*orlistat,* **Xenical®**
C		**Ornex®,** *pseudoephedrine/acetaminophen*
C		*orphenadrine,* **Banflex®, Flexon®, Norflex®**
C		*orphenadrine/aspirin,* **Norgesic®**
C		*orphenadrine/aspirin/caffeine,* **Norgesic®Forte**
X		**Ortho-Cept®-21, Ortho-Cept®-28,** *ethinyl estradiol/desogestrel*
X		**Ortho-Cyclen®-21, Ortho-Cyclen®-28,** *ethinyl estradiol/ norgestimate*
X		**Ortho Dienestrol®,** *dienestrol*
X		**Ortho-Est®,** *estropipate*
X		**Ortho Evra®,** *norelgestromin/ethinyl estradiol*
X		**Ortho-Novum®1/35-21, Ortho-Novum®1/35-28, Ortho-Novum® 777-21, Ortho-Novum®777-28, Ortho-Novum®10/11-21, Ortho-Novum®10/11-28,** *ethinyl estradiol/norethindrone*
X		**Ortho-Novum®1/50-21, Ortho-Novum®1/50-28** *mestranol/ norethindrone*
X		**Ortho Prefest®,** *estradiol/norgestimate*
X		**Ortho Tri-Cyclen®-21, Ortho Tri-Cyclen®-28, Ortho Tri-Cyclen® Lo,** *ethinyl estradiol/norgestimate*
B		**Orudis®, Orudis®KT, Oruvail®,** *ketoprofen*
C		*osalazine,* **Dipentum®**
NR		**Os-Cal®,** *calcium carbonate*
C		*oseltamivir,* **Tamiflu®**
X		**Ovcon®35 Chewable, Ovcon®35-21, Ovcon®35-28, Ovcon®50-21, Ovcon®50-28,** *ethinyl estradiol/norethindrone*
X		**Ovral®-21, Ovral®-28,** *ethinyl estradiol/norgestrel*
X		**Ovrette®,** *norgestrel*
B		*oxacillin,* **Bactocill®, Prostaphlin®**
C		*oxaprozin,* **Daypro®**
D	IV	*oxazepam,* **Serax®**
C		*oxcarbazepine,* **Trileptal®**
B		*oxiconazole,* **Oxistat®**
B		**Oxistat®,** *oxiconazole*
C		**Oxsoralen®, Oxsoralen®Ultra,** *methoxsalen*
C		*oxtriphylline,* **Choledyl®SA**
B		*oxybutynin,* **Ditropan®, Ditropan®XL**
B	II	*oxycodone,* **OxyContin®, OxyFast®, OxyIR®, Percolone®, Roxicodone®**
C	II	*oxycodone/acetaminophen,* **Percocet®, Tylox®**
C	II	*oxycodone/ibuprofen,* **Combunox®**
C	II	*oxycodone/oxycodone terephthalate/aspirin,* **Percodan®, Percodan®-Demi**
B	II	**OxyContin®,** *oxycodone controlled-release*

B	II	**OxyFast®**, *oxycodone immediate-release*
B	II	**OxyIR®**, *oxycodone*
C		*oxymetazoline*, **Afrin®**
C	II	*oxymorphone*, **Numorphan®**, **Opana®**, **Opana®ER**
D		*oxytetracycline*, **Terramycin®**, **Uri-Tet®**
NR		**Oystercal®**, *calcium carbonate*
C	II	**Paladone®**, *hydromorphone*
C		**Palgic®** *carbinoxaminene*
C		**Palgic®-D** *carbinoxamine/pseudoephedrine*
C		**Palgic®DS** *chlorpheniramine/pseudoephedrine*
NR		*palivizumab*, **Synagis®**
B		*palonosetron*, **Aloxi®**
D		**Pamelor®**, *nortriptyline*
C		**Pamine®**, *methscopolamine*
B/D		**Pamprin®-IB**, *ibuprofen*
B		**Panadol®**, *acetaminophen*
C	III	**Pancof®**, *dihydrocodeine/pseudoephedrine/chlorpheniramine*
C	III	**Pancof®EXP**, *dihydrocodeine/pseudoephedrine/guaifenesin*
C	III	**Pancof®PD**, *dihydrocodeine/chlorpheniramine/phenylephrine*
C		**Pancrease®MT**, *pancrelipase*
C		*pancrelipase*, **Cotazym®**, **Cotazym®S**, **Creon®**, **Donnazyme®**, **Kuzyme®**, **Pancrease®MT**, **Ultrase®MT**, **Viokase®**, **Zymase®**
C		**Pandel®**, *hydrocortisone probutate*
C	III	**Panlor®DC, Panlor®SS**, *dihydrocodeine/acetaminophen/caffeine*
C		**Panmist®DM**, *dextromethorphan/pseudoephedrine/guaifenesin*
C		**Panmist®JR**, *pseudoephedrine/guaifenesin*
C		**Panmist®LA**, *pseudoephedrine/guaifenesin*
D		**Panmycin®**, *tetracycline*
C		**Pannaz**, *pseudoephedrinee/chlorpheniramine/methscopolomine*
C		**Pantopon®**, *opium alkaloids hydrochlorides*
B		*pantoprazole*, **Protonix®**
D		**Panwarfin®**, *warfarin*
D		**Paradione®**, *parametkadione*
C		**Paraflex®**, *chlorzoxazone*
C		**Parafon®Forte**, *chlorzoxazone*
C		**Paral®**, *paraldehyde*
C		*paraldehyde*, **Paral®**
D		*parametkadione*, **Paradione®**
C		*parametkasone*, **Haldrone®**
C		**Parcopa®**, *carbidopa/levodopa*
B/D	III	**Paregoric®**, *camphorated tincture of opium*
B		**Parlodel®**, *bromocriptine*
C		**Parnate®**, *tranylcypromine*
C		*paromomycin*, **Humatin®**
D		*paroxetine*, **Paxil®**
D		*paroxetine mesylate*, **Paxil®CR**
C		**Patanol®**, *olopatadine*

B		**Pathocil®**, *dicloxacillin*
D		**Paxil®**, *paroxetine*
D		**Paxil®CR**, *paroxetine mesylate*
D	IV	**Paxipam®**, *halazepam*
B		**PBZ®, PBZ®-SR**, *tripelennamine*
B		**PCE®**, *erythromycin base*
B/D		**PediaCare®Fever Drops**, *ibuprofen*
C		**PediaCare®Infant Decongestant**, *guaifenesin/pseudoephedrine*
C		**PediaCare®Infant Decongestant Plus Cough**, *pseudoephedrine/dextromethorphan*
C		**PediaCare®Cough Cold Liquid**, *pseudoephedrine/Dextromethorphan/chlorpheniramine*
C		**PediaCare®Night Rest Cough, Cold Liquid, PediaCare®Night Rest Cough, Cold Chewables**, *pseudoephedrine/dextromethorphan/chlorpheniramine*
B		**Pediamycin®**, *erythromycin ethylsuccinate*
C		**Pediapred®**, *prednisolone sodium phosphate*
B/D		**PediaProfen®**, *ibuprofen*
C		**Pediatex®**, *carbinoxamine*
C		**Pediatex®-D**, *carbinoxamine/pseudoephedrine*
C		**Pediazole®**, *erythromycin ethylsuccinate/sulfasoxazole*
C		**PediOtic®**, *neomycin/polymixin b/hydrocortisone*
C		**Pediox®**, *carbinoxamine*
C		**PedvaxHIB®**, *haemophilus b conjugated vaccine*
C		**Peganone®**, *ethotoin*
C		**Pegasys®**, *peginterferon alpha-2a*
C		*peginterferon alpha-2a*, **Pegasys®**
C		*peginterferon alfa-2b*, **Peg-Intron®**
C		**Peg-Intron®**, *peginterferon alfa-2b*
B		**Pelamine®**, *tripelennamine*
C		*pemirolast*, **Alamast®**
B		*pemoline*, **Cylert®**
C		*penbutolol*, **Levatol®**
B		*penciclovir*, **Denavir®**
C		**Penetrex®**, *enoxacin*
D		*penicillamine*, **Cuprimine®, Depen®**
B		*penicillin g benzathine*, **Bicillin®, Bicillin®L-A, Permapen®**
B		*penicillin g benzathine/penicillin g procaine*, **Bicillin®C-R**
B		*penicillin g potassium*, **Megacillin®, Pentids®**
B		*penicillin g procaine*, **Crysticillin®AS, Duracillin®, Wycillin®**
B		*penicillin v potassium*, **Betapen®-VK, Ledercillin®VK, Pen-Vee-®K, Robicillin®, V-Cillin-K®, Veetids®**
NR		**Penlac®Nail Laquer**, *ciclopirox topical solution*
C		*pentamidine isethionate*, **Nebupent®**
D	IV	*pentazocine*, **Talwin®**
D	IV	*pentazocine/acetaminophen*, **Talacen®**
C	IV	*pentazocine/aspirin*, **Talwin®Compound**

D	IV	*pentazocine/naloxone*, **Talwin®NX**
B		**Pentids®**, *penicillin g potassium*
D	II	*pentobarbital*, **Nembutal®**
C		**PentoPak®**, *pentoxifylline*
B		*pentosan polysulfate sodium*, **Elmiron®**
C		*pentoxifylline*, **PentoPak®**, **Trental®**
B		**Pen-Vee®-K**, *penicillin v potassium*
B		**Pepcid®, Pepcid®AC, Pepcid®RPD**, *famotidine*
C		**Pepcid®Complete**, *famotidine/CaCO₂/Mg hydroxide*
C/D		**Pepto-Bismol®**, *bismuth subsalicylate*
C	II	**Percocet®**, *oxycodone/acetaminophen*
C	II	**Percodan®, Percodan®-Demi**, *oxycodone/oxycodone/terephthalate/aspirin*
B	II	**Percolone®**, *oxycodone*
B		**Perdiem®**, *psyllium hydrophilic mucoloid*
B		**Periactin®**, *cyproheptadine*
C		**Peri-Colace®**, *docusate/casanthranol*
B		**Peridex®**, *chlorhexidine gluconate*
C		**Peridol®**, *haloperidol*
C/D		*perindopril*, **Aceon®**
B		**PerioGard®**, *chlorhexidine gluconate*
B		**Permapen®**, *penicillin g benzathine*
B		*permethrin*, **Acticin®, Elimite®, NIX**
C		*perphenazine*, **Trilafon®**
C		*perphenazine/amitriptyline*, **Etrafon®, Triavil®**
C		**Persa-Gel®**, *benzoyl peroxide*
B		**Persantine®**, *dipyridamole*
C		**Pertofrane®**, *desipramine*
NR		*petrolatum/cocoa butter/phenylephrine*, **Preparation H®Suppository**
NR		*petrolatum/glycerin/shark liver oil/phenylephrine*, **Preparation H® Ointment**
NR		*petrolatum/lanolin/mineral oil*, **Duratears Naturale®**
NR		*petrolatum/mineral oil*, **Hypotears®, Lacri-Lube®, LacriLube®NP**
NR		*petrolatum/shark liver oil/phenylephrine*, **Preparation®H Cream**
C		**Phazyme®**, *simethicone*
B		**Phenaphen®**, *acetaminophen*
C	III	**Phenaphen®with Codeine #3, #4**, *acetaminophen/codeine*
B		**Phenazodine**, *phenazopyridine*
B		*phenazopyridine*, **Azo Standard®, Phenazodine®, Prodium®, Pyridiate®, Pyridium®, Uristat®, Urodine®, Urogesic®, Vacon®**
C	III	*phendimetrazine*, **Bontril®, Prelu-2®**
C		*phenelzine*, **Nardil®**
C		**Phenergan®**, *promethazine*
C		**Phenergan®DM**, *promethazine/dextromethorphan*
C	III	**Phenergan®w/ Codeine**, *promethazine/codeine*
C		**Phenergan®VC**, *promethazine/phenylephrine*
C	III	**Phenergan®VC w/ Codeine**, *promethazine/codeine/phenylephrine*

C		*pheniramine/pyrilamine/phenyltoloxamine/pseudoephedrine*, **Poly-Histine®-D**
D	II	*phenobarbital*, **Luminal®**, **Phenobarbital®**
C	II	*phenobarbital/hyoscyamine/atropine/scopolamine*, **Donnatal®**
C		*phenolphalein*, **Correctol®**, **Ex-Lax®**, **Feen-A-Mint®**
C		*phenoxybenzamine*, **Dibenzyline®**
C	IV	*phentermine*, **Adipex-P®**, **Fastin®**, **Ionamin®**, **Pro-Fast®HS**, **Pro-Fast®SA Tab 100's**, **Pro-Fast®SR Cap 100's**
C		*phentolamine*, **Regitine®**
D		*phenylbutazone*, **Azolid®**, **Butazolidin®**
C		*phenylephrine*, **Neo-Synephrine®**, **Sinex®**
C		*phenylephrine/brompheniramine*, **Dimetane®Decongestant**
C		*phenylephrine/chlorpheniramine/methscopolamine*, **Duradryl®**
C	III	*phenylephrine/hydrocodone*, **Nalex®DH**
C		*phenylephrine/pyrilamine*, **Ryna®-12**
D		**Phenytek®**, *phenytoin*
D		*phenytoin*, **Dilantin®**, **Phenytek®**
C		**PhisoHex®**, *hexachlorophene*
C		**Phos-Ex®**, **PhosLo®**, *calcium acetate*
C		**Phospholine®Iodide**, *echothiophate*
NR		*phosphorated carbohydrated solution*, **Emetrol®**
C	II	**Phrenilin®**, **Phrenilin®Forte**, *butalbital/acetaminophen*
C		*physostigmine salicylate*, **Isopto Eserine®**
C		*phytonadione*, *vitamin k*, **AquaMEPHYTON®**, **Mephyton®**
C		**Pilocar®**, *pilocarpine*
C		*pilocarpine*, **Isopto Carpine®**, **Pilocar®**, **Pilopine®HS**
C		**Pilopine®HS**, *pilocarpine*
C		*pimecrolimus*, **Elidel®**
C		*pimozide*, **Orap®**
B		*pindolol*, **Visken®**
C		**Pin-X®**, *pyrantel pamoate*
C		*pioglitazone*, **Actos®**
C		*pioglitazone/glimepiride*, **Duetact®**
B		**Pipracil®**, *piperacillin*
B		*piperacillin*, **Pipracil®**
B		*piperacillin/tazobactam*, **Zosyn®**
B		*piperazine*, **Vermizine®**
C		*pirbuterol*, **Maxair®**, **Maxair® Autohaler**
C		*piroxicam*, **Feldene®**
C		**Placidyl®**, *ethchlorvynol*
C		**Plaquenil®**, *hydroxychloroquine*
D		**Platinol®**, *cisplatin*
B		**Plavix®**, *clopidagrel*
X		**Plenaxis®**, *abarelix*
C		**Plendil®**, *felodipine*
C		**Pletal®**, *cilostazol*
X		*plicamycin*, **Mithracin®**

C	pneumococcal 7-valent conjugate vaccine, **Prevnar**®
C	pneumococcal vaccine, **Pneumovax**®**23**, **Pnu-Immune**®**23**
C	**Pneumovax**®**23**, pneumococcal vaccine
C	**Pnu-Immune**®**23**, pneumococcal vaccine
C	**Podo-Ben**®, **Podo-Ben-25**®, podophyllin
C	**Podocon-25**®, podophyllin
C	podofilox, **Condylox**®
C	**Podofin**®, podophyllin
C	podophyllin, **Podo-Ben**®, **Podo-Ben**®**-25**, **Podocon**®**-25**, **Podofin**®
B	**Polaramine**®, dexchlorpheniramine
B	**Polycillin**®, ampicillin
C	**Polycitra**®**-K**, potassium citrate
C	polyethylene glycol, **MiraLax**®
C	poliovirus vaccine, **IPOL**®
NR	polyethylene glycol/propylene glycol, **Systane**®
NR	polyethylene glycol/glycerin/hydroxypropyl methylcellulose, **Visine**®**Tears**
C	**Poly-Histine**®**-D**, pheniramine/pyrilamine/phenyltoloxamine/
C	**Poly-Histine**®**-DM**, dextromethorphan/brompheniramine/
B	polymixin b, **Aerosporin**®
C	polymixin b/bacitracin zinc, **Neomycin**®, **Polysporin**®**Ointment**, **Polysporin**®**Ophthalmic Ointment**
C	polymixin b/bacitracin zinc/neomycin/hydrocortisone, **Cortisporin**®**Ointment**
C	polymixin b/neomycin/hydrocortisone, **Cortisporin**®**Otic**, **Cortisporin**®**Ophthalmic**, **Cortisporin**®**Cream**
B	**Polymox**®, amoxicillin
C	**Poly-Pred**®, prednisolone acetate/neomycin sulfate
C	**Polysporin**®**Ointment**, **Polysporin**®**Ophthalmic Ointment**, polymixin b/bacitracin zinc
D	polythiazide, **Renese**®
C	**Polytrim**®, trimethoprim/polymixin b
NR	polyvinyl alcohol, **Hypotears**®
C	**Ponstan**®, mefenamic acid
C	**Ponstel**®, mefenamic acid
C	**Pontocaine**®, tetracaine
C	ppd, purified protein derivative for tuberculin skin testing, **Aplisol**®, **Tubersol**®
X	**Portia**®, ethinyl estradiol/levonorgestrel
C	posaconazole, **Noxafil**®
A	potassium bicarbonate/potassium citrate, **K-Lyte**®**DS**
C	potassium chloride, **Kaochlor**®, **K-Dur**®, **K-Lor**®, **Klorvess**®, **Klotrix**®, **K-Lyte**®**/Cl**, **K-Norm**®, **K-Tab**®, **Micro-K**®**Extentabs**, **Rum-K**®
C	potassium chloride/potassium citrate, **K-Lyte**®**/DS**
C	potassium citrate, **Polycitra**®**-K**, **Urocit**®**-K**
A	potassium gluconate, **Kaon**®, **Slow-K**®

D		*potassium iodide*, **Thyro-Block**®
B		*povidone-iodine*, **Betadine**®
C		*pramipexole dihydrochloride*, **Mirapex**®
C		*pramlintide*, **Symlin**®
C		**PramOtic**®, *chloroxylenol/pramoxine*
NR		*pramoxine/zinc oxide*, **Anusol**®
C		**Prandin**®, *meglitimide*
X		**Pravachol**®, *pravastatin*
X		*pravastatin*, **Pravachol**®
X		*pravastatin/aspirin*, **Pravigard**®**Pac**
X		**Pravigard**®**Pac**, *pravastatin/aspirin*
D	IV	*prazepam*, **Centrax**®
C		*prazosin*, **Minipress**®
C		*prazosin/polythiazide*, **Minizide**®
A		**PreCare**®, **PreCare**®**Chewables**, *prenatal vitamin*
B		**Precef**®, *ceforanide*
B		**Precose**®, *acarbose*
C		**Pred**®**Forte**, *prednisolone acetate*
C		**Pred**®**-G**, *prednisolone/gentamycin*
C		**Pred**®**Mild**, *prednisolone acetate*
C		*prednicarbate*, **Dermatop**®
C		*prednisolone*, **Delta Cortef**®, **Prelone**®, **Pred Forte**®
C		*prednisolone acetate/neomycin sulfate*, **Poly-Pred**®, **Pred**®**-G**
C		*prednisolone acetate*, **Econopred**®, **Pred**®**Forte**, **Pred**®**Mild**
C		*prednisolone acetate/gentamicin*, **Pred**®**-G**
C		*prednisolone sodium phosphate*, **Hydeltrasol**®, **Inflamase**®**Forte**, **Inflamase**®**Mild**, **Orapred**®, **Orapred**®**ODT**, **Pediapred**®, **Pred**®**Mild**
C		*prednisolone tebutate*, **Hydeltra**®**-TBA**, **Prednisol**®**-TBA**
C		**Prednisol**®**-TBA**, *prednisolone tabulate*
C		*prednisone*, **Deltasone**®, **Meticorten**®, **Orasone**®
C	V	*pregabalin*, **Lyrica**®
X		**Pregnyl**®, *chorionic gonadotropin*
C		**Prelone**®, *prednisolone*
C		**Prelu-2**®, *phendimetrazine*
X		**Premarin**®, **Premarin**®**Vaginal Cream**, *conjugated estrogens*
A		**PremesisRx**®, *prenatal vitamin*
X		**Premphase**®, **Prempro**®, *conjugated estrogens/medroxyprogesterone*
A		*prenatal vitamin*, **Advanced Formula Zenate**®, **Advanced NatalCare**®, **Chromagen**®**OB**, **Citracal**® **Prenatal Rx**, **Citracal**® **Prenatal+DHA**, **Duet by StuartNatal**®, **Duet by StuartNatal**® **Chewables**, **Embrex**®**600**, **Enfamil Natalins**®**Rx**, **NataChew**®, **NataFort**®, **Natalins**®, **Niferex-PN**®, **Niferex**®**-PN Forte**, **NutriNate**®, **PreCare**®, **PreCare**® **Chewables**, **PremesisRx**®, **Prenate**®, **Prenate**®**Advance**, **Prenate**®**GT**, **PrimaCare**®, **StrongStart**®, **StuartNatal**® **Plus 3**, **Ultra NatalCare**®, **Vinate**®**GT**
A		**Prenate**®, **Prenate**® **Advance**, **Prenate**®**Ultra**, *prenatal vitamin*
C		**Preparation H**®**Cream**, *petrolatum/shark liver oil/phenylephrine*

C		**Preparation H®Ointment**, *petrolatum/glycerin/shark liver oil/phenylephrine*
C		**Preparation H®Suppository**, *petrolatum/cocoa butter/phenylephrine*
B		**Prevacid®, Prevacid®Suspension, Prevacid®SoluTab**, *lansoprazole*
B		**Prevacid®NapraPAC**, *lansoprazole/naproxen sodium*
X		**Preven®**, *ethinyl estradiol/levonorgestrel*
C		**Prevnar®**, *pneumococcal 7-valent conjugate vaccine*
B		**Prezista®**, *darunavir*
C		**Priftin®**, *rifapentine*
C		**Prilosec®**, *omeprazole*
A		**PrimaCare®**, *prenatal vitamin*
C		**Primaxin®**, *imipenem/cilastatin*
D		*primidone*, **Mysoline®**
C		**Primsol®**, *trimethoprim*
B		**Principen®**, *ampicillin*
C/D		**Prinivil®**, *lisinopril*
C/D		**Prinzide®**, *lisinopril/hydrochlorothiazide*
C		**ProAmatine®**, *midodrine*
B		**Probampacin®**, *probenecid/ampicillin*
C		**Pro-Banthine®**, *propantheline bromide*
B		*probenecid*, **Benemid®**
B		*probenecid/ampicillin*, **Probampacin®**
C		*procainamide*, **Procan®, Procanbid®, Pronestyl, Pronestyl®SR**
C		**Procan®**, *procainamide*
C		**Procanbid®**, *procainamide*
C		**Procardia®, Procardia®XL**, *nifedipine*
X		**Prochieve®**, *progesterone*
C		*prochlorperazine*, **Compazine®**
C		**Procrit®**, *epoetin alpha*
C		**Proctocort®**, *hydrocortisone*
C		**Proctocream®-HC**, *hydrocortisone/pramoxine*
C		**Proctofoam®-HC**, *hydrocortisone/pramoxine*
C		*procyclidine*, **Kemadrin®**
B		**Prodium®**, *phenazopyridine*
C		**Profasi®HP**, *chorionic gonadotropin*
C	IV	**Pro-Fast®HS, Pro-Fast®SA Tab 100's, Pro-Fast®SR Cap 100's**, *phentermine*
X		*progesterone*, **Crinone®, Prochieve®**
X		*progesterone (micronized)*, **Prometrium®**
C		**Proglycem®**, *diazoxide*
C		**Prohibit®**, *haemophilus b conjugated vaccine (diphtheria toxoid conjugate)*
C		**Prolex®D**, *guaifenesin/phenylephrine*
C	III	**Prolex®DH**, *potassium guaiacolsulfonate/hydrocodone*
C		**Prolixin®**, *fluphenazine*
C		**Prolixin®Decanoate**, *fluphenazine decanoate*
A		**Proloid®**, *thyroglobulin*

C		**Proloprim®**, *trimethoprim*
C	II	**Promacet®**, *butalbital/acetaminophen*
C		*promazine*, **Sparine®**
C		*promethazine*, **Phenergan®**
C	III	*promethazine/codeine*, **Phenergan®w/ Codeine Supp**
C	III	*promethazine/codeine/phenylephrine*, **Phenergan®VC with Codeine**
C		*promethazine/dextromethorphan*, **Phenergan®DM**
C		*promethazine/phenylephrine*, **Phenergan®VC**
X		**Prometrium®**, *progesterone (micronized)*
C	II	**Prominol®**, *butalbital/acetaminophen*
C		**Pronestyl®, Pronestyl®SR**, *procainamide*
D		**Propacil®**, *propylthiouracil*
C		*propantheline bromide*, **Pro-Banthine®**
C		*proparacaine*, **Ophthaine®**
X		**Propecia®**, *finasteride*
B		**Propine®**, *dipivefrin*
C	IV	*propoxyphene*, **Darvon®, Darvon®-N**
C	IV	*propoxyphene/acetaminophen*, **Balacet®, Darvocet®-A500, Darvocet®-N50, Darvocet®-N100, Wygesic®**
D	IV	*propoxyphene/aspirin/caffeine*, **Darvon®Compound-65**
C		*propranolol*, **Inderal®, Inderal®LA, InnoPran®XL**
C		*propranolol/hydrochlorothiazide*, **Inderide®, Inderide®LA**
D		**Propacil®**, *propylthiouracil, ptu*, **Propyl-Thyracil®**
D		**Propyl-Thyracil®**, *propylthiouracil, ptu*
C		**Prosed®EC**, *hyoscyamine sulfate/atropine sulfate/phenyl salicylate/methylene blue/benzoic acid/methenamine (Esprit)*
X	IV	**ProSom®**, *estazolam*
X		**Proscar®**, *finasteride*
B		**Prostaphlin®**, *oxacillin*
D		**ProStep®**, *nicotine transdermal system*
B		**Protonix®**, *pantoprazole*
C		**Protopic®**, *tacrolimus*
D/B		**Protostat®**, *metronidazole*
C		*protriptyline*, **Vivactil®**
C		**Protropin®**, *somatropin*
C	III	**Protuss®**, *hydrocodone/guaiacosulfonate*
C	III	**Protuss®-D**, *guaiacolsulfonate/hydrocodone/pseudoephedrine*
C		**Protuss® DM**, *guaifenesin/pseudoephedrine/dextromethorphan*
C		**Proventil®, Proventil®HFA**, *albuterol*
X		**Provera®**, *medroxyprogesterone*
C		**Provigil®**, *modafinil*
C		**Prozac®, Prozac®Weekly**, *fluoxetine*
B		**Prudoxin®**, *doxepin*
C		*pseudoephedrine*, **Novafed®, PediaCare®Infant Decongestant, Sudafed®, Triaminic®AM**
C		**Psorcon®**, *diflorasone diacetate*
C		*psyllium*, **Fiberall®, Metamucil®**

B		*psyllium hydrophilic mucilloid*, **Effer-Syllium®**, **Hydrocil®**, **Perdiem®**
C		*psyllium, sennosides*, **SennaPrompt®**
B		**Pulmicort®Turbuhaler, Pulmicort®Respules**, *budesonide*
C		*purified protein derivative for tuberculin skin testing, ppd*, **Aplisol®**, **Tubersol®**
C	III	**P-V-Tussin®**, *hydrocodone/pseudoephedrine/chlorpheniramine*
C		**Pyrazinamide®**, *pyrazinamide*
C		*pyrazinamide*, **Pyrazinamide®**
C		*pyrazolopyrimidines*, **Zaleplon®**
C		*pyrantel pamoate*, **Antiminth®**, **Pin-X®**
C		*pyrethrins*, **RID®**
B		**Pyribenzamine®**, *tripelennamine*
B		**Pyridiate®**, *phenazopyridine*
B		**Pyridium®**, *phenazopyridine*
A		*pyridoxine, vitamin b_6*, **Beesix®**, **Hexa-Betalin®**
C		*pyrimethamine*, **Daraprim®**
X	II	**Quadrinal®**, *ephedrine/phenobarbital/theophylline/potassium iodide*
B		*qualadrel*, **Hylorel®**
C		**Qualaquin®**, *quinine sulfate*
X		**Quasense®**, *ethinyl estradiol/levonorgestrel*
X	IV	*quazepam*, **Doral®**
C		**Questran®, Questran®Light**, *cholestyramine*
C		*quetiapine®*, **Seroquel**
C		**Quibron®**, *guaifenesin/theophylline*
C		*quinacrine*, **Atabrine®**
C		**Quinaglute®**, *quinidine gluconate*
C		**Quinamm®**, *quinine sulfate*
C/D		*quinapril*, **Accupril®**
C/D		*quinapril/hydrochlorothiazide*, **Accuretic®**
C		*quinethazone/reserpine*, **Hydromox®R**
C		**Quinidex®**, *quinidine sulfate*
C		*quinidine*, **Duraquin®**, **Quinaglute®**, **Quinidex®**, **Quinora®**
C		*quinine sulfate*, **Novoquinine®**, **Qualaquin®**, **Quinamm®**
C		**Quinora®**, *quinidine*
C		**Quixin®**, *levofloxacin ophthalmic solution*
C		**Qvar®**, *beclomethasone dipropionate*
C		**RabAvert®**, *rabies vaccine (human diploid)*
B		*rabeprazole*, **Aciphex®**
C		*rabies immune globulin (human)*, **Bayrab®**, **HRIG®**, **Hyperab®**, **Imogam®Rabies**
C		*rabies vaccine (absorbed)*, **RVA®**
C		*rabies vaccine, (human diploid cell)*, **HDCV®**, **Imovax®**, **Imovax I.D.**, **RabAvert®**
X		*raloxifene*, **Evista®**
C		*ramelteon*, **Rozerem®**
C/D		*ramipril*, **Altace®**

C		**Ranexa®**, *ranolazine*
B		*ranitidine*, **Zantac®, Zantac®Chewable Tablets, Zantac®Efferdose**
C		*ranitidine bismuth citrate*, **Tritec®**
C		*ranolazine*, **Ranexa®**
B		**Repinex®**, *omeprazole*
C		**Raptiva®**, *efalizumab*
D		**Raudixin®**, *rauwolfia serpentina*
D		*rauwolfia serpentina*, **Raudixin®**
B		**Razadyne®**, *galantamine*
X		**Rebetol®**, *ribavirin*
X		**Rebetron®Combination Therapy**, *ribavirin/interferon alfa-2b (recombinant)*
C		**Recombivax®HB**, *hepatitis b (recombinant)*
C		**Rectacreme®**, *hydrocortisone/lidocaine*
C		**Rectocort®**, *hydrocortisone*
A/C		**Redisol®**, *cyanocobalamin, vitamin b$_{12}$*
C		**Regitine®**, *phentolamine*
B		**Reglan®**, *metoclopramide*
C		**Regranex®Gel**, *becaplermin*
D		**Regroton®**, *chlorthalidone/reserpine*
C		**Relafen®**, *nabumetone*
C		**Relagard®Therapeutic Vaginal Gel**, *acetic acid/oxyquinolone*
C		**Relpax®**, *eletriptan*
B		**Relenza®**, *zanamivir for inhalation*
C		**Remeron®, Remeron®Soltab**, *mirtazepine*
C		**Remicade®**, *infliximab*
B		**Reminyl®**, *galantamine*
D		**Renese®**, *polythiazide*
C		**Renova®**, *tretinoin*
C		**Repetabs®**, *albuterol*
C	III	**Reprexain®**, *hydrocodone/ibuprofen*
C		**Requip®**, *ropinirole*
C		**Rescon®Mx**, *pseudoephedrine/chlorpheniramine/methscopalamine*
C		**Rescriptor®**, *delavirdine mesylate*
C		**Rescula®**, *unoprostone isopropyl*
C		*reserpine*, **Serpasil®**
C		*reserpine/chlorothiazide*, **Diupres®, Hydropres®**
C		*reserpine/hydralazine/hydrochlorothiazide*, **Ser-Ap-Es®**
C		*reserpine/hydroflumethiazide*, *Salutensin*
C		**Respahist®**, *brompheniramine/pseudoephedrine*
C		**Restasis®**, *cyclosporine*
C		**Restylane®**, *hyaluronic acid*
X	IV	**Restoril®**, *temazepam*
C		**Retin-A®**, *tretinoin*
C		**Retrovir®**, *zidovudine, azt*
B		**Revatio®**, *sildenafil*
B		**Revex®**, *nalmefene*

C		**ReVia®**, *naltrexone*
D		**Rheumatrex®**, *methotrexate*
B		**Rhinocort, Rhinocort®Aqua**, *budesonide*
X		*ribavirin*, **Copegus®, Rebetol®, Virazole®**
X		*ribavirin/interferon alfa-2b (recombinant)*, **Rebetron®Combination Therapy**
C		**RID®**, *pyrethrins*
C		**Ridaura®**, *auranofin*
B		*rifabutin*, **Mycobutin®**
C		**Rifadin®**, *rifampin*
C		**Rifamate®**, *rifampin/isoniazid*
C		*rifampin*, **Rifadin®, Rimactane®**
C		*rifampin/isoniazid*, **Rifamate®**
C		*rifampin/isoniazid/pyrazinamide*, **Rifater®**
C		*rifapentine*, **Priftin®**
C		**Rifater®**, *rifampin/isoniazid/pyrazinamide*
C		*rifaxmin*, **Xifaxan®**
C		**Rimactane®**, *rifampin*
C		*rimantadine*, **Flumadine®**
C		*rimexolone*, **Vexol®**
B		**Riomet®**, *metformin*
C		**Riopan®**, *magaldrate*
C		*risedronate*, **Actonel®**
C		**Risperdal®Consta, Risperdal®M-Tab**, *risperidone*
C		*risperidone*, **Risperdal®Consta, Risperdal®M-Tab**
C	II	**Ritalin®, Ritalin®SR**, *methylphenidate*
B		*ritonavir*, **Norvir®**
B		*rivastigmine*, **Exelon®**
C		*rizatriptan*, **Maxalt®, Maxalt®-MLT**
X		**Robatol®**, *ribavirin*
C		**Robaxin®**, *methocarbamol*
D		**Robaxisal®**, *methocarbamol/aspirin*
B		**Robicillin®**, *penicillin v potassium*
B		**Robimycin®**, *erythromycin base*
B		**Robinul®**, *glycopyrrolate*
D		**Robitet®**, *tetracycline*
C		**Robitussin®**, *guaifenesin*
C	III	**Robitussin®A-C**, *guaifenesin/codeine*
C		**Robitussin®-CF**, *guaifenesin/dextromethorphan/ pseudoephedrine*
C	III	**Robitussin®-DAC**, *guaifenesin/pseudoephedrine/codeine*
C		**Robitussin®-DM**, *guaifenesin/dextromethorphan*
C		**Robitussin®-PE**, *guaifenesin/pseudoephedrine*
C		**Rocaltrol®**, *calcitriol*
B		**Rocephin®**, *ceftriaxone*
C		**Roferon®A**, *interferon alfa-2a*
C		**Rogaine®**, *minoxidil*
NR		**Rolaids®**, *dihydroxyaluminum sodium carbonate*

NR		**Rolaids®Extra Strength,** *calcium carbonate*
B		**Rolaids®Sodium Free,** *calcium carbonate/magnesium hydroxide*
C		**Rondec®, Rondec®Chewable, Rondec®Filmtab,** *carbinoxamine/pseudoephedrine*
C		**Rondec®-DM, Rondec®DM Drops,** *carbinoxamine/pseudoephedrine/ dextromethorphan*
C		*ropinirole,* **Requip®**
C		*rosiglitazone,* **Avandia®**
C		*rosiglitazone/glimepiride,* **Avandaryl®**
C		*rosiglitazone/metformin,* **Avandamet®**
X		**Ro-sulfiram®,** *disulfiram*
X		*rosuvastatin,* **Crestor®**
NR		**RotaTeq®,** *rotavirus vaccine (live)*
NR		*rotavirus vaccine (live),* **RotaTeq®**
B		**Rowasa®,** *mesalamine*
C	II	**Roxanol®, Roxanol®Rescudose,** *morphine sulfate*
C	II	**Roxicet®,** *oxycodone/acetaminophen*
B/D	II	**Roxicodone®,** *oxycodone*
C		**Rozerem®,** *ramelteon*
C		*rubella virus vaccine (live),* **Meruvax®II**
A/C		**Rubesol®,** *cyanocobalamin, vitamin b$_{12}$*
A/C		**Rubramin®,** *cyanocobalamin, vitamin b$_{12}$*
B/D		**Rufen®,** *ibuprofen*
C		**Rum-K®,** *potassium chloride*
C		**Ru-Tuss DE®,** *guaifenesin/pseudoephedrine*
C	III	**Rutuss®with Hydrocodone,** *hydrocodone/phenylephrine/ pseudoephedrine/pheniramine/pyrilamine*
C		**RVA®,** *rabies vaccine (absorbed)*
C		**Ryna®-12,** *phenylephrine/pyrilamine*
C		**Rynatan®Tab,** *pseudoephedrine/azatadine*
C		**Rynatan®Ped Susp,** *chlorpheniramine/pyrilamine/phenylephrine*
C		**Rynatuss®,** *carbetapentane/chlorpheniramine/ephedrine/ phenylephrine*
C		**Saizen®,** *somatropin*
C		**Salbutamol®,** *albuterol*
C		**Salflex®,** *salsalate*
NR		*salicylic acid,* **DuoFilm®, DuoPlant®, Keralyt®Gel, Occlusal®-HP, Trans®-Ver-Sal**
NR		*saliva (synthetic),* **Salivert®**
NR		**Salivert®,** *saliva (synthetic)*
C		*salmeterol,* **Serevent®, Serevent®Diskus**
C		*salsalate,* **Disalcid®, Mono-gesic®, Salflex®**
C		**Saluron®,** *hydroflumethaiazide*
C		**Salutensin®,** *reserpine/hydroflumethiazide*
C		**Sanctura®,** *trospium chloride*
C		**Sanorex®,** *mazindol*
C		**Sansert®,** *methysergide*

B		*saquinavir*, **Fortovase**®
B		*saquinavir mesylate*, **Invirase**®
C		**Sarafem**®, *fluoxetine*
C		**Scabene**®, *lindane/benzepine hexachloride*
C		**Scopace**®, *scopolamine*
C		*scopolamine*, **Scopace**®, **Transderm-Scop**®
X		**Seasonale**®, *ethinyl estradiol/levonorgestrel*
X		**Seasonique**®, *ethinyl estradiol/levonorgestrel*
C		**Sebizon**®, *sulfacetamide*
NR		**Sebulex**®, *sulfur/salicylic acid*
D	II	*secobarbital*, **Seconal**®
D	II	**Seconal**®, *secobarbital*
B		**Sectral**®, *acebutolol*
C		*selegiline*, **Atapryl**®, **Carbex**®, **Eldepryl**®, **Emsam**®, **Zelapar**®
C		*selenium sulfide*, **Exsel**®, **Selsun**®, **Selsun**® **Rx**
C		**Selsun**®, **Selsun**®**Rx**, *selenium sulfide*
B		**Semprex**®**-D**, *acrivastine/pseudoephedrine*
C		**Senexon**®, *senna*
C		*senna*, **Black Draught**®, **Senexon**®, **Senokot**®, **Senolax**®
C		**SennaPrompt**®, *psyllium, sennosides*
C		**Senokot**®, *senna*
C		**Senolax**®, *senna*
C		**Sensipar**®, *cinacalcet*
C		**Sensorcaine**®, *bupivacaine*
C		**Septra**®, **Septra**®**DS**, *sulfamethoxazole/trimethoprim*
C		**Ser-Ap-Es**®, *reserpine/hydralazine/hydrochlorothiazide*
D	IV	**Serax**®, *oxazepam*
C		**Serentil**®, *mesoridazine*
C		**Serevent**®**Diskus**, *salmeterol*
C		*sermorelin acetate*, **Geref**®
C		**Seromycin**®, *cycloserine*
X		**Serophene**®, *clomiphene citrate*
C		**Seroquel**®, *quetiapine*
C		**Serostim**®, *somatropin*
D		**Serpasil**®, *reserpine*
C		*sertaconazole*, **Ertaczo**®
C		*sertraline*, **Zoloft**®
C	IV	*sibutramine*, **Meridia**®
B		*sildenafil*, **Viagra**®, **Revatio**®
B		**Silvadene**®, *silver sulfadiazine*
B		*silver sulfadiazine*, **Silvadene**®
C		*simethicone*, **Gas-X**®, **Mylicon**®, **Phazyme**®
C		*simethicone/activated charcoal*, **Flatulex**®
X		*simvastatin*, **Zocor**®
C		**Sinemet**®, **Sinemet**®**CR**, *carbidopa/levodopa*
C		**Sinequan**®, *doxepin*
C		**Sinex**®, *phenylephrine*

B		**Singulair®, Singulair®Chewable,** *montelukast*
B		*sitagliptin,* **Januvia®**
B		**Skelaxin®,** *metaxalone*
C		**Skelid®,** *tiludronate disodium*
C		**Slo-Bid®,** *theophylline*
A/C		**Slo-Niacin®,** *niacin, nicotinic acid, vitamin b₃*
C		**Slo-Phyllin®,** *theophylline*
A		**Slow Fe®,** *ferrous sulfate*
A		**Slow Fe®Plus Folic Acid,** *ferrous sulfate/folic acid*
A		**Slow-K®,** *potassium gluconate*
NR		*sodium chloride,* **Muro®128, Muro®128 Ophthalmic Ointment**
B		*sodium hyaluronate,* **Hyalgan®**
NR		*sodium oxybate,* **Xyrem®**
C		*sodium phosphate/sodium biphosphate,* **Fleet®Enema**
C		*sodium polystyrene sulfonate,* **Kayexalate®**
C		**Solaquin®, Solaquin® Forte, Solaquin®Forte Gel,** *hydroquinone*
B		**Solaraze®,** *diclofenac*
C		**Solarcaine®,** *benzocaine*
C		*solifenacin,* **VESIcare®**
C		**Solu-Cortef®,** *hydrocortisone sodium succinate*
C		**Solu-Medrol®,** *methylprednisolone sodium succinate*
C		**Soma®,** *carisoprodol*
C		**Soma®Compound,** *carisoprodol/aspirin*
C	III	**Soma®Compound with Codeine,** *carisoprodol/aspirin/codeine*
C		*somatrem,* **Protropin®**
C		*somatropin,* **Humatrope®, NordiFlex®, Norditropin®, Nutropin®, Nutropin®AQ, Saizen®, Serostim®**
B		**Sominex®, Sominex® Max Str,** *diphenhydramine*
C		**Somophyllin®, Somophyllin®DF,** *aminophylline, theophylline*
C	IV	**Sonata®,** *zaleplon*
C		**Sorbitrate®, Sorbitrate®SR,** *isosorbide dinitrate*
X		**Soriatane®,** *acitretin*
C		*sotalol,* **Betapace®, Betapace®-AF**
C		*sparfloxacin,* **Zagam®**
C		**Sparine®,** *promazine*
C	II	**Spasmolin®,** *hyoscyamine/atropine/scopolamine/phenobarbital*
C		**Spectazole®,** *econazole*
B		*spectinomycin,* **Trobicin®**
C		**Spectracef®,** *cefditoren pivoxil*
B		**Spectrobid®,** *bacampicillin*
C		**Spiriva®,** *tiotropium (as bromide monohydrate)*
D		*spironolactone,* **Aldactone®**
D		*spironolactone/hydrochlorothiazide,* **Aldactazide®**
C		**Sporanox®,** *itraconazole*
X		**Sprintec®28,** *ethinyl estradiol/norgestimate*
C	IV	**Stadol®,** *butorphanol tartrate*
C		**Stalevo®,** *carbidopa/levodopa/entacapone*

B		**Staphcillin®**, *methicillin*
C		**Starlix®**, *nateglinide*
C		*stavudine*, **Zerit®**
C		**Stelazine®**, *trifluoperazine*
X		**Stilbestrol®**, *diethylstilbestrol*
X		**Stilphostrol®**, *diethylstilbestrol*
B		**Stimate®**, *desmopressin*
D		**Streptomycin®**, *streptomycin*
D		*streptomycin*, **Streptomycin®**
X	III	**Striant®**, *testosterone*
A		**StrongStart®**, *prenatal vitamin*
A		**StuartNatal®Plus 3**, *prenatal vitamin*
C	III	**Suboxone®**, *buprenorphine/naloxone*
C	III	**Subutex®**, *buprenorphine*
C		*succimer*, **Chemet®**
B		*sucralfate*, **Carafate®**, **Sulcrate®**
C		**Sudafed®**, *pseudoephedrine*
C		**Sudal®60/500**, *pseudoephedrine/guafenisen*
C		**Sudal®DM**, *dextromethorphan/guaifenesin*
C		**Sulamyd®**, *sulfacetamide*
C		**Sular®**, *nisoldipine*
C		*sulconazole*, **Exelderm®**
B		**Sulcrate®**, *sucralfate*
C		*sulfacetamide*, **Bleph®-10, Cetamide®, Isopto Cetamide®, Klaron®, Na Sulamyd®, Novacet®, Sebizon®, Sulamyd®**
C		*sulfacetamide/phenylephrine*, **Vasosulf®**
C		*sulfacetamide/prednisolone*, **Blephamide®Liquifilm, Metimyd®, Vasocidin®Ophthalmic Ointment®, Vasocidin®Ophthalmic Solution**
C		*sulfacetamide/sulfur*, **Clinia®, Novacet®Lotion, Rosula®, Sulfacet®-R, Sulfatol®**
C		**Sulfacet®-R**, *sulfacetamide/sulfur*
C		*sulfamethoxazole*, **Gantanol®, Gantanol®DS**
B/D		*sulfamethoxazole/phenazopyridine*, **Azo-Gantanol®**
C		*sulfamethoxazole/trimethoprim*, **Bactrim®, Bactrim®DS, Septra®, Septra®DS**
B/D		*sulfasalazine*, **Azulfidine®, Azulfidine®EN**
C		*sulfanilamide*, **AVC®**
C		*sulfathiazole/sulfacetamide/sulfabenzamide*, **Sultrin®**
C		**Sulfatol®**, *sulfacetamide/sulfur*
C		*sulfinpyrazone*, **Anturane®**
B/D		*sulfisoxazole*, **Gantrisin®, Gantrisin®Ophthalmic Solution**
B/D		*sulfisoxazole/phenazopyridine*, **Azo-Gantrisin®**
B/D		*sulindac*, **Clinoril®**
NR		*sulfur/salicylic acid*, **Sebulex®**
C		**Sultrin®**, *sulfathiazole/sulfacetamide/sulfabenzamide*
C		*sumatriptan*, **Imitrex®, Imitrex®Injectable, Imitrex®Nasal Spray**

B		**Sumox®**, *amoxicillin*
D		**Sumycin®** *tetracycline*
B		**Suprax®Oral Suspension,** *cefixime*
C		**Surfak®,** *docusate calcium/dioctyl calcium sulfosuccinate*
C		**Surmontil®,** *trimipramine*
A		**Surplex®-T,** *vitamin b complex/vitamin c*
C		**Sus-Phrine®,** *epinephrine*
C		**Sustiva®,** *efavirenz*
C		**Symax®SL, Symax®SR,** *hyoscyamine*
C		**Symbicort®,** *budesonide/formoterol*
C		**Symbyax®,** *olanzapine/fluoxetine*
C		**Symlin®,** *pramlintide*
C		**Symmetrel®,** *amantadine*
C		**Synacort®,** *hydrocortisone*
NR		**Synagis®,** *palivizumab*
C		**Synalar®,** *fluocinolone acetonide*
D	III	**Synalgos®-DC,** *dihydrocodeine*
X		**Synarel®,** *nafarelin*
C		**Synemol®,** *fluocinolone acetonide*
C		**Synera®,** *lidocaine/tetracaine*
X		**Syntest®D.S., Syntest®H.S.,** *esterified estrogens/methyltestosterone*
A		**Synthroid®,** *levothyroxine*
C		**Syrophyllin®,** *theophylline*
C		**Syrophyllin®GG,** *theophylline/guaifenesin*
NR		**Systane®,** *polyethylene glycol/propylene glycol*
X		**Tace®,** *chlorotrianisene*
C		**Taclonex®,** *calcipotriene/betamethsone dipropionate*
C		*tacrine,* **Cognex®**
C		*tacrolimus,* **Protopic®**
B		*tadalafil,* **Cialis®**
B		**Tagamet®, Tagamet®HB,** *cimetidine*
D	IV	**Talacen®,** *pentazocine/acetaminophen*
B/D	IV	**Talwin®,** *pentazocine*
C/D		**Talwin®Compound,** *pentazocine/aspirin*
C		**Talwin®NX,** *pentazocine/naloxone*
C		**Tamiflu®,** *oseltamivir*
D		*tamoxifen,* **Nolvadex®**
B		*tamulosin,* **Flomax®**
C		**Tanafed®,** *pseudoephedrine/chlorpheniramine*
B		**Tao®,** *troleandomycin*
D		**Tapazole®,** *methimazole*
C		**Taractan®,** *chlorprothixene*
C/D		**Tarka®,** *trandolapril/verapamil*
C		**Tasmar®,** *tolcapone*
B		**Tavist®, Tavist®-1,** *clemastine*
C		**Tavist®D,** *clemastine/pseudoephedrine*
X		*tazarotene,* **Avage®, Tazorac®**

B		**Tazicef®**, *ceftazidime*
B		**Tazidime®**, *ceftazidime*
X		**Tazorac®**, *tazarotene*
C/D		**Teczem®**, *enalapril/diltiazem*
X		**Tegison®**, *etretinate*
B		**Tegopen®**, *cloxacillin*
D		**Tegretol®, Tegretol® XR**, *carbamazepine*
C		*telithromycin*, **Ketek®**
C/D		*telmisartan*, **Micardis®**
C/D		*telmisartan/hydrochlorothiazide*, **Micardis®HCT**
X	IV	*temazepam*, **Restoril®**
C		**Temovate®**, *clobetasol propionate*
B		**Tempra®**, *acetaminophen*
B		**Tenex®**, *guanfacine*
B		*tenofovir disoproxil fumarate*, **Viread®**
B		*tenofovir disoproxil fumarate/emtricitabine*, **Truvada®**
D		**Tenoretic®**, *atenolol/chlorthalidone*
D		**Tenormin®**, *atenolol*
B	IV	**Tenuate®**, *diethylpropion*
B	IV	**Tepanil®**, *diethylpropion*
C		**Terazol®, Terazol®3, Terazol®7**, *terconazole*
C		*terazosin*, **Hytrin®**
B		*terbinafine*, **Lamisil®, Lamisil®AT**
B		*terbutaline*, **Brethaire®, Brethine®, Bricanyl®**
C		*terconazole*, **Terazol®, Terazol®3, Terazol®7**
C		*teriparatide*, **Forteo®**
D		**Terramycin®**, *oxytetracycline*
C		**Tessalon® Perles**, *benzonatate*
X	III	**Testoderm®, Testostoderm®TTS**, *testosterone*
X	III	*testosterone*, **Androderm®, AndroGel®, Striant®, Testim®, Testostoderm®, Testostoderm®TTS**
X	III	*testosterone cypionate*, **Depo-Testosterone®**
X	III	*testosterone enthanate*, **Delatestryl®**
X	III	**Testred®**, *methyltestosterone*
C		*tetanus immune globulin (human)*, **Baytet®, Hyper-Tet®, TIG®**
C		*tetanus toxoid, dT, Td*
C		*tetracaine*, **Pontocaine®**
D		**Tetracap®**, *tetracycline*
D		*tetracycline*, **Achromycin®, Achromycin®V, Panmycin®, Robitet®, Sumycin®, Tetracap®, Tetracyn®, Topicycline®**
D		**Tetracyn®**, *tetracycline*
C		*tetrahydrozoline*, **Tyzine®, Visine®**
NR		*tetrahydrozoline/polyethylene glycol/povidone/dextran*, **Advanced Relief Visine®**
NR		*tetrahydrozoline/zinc sulfate*, **Visine®AC**
C		**Tetramune®**, *diphtheria/tetanus toxoid/pertussis/haemophilus b conjugate vaccine*

B	**Teva®**, *ticlopidine*
C/D	**Teveten®**, *eprosartan*
C/D	**Teveten®HCT**, *eprosartan/hydrochlorothiazide*
C	**Texacort®**, *hydrocortisone*
C	**Thalitone®**, *chlorthalidone*
C	**Theo-24®**, *theophylline*
C	**Theo-Dur®**, *theophylline*
C	**Theolair®, Theolair®SR**, *theophylline*
C	*theophylline*, **Aerolate®, Syrophyllin®, Slo-Bid®, Slo-Phyllin®, Theo-24, Theo-Dur®, Theolair®, Theolair®SR, Theo-X®, Uni-Dur®, Uniphyl®**
C	*theophylline/guaifenesin*, **Syrophyllin®GG**
C	*theophylline/hydroxizine*, **Marax®**
C	*theophylline ethylenediamine, aminophylline*, **Somophyllin®, Somophyllin®DF**
C	*theophylline/hydroxyzine/ephedrine*, **Marax®**
C	**Theo-X®**, *theophylline*
A	**Theragran®**, *multivitamin*
A	**Theragran®-M**, *multivitamin with minerals*
B	**Theramycin®Z**, *erythromycin base*
C	*thiabendazole*, **Mintezol®**
A	**Thiamine®**, *thiamine, vitamin b₁*
A	*thiamine, vitamin b₁*, **Betalins®, Thiamine®**
X	*thiethylperazine*, **Torecan®**
C	*thioridazine*, **Mellaril®, Mellaril®-S**
C	*thiothixene*, **Navane®**
C	**Thorazine®**, *chlorpromazine*
D	**Thyro-Block®**, *potassium iodide*
A	*thyroglobulin*, **Proloid®**
A	**Thyrolar®**, *liothyronine/levothyroxine*
C	**Tiamate®**, *diltiazem maleate*
C	*tiazabine*, **Gabitril®**
C	**Tiazac®**, *diltiazem*
C	**Ticar®**, *ticarcillin*
C	*ticarcillin*, **Ticar®**
B	*ticarcillin/clavulanate potassium (clavulanic acid)*, **Timentin®**
B	**Ticlid®**, *ticlopidine*
B	*ticlopidine*, **Teva®, Ticlid®**
C	**TIG®**, *tetanus immune globulin (human)*
D	*tigecycline*, **Tygacil®**
B	**Tilade®**, *nedocromil*
C	*tiludronate disodium*, **Skelid®**
B	**Timentin®**, *ticarcillin/clavulanate potassium (clavulanic acid)*
C	**Timolide®**, *timolol/hydrochlorothiazide*
C	*timolol*, **Betimol®, Blocadren®, Istalol®, Timoptic®, Timoptic®XE**
C	**Timoptic®, Timoptic®XE**, *timolol*
C	**Tinactin®**, *tolnaftate*

C		**Tindamax**®, *tinidazole*
C		*tinidazole*, **Tindamax**®
C		*tioconazole*, **Vagistat**®
C		*tiotropium (as bromide monohydrate)*, **Spiriva**®
NR		**Titralac**®, *calcium carbonate*
C		*tizanidine*, **Zanaflex**®
C		**TobraDex**®, *tobramycin/dexamethasone*
B		*tobramycin*, **Nebcin**®, **Tobrex**®
C		*tobramycin/dexamethasone*, **TobraDex**®
B		**Tobrex**®, *tobramycin*
A		*tocopherol, vitamin e*, **Aquasol**®E
C		**Tofranil**®, **Tofranil**®PM, *imipramine*
C		*tolazamide*, **Tolinase**®
C		*tolbutamide*, **Orinase**®
C		*tolcapone*, **Tasmar**®
C		**Tolectin**®, *tolmetin*
C		**Tolinase**®, *tolazamide*
C		*tolmetin*, **Tolectin**®
C		*tolnaftate*, **Aftate**®, **Tinactin**®
C		*tolterodine*, **Detrol**®, **Detrol**®LA
C		**Topamax**®, *topiramate*
C		**Topex Oxy**®, *benzoyl peroxide*
C		**Topicort**®, *desoximetasone*
D		**Topicycline**®, *tetracycline*
C		*topiramate*, **Topamax**®
C		**Toprol**®-XL, *metoprolol*
C		**Topsyn**®, *fluocinonide*
C		**Toradol**®, *ketorolac*
X		**Torecan**®, *thiethylperazine*
D		*toremifene*, **Fareston**®
C		**Tornalate**®, *bitolterol*
B		*torsemide*, **Demadex**®
B		**Totacillin**®, **Totacillin**®-N, *ampicillin*
C		*tramadol*, **Ultram**®, **Ultram**®ER
C		*tramadol/acetaminophen*, **Ultracet**®
C		*tipranavir*, **Aptivus**®
C		**Trandate**®, *labetalol*
C/D		*trandolapril*, **Mavik**®
C/D		*trandolapril/verapamil*, **Tarka**®
C		**Transderm-Nitro**®, *nitroglycerin*
C		**Transderm-Scop**®, *scopolamine*
NR		**Trans-Ver-Sal**®, *salicylic acid*
C	IV	**Tranxene**®, **Tranxene**®-SD, **Tranxene**®-SD Half Strength, *clorazepate*
C		*tranylcypromine*, **Parnate**®
C		**Travatan**®, *travoprost*
C		*trazodone*, **Desyrel**®

C		**Trellium®Plus**, *butalbital/hyoscyamine hydrobromide/phenazopyridine*
C		**Trental®**, *pentoxifylline*
C		**Trental®DM Liquid**, *phenylephrine/dextromethorphan/chlorpheniramine*
C		*tretinoin*, **Avita®, Renova®, Retin-A®**
D		**Trexall®**, *methotrexate*
C		**triact®**, *triamcinolone adetonide*
C		*triamcinolone*, **Aristocort®, Kenalog-E®**
C		*triamcinolone acetonide*, **Aristocort®A, Azmacort®, Kenacort®, Kenalog®Injectable, Kenalog® Lotion, Kenalog® Ointment, Kenalog®Spray, Nasacort®, Nasacort®AQ, Triact**
C		*triamcinolone diacetate*, **Aristocort®Forte**
C		**Triaminic®AM**, *pseudoephedrine*
C		**Triaminic®Sore Throat**, *dextromethorphan/acetaminophen/pseudoephedrine*
C		*triamterene*, **Dyrenium®**
C		*triamterene/hydrochlorothiazide*, **Dyazide®, Maxzide®**
C		**Triavil®**, *perphenazine/amitriptyline*
C		**Triaz®**, *benzoyl peroxide*
X	IV	*triazolam*, **Halcion®**
B		**Trichlorex®**, *trichlorthiazide*
B		*trichlormethiazide*, **Diurese®, Metahydrin®, Naqua®, Niazide®, Trichlorex®**
C		**TriCor®**, *fenofibrate*
C		**Tridesilon®**, *desonide*
X		**Tridione**, *trimethadione*
C		*triethanolamine*, **Cerumenex®**
C		*trifluoperazine*, **Stelazine®**
C		*trifluridine*, **Viroptic®**
C		*trihexyphenidyl*, **Artane®**
C		**Trilafon®**, *perphenazine*
C		**Trileptal®**, *oxcarbazepine*
X		**Tri-Levlen®-21, Tri-Levlen®-28**, *ethinyl estradiol/levonorgestrel*
C		**Trilisate®**, *choline magnesium trisalicylate*
C		**Tri-Luma®**, *hydroquinone/fluocinolone/tretinoin*
X		*trimethadione*, **Tridione®**
C		*trimethoprim*, **Primsol®, Proloprim®, Trimpex®**
C		*trimipramine*, **Surmontil®**
B		**Trimox®**, *amoxicillin*
C		**Trimpex®**, *trimethoprim*
C		**Trinalin®Repetabs**, *pseudoephedrine/azatadine*
X		**Tri-Norinyl®-21, Tri-Norinyl®-28**, *ethinyl estradiol/norethindrone*
C		**Trinsicon®**, *multivitamin*
C		*trioxsalen*, **Trisoralen®**
C		**Tripedia®**, *diphtheria/tetanus toxoids/acellular pertussis vaccine (absorbed)*

B		*tripelennamine*, **PBZ®, PBZ-SR®, Pelamine®, Pyribenzamine®**
X		**Triphasil®-21, Triphasil-28**, *ethinyl estradiol/levonorgestrel*
C		*triprolidine/pseudoephedrine*, **Actifed®Cold & Allergy**
C	III	*triprolidine/pseudoephedrine/codeine*, **Actifed®with Codeine**
C		**Trisoralen®**, *trioxsalen*
X		**Tri-Sprintec®28**, *ethinyl estradiol/norgestimate*
C		**Tritec®**, *ranitidine bismuth citrate*
C		*trivalent inactivated influenza subvirion vaccine*, **Fluzone®, Fluzone® Preservative-Free: Adult Dose, Fluzone®Preservative-Free: Pediatric Dose**
C		*trivalent oral polio vaccine*, **Orimune®**
A		**Tri-Vi-Flor®**, *multivitamin*
X		**Trivora®-21, Trivora®-28**, *ethinyl estradiol/levonorgestrel*
C		**Trizivir®**, *abacavir/lamivudine/zidovudine*
B		**Trobicin®**, *spectinomycin*
B		*troleandomycin*, **Tao®**
C		*trospium chloride*, **Sanctura®**
C		*trovafloxacin*, **Trovan®**
C		**Trovan®**, *trovafloxacin*
C		**Trovan®IV**, *alatrovafloxacin*
C		**Trusopt®**, *dorzolamide*
B		**Truvada®**, *tenofovir disoproxil fumarate/emtricitabine*
C		**Tubersol®**, *ppd, purified protein derivative for tuberculin skin test*
NR		**Tucks®**, *witch hazel*
D	II	**Tuinal®**, *amobarbital/secobarbital*
NR		**Tums®, Tums®E-X**, *calcium carbonate*
C		**Turbinaire®**, *dexamethasone*
C	III	**Tussend®**, *hydrocodone/pseudoephedrine*
C	III	**Tussionex®**, *hydrocodone polistirex/chlorpheniramine polistirex*
C		**Tussi®-Organidin**, *guaifenesin*
C	III	**Tussi®-Organidin NR**, *guaifenesin/codeine*
C		**Tuss®-Ornade**, *caramiphen/pseudoephedrine*
C		**Tussi®12**, *carbetapentane/chlorpheniramine*
C		**Tussi®12D, Tussi®12D S**, *carbetapentane/pyrilamine/phenylephrine*
C		**Twinrix®**, *hepatitis a inactivated/hepatitis b surface antigen (recombinant) vaccine*
D		**Tygacil®**, *tigecycline*
B		**Tylenol®**, *acetaminophen*
C	III	**Tylenol®#1, #2, #3, #4**, *acetaminophen/codeine*
B		**Tylenol®PM**, *acetaminophen/diphenhydramine*
C	II	**Tylox®**, *oxycodone/acetaminophen*
C		**Typhin Vi®**, *typhoid vi polysaccharide*
C		*typhoid vi polysaccharide*, **Typhin Vi®**
C		**Tysabri®**, *natalizumab*
C		**Tyzine®**, *tetrahydrozoline*
C		**U-Cort®**, *hydrocortisone acetate*
B		**Ultracef®**, *cefadroxil*

C		**Ultracet®**, *tramadol/acetaminophen*
C		**Ultram®, Ultram®ER** *tramadol*
A		**Ultra NatalCare®**, *prenatal vitamin*
C		**Ultrase®MT**, *pancrelipase*
C		**Ultravate®**, *halobetasol propionate*
B		**Unasyn®**, *ampicillin/sulbactam*
NR		*undecylenic acid*, **Desenex®**
A		**Uni-Cap®**, *multivitamin*
C		**Uni-Dur®**, *theophylline*
B		**Unipen®**, *nafcillin*
C		**Uniphyl®**, *theophylline*
C/D		**Uniretic®**, *moexipril/hydrochlorothiazide*
B		**Unisom®Sleepgels, Unisom® Sleeptabs**, *diphenhydramine*
C	III	**Unituss®HC**, *hydrocodone/phenylephrine/chlorpheneramine*
C/D		**Univasc®**, *moexipril*
C		*unoprostone isopropyl*, **Rescula®**
C		*urea cream*, **Carmol®40, Keratol® 40**
C		**Urecholine®**, *bethanechol*
C		**Urex®**, *methenamine hippurate*
C		**Urimax®**, *methenamine/salicylate/methylene blue/ hyoscyamine sulfate/benzoic acid/atropine sulfate/hyoscyamine*
C		**Urised®**, *methenamine/sodium biphosphate/phenyl salicylate/ methylene blue/hyoscyamine sulfate*
B		**Urispas®**, *flavoxate*
B		**Uristat®**, *phenazopyridine*
D		**Uri-Tet®**, *oxytetracycline*
C		**Urocit-K®**, *potassium citrate*
B		**Urodine®**, *phenazopyridine*
B		**Urogesic®**, *phenazopyridine*
B		**UroXetral®**, *alfuzosin*
B		*ursodiol*, **Actigall®**
B		**Utimox®**, *amoxicillin*
C		*vaccina virus vaccine (dried calf lymph type)*, **Dryvax®**
C		**Vacon®**, *phenylephrine*
C		**Valcyte®**, *valgancidovir*
C		*valgancidovir*, **Valcyte®**
X		**Vagifem®**, *estradiol*
C		**Vagistat®**, *tioconazole*
B		*valacyclovir*, **Valtrex®**
B		**Valadol®**, *acetaminophen*
C		**Valisone®**, *betamethasone valerate*
D	IV	**Valium®**, *diazepam*
D		*valproic acid*, **Depakene®**
C/D		*valsartan*, **Diovan®**
C/D		*valsartan/hydrochlorothiazide*, **Diovan®HCT**
B		**Valtrex®**, *valacyclovir*
C		**Vancenase®, Vancenase®AQ**, *beclomethasone dipropionate*

		monohydrate
C		**Vancerase®, Vancerase®AQ,** *beclomethasone*
C		**Vanceril®, Vanceril®DS,** *beclomethasone dipropionate monohydrate*
C		**Vancocin®, Vancocin®Oral Solution, Vancocin®Pulvules,** *vancomycin*
C		*vancomycin,* **Vancocin®, Vancocin®Oral Solution, Vancocin® Pulvules**
B		**Vandazole®,** *metronidazole*
C		**Vaniqa®,** *eflornithine*
C		**Vanos®,** *fluocinonide*
C		**Vanoxide®HC,** *benzoyl peroxide/hydrocortisone*
B		**Vantin®,** *cefpodoxime proxetil*
C		**Vaponefrin®,** *epinephrine (racemic)*
C		**Vaqta®,** *hepatitis a vaccine*
B		*vardenafil,* **Levitra®**
C		*varenicline,* **Chantix®**
C		*varicella virus vaccine (live),* **Varivax®**
C		**Varivax®,** *varicella virus vaccine (live)*
C/D		**Vascor®,** *bepridil*
C/D		**Vaseretic®,** *enalapril/hydrochlorothiazide*
C		**Vasocidin®Ophthalmic Ointment, Vasocidin®Ophthalmic Solution,** *sulfacetamide/prednisolone*
C		**Vasocon®-A,** *naphazoline*
C		**Vasosulf®,** *sulfacetamide/phenylephrine*
C/D		**Vasotec®,** *enalapril*
B		**V-Cillin-K®,** *penicillin v potassium*
B		**Veetids®,** *penicillin v potassium*
B		**Velcade®,** *bortezomib*
X		**Velivet®,** *ethinyl estradiol/desogestrel*
B		**Velosef®,** *cephradine*
C		*venlafaxine,* **Effexor®, Effexor®XR**
C		**Ventolin®,** *albuterol*
C		*verapamil,* **Calan®, Calan®SR, Covera®-HS, Isoptin®, Isoptin®SR, Verelan®**
C		**Verelan®,** *verapamil*
B		**Vermizine®,** *piperazine*
C		**Vermox®,** *mebendazole*
NR		**Verrusol®,** *cantharidin*
C		**VESIcare®,** *solifenacin*
C		**Vexol®,** *rimexolone*
D		**Vfend®,** *voriconazole*
X		**Viadur®,** *leuprolide*
B		**Viagra®,** *sildenafil*
D		**Vibramycin®, Vibra-Tab®,** *doxycycline*
C	III	**Vicodin®, Vicodin®ES, Vicodin®HP,** *hydrocodone/acetaminophen*
C	III	**Vicodin®Tuss,** *guaifenesin/hydrocodone*
A		**Vicon®Forte,** *multivitamin*

C	III	**Vicoprofen®,** *hydrocodone/ibuprofen*
C		*vidarabine,* **Vira-A®**
D		**Vidaza®,** *azactidine*
B		**Videx®, Videx®EC,** *didanosine*
C		**Vigamox®,** *moxifloxacin*
A		**Vinate®GT,** *prenatal vitamin*
C		**Viokase®,** *pancrelipase*
C		**Vira-A®,** *vidarabine*
B		**Viracept®,** *nelfinavir*
C		**Viramune®,** *nevirapine*
X		**Virazole®,** *ribavirin*
B		**Viread®,** *tenofovir disopoxil fumarate*
X	III	**Virilon®,** *methyltestosterone*
C		**Viroptic®,** *trifluridine*
NR		**Visine®,** *tetrahydrozoline*
NR		**Visine®AC,** *tetrahydrozoline/zinc sulfate*
NR		**Visine®L-R,** *oxymetazoline*
B		**Visken®,** *pindolol*
C		**Vistaril®,** *hydroxyzine*
C		**Vistide®,** *cidofovir*
A		*vitamin a palmitate,* **Aquasol®A**
A/C		*vitamin b_{12}, cyanocobalamin,* **Nascobal®, Redisol®**
A		*vitamin b complex/vitamin c,* **Surplex-T®**
C		**Vivactil®,** *protriptyline*
X		**Vivelle®, Vivelle Dot®,** *estradiol transdermal system*
C		**Vivitrol®,** *naltrexone*
D		**Vivox®,** *doxycycline*
C		**Volmax®,** *albuterol*
B		**Voltaren®, Voltaren®Ophthalmic Solution, Voltaren®-XR,** *diclofenac*
C		**Vontrol®,** *diphenidol*
D		*voriconazole,* **Vfend®**
C		**Vosol®,** *acetic acid*
C		**Vosol®HC,** *acetic acid/hydrocortisone*
C		**Vospire®ER,** *albuterol*
C		**Vytone®,** *hydrocortisone/iodoquinol*
X		**Vytorin®,** *ezetimibe/simvastatin*
D		*warfarin,* **Coumadin®, Panwarfin®**
B		**Welchol®,** *colesevelam*
B		**Wellbutrin®, Wellbutrin®SR, Wellbutrin®XL,** *bupropion*
C		**Wellcovorin®,** *leucovorin*
C		**Wellferon®,** *interferon alfa-2b*
C		**Westcort®,** *hydrocortisone valerate*
X		**Wigraine®,** *ergotamine/caffeine*
NR		*witch hazel,* **Tucks®**
B		**Wycillin®,** *penicillin g procaine*
C	IV	**Wygesic®,** *propoxyphene/acetaminophen*

B		**Wymox®**, *amoxicillin*
C		**Wytensin®**, *guanabenz*
C		**Xalatan®**, *latanoprost*
D	IV	**Xanax®, Xanax®XR**, *alprazolam*
D		**Xeloda®**, *capecitabine*
B		**Xenical®**, *orlistat*
C		**Xibrom®**, *brofenac*
C		**Xifaxan®**, *rifaxmin*
B		**Xolair®**, *omalizumab*
C		**Xopenex®**, *levalbuterol*
B		**Xylocaine®Injectable, Xylocaine®Viscous Solution**, *lidocaine*
NR		**Xyrem®**, *na oxybate*
X		**Yasmin®, Yaz®**, *ethinyl estradiol/drospirenone*
NR		**Yocon®**, *yohimbine*
C		**Yodoxin®**, *diiodohydroxyquin, iodoquinol*
NR		*yohimbine*, **Yocon®**
C		**Zaditor®**, *ketotifen*
B		*zafirlukast*, **Accolate®**
C		**Zagam®**, *sparfloxacin*
C		*zalcitabine*, **Hivid®**
C	IV	*zaleplon*, **Sonata®**
C		**Zanaflex®**, *tizanidine*
B		*zanamivir for inhalation*, **Relenza®**
B		**Zantac®, Zantac®Chewable Tablets, Zantac®Efferdose** *ranitidine*
D		**Zarontin®**, *ethosuximide*
B		**Zaroxolyn®**, *metolazone*
C		**Zatidor®**, *ketotifen fumarate*
C		**Z-Cof®DM**, *guaifenesin/dextromethorphan/pseudoephedrine*
C		*zdu, zidovudine,* **Retrovir®**
C		**Zebeta®**, *bisoprolol fumarate*
C	II	**Zebutal®**, *butalbital/acetaminophen/caffeine*
B		**Zegerid®**, *omeprazole/na bicarbonate*
C		**Zelapar®**, *selegiline*
A		**Zenate®Advanced Formula**, *prenatal vitamin*
C		**Zephrex®LA**, *guaifenesin/pseudoephedrine*
C		**Zerit®**, *stavudine*
C/D		**Zestoretic®**, *lisinopril/hydrochlorothiazide*
C/D		**Zestril®**, *lisinopril*
C		**Zetar®, Zetar®Shampoo**, *coal tar*
C		**Zetia®**, *ezetimibe*
C		**Ziac®**, *bisoprolol/hydrochlorothiazide*
C		**Ziagen®**, *abacavir*
C		*zidovudine, zdu,* **Retrovir®**
C		*zileuton,* **Zyflo®**
B		**Zinacef®**, *cefuroxime*
C		*ziprasidone,* **Geodon®**
B		**ZithPed Syr®**, *azithromycin*

B		**Zithromax®, Zithromax®Tri-Pak, Zmax®**, *azithromycin*
B		**Zmax®**, *azithromycin*
X		**Zocor®**, *simvastatin*
C		**ZoDerm®**, *benzoyl peroxide*
X		**Zoladex®**, *goserelin*
D		*zoledronic acid*, **Zometa®**
B		**Zolicef®**, *cefazolin*
C		*zolmitriptan*, **Zomig®, Zomig®-ZMT**
C		**Zoloft®**, *sertraline*
B	IV	*zolpidem*, **Ambien®**
D		**Zometa®**, *zoledronic acid*
C		**Zomig®, Zomig®ZMT**, *zolmitriptan*
B		**Zonalon®**, *doxepin*
C		**Zonegran®**, *zonisamide*
C		*zonisamide*, **Zonegran®**
NR		**Zostrix®, Zostrix®HP**, *capsaicin*
B		**Zosyn,®** *piperacillin/tazobactam*
C		**Zoto®-AC**, *chloroxylenol/hydrocortisone/pramoxine*
X		**Zovia® 1/35-21, Zovi®a 1/35-28, Zovia® 1/50-21, Zovia® 1/50-28**, *ethinyl estradiol/ethynodiol diacetate*
C		**Zovirax®**, *acyclovir*
B		**Zyban®**, *bupropion*
C	III	**Zydone®**, *hydrocodone/acetaminophen*
C		**Zyflo®**, *zileuton*
C		**Zylet®**, *loteprednol/tobramycin /tobramycin*
C		**Zyloprim®**, *allopurinol*
C		**Zymase®**, *pancrelipase*
C		**Zyprexa®, Zyprexa®Zudis**, *olanzapine*
B		**Zyrtec®, Zyrtec® Chewable Tablets**, *cetirizine*
C		**Zyrtec®-D 12 Hour**, *cetirizine/pseudoephedrine*
C		**Zyvox®**, *linezolid*

Amelie's Antibiotic Cards

- ✓ Invaluable prescribing information
- ✓ Arranged by bugs, drugs, and treatment
- ✓ Makes understanding antibiotics a snap!

Pediatric Dosage Cards

- ✓ Set of 6 cards arranged by antibiotic class
- ✓ Pediatric dosage calculated by weight and concentration
- ✓ Never calculated a dose again!!

Advanced Practice Education Associates
103 Darwin Circle, Lafayette, LA 70508

____ Set of *Amelie's Antibiotic Cards* for $19.00 (includes packaging).

____ Set of *Pediatric Dosage Cards* for $13.00 (includes packaging).

____ Set of *Amelie's Antibiotic Cards* and *Pediatric Dosage Cards* for $31.00 (includes packaging).

Payment: ☐ Check ☐ VISA ☐ MasterCard ☐ AMEX ☐ Discover

Credit Card Number:_____

Name on card: _____ Exp. Date: _____/_____

Shipping Address:
Name_____

Address_____

City _____ State _____ Zip _____

Please allow 2-3 weeks for delivery. Prices and availability subject to change without notice.

Advanced Practice Education Associates
http://www.apea.com
1-800-899-4502

Advanced Practice Education Associates
Presents

Family Nurse Practitioner
Certification Prep Exams

By
Amelie Hollier, MSN, APRN-BC, FNP
Mari J. Wirfs, MN, PhD, APRN-BC, FNP

Family Nurse Practitioner Certification Prep Exams are for FNP students preparing for the AANP or ANCC certification exam. *Family Nurse Practitioner Certification Prep Exams* contains 1000 multiple choice review questions, including over 400 subject-specific questions *plus* four-150 question practice examinations. Answers **and rationales** are included with each question and arranged in an easy to use format. Questions are written to give students an idea of the format and subject areas to expect on the exam and to help identify students' strengths and areas needing further attention.

••

Advanced Practice Education Associates
103 Darwin Circle, Lafayette, LA 70508

Please send _____ Copy of *Family Nurse Practitioner Certification Prep Exams* for $44.95 (includes packaging).

Please send _____ COMBO PACKAGE: *Adult and Family Nurse Practitioner Certification Review Book* and *Family Nurse Practitioner Certification Prep Exams* for $97.90 (includes packaging).

Payment: ☐ Check ☐ VISA ☐ MasterCard ☐ AMEX ☐ Discover

Credit Card Number:_____

Name on card: _____ Exp. Date: _____/_____

<u>Shipping Address:</u>
Name_____

Address_____

City _____State _____Zip _____

Please allow 2-3 weeks for delivery. Prices and availability subject to change without notice.

Advanced Practice Education Associates
http://www.apea.com
800-899-4502

Advanced Practice Education Associates
Presents
Adult and Family Nurse Practitioner
Certification Review Book
By
Amelie Hollier, MSN, APRN-BC, FNP

Adult and Family Nurse Practitioner Certification Review Book is written for ANP and FNP students preparing for the AANP or ANCC certification exam. This study guide offers a comprehensive review of all common diseases arranged by body system, growth and development, and professional issues. Chapters are organized by subjects and diseases in an outline format to facilitate studying and reinforce learning of similar subject areas. Considerations for treating adult, pediatric, pregnant, and lactating patients are integrated throughout the book eliminating the need for multiple books for each area.

Great clinical guideline reference for the **practicing NP**!

••

Advanced Practice Education Associates
103 Darwin Circle, Lafayette, LA 70508

Please send _____ Copy of *Adult and Family Nurse Practitioner Certification Review Book* for $54.95 (includes packaging).

Please send _____ COMBO PACKAGE: *Adult and Family Nurse Practitioner Certification Review Book* and *Family Nurse Practitioner Certification Prep Exams* for $97.90 (includes packaging).

<u>Payment:</u> ☐Check ☐VISA ☐MasterCard ☐AMEX ☐Discover

Credit Card Number:_____

Name on card: _____ Exp. Date: _____/_____

<u>Shipping Address:</u>
Name_____

Address_____

City _____ State _____ Zip _____

Please allow 2-3 weeks for delivery. Prices and availability subject to change without notice.

Advanced Practice Education Associates
http://www.apea.com
1-800-899-4502